Brain Activation and CBF Control

Brain Activation and CBF Control

Proceedings of the Satellite meeting on Brain Activation and Cerebral Blood Flow
Control, held in Tokyo, Japan 5-8 June 2001

Editors:

M. Tomita
Department of Neurology.
School of Medicine Keio University Tokyo, Japan

I. Kanno
Department of Radiology and Nuclear Medicine.
Akita Research Institute of Brain and Blood Vessels Akita, Japan

E. Hamel
McGill University, Montreal Neurological Institute, Montreal, Quebec, Canada

ELSEVIER
Amsterdam – Boston – London – New York – Oxford – Paris – San Diego – San Francisco – Singapore – Sydney – Tokyo

ELSEVIER SCIENCE B.V.
Sara Burgerhartstraat 25
P.O. Box 211, 1000 AE Amsterdam, The Netherlands

First edition 2002
Second impression 2002

Library of Congress Cataloging-in-Publication Data
International Symposium "Brain Activation and CBF Control" (2001: Tokyo, Japan)
  Brain Activation and CBF Control: proceedings of the Satellite meeting on Brain
  Activation and Cerebral Blood Flow Control, held in Tokyo, Japan 5-8 June 2001/ editors,
  M. Tomita, I. Kanno, E. Hamel.
    p. cm.-- (International congress series; 1235)
  "Selected papers presented at the International Symposium" Brain Activation and CBF
  Control" which was held at Tokyo Big Sight on June 5-8 June, 2001, as a Satellite Symposium
  of the 20th International Symposium on Cerebral Blood Flow, Metabolism and Function,
  Taipei, June 10-13, 2001"-- Intro.
  Includes bibliographical references and index.
  ISBN 0-444-50874-0
  1. Cerebral circulation--Congresses. 2. Brain stimulation--Congresses. 3. Brain--
  Metabolism--Congresses. I. Tomita, M. (Minoru). II. Kanno, I. (Iwao) III. Hamel, E. (Edith)
  IV. Title. V. Series.

  QP108.5.C4 1567 2002
  612.8'25--dc21

                                                            2002069263

British Library Cataloguing in Publication Data
Brain activation and CBF control: proceedings of the satellite meeting on brain activation
  and cerebral blood flow control, held in Tokyo, Japan 5-8 June 2001. – (International congress
  series; 1235)
  1. Cerebral circulation - Congresses
  I. Tomita, M. (Minoru). II. Kanno, I. III. Hamel, E. 616.8'1

  ISBN 0444508740

International Congress Series No. 1235
ISBN: 0-444-50874-0
ISSN: 0531-5131

Preface

This book contains selected papers presented at the International Symposium "Brain Activation and CBF Control" which was held at Tokyo Big Sight on June 5-8, 2001, as a Satellite Symposium of The 20th International Symposium on Cerebral Blood Flow, Metabolism and Function, Taipei, June 10-13, 2001 (Brain 01). The focus of this Symposium was centered on the old and yet always new problem of why flow increases when neurons are activated. The underlying rationale for this flow increase is considered to be that when neurons are activated with function, they need to recover immediately for the next function. To meet this requirement, the microvascular flow close to the neurons needs to be increased in order to carry in nutritional substances and transport away waste products. However, the sequential process of function/metabolism/flow coupling still remains enigmatical, with the least known points being how the pertinent capillary flow is increased by activated neurons, and how the glial cells intervene in the capillary flow regulation by neurons. Elucidation of the precise mechanisms involved is not only of scientific interest, but also of clinical importance for treating conditions such as migraine, and various brain pathologies such as cerebral ischemia, which would be a result of insufficient flow for neuronal recovery.

We believe that the progress of science thrives on conflicts and compromises between old concepts and new challenges, and the integration of specialized concepts derived from different disciplinary viewpoints. To this end, for the present Symposium, we adopted the modified "Tbilisi format" developed by Professor George Mchedlishvili. This includes the following elements: categorization of the problem, selection of experts, presentation of introductory remarks, round-table discussions, recordings of the points raised by speakers immediately after they make their comments despite the inconvenience, and editing of all the collected records. Invited authorities and promising young scientists as well as selected participants from different disciplines were convened in a single hall so that all attendants had an opportunity to share in the enthusiastic exchanges generated by the on-site discussions. Categories were selected from three standpoints: 1) brain imaging of function/metabolism/flow by sophisticated methods which have recently achieved a quantum leap through their ever-increasing resolution (organized by Iwao Kanno), 2) mediators released from neurons, nerves, blood, vascular and perivascular cells targeting the microvasculature (organized by Edith Hamel), and 3) functioning microcirculation and its overfunction/failure during neuronal depolarization (organized by Minoru Tomita). The present book therefore consists of introductory remarks and three chapters. Following Chapter 1 (Introductory Remarks by Professor Peter Gaehtgens and Professor Marcus Raichle), Chapter 2 (Brain Imaging) covers the methodology used for measuring signals related to the metabolic and hemodynamic changes induced by neuronal activation. It also discusses the physiological interpretation and possible mechanisms of neuron-blood vessel coupling through the presentation of macroscopic/microscopic and quantitative/qualitative measurements of blood flow, oxygen metabolism, (de)oxy-hemoglobin, and the oxygen-glucose index as measured by optical imaging/near infrared spectroscopy, positron emission tomography (PET) and magnetic resonance imaging (MRI). In particular, aspects of the microcirculation related to the blood oxygenation level dependent (BOLD) contrast seen on functional MRI are considered. Chapter 3 (Mediators) covers not only the mediators released from active neurons but also the mediators from nerves, red blood cells, endothelial cells and perivascular cells to achieve a harmonious and self-consistent flow regulation in the local tissue. In relation to the rapidity of regulation, gaseous substances (NO, O_2, CO_2, and CO) occupy some part of this chapter, since they penetrate biological membranes very easily. However, flow changes occurring within the order of milliseconds after neuronal activation seem to be much faster than gas diffusion. Consideration is also given to a novel pathway for vasodilatation through the release of epoxyeicosatrienoic acids from arachidonic acid by p450 epoxygenases. The topics are extended to touch on the role of glial cells in neurovascular regulation. Finally, Chapter 4 (Microcirculation) is limited to spreading depression (cortical spreading depression, anoxic depolarization, periinfarct depolarization, etc.) and concomitant microcirculatory changes for examining the coupling between neuronal states and vascular reactions. The above categorization of topics was, however, made just for convenience, and some themes are interwoven among the three chapters. During the actual sessions, we engaged in interdisciplinary discussions, exchanging new information and spending ample time as appropriate following each presentation. These lively on-site discussions were summarized and, where relevant, have been inserted at the appropriate positions after the state-of-the-art articles comprising book. Readers can therefore enjoy many of the outspoken comments made during the course of the Symposium.

This book provides a valuable source of up-to-date information about "neurovascular coupling". It represents a useful and stimulating reference for medicine-oriented people, students, postgraduates and established investigators working in the field. The articles and on-site multidisciplinary discussions will undoubtedly open up new and exciting challenges for organizing fundamental research, and for developing solutions to practical problems. Although the book has been edited largely with individual specialists in mind, we do believe that it will prove useful for those from other disciplines who desire an overview of this specific branch of medicine. We hope the volume will contribute to an increased understanding and mutual cooperation among scientists throughout the world who have a similar target but work from different standpoints.

Throughout the Symposium and the preparation of the final book, we have had continued recourse to the work and expertise of the many people who have contributed to the questions and answers. We would like to express our indebtedness to all those whose have aided us in the publication of this book. In particular, we owe much to Mr. Kazuo Inokuchi for his financial support, Professor Akio Sato for his invaluable suggestions, Ms. Yoko Asano for her devoted assistance with the Symposium, and Ms. Karena Grundy, Mr. Rol James and their colleagues at Elsevier Science, B.V. for their fine work. Finally, we would like to acknowledge that part of the Mihara Prize, awarded to Minoru Tomita in 2002 for his contribution to the field of stroke, was used to help support the publication of these proceedings.

Minoru Tomita
Iwao Kanno
Edith Hamel
Tokyo, June 2001

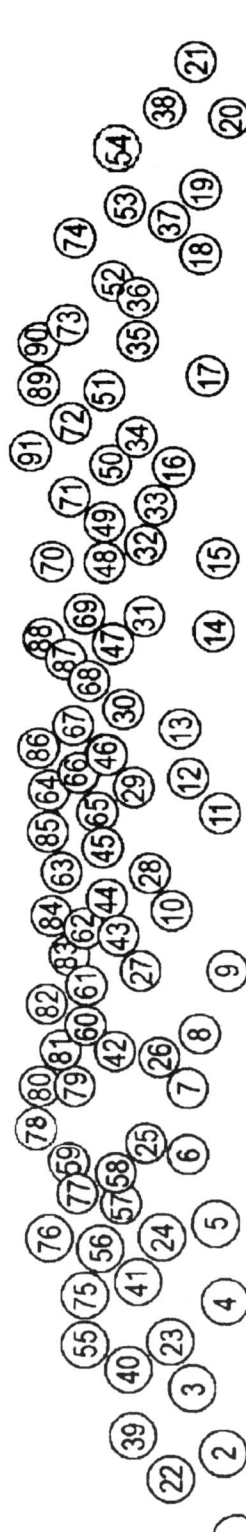

Group photo

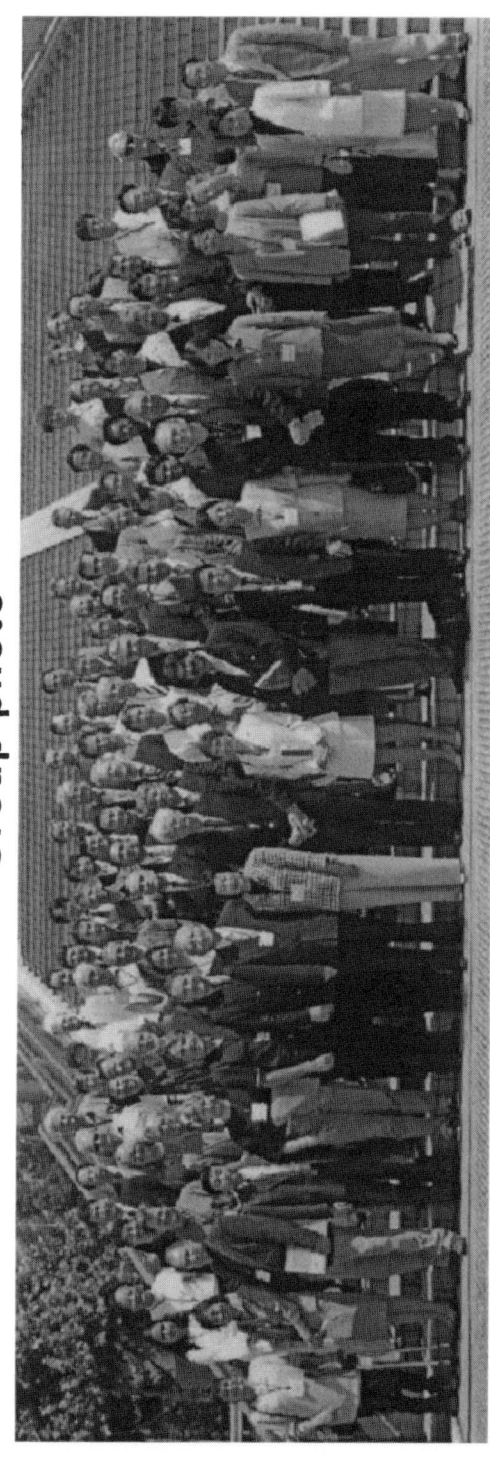

1: Lindauer, Ute; 2: Asano, Yoko; 3: Grinvald, Amiram; 4: Takeda, Hidetaka; 5: Rasmussen, Tina; 6: Andrew, David; 7: Kempski, Oliver; 8: Tomita, Minoru; 9: Tomita, Noriko; 10: Gaehtgens, Peter; 11: Hamel, Edith; 12: Tamura, Mamoru; 13: Kalaria, Raj N.; 14: Tanahashi, Norio; 15: Hotta, H.; 16: Harder, David; 17: Takiyama, Yoko; 18: Rajagopalan, Uma; 19: Pinard, Elisabeth; 20: Kanno, Keiko; 21: Kanno, Iwao; 22: Nageswari, Kolammal; 23: Buxton, Richard; 24: Paulson, Olaf B.; 25: Raichle, Marcus; 26: Caesar, Kirsten; 27: Heiss, Wolf-Dieter; 28: Naritomi, Hiroaki; 29: Busija, David; 30: Traystman, Richard J.; 31: Busch, Elmar; 32: Kida, Ikuhiro; 33: Hyder, Fahmeed; 34: Sato, Akio; 35: Pearce, William; 36: Musha, Takashi; 37: Uchida, S.; 38: Fukuda, Mitsuhiro; 39: Tanifuji, Manabu; 40: Kim, Seong-Gi; 41: Krause, Diana; 42: Seylaz, Jacques; 43: Kobari, Masahiro; 44: Sakoh, Masaharu; 45: Jones, Stephen; 46: Bryan, Robert; 47: Giza, Christopher C.; 48: Glenn, Thomas C.; 49: Matsuura, Tetsuya; 50: Toussaint, Paule-Joanna; 51: Ureshi, Masakatsu; 52: Iadecola, Constantino; 53: Nogawa, Shigeru; 54: Shulman, Robert; 55: Kumura, Eiji; 56: Gjedde, Albert; 57: Pellerin, Luc; 58: Law, Ian; 59: Badaut, Jerome ; 60: Watanabe, Manabu; 61: Lauritzen, Martin; 62: Suzuki, Norihiro; 63: Kuschinsky, Wolfgang; 64: Fukuuchi, Yasuo; 65: Bonvento, Gilles; 66: Nemoto, Edwin; 67: Kent, Thomas A.; 68: Ogawa, Seiji; 69: Huege, Steffen; 70: Ances, Beau M. R.; 71: Asai, Satoshi; 72: Dietrich, Hans; 73: Musha, Takashi; 74: Horiuchi, Tetuyoshi; 75: Sasaki, Yasuto; 76: Anderson, Robert; 77: Schmidt, Kathleen C.; 78: Graf, Rudolf; 79: Strong, Anthony; 80: Schiszler, Istvan; 81: Araki, Nobuo; 82: Yamauchi, Hiroshi; 83: Hayashi, Takuya; 84: Sándor, Péter; 85: Dirnagl, Ulrich; 86: Benyó, Zoltán; 87: Greenberg, Joel H.; 88: Schwindt, Wolfram; 89: Petzold, Gabor; 90: Dreier, Jens P.; 91: Kleinfeld, David

Brain activation and CBF control, June 5-8, 2001 at Tokyo Big Sight

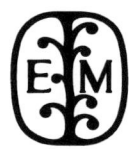

International Congress Series 1235 (2002) xi–xvii

List of Active Participants

Beau M.R. Ances,
Department of Neurology,
University of Pensylvania,
Philadelphia, USA

Robert Anderson,
T M Sundt Jr. Neurosurgical
Research Laboratory,
Department of Neurosurgery,
Mayo Foundation, Rochester,
Minnesota, USA

David Andrew,
Department of Anatomy & Cell Biology,
Queen's University,
Ontario, Canada

Naoki Aoyama,
UCLA, Los Angeles, California, USA

Satoshi Asai,
Nihon University School of Medicine,
Department of Pharmacology,
Tokyo, Japan

Jerome Badaut,
Neurosurgery Department,
CHUV, Lausanne, Switzerland

Peter Bandettini,
Unit on Functional Imaging Methods,
Laboratory of Brain and Cognition,
National Institute of Mental Health,
Bethesda, Maryland, USA

Zoltan Benyo,
Institute of Human Physiology and
Clinical Experimental Research,
Semmelweis University,
Budapest, Hungary

Gilles Bonvento,
CNRS, UFR Lariboisiere-Saint-Louis
Universite, Paris, France

Robert Bryan,
Department of Anesthesiology,
Baylor College of Medicine,
Houston, Texas, USA

Elmar Busch,
Department of Neurology,
University of Essen, Essen, Germany

David Busija,
Depts. Physiol. and Pharmacol.,
Bowman Gray School of Med.,
Wake Forest Univ.,
Medical Center Boulevard,
North Carolina, USA

Richard Buxton,
Department of Radiology,
UCSD Medical Center,
San Diego, California, USA

Kirsten Caesar,
Copenhagen University,
Copenhagen, Denmark

Kang Cheng,
Riken Brain Science Institute,
Saitama, Japan

Arnaud Courtois,
Charge de mission,
Medecine, Pharmacy, Biotechnology,
French Embassy, Tokyo, Japan

Hans Dietrich,
Department of Neurological Surgery,
Washington University,
School of Medicine,
St. Louis, Missouri, USA

Ulrich Dirnagl,
Experimentelle Neurologie,
Universitätsklinium Charite,
Berlin, Germany

Jens P. Dreier,
Department of Experimental Neurology,
Charité, Humboldt University,
Berlin, Germany

Yasutaka Fujita,
Ohtsuka Pharmaceutical Factory, Inc.,
Tokushima, Japan

Mitsuhiro Fukuda,
Riken Brain Science Institute,
Saitama, Japan

Yasuo Fukuuchi,
Department of Neurology,
School of Medicine, Keio University,
Tokyo, Japan

Peter Gaehtgens,
Free University of Berlin,
Department of Physiology,
Berlin, Germany

Christopher C. Giza,
Division of Neurosurgery,
UCLA School of Medicine,
Los Angeles, CA, USA

Albert Gjedde,
PET Center, Aarhus Universit Hospital,
Denmark

Thomas C. Glenn,
Cerebral Blood Flow Laboratory,
Division of Neurosurgery,
UCLA, California, USA

Eugene V. Golanov,
Division. of Neurobiology,
Weil Medical College Cornell University,
New York, USA

Rudolf Graf,
Max-Planck-Institut für neurologische
Forschung, Universitätsklinik,
Köln, Germany

Joel H. Greenberg,
Cerebrovascular Research Center,
Department of Neurology,
University of Pennsylvania,
Philadelphia, USA

Amiram Grinvald,
The Grodetsky Center for Research,
Dept. of Neurobiology,
The Weizmann Institute of Science,
Rehovot, Israel

Munetaka Haida,
Department of Neurology,
Tokai University School of Medicine,
Kanagawa, Japan

John M. Hallenbeck,
NINDS/NIH/ Stroke Branch,
Bethesda, Maryland, USA

Edith Hamel,
Montreal Neurological Institute,
McGill University,
Montreal, Quebec, Canada

David Harder,
Cardiovascular Research Center,
Medical College of Wisconsin,
Milwaukee, WI, USA

Takuya Hayashi,
Department of Neurology,
Kyoto Graduate School of Medicine,
Kyoto, Japan

Wolf-Dieter Heiss,
Max-Planck-Institut für neurologische
Forschung, Universitätsklinik,
Köln, Germany

Rick Hoge,
Deparment of Radiology,
Massachusetts General Hospital
NMR Center, Charlestown,
Massachusetts, USA

Masahiro Horiuchi,
Division of Neurology,
Department of Internal Medicine,
St. Marianna University
School of Medicine,
Kanagawa, Japan

Tetuyoshi Horiuchi,
Department of Neurosurgery,
Shinsyu University,
Nagano, Japan

Harumi Hotta,
Department of the Autonomic
Nervous System, Tokyo
Metropolitan Institite of Gerontology,
Tokyo, Japan

Huege, Steffen
Department of Neurology,
University of Essen, Germany

Fahmeed Hyder,
Department of Diagnostic Radiology,
Yale University, CT, USA

Constantino Iadecola,
Department of Neurolology,
University of Minneapolis Medical School,
Minneapolis, USA

Stephen Jones,
Dept. of Anesthesiology,
Allegheny General Hospital,
Pittsburgh, USA

Raj N. Kalaria,
Wolfson Research Centre,
Institute for the Health of the Elderly,
Newcastle General Hosp. and
Univ. of Newcastle upon Tyne, UK

Iwao Kanno,
Division of Radiology &
Nuclear Medicine,
Research Institute of Brain &
Blood Vessels, Akita, Japan

Takeshi Kawase,
Department of Neurosurgery,
School of Medicine, Keio University,
Tokyo, Japan

Oliver Kempski,
Inst. Neurosurgical Pathophysiology,
Johannes Gutenberg-University,
Mainz, Germany

Thomas A. Kent,
A. University of Texas Medical Branch,
Department. of Neurology, Galveston,
Texas, USA

Ikuhiro Kida,
Yale University,
Magnetic Resonance Center,
New Haven, Connecticut, USA

Kim, Seong-Gi
Center for Magnetic Resonance Research,
Department of Radiology,
University of Minnesota Medical School,
Minneapolis, USA

David Kleinfeld,
Department of Physics,
University of California,
California, USA

Masahiro Kobari,
Department of Neurology,
Tachikawa Hospital, Tokyo, Japan

Diana Krause,
Department of Pharmacology,
College of Medicine,
University of California at Irvine,
California, USA

Eiji Kumura,
Osaka Prefectural Nakakawachi
Medical Center, Osaka, Japan

Wolfgang Kuschinsky,
Physiologisches Institut,
Der Universität Heidelberg,
Heidelberg, Germany

Lauritzen, Martin
Departmenrt of Clinical Neurophysiology,
Glostrup Hospital, Denmark

Ian Law,
Neurobiology Research Unit,
PET and Cyclotron Unit,
Rigshospitalet, Copenhagen, Denmark

Tony Lee,
Southern Illinois University
School of Medicine, Springfield, USA

Ute Lindauer,
Department of Experimental Neurology,
Charite Hospital, Berlin, Germany

Takeshi Maeda,
Department of Neurosurgery,
Nihon University, School of Medicine,
Tokyo, Japan

Kenneth Maiese,
Neurology, Univ. Health Center,
Wayne State University
School of Medicine, Detroit, USA

Tetsuya Matsuura,
Deparment of Radiology and
Nuclear Medicine,
Akita Research Institute of Brain and
Blood Vessels, Akita, Japan

Takashi Musha,
Drug discovery research laboratories,
Eisai Co., Ltd., Ibaraki, Japan

Kolammal Nageswari,
Department of Vascular Physiology,
National Cardiovascular
Center Research Institute, Osaka, Japan

Tadashi Nariai,
Neurosurgery, Department of Brain
Medical Science, Graduate School Tokyo
Medical & Dental University,
Tokyo, Japan

Naritomi, Hiroaki
Cerebrovascular Division,
National Cardiovascular Center,
Osaka, Japan

Edwin Nemoto,
Department of Neurological Surgery,
Presbyterian Univ. Hospital,
Pittsburgh, USA

Shigeru Nogawa,
Department of Neurology,
School of Medicine, Keio University,
Tokyo, Japan

Seiji Ogawa,
Biological Computation Research,
Bell Laboratories, Lucent Technologies,
New Jersey, USA

Minoru Ohtsuka,
Fujusawa Pharmaceutical Co., Ltd.,
Osaka, Japan

Taisuke Otsuki,
Department of Neurosurgery,
National Center of Neurology and
Psychiatry, Tokyo, Japan

Paulson B. Olaf
The Neurobiology Research Unit,
Copenhagen University Hospital,
Copenhagen, Denmark

William Pearce,
Depts of Physiol. and Pharmacol.,
Center for Perinatal Biology, Loma Linda
University School of Medicine,
California, USA

Luc Pellerin,
Instutut de Physiologie et Lab. de
Recherche du Service de Neurilogie,
Universite de Lausanne, Switzerland

Pelligrino A. Dale
Department of Anesthesiology,
Neuroanesthesia Research Laboratory,
University of Illinois at Chicago,
Chicago, USA

Gabor Petzold,
Department of Experimental Neurology,
Charite Hospital, Berlin, Germany

Elisabeth Pinard,
UFR Lariboisiere-Saint-Louis Universite,
Paris, France

Marcus Raichle,
Washington University School of
Medicine, St. Louis, Missouri, USA

Uma Rajagopalan
Riken Brain Science Institute,
Saitama, Japan

Tina Rasmussen,
Department of Control Engineering,
Institute of Electronic Systems,
Aalborg University, Aalborg, Denmark

Fumihiko Sakai,
Department of Internal Medicine,
Kitasato University, Kanagawa, Japan

Masaharu Sakoh,
Department of Neurological Surgery,
Ehime University School of Medicine,
Ehime, Japan

Péter Sándor,
Clinical Research Department and
Institute of Human Physiology,
Semmelweis University,
Faculty of Medicine, Hungary

Yasuto Sasaki,
Laboratory of Physiology,
Faculty of Nutrition,
Kobe Gakuin University, Hyogo, Japan

Akio Sato,
University of Human Arts and Sciences,
Tokyo, Japan

Istvan Schiszler,
Department of Neurology,
School of Medicine, Keio University,
(Torokbalint, Hungary)

Kathleen C. Schmidt,
National Institute of Mental Health,
Bethesda, Maryland, USA

Wolfram Schwindt,
Max Planck Institute for Neurological
Research, Köln, Germany

Jacques Seylaz,
Laboratoire de Rechershes
Cerebrovasculaires, Paris, France

Sadatomo Shimojo,
Institute of Medical Science,
St. Marianna Univ., School of Med.,
Kanagawa, Japan

Yukito Shinohara,
Department of Neurology,
Tokai University School of Medicine,
Kanagawa, Japan

Anthony Strong,
Department of Neurosurgery,
King's College Hospital, London, UK

Makoto Suematsu,
Deparment of Biochemistry,
School of Medicine,
Keio University,
Tokyo, Japan

Norihiro Suzuki,
Deptartment of Medicine,
Neurology, Kitasato University,
Kanagawa, Japan

Kazuji Takahashi,
Department of Neurology,
National Tokyo Medical Center,
Tokyo, Japan

Shin-ichi Takahashi,
Urawa Municipal Hospital,
Urawa, Saitama, Japan.

Hidetaka Takeda,
Deptartment of Neurology,
School of Medicine, Keio University,
Tokyo, Japan

Yoko Takiyama,
Department of Internal Medicine,
School of Medicine,
Kitasato University,
Kanagawa, Japan

Akira Tamura,
Teikyo University School of Medicine,
Tokyo, Japan

Mamoru Tamura,
Biophysics Laboratory,
Research Institute for Electronic Science,
Hokkaido University, Sapporo, Japan

Norio Tanahashi,
Department of Neurology,
School of Medicine, Keio University,
Tokyo, Japan

Kotaro Tanaka,
Department of Neurology,
School of Medicine, Keio University,
Tokyo, Japan

Manabu Tanifuji,
Laboratory for Integrative Neural System,
Brain Science, Institute,
Riken, Saitama, Japan

Minoru Tomita,
Department of Neurology,
School of Medicine, Keio University,
Tokyo, Japan

Yutaka Tomita,
Department of Neurology,
Saitama Municipal Hospital,
Saitama-city, Saitama, Japan

Paule-Joanna Toussaint,
Division of Radiology &
Nuclear Medicine,
Research Institute of Brain &
Blood Vessels, Akita, Japan

Richard J. Traystman,
Anesthesiology/Critical Care Medicine,
The Johns Hopkins Medical Institutions,
Baltimore, Maryland, USA

Masakatsu Ureshi,
Division of Radiology &
Nuclear Medicine, Research Institute of
Brain & Blood Vessels, Akita, Japan

Arno Villringer,
Neurology, Charite, Humboldt-University,
Berlin, Germany

Allen Waggoner,
Riken Brain Science Institute,
Saitama, Japan

Manabu Watanabe,
Osaka Minami National Hospital,
Osaka, Japan

Takenori Yamaguchi,
National Cardiovascular Center,
Osaka, Japan

Hiroshi Yamauchi,
Research Institute, Shiga Medical Center,
Moriyama, Shiga, Japan

Midori Yenari,
Dept of Neurosurgery,
Stanford University, Stanford, USA

Masako Yokoyama,
Mitsukoshi health and welfare
foundation clinic, Tokyo, Japan

Contents

Oxygen Delivery and Microcirculation

Regulatory factors and microcirculation

Opening Lectures

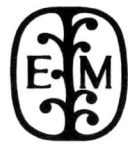

International Congress Series 1235 (2002) 3–13

Microcirculation—historical background and conceptual update

Peter Gaehtgens[*]

Department of Physiology, Freie Universität Berlin, Arnimallee 22, 14195 Berlin, Germany

During the last two or three decades, we have witnessed remarkable progress in our understanding of the biophysics, physiology, and pathophysiology of the terminal circulation. The evolution of experimental methodology and thus of conceptual analysis has advanced during this period from a more descriptive, qualitative stage (largely based on the use of intravital microscopy) through a period of mathematical analysis (employing computer modelling), to develop the concept of the microvascular network as a fundamental hemodynamic and functional unit. Finally, to the current focus on cellular and molecular interaction between blood, the vessel wall, and tissue components (by application of molecular biology). While these changes of perspective were driven by the development of methodology, a complete picture of the object of study appeared to exist at all stages of this evolution in spite of the remaining discrepancies and questions. It is, however, not clear whether the transition from one period to another has allowed us to understand better or only to know more.

Having arrived at the level of single molecules and molecular interactions, we must obviously return to an integrated view which will obviously remind us that micro-circulation is connected to macrovessels, which were for some time considered to serve as supply conduits without a significant biological contribution to the regulation of blood flow to tissues. It is clear, however, that this is not true, since apart from the relevance of these conduits under conditions of pathology (e.g., atherosclerosis), the conducted trans-mission of signals affecting vascular tone as well as flow-or-shear-dependent adjustment of conduit resistance are indeed relevant for even physiological supply regulation. Furthermore, we know that this is particularly relevant when considering conditions in which the dilation reserve of the microvessels has been fully recruited, such that the

[*] Tel.: +49-30-84-45-16-31; fax: +49-30-84-45-16-34.
E-mail address: pgae@zedat.fu-berlin.de (P. Gaehtgens).

normally low fraction of resistance residing in the conduit vessels becomes a determinant component of the blood supply.

As far as blood flow regulation in the small vessels embedded in the tissue is concerned, we are far from having arrived at the end of attempts to unravel the complex interplay of components, in fact, the complexity of this interplay becomes greater as more and more data are accumulated. New mechanisms have been brought to light such as, e.g., endothelium-dependent adjustment of vascular tone or longitudinal communication along microvessels using electronic conduction of signals spreading through a vascular network. Numerous transmitters, signal molecules, mediators, agonists and modulators have been identified, most notably the family of eicosanoids, nitrogen oxide, the various ion channels or receptor molecules, and now, we are down at the level of the genes. All of these represent a complex network of mechanisms, the concerted action of which, we do not at the present moment fully understand.

Yet, the facts are as simple as they were 150 years ago, when J. Gaskell in the 19th century first came up with the very convincing idea: As a tissue is activated and its metabolism increased, the products of this metabolism initiate the resulting vascular dilatation. Today, on our way into the 21st century and on occasion of a Symposium on "Brain Activation and CBF Regulation", it must be permitted to ask: Do we understand better or do we only know more?

A similar picture seems to exist with respect to the mechanisms, which have been held responsible for pathophysiological disturbances of microvascular blood flow distribution and tissue supply. In sequence, red cell aggregation, rigidification of red cells, action of precapillary sphincters, anomalous blood viscosity and hemoconcentration, microembolization by platelet aggregates, interstitial hyperosmolality, leukocyte adhesion, and local endothelial cell swelling have been identified in animal experiments, shown to be relevant in clinical patients, and used as a starting point for the design of therapeutic interventions. However, the identification of the one all-important mechanism or even a clear hierarchy of mechanisms has not yet been achieved. Does an all-important mechanism of a hierarchy of mechanisms exist at all? When prostaglandins, potassium, nitric oxide, pH, or adenosine were identified, we have settled with the idea of a cocktail and learned to accept 'complexity' as a constitutive system property. Is complexity still the concept in the era of molecules and receptor proteins, or will the genes take us back to a fundamental and unifying mechanism? These are the questions of tomorrow, however, I have been given the task to look back.

However, even complex systems follow rules. Therefore, in order to understand the rules, we must understand the structures to which these rules apply. In one very important aspect, our understanding of the vascular system has fundamentally changed due to the experimental evidence accumulated, and I want to address this in more detail. In all physiology textbooks, we find illustrations providing a hydraulic description of the cardiovascular system (Fig. 1) showing a high-pressure, high-resistance arterial supply system and a low-pressure, low-resistance venous drainage system. Between these two, the functionally most important exchange compartment is located in which pressure is roughly similar to and in balance with the plasma oncotic pressure, thus guaranteeing equilibrium in the volume distribution between the extra- and intravascular compartments. In line with this basic concept, we also learn from textbooks that the pressure continuously falls from

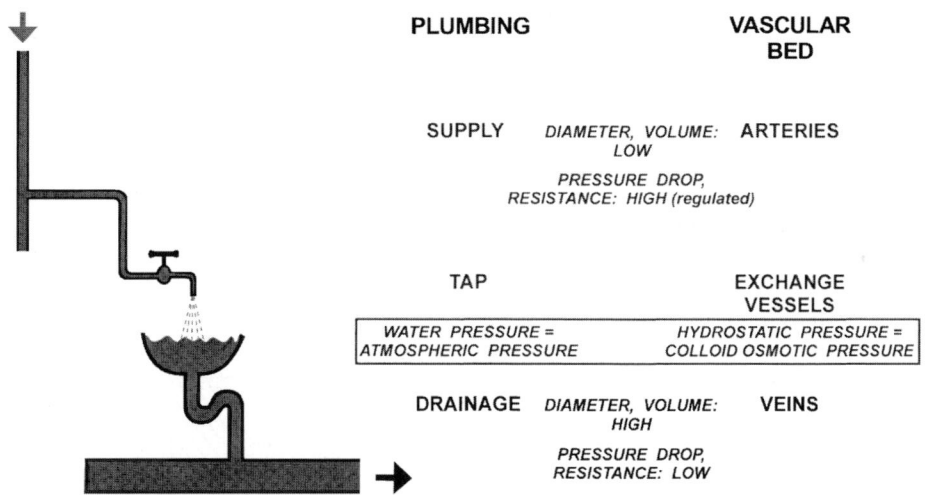

Fig. 1. Schematic representation of the hydraulic characteristics of the vascular system.

the left ventricle through the capillaries towards the right ventricle, and this pressure profile reflects the characteristic distribution of total cross-sectional area, which maximizes somewhere in the post-capillary vessels. This pressure profile had already been calculated and predicted long ago from the first anatomic data on the number and cross-section of blood vessels, and in this calculation, the microcirculation was treated as a simple symmetric branching system. Thus, the prediction obtained was confirmed some decades later when direct pressure measurements in the microvessels became possible, a confirmation which is very satisfying when predictions derived from the first principles are confirmed by measurements.

However, single values of capillary pressure were also obtained which substantially deviate from the general trend, and the frequency distribution of the capillary pressures seen in a synopsis of many measurements (Fig. 2) exhibits a very wide distribution [1]. In addition, single capillary pressures may differ by a factor of up to 3, and the coefficient of variation of the accumulated data set is in the order of 20%. Obviously, it is not correct to regard as the overall analysis suggested any single capillary as a characteristic point along an arteriovenous pathway, at which the high-resistance section has consistently been passed: In fact, the high resistance may still have to be overcome downstream of the considered capillary. This observation is, of course, very relevant, e.g., for the analysis of the overall capillary exchange, since the other parameters in Starling's equation for fluid exchange would not easily make up for the high intra-capillary pressure and a filtration/absorption equilibrium along the flow pathway may thus be very unlikely to occur.

As the years went by, considerable variability indeed turned out to be a characteristic feature of practically all parameters, which became accessible to quantitative measurement. Capillary hematocrit data exhibit an extreme scatter for any category of microvessels, and transit times of both red cells and plasma through microvascular networks also indicate substantial dispersion. Indeed, two red cells entering an arteriole at the same instant of time will immediately be separated and never meet again. This fact which

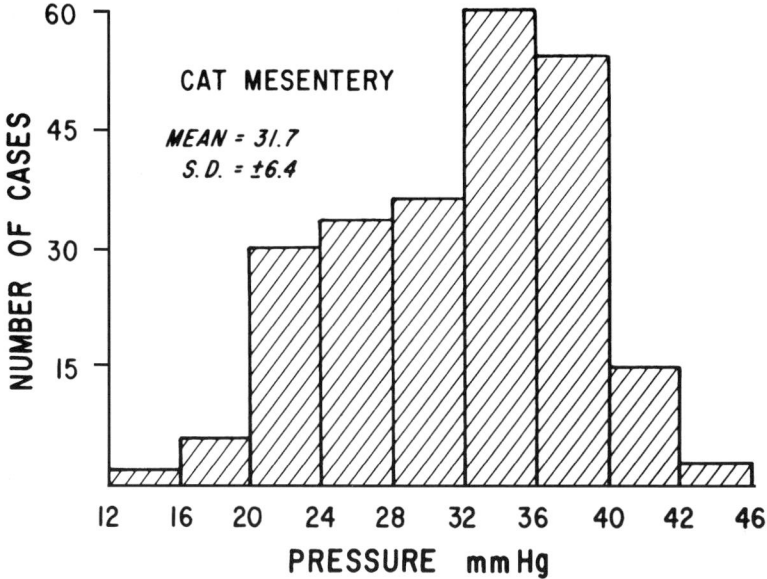

Fig. 2. Frequency distribution of capillary pressures obtained by direct measurements in the cat mesentery. From Zweifach [1].

guarantees the effective mixing of blood constituents during passage through the micro-circulation is obvious to everybody who has ever seen a fluorescence angiogram of the retina. On the whole, the analysis of microvascular networks over the years has brought about a stunning degree of heterogeneity as documented by very large coefficients of variation, for almost all parameters measured (Fig. 3). However, these findings certainly do not agree with the conceptual view of the hydraulic engineer who, in making predictions of the pressure profile in the cardiovascular system, treated the terminal vascular bed as a symmetric branching network.

Heterogeneity must obviously have a basis in morphology and topology, and indeed, the length of arteriovenous pathways is widely dispersed within one microvascular bed. In principle, this is also true for the "macrocirculation" where coronary and femoral circuits differ significantly in length and thus transit times, also guaranteeing good mixing. Of course, structural heterogeneity of the microvascular network can be quantified too, and such data have shown that it is not only the geometric features of the network, but also its topology, which contribute to heterogeneity. From the analysis of the branching mode in the arteriolar and venular trees of the rat mesentery, which is based on so-called generation numbers and their resulting frequency distribution, two conclusions can be made. First, generation numbers in both the arterial and venous trees of the microcirculation show a rather wide distribution. Second, arterial and venous generation numbers are positively correlated. This is evidence of a characteristic topological structure of these networks (Fig. 4), which accentuates the existing differences in morphological length between the pathways by connecting arterial and venous trees so that the shortest arterial pathway is

Heterogeneity of vessel segment parameters; 7 networks, 3129 segments (*: 3 networks, 1321 segments)

	ARTERIOLES		CAPILLARIES		VENULES	
	AVG	C.V.	AVG	C.V.	AVG	C.V.
GENERATION	10.24	0.43	11.96	0.37	13.92	0.44
DIAMETER (μm)	13.29	0.41	8.72	0.28	20.63	0.53
LENGTH (μm)	337.8	0.83	424.8	0.65	334.6	0.82
HEMATOCRIT	0.29	0.41	0.23	0.60	0.31	0.41
VELOCITY* (mm/s)	2.03	0.84	0.85	0.99	1.07	0.65
VOLUME FLOW (nl/min)	28.03	2.23	3.11	1.76	40.98	1.86
RBC FLOW (nl/min)	12.28	2.22	1.15	1.92	18.23	1.86
SHEAR RATE (Diam/s)	147.1	0.92	103.2	1.62	61.9	0.97
PRESSURE above outflow (mmHg)	26.44	0.56	13.92	0.64	8.99	0.60
PRESSURE GRADIENT (mmHg/mm)	23.16	1.57	24.62	2.00	6.51	1.75
	ARTERIOLAR		TOTAL		VENULAR	
A-V PATHLENGTH* (mm)	2.46	0.48	6.16	0.45	3.58	0.56
A-V TRANSIT TIME* (s)	1.07	0.78	3.64	0.69	2.63	0.75

Fig. 3. Mean values and coefficients of variation of various parameters determined in arteriolar, capillary, and venular segments of the rat mesentery. After Ref. [2].

connected to the shortest venous pathway. This mode of connection, of course, increases the heterogeneity of the passage even further.

In two-dimensional tissues, a geometrically and topologically heterogeneous structure inevitably generates a typical spatial distribution pattern (Fig. 5), because of the requirement that the growth of networks must be space (or area) filling. As a result, all hemodynamic or functional parameters, such as capillary pressures, flows, hematocrits or oxygen partial pressures, will also be spatially distributed in a characteristic pre-determined manner. This provides a supply heterogeneity, which can only be compensated for if an active control of microvascular resistance were to exist in the upstream arterioles of any single arteriovenous pathway. Such a control mechanism may, of course, be time-dependent, such as that provided by vasomotion activity typically seen in some tissues to shift blood flow between different tissue regions.

On the whole, these findings demonstrate that the microcirculation represents a system, which is not only geometrically nonuniform, but also topologically and functionally strongly heterogeneous. This view represents a significant conceptual step from the simplified idealization of the cardiovascular system existing previously, and it leads to significant conclusions with respect to the functional behaviour of microcirculation. Heterogeneous microvascular systems will, for instance, not show a linear relationship between blood flow and exchange function, particularly if exchange is diffusion limited and therefore dependent on convective flow, as is the case for many physiologically relevant constituents of the blood. It is therefore not surprising that tissue PO_2 is so heterogeneously distributed as also shown repeatedly for the cerebral cortex.

In the face of a given morphological heterogeneity, functional heterogeneity can be even further aggravated, and this we believe, explains many observations in pathophysio-

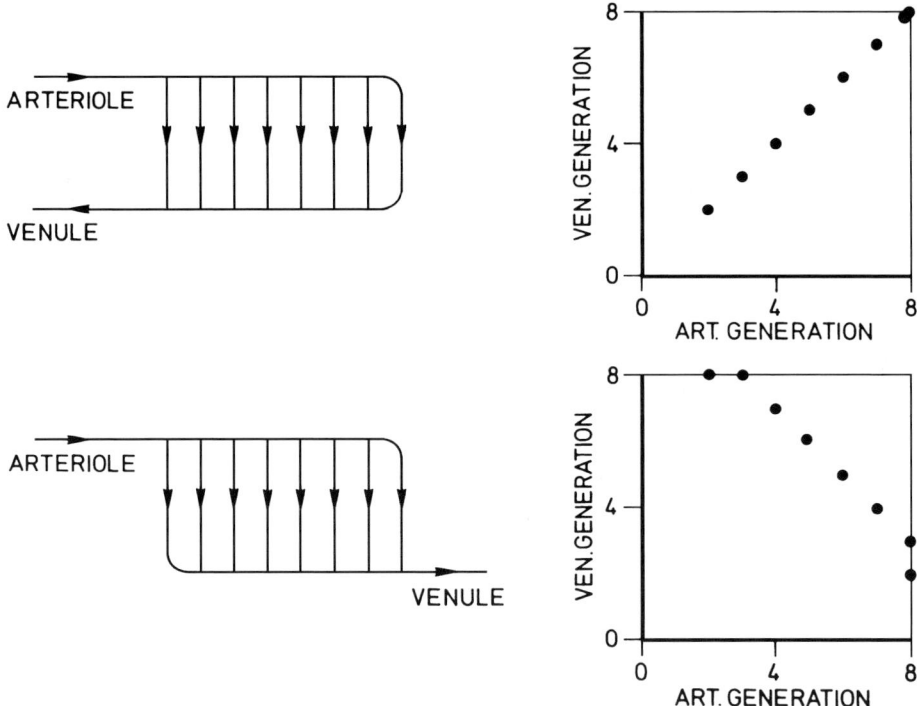

Fig. 4. Two topological types of connection between the arterial and venous trees of a microvascular network and the corresponding correlation between arterial and venous generation numbers of the capillary segments. This upper topological type is observed in mesenteric networks. After Ref. [3].

logical conditions in which the exchange function is more severely impaired than expected on the basis of blood flow. This example was observed in working skeletal muscle rat mesenteric networks in which microsphere embolization caused a loss of contractile power and O_2-consumption, which by far exceeded that seen following hemodilution or arterial occlusion at comparable levels of the overall reduction in O_2 availability. Similarly, experiments in which ADP-infusion was used to induce microembolization by platelet aggregates in the exercising gastrocnemius muscle (Fig. 6) did not only show a gradual reduction in blood flow and contractile power because of the cumulative obstruction of arteriovenous pathways by platelets, but a more important factor was the associated inability of the muscle to utilize the available oxygen, as evidenced by the elevation of venous O_2-saturation functionally speaking "luxury" perfusion. Furthermore, intensified heterogeneity had developed.

With such information in the background, we are very careful when interpreting observations suggesting phenomenologically similar behaviour at the macro- and micro-circulatory level, such as during reactive hyperaemia (Fig. 7). We know that such a similarity is not seen systematically and many grossly different reaction patterns to the same stimulus are observed within a given capillary bed, even post-ischemic vaso-constriction has been observed in single vessels. This indicates that heterogeneity is also

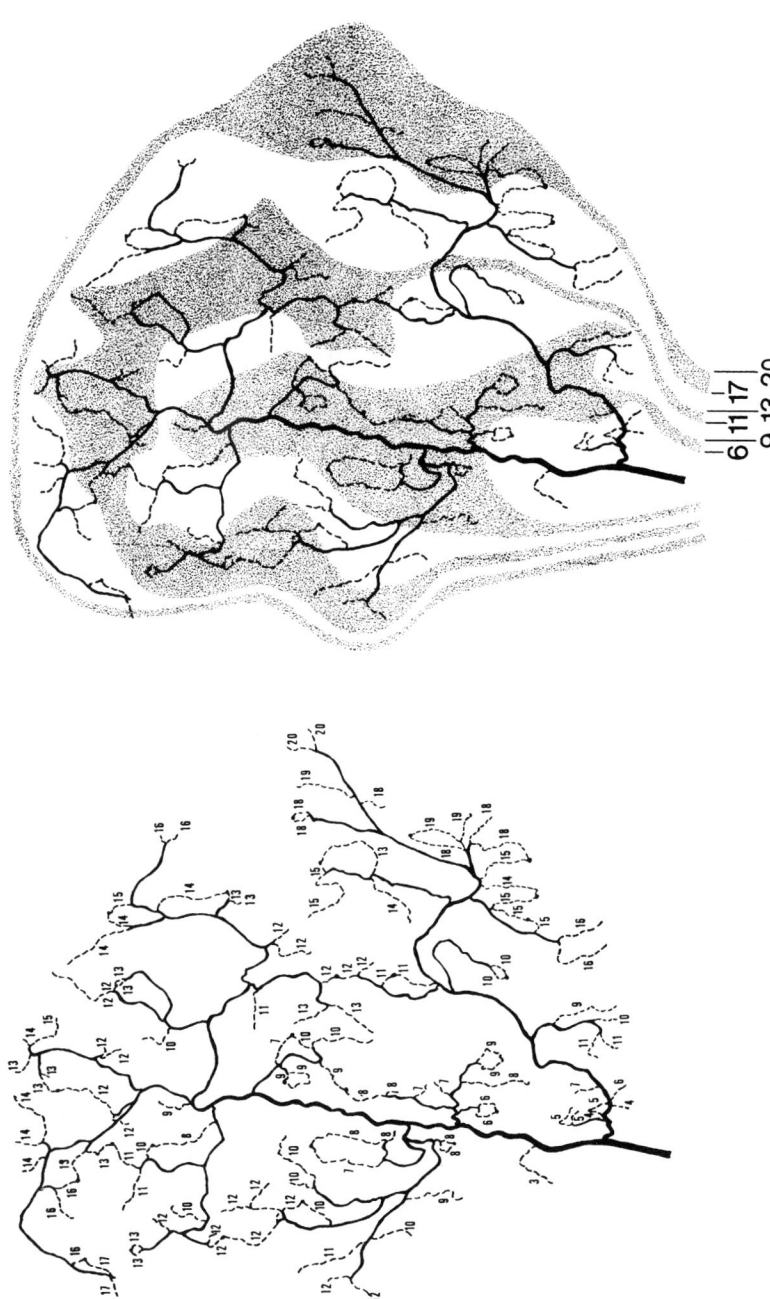

Fig. 5. Spatial distribution pattern of capillary segments according to their generation number. Topologically "early" capillary ramifications are observed near the inflow vessel of the network; "late" capillary ramifications are located in the network periphery. In terms of blood supply, the resulting distribution pattern results in "preferred" and "disadvantaged" tissue areas.

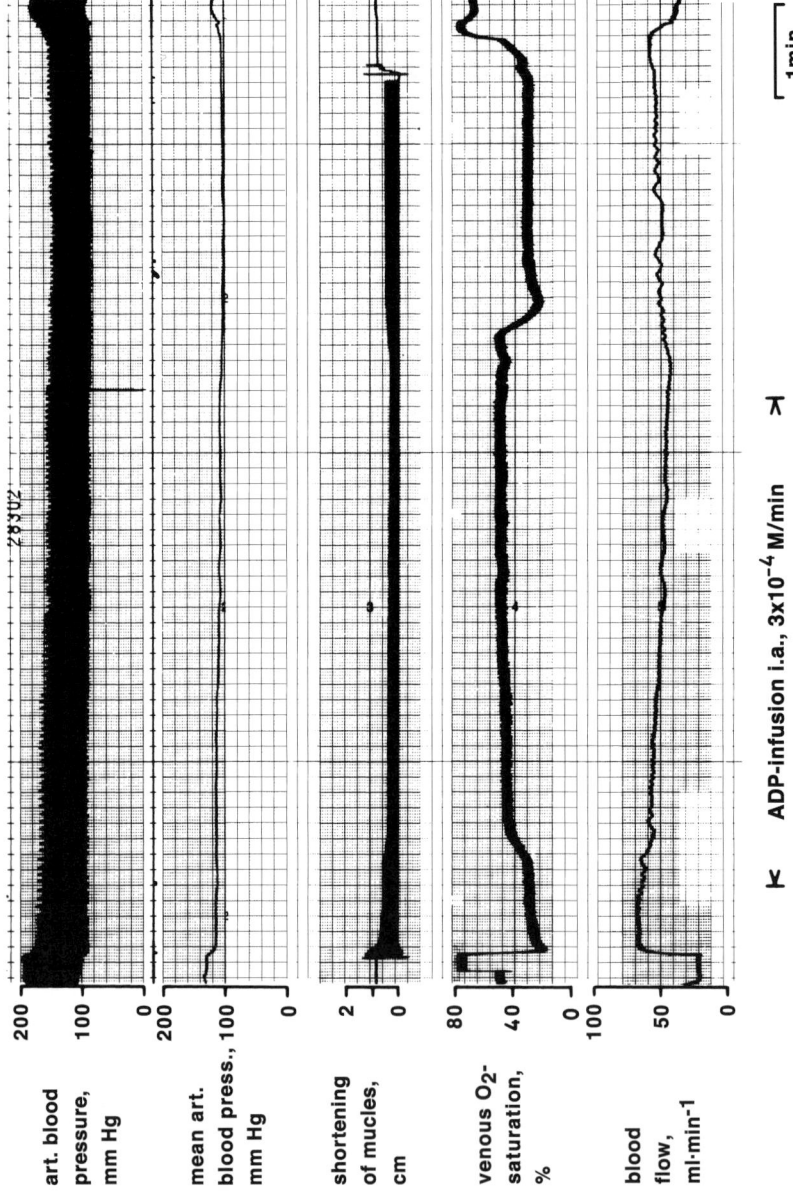

Fig. 6. Blood flow, contractile power, and venous O_2-saturation of an exercising canine gastrocnemius muscle during intra-arterial ADP-infusion. ADP causes aggregation of the platelets in the perfused blood and thus microembolization of the tissue microvessels. After Ref. [4].

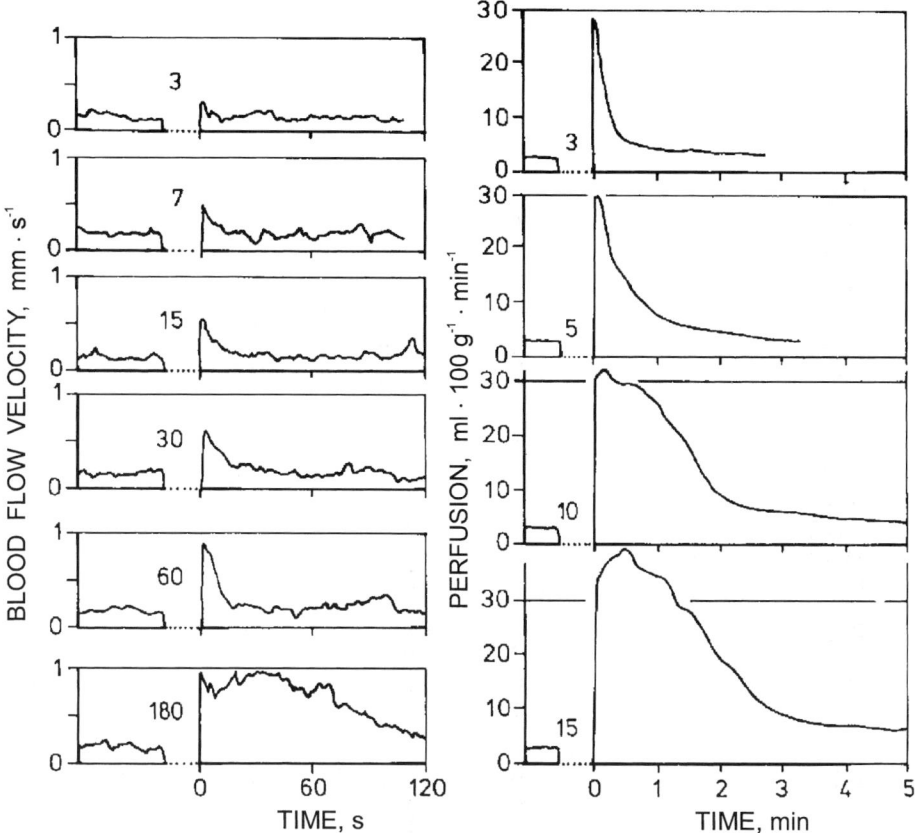

Fig. 7. Reactive hyperaemia as observed in a single capillary (left) and the human forearm (right) after ischemic periods of different durations (left: in seconds, right: in minutes). The left capillary tracings were selected for similarity from a group of capillaries, which showed very different behaviour. After Refs. [5] and [6].

present at the functional level and does not only result from the structural characteristics of a complex vascular network.

While we do not presently understand the reasons for such differences in functional behaviour, we do understand that the system as a whole is clearly heterogeneous yielding nonlinear effects that are functionally relevant. Several interesting questions have been brought up as a result of this insight.

On the one hand, a very old question still remains unsolved, how is it possible that the normally very close adaptation between tissue demand and blood supply can be achieved with such remarkable perfection? Cardiac output in exercise increases linearly and in proportion to the overall O_2-consumption over a range of almost 5–10 fold, and it is only in the uppermost range of maximal physical performance that this relationship does not hold. This also holds for isolated tissues, and mechanisms must therefore be present which precisely adjust vascular tone and thus tissue supply to metabolism. Even in the era of molecular biology, we are still not, I believe, in a position to know, or fully understand and explain this long-known observation.

On the other hand, it is interesting to speculate why the mechanisms determining vessel growth and network development lead to and maintain structural heterogeneity over time. We must realize that the vessel architecture existing at any one time is not fixed but results from continuous adaptation by both formation and disappearance of vessels. Since even in the mature microvasculature, some degree of vessel formation always occurs (Fig. 8), we should try to learn not only the molecular programmes, but the principle of how newly formed vessels know where to join and combine with existing ones to form a complex network which is not only functionally heterogeneous, but even specific for the tissue in which it exists. Furthermore, since dimensions and wall structure of all blood vessels constantly adapt to the local physical conditions of distension and shear stress, the question arises whether the heterogeneity of the microcirculation represents either an unavoidable consequence of vascular renewal, or even an advantage, which we are so far not aware of.

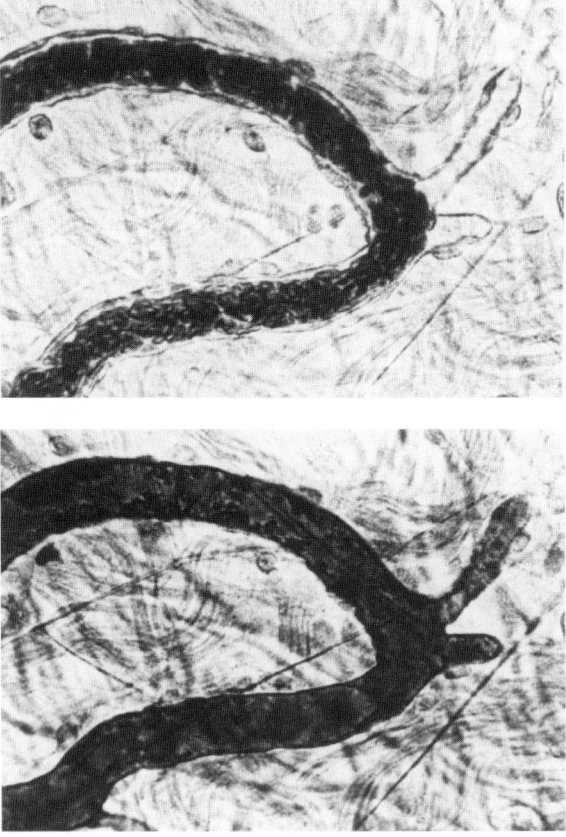

Fig. 8. Capillary sprout as observed in the rat mesentery. The sprout is not perfused with red cells and therefore not easily recognized (top), but becomes evident when the vessels are filled with a dye.

Our comprehensive understanding of microcirculation has meant that significant progress has been made in the last decades by allowing us to understand that the peripheral ramification of the cardiovascular system is in itself geometrically, topologically, and functionally heterogeneous and nonuniform. Thus, significantly adding to the nonlinearity of the macrocirculation. The search for answers to the interesting questions of angiogenesis, vascular adaptation and network renewal will be that of years to come, and the combination of molecular biology and computer modelling will again form the methodical basis of this search. It is only then that a full understanding of the circulatory system as a whole can be expected.

References

[1] B.W. Zweifach, Quantitative studies of microcirculatory structure and function: II. Direct measurement of capillary pressure in splanchnic mesenteric vessels, Circ. Res. 34 (1974) 858–866.

[2] A.R. Pries, T.W. Secomb, P. Gaehtgens, Structure and hemodynamics of microvascular networks: heterogeneity and correlations, Am. J. Physiol. 269 (1995) H1713–H1722.

[3] K. Ley, A.R. Pries, P. Gaehtgens, Topological structure of rat mesenteric microvessel networks, Microvasc. Res. 32 (1986) 315–332.

[4] K.U. Benner, P. Gaehtgens, S. Schickendantz, Hemodynamic and functional consequences of intravascular platelet aggregation in skeletal muscle, Microvasc. Res. 9 (1975) 310–316.

[5] R.E. Klabunde, P.C. Johnson, Reactive hyperemia in capillaries of red and white skeletal muscle, Am. J. Physiol. 232 (1977) H411–H417.

[6] G.C. Patterson, R.F. Whelan, Reactive hyperaemia in the human forearm, Clin. Sci. 14 (1955) 197–211.

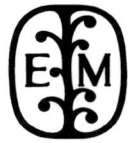

International Congress Series 1235 (2002) 15–20

The circulatory and metabolic correlates of functional activity

Marcus Raichle

Washington University School of Medicine, 4525 Scoh Ave-E. Campus Box #8225, 63110 St. Louis, MO, USA

Thank you very much Dr. Kanno and Dr. Tomita for the gracious invitation to participate in this meeting. What I'd like to do is present some personal impressions of the state of our knowledge of the circulatory and metabolic correlates of functional activity and some directions that might be considered for future research.

To begin let me give you my definition of an activation response viewed in metabolic and circulatory terms [1]. Everybody in this room knows this by heart. When the brain is physiologically stimulated say, for example by a visual stimulus, we get a remarkably reliable increase in blood flow, which as many of you know, we have known about for well over a hundred years [2].

What is also the case although to a variable degree depending upon who has measured it, is that we get an increase in oxygen consumption which is conspicuous because it is so much less than the increase observed in the blood flow [3,4]. The other element of the activation response, which I'm going to emphasize because it tends to get overlooked, is that we also get an increase in glucose utilization that parallels rather nicely the increase in blood flow both in spatial extent and magnitude. Often when we discuss why the blood flow increases and what that has to do with oxygen delivery and consumption, we tend to overlook the increase in glucose consumption, which is always present and exceeds the increase in oxygen consumption. So I would like to comment about this.

The demonstration that glucose consumption increases in parallel with blood flow is not restricted to measurements with PET with their inherent spatial inaccuracies, but has been seen in several laboratories using tissue autoradiographic techniques [5,6].

In all of this work including our own, I'm just struck by the fact that we see an increase in blood flow and an increase in glucose utilization that in magnitude and spatial extent are very much the same. So, any explanation of why the blood flow is going up when neuronal activity increases from the baseline must account for the fact that blood flow and glucose utilization together increase much more than does the oxygen consumption.

E-mail address: marc@npg.wustl.edu (M. Raichle).

Now, while we don't have a complete explanation for the metabolic and circulatory findings, people like Pierre Magistretti and his colleagues have articulated one attractive hypothesis [7]. Their work has been complimented by the work of the Shulman group at Yale [8]. Their formulation calls attention to the intimate relationship between the astrocyte and the adjacent neuron and the critical role played by the astrocyte in removing glutamate, the brain's primary excitatory neural transmitter, from the synapse. What emerges from this work is that glycolysis plays an important role in providing the energy for the uptake of glutamate from the synapse and its conversion to glutamine during brief increases in neuronal activity. In the steady state, there is still a coupling between oxidative metabolism.

What's interesting about this hypothesis is that it provides an explanation for the sudden increase in glycolysis. It is taking place in astrocytes adjacent to the neurons that have increased their activity. Furthermore, it probably involves an increased utilization of glycogen, which, in the brain, is strikingly localized in astrocytes.

The preferential localization of glycogen in astrocytes is obviously not occurring by accident. It provides a very immediate source of energy for a very important process. A simple-minded way that I have come to think about this is to equate the metabolic activities within the astrocyte to those in the skeletal muscle. And that is, when you run a marathon, in order to get through that 26 plus miles, you are obligated to oxidize glucose fully for its energy. We all know that the complete oxidation of glucose provides an enormous amount of ATP as compared to glycolysis alone (i.e. 32 molecules of ATP versus 2 molecules of ATP for glycolysis alone). On the other hand, if you are sprinting 100 m, energy is needed immediately. Under these circumstances, glycolysis is used preferentially. The reason for this is that glycolysis is much faster in producing ATP than is oxidative phosphorylation. Thus, glycolysis as a source of energy fits very nicely with a circumstance in which there is a sudden and rapid increase in energy requirements. Which is precisely what is going on at the synapse when the brain, in a matter of milliseconds, goes from one level of neuronal activity to another.

Now one of the things that has been missing for me in many of the discussions that I've been listening to is the whole issue of time. We talk about the BOLD signal and oxygen delivery, but we seem to lose sight of the fact that changes in blood flow commence 1–2 s after the onset of increased neuronal activity and do not peak for many seconds thereafter [9–11]. For brief changes in neuronal activity, the brain is over and done with the process before the vascular response ever occurs. Any delivery of additional oxygen at that point seems to me to be irrelevant. The system supporting the added energy demands of activation must deliver energy in milliseconds. The astrocyte is well equipped to perform this function because it contains an immediate source of energy in the form of glycogen. Thus, I would submit that the best current cell biology hypothesis concerning the generation of the so-called BOLD signal centers on the activities within the astrocyte and how it supports sudden changes in neuronal activity by employing glycolysis for energy production.

Why then, if not to deliver oxygen, does the blood flow increase? I don't have an answer, but I have some thoughts about what it might not be. Many say even now that blood flow increases support and increased oxygen demand. This seems unlikely to me simply because the increased blood flow is not going to occur in a timely fashion. But I would also suggest to you that increased oxygen delivery to the brain is probably not even needed under these circumstances. Models that have been discussed about oxygen delivery to the brain have often overlooked the fact that the brain is not devoid of oxygen. In fact, there is oxygen in the brain, and there is a flux not only of oxygen from the blood out, but from the brain back, as Rick Buxton mentioned at this meeting and as we have recently published [12]. Still I think some people harbor the notion that there is no oxygen reserve in the brain, or it is so low to be nearly immeasurable. I would suggest to you that is not the case.

It would seem to me that evidence suggests a margin for safety, which you might expect any sensibly, designed system as heavily dependent on oxygen for its very high *baseline* metabolic rate, to incorporate. There are data published back in 1968 [13] in which it was shown that as you begin to lower the oxygen content of the blood, you do not increase the blood flow until you get to a PaO_2 level of about 35 mm Hg. These important data clearly suggest that the small incremental increases in oxygen consumption that have been attributed to brain activation would be easily accommodated by existing brain oxygen reserves without any need to increase blood flow. So we might have suspected as early as these observations that the brain has a margin of error to deal with the fact that it has a vascular system which is just simply too slow to respond to the transients.

We have recently tested this hypothesis in an experiment that looked at the effect of graded hypoxia on the response to visual stimulation but keeping arterial PaO_2 above the level known to produce increases in blood flow [12]. There was no augmentation of blood flow to visual stimulation despite significant reductions of arterial blood oxygen content. So, unless one gets to a critical level of brain oxygenation, it seems to me that the increase in blood flow we observe with brain activation is not either designed to nor does aid increased oxygen delivery.

Now the other possibility might be that the blood flow increase is designed to replenish the glucose that might be used either directly or by way of glycogen. I know of only one experiment that has directly assessed this possibility [14]. This was done by my colleague Bill Powers and some of his associates a number of years ago. They used step hypoglycemia and looked at the blood flow response to somatosensory stimulation. There was absolutely no relationship between the level of blood glucose and the magnitude of the somatosensory evoked response. Together, these data [12–14] suggest that the blood flow response associated with brain activation is neither geared to oxygen delivery nor to glucose delivery to the site.

So it strikes me that we do need to consider other alternative explanations for the activation-induced increase in blood flow and consider not only what is being delivered but what might be removed, or how constituents of the system might be modulated by these changes in blood flow (e.g. see Ref. [15]). I don't believe we know nor have a good explanation for the change in blood flow.

Should we abandon functional imaging while waiting for the explanation? I, for one, will not. Why not? Because blood flow, whatever its cause, has a most remarkable and intimate relationship to the neuronal activity in the brain. This relationship permits us to go forward with functional brain imaging while, in parallel, we pursue answers to the challenging question of why the blood flow changes. Ultimately, however, understanding exactly how such signals arise will enrich our use of blood flow based imaging signals to explore the functions of the human brain in health and disease.

In the remainder of this talk, I want to turn to another issue. The human brain is just 2% of the entire body weight, yet it receives 11% of the cardiac output, and accounts for 20% of the body's oxygen consumption. And yet, cognitive activations, for example those elicited by researchers looking at memory and language, produce relatively small changes in blood flow and the BOLD signal. As a consequence, these localized cognitive activations produce no measurable overall changes in overall brain blood flow and metabolism [16]. So cognitive activations sit inconspicuously on the top of an enormous level of metabolic activity that is going on in the brain at all times. Yet, little attention has been directed to the potential *functional* significance of this large energy consumption. So the question I pose is, why does the brain command such a high fraction of the body's resources when functions cognitive neuroscientists study, that is activations, demand so little?

One important clue is that synaptic activity including the recycling of neurotransmitters in the brain at its baseline (and I'll come to what I mean by that in a minute) may account for a sizeable fraction of this large energy consumption by the brain in the resting state [11,17–19]. That to me means that this has functional implications [1]. The nervous system is not idle when you are not "using it" in the pursuit of some type of goal directed behavior but, rather, it is doing a sizeable amount of brainwork.

So how might we define a physiological baseline for the brain, and, if we can define it, what functional significance might this baseline state possess? I define the baseline in metabolic terms and assert that it is the absence of activation as I have defined it earlier in this talk and elsewhere [1].

If we then turn to the human brain and look at it in a state that involves simply lying in a scanner (and you can have your eyes closed, you can have your eyes open and looking a fixation point, or simply passively viewing a stimulus—but the data to which I will refer [1] involves lying with your eyes closed) what we observe is an almost perfect match between blood flow and oxygen consumption. As a result, the OEF is uniform throughout the brain. In this state, there is a conspicuous lack of activation by the definition I have proposed [1].

Hence, I would suggest that while resting quietly, the brain has accommodated a basic modal level of neuronal activity by matching its blood flow and oxygen consumption in a very precise manner. One deviation does exist in this spatial uniformity of the OEF in the resting state and this occurs in the visual cortex where there is an increase in the OEF. This is not a new observation, having been made almost 20 years ago when OEF maps were first produced [20]. And yet, little comment was ever made of it. What it suggests is that visual cortices are actually deactivated in the eyes-closed-awake state and that their baseline in fact involves eyes open.

So, what might reside in this baseline state in terms of functional activities? I think that we have some clues about how to begin this process. They have emerged very uniquely in the field of functional brain imaging. And they are in the form of deactivations from the baseline [1,21]. What is remarkable about these deactivations is that one routinely sees them consistently in the same areas despite the nature of the cognitive task being undertaken. Thus, while accompanying activations vary tremendously with the task demands these deactivations remain consistent. What it suggests is a specific set of regions that obviously must instantiate specific functions that must be attenuated from the baseline state during goal directed behaviors. This perspective allows us to begin the process of unraveling the functionality of the baseline activity of the brain [1,22].

From the perspective of those concerned with understanding the relationship between oxygen consumption and blood flow during functionally induced changes in brain activity, there is an important point to be made. These decreases are seen with both PET and functional magnetic resonance imaging or fMRI. Thus, the BOLD signal of fMRI can increase (activation) as well as decrease (deactivation) from the baseline as defined using the OEF and PET [1]. Because the BOLD signal is dependent upon a change in the OEF [23] this provides evidence for an increase in the OEF with deactivation. Thus, as we try to understand the relationship between blood flow and neuronal activity we must incorporate in to our thinking the fact that deviations from the baseline activity of the brain caused by changes in neuronal activity in either direction (i.e. increases or decreases) alter the baseline relationship between oxygen consumption and oxygen delivery. Any complete theory purporting to explain the relationship between brain hemodynamics and metabolism and changes in neuronal activity must account for this fact. Presently, no theory does so.

I will close with what I would consider a somewhat nostalgic reflection. My scientific life began in the world of cerebral blood flow and metabolism yet I now find myself largely in the field of cognitive neuroscience. Coming to a meeting like this, I realize that the intellectual gap between the people trying to understand the signals generated by neuronally induced changes in blood flow and metabolism in the brain and the people using such signals to understand how the human brain work is large and counter-productive. I am convinced that combining the insights from studies of brain circulation and metabolism, in particular, and neuroscience in general with those from cognitive neuroscience is the most productive course to follow. This meeting is certainly an important element in such a process.

References

[1] M.E. Raichle, A.M. MacLeod, A.Z. Snyder, W.J. Powers, D.A. Gusnard, G.L. Shulman, A default mode of brain function, Proceedings of the National Academy of Sciences of the United States of America 98 (2001) 676–682.

[2] M.E. Raichle, A brief history of human functional brain mapping, in: A.W. Toga, J.C. Mazziotta (Eds.), Brain Mapping. The Systems, Academic Press, San Diego, 2000, pp. 33–75.

[3] P.T. Fox, M.E. Raichle, Focal physiological uncoupling of cerebral blood flow and oxidative metabolism during somatosensory stimulation in human subjects, PNAS 83 (1986) 1140–1144.

[4] P.T. Fox, M.E. Raichle, M.A. Mintun, C. Dence, Nonoxidative glucose consumption during focal physiologic neural activity, Science 241 (1988) 462–464.

[5] M. Ueki, F. Linn, K.-A. Hossmann, Functional activation of cerebral blood flow and metabolism before and after global ischemia of rat brain, Journal of Cerebral Blood Flow and Metabolism 8 (1988) 486–494.

[6] T.A. Woolsey, C.M. Rovainen, S.B. Cox, M.H. Henegar, G.E. Liang, D. Liu, Y.E. Moskalenko, J. Sui, L. Wei, Neuronal units linked to microvascular modules in cerebral cortex: response elements for imaging the brain, Cerebral Cortex 6 (1996) 647–660.

[7] P.J. Magistretti, L. Pellerin, D.L. Rothman, R.G. Shulman, Energy on demand, Science 283 (1999) 496–497.

[8] R.G. Shulman, F. Hyder, D.L. Rothman, Cerebral energetics and the glycogen shunt: neurochemical basis of functional imaging, PNAS 98 (2001) 6417–6422.

[9] G.M. Boynton, S.A. Engel, G.H. Glover, D.J. Heeger, Linear systems analysis of functional magnetic resonance imaging in human V1, Journal of Neuroscience 16 (1996) 4207–4221.

[10] D. Malonek, A. Grinvald, Interactions between electrical activity and cortical microcirculation revealed by imaging spectroscopy: implications for functional brain mapping, Science 272 (1996) 551–554.

[11] N.K. Logothetis, J. Pauls, M. Augath, T. Trinath, A. Oeltermann, Neurophysiological investigation of the basis of the fMRI signal, Nature 411.

[12] M.A. Mintun, B.N. Lundstrom, A.Z. Snyder, A.G. Vlassenko, G.L. Shulman, M.E. Raichle, Blood flow and oxygen delivery to human brain during functional activity: theoretical modeling and experimental data, PNAS 98 (2001) 6859–6864.

[13] S. Shimojyo, P. Scheinberg, K. Kogure, O.M. Reinmuth, The effect of graded hypoxia upon transient cerebral blood flow and oxygen consumption, Neurology 18 (1968) 127–133.

[14] W.J. Powers, I.B. Hirsch, P.E. Cryer, Effect of stepped hypoglycemia on regional cerebral blood flow response to physiological brain activation, American Journal of Physiology 270 (1996) H554–H559 (Heart Circ Physiology 39).

[15] D.A. Yablonskiy, J.J. Ackerman, M.E. Raichle, Coupling between brain temperature and oxidative metabolism during prolonged visual stimulation, PNAS 97 (2000) 7603–7608.

[16] L. Sokoloff, R. Mangold, R. Wechsler, C. Kennedy, S.S. Kety, The effect of mental arithmetic on cerebral circulation and metabolism, Journal of Clinical Investigation 34 (1955) 1101–1108.

[17] W.J. Schwartz, C.B. Smith, L. Davidsen, H. Savaki, L. Sokoloff, M. Mata, D.J. Fink, H. Gainer, Metabolic mapping of functional activity in the hypothalamo-neurohypophysial system of the rat, Science 205 (1979) 723–725, Washington, DC.

[18] M. Mata, D.J. Fink, H. Gainer, C.B. Smith, L. Davidsen, H. Savaki, W.J. Schwartz, L. Sokoloff, Activity-dependent energy metabolism in rat posterior pituitary primarily reflects sodium pump activity, Journal of Neurochemistry 34 (1980) 213–215.

[19] J. Astrup, P.M. Sorensen, H.R. Sorensen, Oxygen and glucose consumption related to Na+–K+ transport canine brain, Stroke 12 (1981) 726–730.

[20] J.C.L.-G.P. Baron, P. Collard, C. Crouzel, G. Mestelan, M.G. Bousser, Noninvasive measurement of blood flow, oxygen consumption, and glucose utilization in the same brain regions in man by positron emission tomography: concise communication, Journal of Nuclear Medicine, (1982) 391–399.

[21] G.L. Shulman, J.A. Fiez, M. Corbetta, R.L. Buckner, F.M. Miezin, M.E. Raichle, S.E. Petersen, Common blood flow changes across visual tasks: II. Decreases in cerebral cortex, Journal of Cognitive Neuroscience 9 (1997) 648–663.

[22] D.A. Gusnard, M.E. Raichle, Searching for a baseline: functional imaging and the resting human brain, Nature Reviews Neuroscience 2 (2001).

[23] M.E. Raichle, Behind the scenes of functional brain imaging: a historical and physiological perspective, Proceedings of the National Academy of Sciences of the United States of America 95 (1998) 765–772.

Brain Imaging

Hemodynamic models and BOLD signal

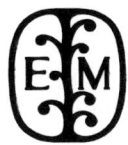

International Congress Series 1235 (2002) 23–32

Coupling between CBF and CMRO$_2$ during neuronal activity

Richard B. Buxton[*]

Department of Radiology, University of California at San Diego Medical Center, 200 West Arbor Drive, San Diego, CA 92103, USA

Abstract

The central idea of the oxygen limitation model is that the oxygen extraction fraction E must decrease during neuronal activation, so a large change in cerebral blood flow (CBF) is required to support a small change in the cerebral metabolic rate of O$_2$ (CMRO$_2$). The model is expanded here to show that maintaining mitochondrial pO_2 at a constant non-zero level during activation, so that O$_2$ availability does not become limiting for CMRO$_2$, still requires the fractional CBF change to be several times larger than the CMRO$_2$ change. Furthermore, the expanded model also allows for a brief initial increase in E at stimulus onset with a corresponding transient dip in cytoplasm and mitochondrial pO_2. However, because the tissue pO_2 must increase to support a higher CMRO$_2$, the tissue O$_2$ content itself would be an ambiguous signal for regulating CBF. For this reason, although the function served by a large CBF increase may be to support CMRO$_2$, the tissue O$_2$ content itself is probably not the key factor for regulation of CBF. © 2002 Elsevier Science B.V. All rights reserved.

Keywords: Cerebral blood flow (CBF); Cerebral metabolic rate of oxygen (CMRO$_2$); Oxygen limitation model; Neurovascular coupling

1. Introduction: why does blood flow increase more than oxygen metabolism with neuronal activation?

The brain is normally maintained in a state far from equilibrium, so that neural activity in the form of ionic shifts and neurotransmitter release at the synapse proceeds in a thermodynamically downhill fashion. However, the ionic gradients degraded by neural activity must be restored and neurotransmitter molecules repackaged, and this requires

---

[*] Tel.: +1-619-543-2953; fax: +1-619-543-3736.
E-mail address: rbuxton@ucsd.edu (R.B. Buxton).

0531-5131/02 © 2002 Elsevier Science B.V. All rights reserved.
PII: S0531-5131(02)00169-3

energy metabolism. Cerebral blood flow (CBF) serves both to deliver glucose and oxygen, the metabolic substrates that fuel the brain, and to carry away the waste products of metabolism, carbon dioxide and heat [1]. For this reason it is not surprising that focal increases in CBF closely follow neural activity. But what has been surprising, and is still not well understood, is that CBF increases much more than the cerebral metabolic rate of oxygen ($CMRO_2$) [2]. With a modest increase in oxygen metabolism, but a much larger increase of CBF, less oxygen is removed from each gram of blood as it traverses the capillary bed. In other words, the seemingly paradoxical result is that the oxygen extraction fraction E is *reduced* with activation.

Functional neuroimaging to map patterns of brain activation is based on these changes in CBF and energy metabolism, so the nature of the coupling between neural activity and energy metabolism is critical for the interpretation of these imaging studies. In particular, the reduction of E with activation is the primary physiological effect underlying functional magnetic resonance imaging (fMRI) based on the blood oxygenation level dependent (BOLD) effect [3,4]. Yet the functions and mechanisms of neurovascular coupling that produce this effect are still poorly understood. In wrestling with these issues we must address two critical questions: (1) What is the function served by a flow increase that is much larger than the oxygen metabolism increase? (2) What are the mechanisms that accomplish the coupling of neural activity to CBF? These two questions make an important distinction, as the arguments presented in this paper will emphasize. The hypothesis elaborated here is that under normal physiologic conditions a large change in CBF is required to support a small change in $CMRO_2$, but the mechanism producing this "coupling" is most likely *not* directly related to tissue oxygenation.

2. The oxygen limitation model

The apparent mismatch of the changes in CBF and $CMRO_2$ was originally described as an uncoupling of the two processes [2], but in the last few years an alternative explanation for this phenomenon has been developed based on the idea that oxygen delivery is limited at rest [5–8]. In the context of this oxygen limitation model the large increase in CBF is required to support the smaller increase of oxygen metabolism. The model is based on experiments showing two effects: (1) at rest a large fraction of the delivered oxygen never leaves the capillary, but nearly all of the oxygen that does enter the extravascular tissue space is metabolized [9]; and (2) CBF increases by increasing capillary velocity rather than by opening new capillaries (i.e., there is no capillary recruitment) [10]. The implications of these results can be viewed in two complementary ways, based either on the dynamics of oxygen extraction or on a more passive view of oxygen diffusing from capillaries to mitochondria down a concentration gradient.

From the dynamic view, the limited extraction of oxygen at rest means that the probability of an O_2 molecule leaving the capillary is strongly dependent on the capillary transit time. Without capillary recruitment, the transit time must decrease as CBF increases, so the probability of extraction must decrease [6]. If the net extraction E is close to the unidirectional extraction (i.e., nearly all of the extracted O_2 is metabolized), then E must decrease with increased CBF. The steady-state $CMRO_2$ is always proportional to the product of CBF and E, so if E decreases when CBF increases, the change in CBF must be large in order to produce a more modest increase of the product of E and CBF.

From the view of diffusion down a concentration gradient, oxygen diffuses from a high concentration in the capillary to a low concentration in the mitochondria. If the net extraction is nearly equal to the unidirectional extraction, then backflux of O_2 from tissue to capillary must be small, implying that the tissue pO_2 is near zero. With no capillary recruitment the diffusion distance from capillary to mitochondria is fixed, so to increase the O_2 flux either the mean capillary pO_2 must be increased or the mitochondrial pO_2 must be decreased. If the mitochondrial pO_2 is already near zero, then the only option is to raise capillary pO_2. And to raise the mean capillary pO_2 the venous O_2 content must be increased, and this means that E must decrease. At steady-state the product of E and CBF must match this increased flux from capillary to mitochondria, so again CBF must increase by a larger amount to overcome the decrease of E.

3. Tissue oxygenation is not a reliable signal for regulation of CBF

By either argument, the picture presented by the oxygen limitation model is that the local oxygen extraction fraction E must decrease in order to raise $CMRO_2$. An important consequence of this is that the average tissue O_2 content must rise, as discussed more fully below. The average tissue pO_2 must lie somewhere between the mitochondrial pO_2, which is very low, and the plasma pO_2 that increases. This increase of tissue pO_2 with activation can be misinterpreted as evidence that oxygen is being delivered in excess of what is needed. Instead, by this model such an increase is required to make possible an increase of $CMRO_2$.

This requirement for increased tissue oxygenation with activation makes it unlikely that tissue pO_2 could serve as the primary signal for controlling CBF. For example, consider a mechanism that senses tissue pO_2 and adjusts CBF to maintain it at a constant level, so that if tissue pO_2 increases, CBF is reduced to restore tissue pO_2 to its set point. Such a mechanism would work to compensate for fluctuations in CBF with a constant demand for $CMRO_2$, but it would not work for adjusting to a new level of demand for $CMRO_2$. In the context of the oxygen limitation model, increased $CMRO_2$ requires an increase of tissue oxygenation, and so this mechanism would tend to counteract the necessary increase of CBF. This means that although the postulated function served by a large increase in CBF is to support oxygen delivery to tissue, the mechanism for control of CBF may not involve oxygen content at all.

This scenario could explain some of the results obtained with non-physiological manipulations such as hypercapnia. With increased inspired CO_2, CBF increases substantially while $CMRO_2$ remains constant. In this case oxygen *is* delivered in excess of what is required, yet neural activation on top of the hypercapnia produces a large increase in CBF comparable to the increase at normocapnia. This could occur if the regulation of CBF is independent of oxygen availability, and the chemical agents that do mediate CBF changes have additive effects [11]. For example, the arteriolar dilation due to chemical agents released through elevated neuronal activity may be tuned to provide (under physiologic conditions) the necessary flow increase to support the increase in oxidative metabolism associated with the increased neural activity. Then during hypercapnia these vasodilatory effects add to those induced by changes in extravascular pH due to the elevated CO_2 levels to produce a large change in CBF that is not strictly necessary for increasing $CMRO_2$.

4. Is there a buffer of oxygen availability?

In our original mathematical model for the effects of limited oxygen delivery we assumed the extreme form of equal unidirectional and net extraction fractions, and the prediction of that model was that the fractional change in CBF would need to be about five times larger than the fractional change in $CMRO_2$ [6]. Measurements in the awake human brain with positron emission tomography (PET) and calibrated fMRI have found this ratio to lie in the range 2–6 [2,12–14], so the predicted ratio lies near the high end of the experimental results. However, this form of the model is undoubtedly too simple. Other factors can influence the diffusibility of O_2, such as capillary dilation and shifts of the binding curve of

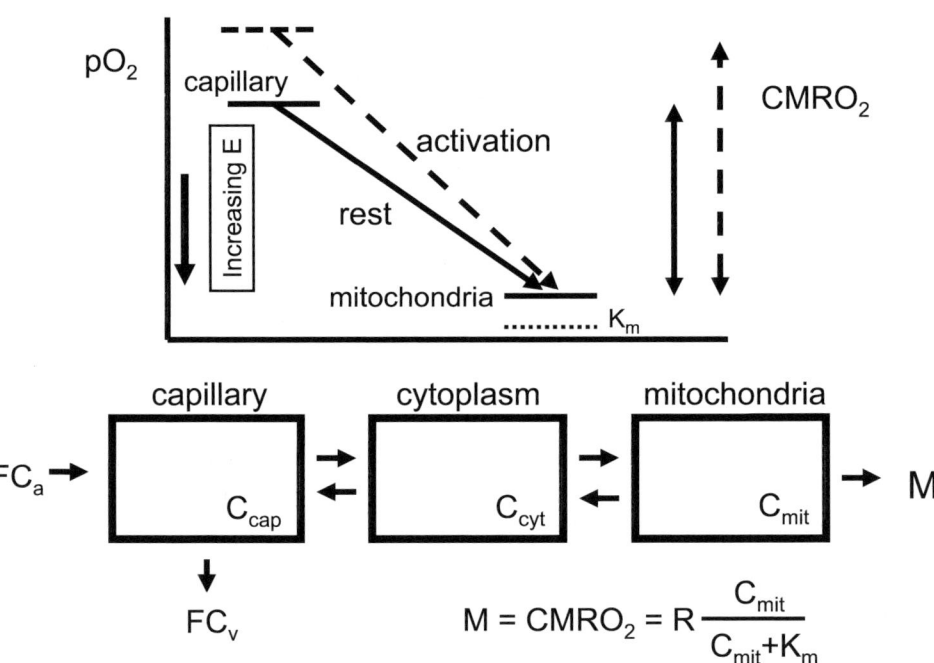

Fig. 1. Modified form of the oxygen limitation model with the requirement that during activation mitochondrial pO_2 is maintained at a constant level higher than K_m, the level at which O_2 availability would become limiting for $CMRO_2$. Then with activation the average capillary pO_2 must increase to increase the O_2 gradient from capillary to mitochondria, and so the oxygen extraction E must decrease (top). This can be modeled in a simple way with a pseudo-compartmental model that takes into account the O_2/hemoglobin binding curve (bottom). In this model, the parameter F controls O_2 delivery and the parameter R controls O_2 demand, and if R increases before F the model produces a transient increase of E and a dip in tissue pO_2 (the "initial dip" phenomenon).

O_2 and hemoglobin, and these effects should be included in the modeling [7]. An increase of diffusivity through these mechanisms would soften the requirement for the CBF increase, but detailed modeling of these effects in this context has not been reported.

Furthermore, in the original simple form of the oxygen limitation model the assumption of equal unidirectional and net extraction fractions is equivalent to assuming no backflux of O_2 and a tissue pO_2 of zero. This is certainly an oversimplification, and is incompatible with two observations. First, studies of the oxidation state of cytochrome oxidase indicate that at rest oxygen concentration is not a limiting factor in determining the rate of oxidative metabolism in the mitochondria [15], which we would certainly expect to be the case if the mitochondrial pO_2 is really zero. Second, studies of the fast response to activation using optical techniques [16–18] and fMRI [19,20] suggest that there may be an early increase of oxygen extraction prior to the larger decrease. This "initial dip" (so-called because it would appear as a dip of the BOLD signal) is still controversial [6,21], but if it is indeed an early increase of E that would be incompatible with strictly limited oxygen delivery.

These observations can be reconciled with the oxygen limitation model if the mitochondrial pO_2 is greater than zero but still significantly less than the average capillary pO_2, and the blood flow increase serves to maintain a constant mitochondrial oxygen tension (Fig. 1). In this case, the mitochondrial pO_2 would be held at a high enough level that O_2 availability would not become limiting in the mitochondria. In short, the tissue pO_2 would constitute a buffer that is normally not used with physiological activation, but which could come into play under some conditions at the beginning of stimulation or in hypoxia. However, the oxygen delivery is still fundamentally limited, in the sense that maintenance of this mitochondrial pO_2 requires a steady flux of O_2 from the capillaries. Variability of this oxygen buffer (e.g., through alterations of inspired oxygen content or resting CBF) is a possible source of the variability between laboratories of detection of the initial deoxygenation [17].

5. Expanding the oxygen limitation model

To put these ideas on a more quantitative footing we explored the consequences of non-zero mitochondrial pO_2 with the model shown in Fig. 1. A more elaborate model for these effects is under development by the Sheffield group (J. Mayhew, personal communication), but the compartmental model in Fig. 1 will serve to illustrate the basic ideas. Oxygen transport and metabolism is modeled with three compartments representing blood, cytoplasm, and mitochondria. The cytoplasm compartment is meant to represent everything that is not blood or mitochondria. Flow (F) delivers O_2 in arterial blood and carries away O_2 in venous blood. Oxygen enters the tissue compartment in proportion to the average plasma pO_2 in the capillary. Average capillary pO_2 was calculated with a numerical expression for the O_2/hemoglobin saturation curve [22] and the assumption that the O_2 content of blood varies linearly from the arterial value to the venous value. Backflow from the cytoplasm compartment to the capillary was taken to be proportional to the cytoplasm concentration. Similarly, the fluxes between the cytoplasm and mitochondrial compartments were proportional to the respective concentrations. Finally, the metabolic consumption of O_2 was assumed to depend on the mitochondrial O_2 concentration with a simple Michaelis–Menten form (see Fig. 1), with K_m indicating the concentration at which oxygen metabolism begins to be compromised. In this way the demand for oxygen metabolism is represented by the parameter R, and as long as the mitochondrial concentration is much greater than K_m this demand can be met. But if the concentration drops to the level K_m, the achieved $CMRO_2$ will be less than R. This is undoubtedly an oversimplification of the kinetics of O_2 metabolism in the mitochondria, but it serves to bring in the idea of how O_2 metabolism at the mitochondrial level can be independent of O_2 concentration provided the latter is maintained at a high enough level.

For these calculations the assumed resting values were a cytoplasmic pO_2 of 20 mm Hg, a mitochondrial pO_2 of 5 mm Hg, a K_m value of 1 mm Hg, and a resting net extraction $E=0.4$. With these assumptions the values of the first order rate constants connecting the compartments and the parameter R were set by requiring the steady-state flux through the system to be equal to EFC_a, where C_a is the assumed arterial concentration. With these parameters set, we can calculate the flow change (F) required to maintain a constant mitochondrial pO_2 while still supporting a given change in R (i.e., a given change in $CMRO_2$). Fig. 2 shows that the required fractional flow change is about four times larger than the fractional change in $CMRO_2$. Note also that the cytoplasm pO_2 increases monotonically with the increase in $CMRO_2$. Other calculations with cytoplasm pO_2 in the range 20–30 mm Hg and mitochondrial pO_2 in the range 5–10 mm Hg yield similar results.

We can also use this model to begin to explore the fast response in the dynamics of CBF and $CMRO_2$. In this model, there are two key parameters: F, which governs the supply of oxygen, and R, which governs the demand for oxygen. By specifying independent time

Steady-state changes in CBF, $CMRO_2$ and tissue pO_2

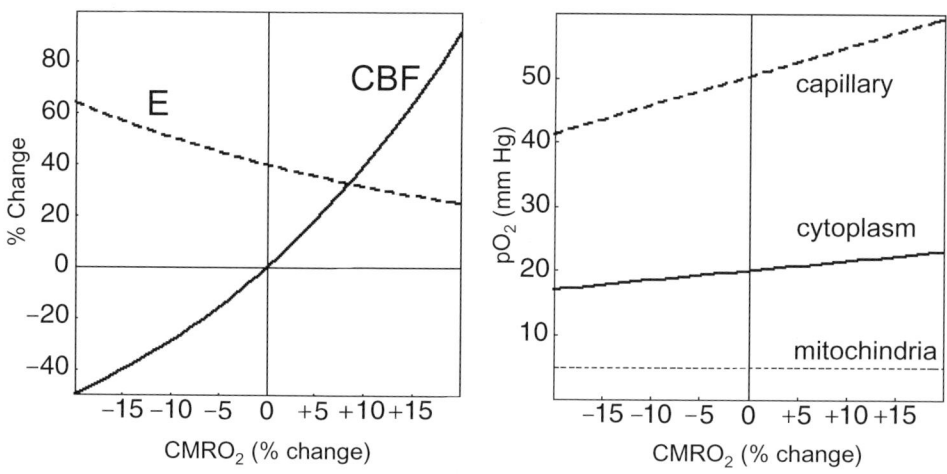

Fig. 2. Steady-state calculations based on the model in Fig. 1 showing the changes in CBF and E required to support a given increase in $CMRO_2$ while maintaining constant mitochondrial pO_2 (left). Cytoplasm and average capillary pO_2 values vary linearly with $CMRO_2$ (right).

courses for $F(t)$ and $R(t)$, we examined how the net oxygen extraction E and the tissue oxygen levels vary with time. In each of these numerical experiments the two dynamic quantities were varied in a smooth step from the resting level to the activated level. If $F(t)$ and $R(t)$ are synchronous, then E exhibits a smooth decrease, while if $R(t)$ precedes $F(t)$ by 2 s there is an initial increase in E prior to the decrease, and an initial drop in cytoplasm and mitochondrial pO_2 (data not shown). Other calculations indicate that the magnitude of the initial increase of E is enhanced if the resting O_2 extraction is reduced. Thus, the initial increase of E is affected by two factors which could be altered by different experimental preparations: (1) the relative timing of the increases in F and R, and (2) the "resting" value of E.

6. Conclusions

The argument presented here is that it is advantageous to the organism for the mitochondrial pO_2 to be maintained at a constant level during physiological activation, so that O_2 availability does not become a limiting factor in satisfying the demand for increased $CMRO_2$. To do this, the average tissue pO_2 must increase and the oxygen extraction fraction E must decrease, so the fractional change in CBF must be several times larger than the fractional change in $CMRO_2$ with activation. However, while the proposed *function* of the large CBF increase is to support the smaller $CMRO_2$ increase, it is likely that the *mechanism* that controls CBF does not depend on the tissue pO_2 at all. For this reason, under non-physiological manipulations the CBF and $CMRO_2$ responses to activation may differ significantly from the normal physiologic response (e.g., the CBF increase with activation under hypercapnia). Furthermore, the reported initial increase of E at stimulus onset could reflect a brief uncoupling of CBF and $CMRO_2$ due to slightly different time courses for the increase of O_2 demand and O_2 supply. However, the fact that this "initial dip" is so brief reinforces the proposed idea of a general close coupling of CBF and $CMRO_2$ during activation.

2.1.1.8. On-Site Discussion

2.1.1.8.1. *Question: (Iadecola)* How about glucose? Glucose consumption increases with activation. How is it regulated?

Answer: (Buxton) The delivery of glucose is not as limited as the delivery of oxygen. About half of the glucose that leaves the capillary is not metabolized, and simply diffuses back to the blood and is carried away by venous flow. So, in principle this would make it possible to increase glucose consumption quickly without having to wait for a CBF increase.

2.1.1.8.2. *Question: (Harder)* PO_2 may not be limiting—rather other factors which regulate electron transfer.

Answer: (Buxton) I agree, and this is the argument that I am trying to make. pO_2 in the mitochondria will not be limiting if it is maintained at a sufficiently high level. But in order to maintain it at this level, the CBF must increase about four times more than the $CMRO_2$ to support the flux of oxygen from capillary to mitochondria.

2.1.1.8.3. Question: (Gjedde) As all mitochondria are not at the same distance from the capillary, how are the "controlling" mitochondria defined, and is it possible that the "dip" is generated by mitochondria not at the end of the diffusion path?

Answer: (Buxton) The heterogeneity of oxygen delivery is certainly a factor that has not been taken into account. I can imagine that the mitochondria nearest the capillary would have the largest effect on altering the pO_2 near the capillary. And this would alter the back flux of oxygen, which could contribute to the initial dip.

2.1.1.8.4. Question: (Traystman) How can mitochondrial pO_2 be the limiting factor in your "limitation model" when mitochondria are known to function at pO_2s of as low as 1 mm Hg? It would seem that mitochondrial pO_2 cannot be the limiting factor here.

Answer: (Buxton) I agree. I am saying that mitochondrial pO_2 is not limiting in the healthy brain because it is maintained at a level much higher than KID. But even if pO_2 is 10 times KID, the amount of oxygen present in the mitochondria would fuel $CMRO_2$ for less than a second. So in order to maintain the pO_2 well above KID, the flux of oxygen into the mitochondria must increase as $CMRO_2$ increases. But to increase that flux with constant mitochondrial pO_2 requires capillary pO_2 to increase, and this requires the oxygen extraction to drop and the flow must increase substantially.

2.1.1.8.5. Question: (Jones) There are two issues concerning oxygen that might be important to consider when a lumped model such as the one. You propose: (1) The substantial pre-capillary extraction of O_2 as described by Popel et al. [Am. J. Physiol. Heart Circ. Physiol. 1989; 256: H921]; and (2) the well-known heterogeneity of brain tissue pO_2. Both of these effects make a lumped compartmental model of brain O_2 seem similar to putting a "compartmental box" over the entire USA to use for weather modeling.

Answer: (Buxton) Compartmental models are useful when our primary interest is to model net fluxes, how much oxygen comes in, how much goes back out, and how much is metabolized. A more detailed model that takes into account the true heterogeneity of the tissue would still have to produce net fluxes that satisfy mass balance. So, treating the USA as a single compartment might not be too bad if you are only interested in measuring the net flux of air in and out. These issues of heterogeneity and pre-capillary oxygen extraction are certainly important for a full understanding of how oxygen gets in and is metabolized, but I think that a more complex model will still have to show the same effects of oxygen limitation that already come through in the simple compartmental model.

2.1.1.8.6. Question: (Nemoto) (1) Have you considered the Bohr effect in causing on increase in cerebral capillary pO_2? (2) The central of CBF in relation to neural activation should also consider the role of neurohumoral factors that are involved in both neural activation and cerebrovascular control.

Answer: (Buxton) (1) Not in these calculations, and that is a good point. There are several factors that could aid in getting oxygen out of the capillary, including the shift of the oxygen/hemoglobin binding curve and possibly capillary dilation. These factors would soften the requirement for a larger increase of CBF than $CMRO_2$, possibly from the factor of 4 calculated here to a factor of $2-3$, but we have not yet done those calculation. (2) That would be a good idea. But my main argument here is related to the function served by a large increase in CBF, rather than the mechanism that produces the change.

2.1.1.8.7. **Question: (Tamura)** The K_m value of cytochrome oxidase against oxygen is around 10^{-7} M. Thus, under the normoxic/condition, cytochrome oxidase is fully oxidized suggesting that oxygen is enough supplied from circulatory system. We could not detect the redox change of cytochrome oxidase during the activation by near infrared photometry. The drop of oxygen tension around mitochondria may not trigger the increase in blood flow. Other mechanism might be present.

Answer: (Buxton) Your observation supports the picture I am trying to describe, that mitochondrial pO_2 is maintained at a high enough level so that there will not be any redox changes with activation. But I do not think average tissue pO_2 would be a good signal for regulating flow, for the reasons discussed earlier. The calculation that showed an initial decrease in mitochondrial pO_2 were meant to show how the "initial dip" could occur as a transient phenomenon if the oxygen demand increases more rapidly than the oxygen supply. I did not mean to suggest that such a dip is required or that it would be a trigger for the CBF increase.

2.1.1.8.8. **Comment: (Tomita)** I would like to make a point concerning gas diffusion through living tissue. Gotoh et al. reported that oxygen transport is several times faster in living tissue than in dead tissue [Exp. Neurol. 1961; 4: 48]. MacDougall and McCabe noted that the diffusion of gas was greatly enhanced in living tissue slices [Nature 1967; 215]. We found that the diffusion of hydrogen gas and oxygen gas in a living cell (C6) suspension was considerably facilitated when compared with that in the dead cell suspension [Adv. Exp. Med. Biol. 1999; 471: 741 and CBF&M 1991; 11(suppl 2), 8471]. The facilitation was living cell population dependent. It is likely that when neurons are activated the diffusion of oxygen from capillary to the neurons will be facilitated.

Acknowledgements

Support for this work was provided by NIH grant NS-36722.

References

[1] B.K. Siesjo, Brain Energy Metabolism, Wiley, New York, 1978.
[2] P.T. Fox, M.E. Raichle, Focal physiological uncoupling of cerebral blood flow and oxidative metabolism during somatosensory stimulation in human subjects, Proc. Natl. Acad. Sci. U. S. A. 83 (1986) 1140–1144.
[3] K.K. Kwong, J.W. Belliveau, D.A. Chesler, I.E. Goldberg, R.M. Weisskoff, B.P. Poncelet, D.N. Kennedy, B.E. Hoppel, M.S. Cohen, R. Turner, H.-M. Cheng, T.J. Brady, B.R. Rosen, Dynamic magnetic resonance imaging of human brain activity during primary sensory stimulation, Proc. Natl. Acad. Sci. U. S. A. 89 (1992) 5675–5679.
[4] S. Ogawa, D.W. Tank, R. Menon, J.M. Ellermann, S.-G. Kim, H. Merkle, K. Ugurbil, Intrinsic signal changes accompanying sensory stimulation: functional brain mapping with magnetic resonance imaging, Proc. Natl. Acad. Sci. U. S. A. 89 (1992) 5951–5955.

[5] A. Gjedde, S. Ohta, H. Kuwabara, E. Meyer, Is oxygen diffusion limiting for blood–brain transfer of oxygen? In: Lassen, Ingvar, Raichle, Friberg (Eds.), Brain Work and Mental Activity, Munksgaard, Copenhagen, 1991, pp. 177–184.

[6] R.B. Buxton, L.R. Frank, A model for the coupling between cerebral blood flow and oxygen metabolism during neural stimulation, J. Cereb. Blood Flow Metabol. 17 (1997) 64–72.

[7] F. Hyder, R.G. Shulman, D.L. Rothman, A model for the regulation of cerebral oxygen delivery, J. Appl. Physiol. 85 (1998) 554–564.

[8] A. Gjedde, P.H. Poulsen, L. Ostergaard, On the oxygenation of hemoglobin in the human brain, Adv. Exp. Med. Biol. 471 (1999) 67–81.

[9] I.G. Kassissia, C.A. Goresky, C.P. Rose, A.J. Schwab, A. Simard, P.M. Huet, G.G. Bach, Tracer oxygen distribution is barrier-limited in the cerebral microcirculation, Circ. Res. 77 (1995) 1201–1211.

[10] U. Gobel, H. Theilen, W. Kuschinsky, Congruence of total and perfused capillary network in rat brains, Circ. Res. 66 (1990) 271–281.

[11] R.B. Buxton, Commentary: the elusive initial dip, NeuroImage 13 (2001) 953–958.

[12] R.J. Seitz, P.E. Roland, Vibratory stimulation increases and decreases the regional cerebral blood flow and oxidative metabolism: a positron emission tomography (PET) study, Acta Neurol. Scand. 86 (1992) 60–67.

[13] T.L. Davis, K.K. Kwong, R.M. Weisskoff, B.R. Rosen, Calibrated functional MRI: mapping the dynamics of oxidative metabolism, Proc. Natl. Acad. Sci. U. S. A. 95 (1998) 1834–1839.

[14] R.D. Hoge, J. Atkinson, B. Gill, G.R. Crelier, S. Marrett, G.B. Pike, Linear coupling between cerebral blood flow and oxygen consumption in activated human cortex, Proc. Natl. Acad. Sci. U. S. A. 96 (1999) 9403–9408.

[15] R. Springett, M. Wylezinska, E.B. Cady, M. Cope, D.T. Delpy, Oxygen dependency of cerebral oxidative phosphorylation in newborn piglets, J. Cereb. Blood Flow Metabol. 20 (2000) 280–289.

[16] D. Malonek, A. Grinvald, Interactions between electrical activity and cortical microcirculation revealed by imaging spectroscopy: implications for functional brain mapping, Science 272 (1996) 551–554.

[17] J. Mayhew, D. Johnston, J. Berwick, M. Jones, P. Coffey, Y. Zheng, Spectroscopic analysis of neural activity in brain: increased oxygen consumption following activation of barrel cortex, Neuroimage 12 (2000) 664–675.

[18] I. Vanzetta, A. Grinvald, Increased cortical oxidative metabolism due to sensory stimulation: implications for functional brain imaging, Science 286 (1999) 1555–1558.

[19] R.S. Menon, S. Ogawa, J.P. Strupp, P. Anderson, K. Ugurbil, BOLD based functional MRI at 4 tesla includes a capillary bed contribution: echo-planar imaging correlates with previous optical imaging using intrinsic signals, Magn. Reson. Med. 33 (1995) 453–459.

[20] E. Yacoub, X. Hu, Detection of the early decrease in fMRI signal in the motor area, Magn. Reson. Med. 45 (2001) 184–190.

[21] I. Vanzetta, A. Grinvald, Commentary: evidence and lack of evidence for the initial dip in the anesthetized rat: implications for human functional brain imaging, NeuroImage 13 (2001) 959–967.

[22] D.G. Buerk, E.W. Bridges, A simplified algorithm for computing the variation in oxyhemoglobin saturation with pH, pCO_2, T and DPG, Chem. Eng. Commun. 47 (1986) 113–124.

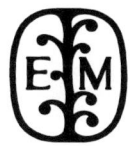

International Congress Series 1235 (2002) 33–38

Flow-metabolism regulation during brain activation and respiratory manipulations

Richard Hoge [a,*], Jeff Atkinson [b], Brad Gill [b], Gerard Crelier [b], Sean Marrett [c], Bruce Pike [b]

[a]*Massachusetts General Hospital NMR Center, Building 149, 13th Street, Charlestown, MA 02129, USA*
[b]*Montreal Neurological Institute, Montreal, QC, Canada*
[c]*US National Institutes of Health, Bethesda, MD, USA*

Abstract

Flow-metabolism coupling was examined in awake human volunteers during graded focal brain activation and during graded exposure to CO_2, a systemic vasodilator. Data acquired during activation with arterial CO_2 levels stabilized to normal values suggest an invariant flow-metabolism coupling relationship, but CO_2-related variations in cerebral blood flow combined additively with activation-related flow responses, with negligible interaction between focal and systemic effects. These findings are inconsistent with the existence of a strictly homeostatic feedback scheme for the regulation of cerebral blood flow, and support the existence of multiple independent pathways of cerebrovascular control. © 2002 Elsevier Science B.V. All rights reserved.

Keywords: Metabolism, Perfusion; Brain; MRI; Hypercapnia

1. Introduction

Metabolic responses during brain activation are of interest as potential markers for neuronal activation, as processes which may be affected by ischemia, and as a fundamental aspect of cellular function in the brain. Recent attention has been focused on the oxidative metabolic response, with much previous work aimed at determining the degree to which

Abbreviations: BOLD, blood oxygenation level dependent; B_0, static magnetic field strength of imager; CBF, cerebral blood flow; $CMRO_2$, cerebral metabolic rate of oxygen consumption; EPI, echo planar imaging; IR, inversion recovery; TE, echo time; TI, inversion time.
* Corresponding author. Tel.: +1-617-726-8790; fax: +1-617-726-7422.
E-mail address: rhoge@nmr.mgh.harvard.edu (R. Hoge).

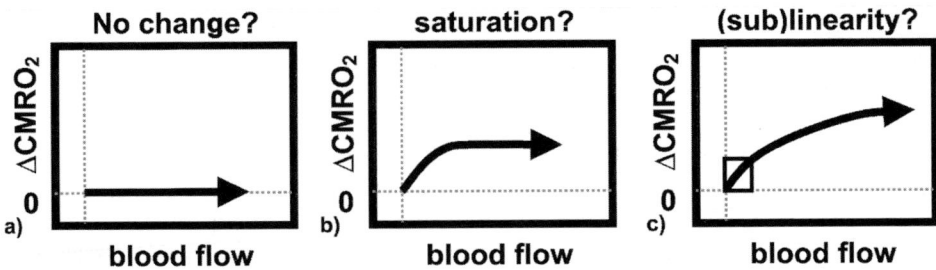

Fig. 1. Three possible flow/metabolism coupling scenarios: (a) no change in $CMRO_2$ with increasing blood flow; (b) increases in $CMRO_2$ with saturations; (c) monotonic sublinearity, which would encompass near-linearity over some limited range (denoted by box in the figure).

the cerebral metabolic rate of oxygen consumption ($CMRO_2$) increased during specific sensory stimulation conditions [1–3]. We have sought to extend this knowledge by measuring increases in both $CMRO_2$ and cerebral blood flow (CBF) during systematically graded neuronal activation in conscious human volunteers [4]. Our main objective has been to identify which of several possible flow-metabolism coupling scenarios, illustrated in Fig. 1, might apply during graded activation. We have also examined flow responses to metabolically demanding neuronal stimuli in combination with systemic vasodilators such as CO_2. The objective in the latter analysis was to determine whether activation-related components of the flow response were adjusted to attain a specific target flow level during a given neuronal state, consistent with homeostatic regulation.

2. Methods

Primary visual cortex was identified in human subjects using phase-encoded retinotopic mapping [5]. BOLD and relative flow responses in this region were then simultaneously recorded during graded visual stimulation. Gradation of visual stimulus potency was achieved by systematically increasing the contrast modulation amplitude of the patterns used, which were each presented for a three minute interval bracketed by baseline periods (1 min pre and 2 min post). The stimuli used were designed to selectively activate different visual pathways and included a red uniform field changed to isoluminant grey and back at 3 Hz, a high spatial-frequency (4 cycle/°) squarewave grating drifted across the visual field at 1°/s at varied orientations, and radial checkerboard patterns with color and luminance contrast, modulated in a temporal squarewave at different frequencies (1–8 Hz). The first two patterns have been reported to selectively activate regions with different levels of the aerobic metabolic enzyme cytochrome oxidase [6], while the checkerboard patterns are non-specific stimuli. BOLD and perfusion responses were also measured during graded hypercapnia, as a calibration procedure [7] to establish the BOLD/perfusion relationship at baseline $CMRO_2$. Steady-state responses (>60 s post-transition) were averaged across subjects ($n=12$) and graphs of $\Delta\%BOLD$ vs. $\Delta\%CBF$ were generated. A mathematical model of the BOLD signal [7,8] was used to translate BOLD-CBF data into

CBF/CMRO$_2$ coupling relationships. Simultaneous BOLD and relative CBF signals were recorded using a modified FAIR EPI acquisition (B$_0$/TI/TE=1.5 T/900 ms/20 ms) with T$_2$*-weighted (BOLD) EPI acquisitions (TE=50 ms) interleaved between the two IR acquisitions. In one set of experiments, flow increases were recorded at four levels of graded hypercapnia (up to 5 mm Hg increase in four equal steps) during a baseline visual state, and also with imposition of a moderate visual stimulus (25% contrast checkerboard pattern) during a second set of graded hypercapnia intervals. This permitted interactions between focal, neuronally driven flow increases and global, CO$_2$-related effects to be studied. All hypercapnic intervals lasted 3 min, and when visual stimulation was performed it was applied only during the period of CO$_2$/air inhalation. Thus all flow responses were normalized to the same baseline state-normocapnia with viewing of a uniform grey display.

3. Results

Fig. 2a shows BOLD vs. perfusion data for graded hypercapnia and for graded visual stimulation, with curves corresponding to different levels of relative CMRO$_2$ (iso-CMRO$_2$ contours) plotted by fitting the model mentioned above to the graded hypercapnia data. While the BOLD/perfusion relationships for graded hypercapnia and graded visual stimulation were significantly different, all visually evoked responses lay in a single well-defined cluster. Transforming Fig. 1a into a plot of flow-metabolism coupling, by solving the fitted model for CMRO$_2$ at the measured data points, resulted in the graph shown in Fig. 2b. Percent changes in perfusion and oxygen consumption were found to be linearly coupled in a consistent ratio of approximately 2:1. In the subsequent experiment, in which stimulation-induced flow/metabolism coupling was examined during simulta-

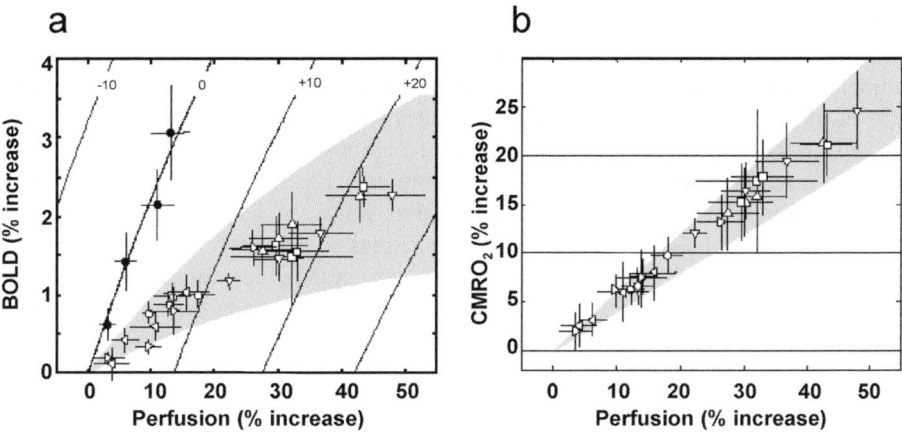

Fig. 2. (a) BOLD signal increase as a function of blood flow increase during graded hypercapnia (●) and graded visual stimulation with various stimuli (◁▷○▽△□). (b) Percent changes in oxidative metabolism as a function of percent change in blood flow.

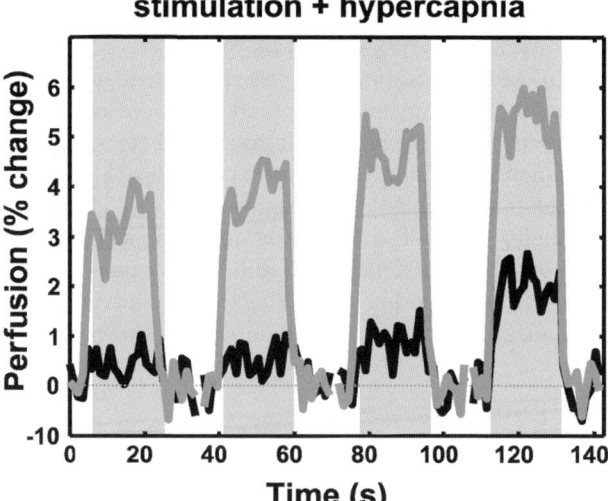

Fig. 3. Flow responses to four levels of graded hypercapnia (black) and graded hypercapnia with exposure to a visual stimulus during hypercapnic interval (grey). The visually evoked component of the flow increase does not change significantly, in spite of the CO_2-induced flow increases. This observation is inconsistent with a feedback-driven control mechanism in which blood flow is regulated to maintain a specific level of tissue oxygenation.

neously imposed hypercapnically induced global flow changes, the global effects combined additively with the effects observed during stimulation at normocapnia, leading to departures from the relationship depicted in Fig. 2b. Signals recorded during this experiment are shown in Fig. 3.

4. Conclusion

In primary visual cortex, steady-state perfusion and oxygen consumption responses appeared to be linearly coupled. Although the visual stimulus types were designed to selectively activate different sub-populations of neurons in V1, including tissue such as the cytochrome oxidase blobs, there were no stimulus specific variations in the slope of the flow/metabolism coupling relationship. It was, however, noted that in general those stimuli consisting of more specific forms of visual information (e.g. diffuse colored fields with no luminance contrast and no spatial structure *or* very high spatial frequency gratings with luminance contrast but no color variations) produced smaller metabolic and flow effects than stimuli such as checkerboard patterns with both luminance and color contrast plus a broad range of spatial frequency content. This may be due simply to the larger number of V1 neurons that are likely to be excited by such non-specific stimuli.

The most potent stimulus patterns employed (high contrast radial checkerboard patterns at high temporal modulation frequencies) did not appear to produce any significant departure from linearity with the flow increases. From this, it might be concluded that physiological stimulation of the visual system is not capable of driving affected neurons to the point where their aerobic metabolic capabilities are exceeded. However, it is also possible that the mechanisms driving flow and metabolism attain maximal values, but in tandem.

The experiments investigating the combination of perfusion increases evoked by blood gas changes and neuronal activation are not consistent with regulation via a feedback mechanism in which substrate availability is monitored to sustain a specific neuronal state. Rather they are suggestive of two independent control mechanisms that do not interact significantly, at least under the conditions of the present experiments.

2.1.2.6. On-Site Discussion

2.1.2.6.1. *Question: (Dirnagl)* What is the evidence that CO_2 is an inert stimulus to raise CBF? Are there possible effects on $CMRO_2$, sympathetic or parasympathetic nerve system, etc.?

Answer: (Hoge) Available evidence for autonomic stimulation and metabolic increases during hypercapnia indicates that these effects become insignificant at the low levels of arterial CO_2 employed in this study, in which increases in end-tidal CO_2 were not greater than 5 mm Hg. Subjects were also free to increase tidal volume and accelerate breathing rate during CO_2 inhalation, which prevented the autonomic activation that occurs in mechanically ventilated animals that are not allowed to react to the increased respiratory drive. Even under more strenuous hypercapnic protocols, the structures that have been found to undergo increased metabolism are those brain regions involved in response to noxious stimuli, such as the limbic and paralimbic systems. The primary visual area sampled in the present study plays no role in processing such stimuli, and is therefore not likely to undergo metabolic increase due to mild hypercapnia.

2.1.2.6.2. *Comment: (Raichle)* Measurements of regional O_2 concentration may not be sensitive enough to detect the "typical" signals of interest to people doing functional imaging in cognitive neuroscience.

Response: (Hoge) The feasibility of using a physiological index such as $CMRO_2$ as a marker for neuronal activation depends ultimately on whether that process increases monotonically with the degree of neuronal electrical activity. The question of whether changes evoked by subtle tasks or stimuli are large enough to detect depends on the precision and stability of available imaging technology. Our preliminary experiments at 1.5 T using an off-the-shelf RF receive coil have demonstrated that the changes in oxidative metabolism produced by high-contrast visual stimulation are well above the threshold of detectability even with standard clinical hardware, and more importantly have indicated that $CMRO_2$ does increase monotonically with neuronal activity over a large range of stimulation levels. Using a higher magnetic field strength and recently available high-performance phased-array coil technology, the sensitivity should be considerably higher and the improvement in specificity of a metabolic marker should be of interest to cognitive neuroscience investigators who may wish to perform studies in which task-related respiratory modulation produces confounding global blood flow changes.

References

[1] P.T. Fox, M.E. Raichle, Focal physiological uncoupling of cerebral blood flow and oxidative metabolism during somatosensory stimulation in human subjects, Proc. Natl. Acad. Sci. U. S. A. 83 (4) (1986) 1140–1144.

[2] I. Vanzetta, A. Grinvald, Increased cortical oxidative metabolism due to sensory stimulation: implications for functional brain imaging, Science 286 (5444) (1999) 1555–1558.

[3] J.B. Mandeville, et al., MRI measurement of the temporal evolution of relative CMRO(2) during rat forepaw stimulation, Magn. Reson. Med. 42 (5) (1999) 944–951.

[4] R.D. Hoge, et al., Linear coupling between cerebral blood flow and oxygen consumption in activated human cortex, Proc. Natl. Acad. Sci. U. S. A. 96 (16) (1999) 9403–9408.

[5] M.I. Sereno, et al., Borders of multiple visual areas in humans revealed by functional magnetic resonance imaging, Science 268 (5212) (1995) 889–893.

[6] R.B. Tootell, et al., Functional anatomy of macaque striate cortex: III. Color, J. Neurosci. 8 (5) (1988) 1569–1593.

[7] T.L. Davis, et al., Calibrated functional MRI: mapping the dynamics of oxidative metabolism, Proc. Natl. Acad. Sci. U. S. A. 95 (4) (1998) 1834–1839.

[8] R.D. Hoge, et al., Investigation of BOLD signal dependence on cerebral blood flow and oxygen consumption: the deoxyhemoglobin dilution model, Magn. Reson. Med. 42 (5) (1999) 849–863.

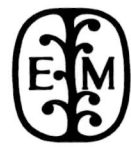

International Congress Series 1235 (2002) 39–47

Spatial specificity of CBF and BOLD responses induced by neural activity

Seong-Gi Kim*, Timothy Q. Duong, Dae-Shik Kim,
Tsukasa Nagaoka, Noam Harel

*Center for Magnetic Resonance Research, University of Minnesota Medical School,
2021 6th St. SE, Minneapolis, MN 55455, USA*

Abstract

Functional magnetic resonance imaging (fMRI) has been widely utilized for imaging brain functions. However, the extent of the fMRI response around the active sites, at sub-millimeter columnar resolution, remains poorly understood. We have investigated spatial specificity of conventional positive blood-oxygenation level dependent (BOLD), early negative BOLD, and perfusion-based fMRI by using a well-established feline orientation column model. The conventional positive BOLD signal is widespread and diffused due to large venous vessel contributions. However, both the early negative BOLD and cerebral blood flow (CBF) responses are specific to individual cortical columns. Thus, hemodynamic-based fMRI can indeed be used to map individual functional columns if large vessel contributions can be minimized. © 2002 Elsevier Science B.V. All rights reserved.

Keywords: Functional MRI; Brain mapping; Perfusion; Cerebral blood flow; Dip

1. Introduction

Recently introduced functional magnetic resonance imaging (fMRI) has the capability to noninvasively visualize brain functions at system level with unprecedented spatio-temporal resolution. Whole brain functional imaging with spatial resolution of a few millimeters to a centimeter can be readily achieved. With growing interest in obtaining high-resolution functional maps, determining intrinsic spatial specificity and resolution of

Abbreviations: fMRI, functional magnetic resonance imaging; BOLD, blood-oxygenation level dependent; CBF, cerebral blood flow.
  * Corresponding author. Tel.: +1-612-626-2001; fax: +1-612-626-2004.
  E-mail address: kim@cmrr.umn.edu (S.-G. Kim).

fMRI becomes critically important. However, the response function of the stimulus-evoked hemodynamic response remains poorly understood. Furthermore, the most widely used blood-oxygenation level dependent (BOLD) fMRI methodology [1] is sensitive to (large) draining veins [2,3], which can run several centimeters in length from neuronally active regions, degrading an effective spatial resolution of fMRI.

To improve spatial specificity of hemodynamic-based fMRI, Malonek and Grinvald [4] suggested the use of the early negative BOLD signal (sometimes referred to as "dip") which is presumably due to an increase in oxygen consumption without concomitant cerebral blood flow (CBF) increase within a few seconds after the onset of stimulus. Based on their optical imaging studies [4], a *biphasic* BOLD signal change is expected where an initial early increase of local deoxyhemoglobin (i.e., a decrease in fMRI signal) is followed by a subsequent decrease of deoxyhemoglobin contents (i.e., an increase of fMRI signal) (see Fig. 1). The former predominantly indicates a metabolic response, which is co-localized to neural active area, while the latter is a hemodynamic response, which may be widespread relative to neuronally active regions [4].

To investigate spatial specificity of conventional BOLD, dip, and CBF responses, we used a well-established cat orientation column model where the periodicity of cortical columns in area 18 is 1.1–1.4 mm and the average size of the column is ~500 μm, as demonstrated by the 2-deoxyglucose (2-DG) mapping technique and intrinsic optical imaging [5,6]. BOLD and CBF responses were obtained by using conventional gradient-echo BOLD and perfusion-based flow-sensitive alternating inversion recovery (FAIR) techniques [7], respectively.

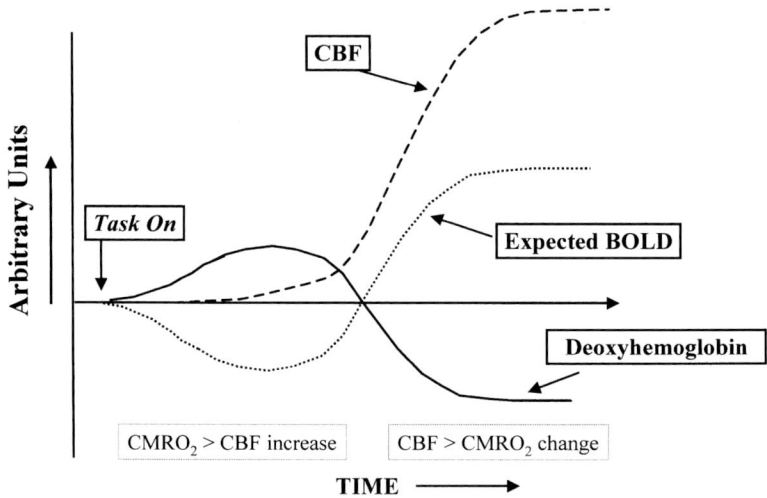

Fig. 1. Hypothetical hemodynamic responses induced by neural activity. Assuming that oxygen consumption change is immediate following the stimulation onset, change of deoxyhemoglobin content is interrelated to that of CBF response. Until the CBF response matches to the oxygen consumption change (CMRO$_2$), deoxyhemoglobin content increases (i.e., the early negative BOLD signal). Later when the CBF response overcompensate the oxygen consumption, deoxyhemoglobin content decreases (i.e., the positive BOLD signal).

2. Methods

2.1. Animal preparations

Detail experimental procedures were described elsewhere [8–10]. In brief, female adolescent cats (0.5–1.1 kg) were treated with atropine sulfate (0.05 mg/kg, i.m.) and anesthetized with a ketamine (10–25 mg/kg) and xylazine (2.5 mg/kg) cocktail (i.m.). Following oral intubation, the animal was mechanically ventilated using a Harvard ventilator ($\sim$25–35 stroke/min, 15–30 ml/stroke) under isoflurane anesthesia (1.0–1.3% v/v) in a 70:30 N_2O/O_2 mixture. End tidal CO_2 was kept at physiological level (3.4–4.0%). The animal's temperature was maintained at 38 ± 1 °C.

2.2. Stimulation paradigm

Binocular visual stimuli consisted of high-contrast, *moving* square-wave gratings (0.15 cycle/degree, 2 c/s) of four different orientations (0°, 45°, 90°, 135°). *Stationary* gratings of identical spatial frequency and orientation were presented during the control period. This stimulus was optimized to activate orientation-selective neurons in area 18 [11].

2.3. MR experiments

MR experiments were performed on a 4.7-T/40-cm horizontal magnet (Oxford Magnet, Oxford, UK), equipped with a homebuilt 15-G/cm gradient and an INOVA console (Varian, Palo Alto, CA). After placing the animal in a cradle, a small surface coil of 1.6-cm diameter was placed on top of the cat brain. A single oblique slice, $\sim$500 μm below the cortical surface, was chosen to target the columnar structure in area 18 with minimal superficial vessel contamination as shown previously [8–10].

BOLD fMRI studies were performed using a single-shot, gradient-echo EPI technique [8,9]. The parameters were echo time=32 ms, repetition time (TR)=0.5 s, data matrix= 64×64, field of view=2.0×2.0 cm^2, slice thickness=2 mm, and flip angle=40°. For each BOLD fMRI measurement, a total of 160 images were acquired, with 60 images prestimulation, 20 images during stimulation, and 80 images poststimulation. CBF measurements were performed using the FAIR technique [10]. Paired images were acquired, one with slice selective inversion and the other non-slice selective inversion. Single-shot, gradient-echo echo-planar images were acquired with the following parameters: TR=3.0 s, inversion delay=1.5 s, and flip angle=90°. All other parameters were the same as those used in BOLD measurements. The slice selective inversion slab was 5 mm thick. Seventy pairs of images were acquired during a three-epoch stimulus paradigm. Each epoch consisted of 10 controls (60 s) and 10 stimulated images. At the end of three epochs, 10 control images were additionally acquired.

2.4. Data analysis

Repeated BOLD and CBF measurements of the same orientation stimulus were averaged before further analysis. CBF images were obtained by pair-wise pixel-by-pixel subtraction of the non-slice selective images from the slice selective images [7]. BOLD and CBF activation maps were computed on a pixel-by-pixel basis using a cross-correlation method. Details have been described elsewhere [8–10].

3. Results and discussion

3.1. Spatial specificity of the conventional positive BOLD signal

Fig. 2 shows conventional BOLD functional maps obtained during stimulation with four different orientations (0°, 45°, 90°, 135°). Activation predominantly lies within

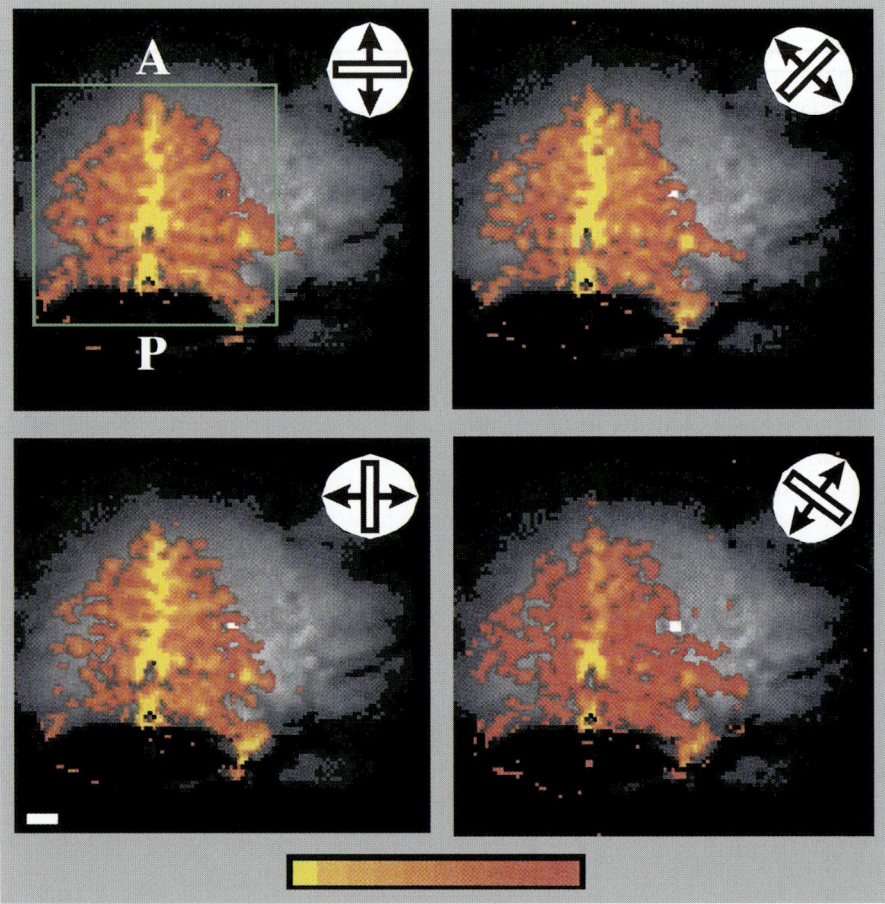

Fig. 2. Conventional positive BOLD fMRI maps during stimulation with moving gratings of four different orientations (0°, 45°, 90°, 135°) in a single animal. A green ROI roughly indicates area 18 in both hemispheres. A color bar indicates a cross-correlation value from 0.3 (red) to 0.8 (yellow). The highest signal change is located at the sagittal sinus. A: anterior; P: posterior; white scale bar: 1 mm.

cortical area 18 (roughly marked by a green box), which corresponds to the primary visual cortex. However, the highest signal change is located at the sagittal sinus [8]. The conventional BOLD signal change is not specific to active orientation columns. In fact, all four activation maps obtained in response to moving gratings of four different orientations yielded similar spatial distributions that were hardly distinguishable from each other (Fig. 2). This result is consistent with the recent optical spectroscopy study [4].

3.2. Spatial specificity of the early negative BOLD signal

In order to examine whether the biphasic BOLD response predicted by optical imaging studies [4] is observed, time courses were obtained from entire area 18 at two different physiological conditions in the same animal (Fig. 3). Dynamics of the BOLD signal changes is closely dependent on an arterial pCO_2; the dip was not observed at a pCO_2 level of ~ 30 mm Hg, while the dip was clearly observed at a pCO_2 level of ~ 40 mm Hg. Thus, animal physiological condition was adjusted for maximizing the magnitude of the dip (i.e., setting pCO_2 level of 35–40 mm Hg). Typically, the dip reaches a minimum of ~ −0.2– −0.4% at ~ 3 s after the stimulus onset. The maximum positive signal change occurs ~ 10 s following the stimulus onset.

To investigate spatial specificity of the early negative BOLD signal, the early negative BOLD functional maps were generated using images acquired at 0.5–2.0 s following the onset of stimulation [5,6]. In contrast to the conventional statistical maps, the early (0.5– 2.0 s) negative map showed predominantly patchy activation patterns in area 18 but not around the sinus (Fig. 3B). These patchy patterns appeared to be column-like based on column size and spacing. The average cluster size of the activated pixels was ~ 300–500 μm and the distance between neighboring pixel clusters was ~ 1.3±0.2 mm [8], consistent with the dimensions of orientation columns visualized with the 2-DG technique (~ 500 μm and ~ 1.1–1.4 mm, respectively [5]). The clustered pixels are irregularly

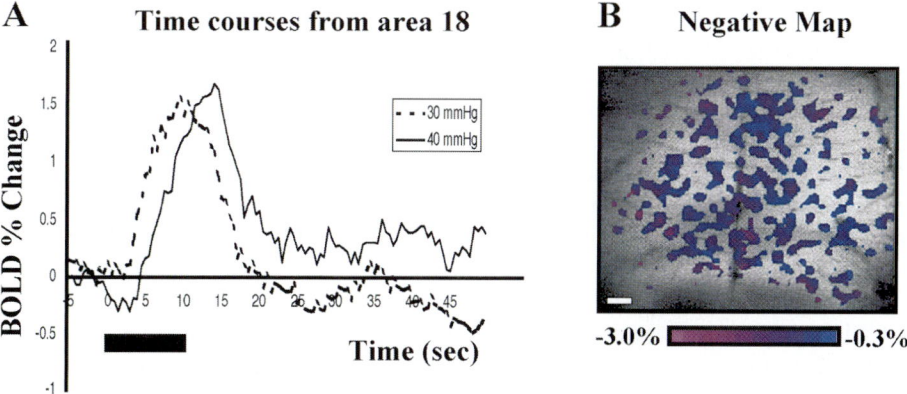

Fig. 3. (A) Dependence of the BOLD response on physiological conditions. BOLD responses were obtained from entire area 18 in the same animal at pCO_2 levels of 30 and 40 mm Hg. The stimulus duration is marked by the black box. (B) Improvement of spatial specificity of the dip. Functional map was generated by using the first 2-s of early negative BOLD (dip) signal. The scale indicates the negative percent change. Scale bar: 1 mm.

shaped, also consistent with those observed using the 2-DG and optical imaging methods [5,6]. The late (2.5–4.0 s) negative map shows that the active areas have moved toward the region of the sagittal sinus (9). These observations suggest that the regional accumulations of deoxyhemoglobin in active tissue were dynamically drained from capillaries into venules and veins.

Since the activation maps constructed by the early negative segment showed patchy patterns that are consistent with columnar organization, further analysis was performed to evaluate their veracity. Activation maps were generated for two orthogonal orientation stimuli (i.e., $0°$ and $90°$ or $45°$ and $135°$). Based on the optical imaging and single-unit recording data [6,12], functional maps of two orthogonal orientations should be complementary. Our data based on the early dip show that functional maps of two orthogonal orientations were indeed occupied at complementary cortical territory [8], suggesting that the map based on the early dip is genuine.

Although the dip has been successfully applied for mapping columnar structures in anesthetized animals [8,9], this approach poses several challenges because it has small percent changes and requires high spatial and temporal resolution. Consequently, the early dip has small overall contrast-to-noise ratio and is highly susceptible to physiological fluctuations and basal physiological condition (see Fig. 3A). Thus, this technique cannot be easily applied to human columnar mapping.

3.3. Spatial specificity of the CBF response

The BOLD signal originates from the overcompensated CBF response, and thus, maps based on both signals can be similar if their anatomical sources are the same. However, the conventional gradient-echo BOLD signal arises from the venous side including large draining veins, while the CBF signal comes from small arterioles and capillaries [7,13]. Thus, it is interesting to examine whether the delayed positive CBF map is similar to the delayed positive BOLD map. Fig. 4 shows one representative CBF map of the cat visual cortex obtained following visual presentation of a single orientation stimulus. Increased CBF activity was observed predominantly in tissue area, avoiding the superior sagittal sinus. Most importantly, the CBF functional map shows patchy layouts with semi-regular cluster shapes, a prominent topological characteristic of orientation columns as observed using 2-DG, optical imaging and the early negative BOLD techniques [5,6,8,9]. This is in marked contrast to the delayed positive BOLD response where large draining vessels were heavily labeled and the mapping signals appeared too diffuse for resolving the patchy layouts (see Fig. 2). The spacing between CBF-responded clusters was 1.1 ± 0.2 mm ($n=14$) [10], consistent with those obtained by using 2-DG [5], optical imaging [6], and early negative BOLD [8,9]. The average full-width at the half maximum of the clusters of this CBF map was estimated to be 470 μm [10]. Also, functional maps at columnar resolution based on the CBF signals were corresponded to those based on the early dip, and highly reproducible under repeated measures [10]. Furthermore, CBF maps of two orthogonal stimuli were found to be spatially complementary. This finding suggests that stimulus-evoked CBF response is spatially localized to individual sub-millimeter cortical orientation columns. This observation contradicts previous findings based on optical imaging and the delayed positive BOLD measurements. This is because these techniques

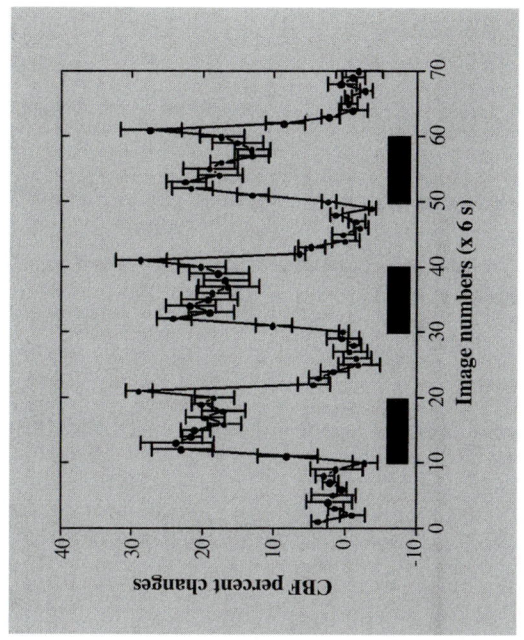

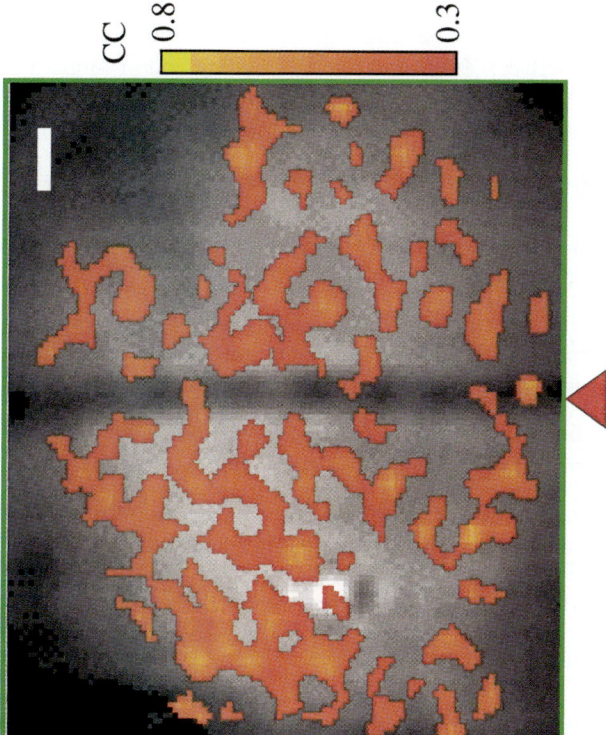

Fig. 4. CBF-based functional map during a single orientation stimulus and its time course. An arrowhead indicates the position of the midline. A color bar shows a cross-correlation value. Scale bar=1 mm. Time course was obtained from active pixels. Boxes underneath the time course indicate 1-min long stimulation periods.

are susceptible to large draining vessel contamination. Therefore, CBF fMRI could offer a superior method to map columnar organizations.

4. Conclusion

Hemodynamic-based functional imaging techniques can be used for sub-millimeter column-resolution brain mapping if large vascular contribution is minimized. Large vascular contribution can be suppressed by using the early negative BOLD, CBF, and other methods such as spin-echo BOLD technique at high field.

2.1.3.7. On–Site Discussion

2.1.3.7.1. *Question: (Fukuda)* Does the signal in perfusion-based MRI mainly come from capillaries or arterioles?

Answer: (Kim) Most perfusion-weighted signal originates from capillaries and tissue. Based on our preliminary diffusion-weighted fMRI data, 80–90% of signal originates from capillary and tissue.

2.1.3.7.2. *Question: (Grinvald)* In optical imaging experiment the dip is highly localized CBF and CBV are not. This was not the case with fMRI. Can you explain the difference?

Answer: (Kim) This issue has to be investigated further. Potential differences are (1) different signal sources between fMRI and optical imaging and/or fundamental difference between CBF and CBV regulation. It should be noted that intrinsic optical imaging measures total hemoglobin (CBV) or deoxyhemoglobin contents, not CBF.

2.1.3.7.3. *Question: (Bandettini)* Of course you are aware of other techniques that do not attempt to remove the vascular contribution, those of Menon et al. in mapping ocular dominance columns (J. Neurophysiol. 1997; 77: 2780). These use the positive BOLD response and perform left vs. right eye subtraction.

Answer: (Kim) As long as you can remove vascular contribution, the resultant map should be specific to a columnar level. Thus, I expect that the subtraction method can be workable. Subtraction will remove non-specific large vessel contribution.

2.1.3.7.4. *Question: (Hoge)* Flow technique using late response permits use in activations where it is not possible/meaningful to impose step input.

Answer: (Kim) Yes, you can use late positive CBF signals, not transient signal. Thus, it is not practical to use this technique which requires high temporal resolution such as event-related fMRI.

Acknowledgements

This work was supported by the National Institutes of Health (RR08079, NS38295, NS40719).

References

[1] S. Ogawa, T.-M. Lee, A.S. Nayak, P. Glynn, Oxygenation-sensitive contrast in magnetic resonance image of rodent brain at high magnetic fields, Magn. Reson. Med. 14 (1990) 68–78.

[2] R.S. Menon, S. Ogawa, D.W. Tank, K. Ugurbil, 4 Tesla gradient recalled echo characteristics of photic stimulation-induced signal changes in the human primary visual cortex, Magn. Reson. Med. 30 (1993) 380–386.

[3] S.-G. Kim, K. Hendrich, X. Hu, H. Merkle, K. Ugurbil, Potential pitfalls of functional MRI using conventional gradient-recalled echo techniques, NMR Biomed. 7 (1/2) (1994) 69–74.

[4] D. Malonek, A. Grinvald, Interactions between electrical activity and cortical microcirculation revealed by imaging spectroscopy: implication for functional brain mapping, Science 272 (1996) 551–554.

[5] S. Lowel, B. Freeman, W. Singer, Topographic organization of the orientation column system in large flat-mounts of the cat visual cortex: a 2-deoxyglucose study, Exp. Brain Res. 71 (1988) 33–46.

[6] A. Grinvald, E. Leike, R.D. Frostig, C.D. Gillbert, T.N. Wiesel, Functional architecture of cortex revealed by optical imaging of intrinsic signals, Nature 324 (1986) 361–364.

[7] S.-G. Kim, Quantification of relative cerebral blood flow change by flow-sensitive alternating inversion recovery (FAIR) technique: application to functional mapping, Magn. Reson. Med. 34 (1995) 293–301.

[8] D.-S. Kim, T.Q. Duong, S.-G. Kim, High-resolution mapping of iso-orientation columns by fMRI, Nat. Neurosci. 3 (2000) 164–169.

[9] T.Q. Duong, D.-S. Kim, K. Ugurbil, S.-G. Kim, Spatio-temporal dynamics of the BOLD fMRI signals: toward mapping submillimeter columnar structures using the early negative response, Magn. Reson. Med. 44 (2000) 231–242.

[10] T.Q. Duong, D.-S. Kim, K. Ugurbil, S.-G. Kim, Localized cerebral blood flow response at sub-millimeter columnar resolution, Proc. Natl. Acad. Sci. 98 (2001) 10904–10909.

[11] J.A. Movshon, I.D. Thompson, D.J. Tolhurst, Spatial and temporal contrast sensitivity of neurons in areas 17 and 18 of the cat's visual cortex, J. Physiol. 283 (1978) 101–120.

[12] D. Hubel, T. Wiesel, Receptive fields, binocular interactions and functional architecture in the cat's visual cortex, J. Physiol. (London) 160 (1962) 106–154.

[13] S.-G. Kim, N.V. Tsekos, Perfusion imaging by a flow-sensitive alternating inversion recovery (FAIR) technique: application to functional mapping, Magn. Reson. Med. 37 (1997) 425–435.

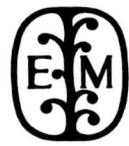

International Congress Series 1235 (2002) 49–56

Activated areas found by BOLD, CBF, CBV and changes in CMRO$_2$ during somatosensory stimulation do not co-localize in rat cortex

W. Schwindt, M. Burke, M. Hoehn[*]

Max-Planck-Institut für neurologische Forschung, Gleueler Str. 50, 50931 Köln, Germany

Abstract

The two presently used methods for functional magnetic resonance imaging (fMRI), blood oxygen level dependent (BOLD) and perfusion-weighted imaging (PWI), depict the hemodynamic response to increased neuronal activity and in consequence, are only indirect parameters. In order to get a more direct mapping of brain activation, we have developed an approach exclusively based on MRI: this method allows the spatially resolved estimation of changes in oxygen consumption ($\Delta CMRO_2$) from changes in the BOLD, signal intensity in perfusion-weighted images (SI_{PWI}) and cerebral blood volume (CBV). As a model, the somatosensory activation after electrical forepaw stimulation was used in α-chloralose anaesthetized rats ($n=5$). A center-of-mass analysis of the BOLD, SI_{PWI} or CBV derived activation maps, revealed that the centers of activation do not co-localize: e.g., centers of the BOLD-and SI_{PWI}-maps were separated by 1.0 ± 0.2 mm. The closest match with the estimated $\Delta CMRO_2$ was found for maps derived from SI_{PWI}. Tissue with increased perfusion encloses areas with and without increased neuronal activity. In areas with increased neuronal activity, the concentration of paramagnetic deoxyhemoglobin is higher than in areas with an increased perfusion but without higher neuronal activity, resulting in a higher BOLD-dependent signal gain in the latter areas. We conclude that merely BOLD-based fMRI may give misleading results for the exact localization of areas of increased neuronal activity. In addition, perfusion-weighted imaging better represents areas of brain activation. © 2002 Elsevier Science B.V. All rights reserved.

Keywords: Functional magnetic resonance imaging; Functional activation; Oxidative metabolism; Cerebral blood volume; Cerebral blood flow; BOLD

[*] Corresponding author. Tel.: +49-221-4726-315/336; fax: +49-221-4726-337.
E-mail addresses: WSchwindt@mpin-koeln.mpg.de (W. Schwindt), Burke@mpin-koeln.mpg.de (M. Burke), Mathias@mpin-koeln.mpg.de (M. Hoehn).

0531-5131/02 © 2002 Elsevier Science B.V. All rights reserved.
PII: S 0 5 3 1 - 5 1 3 1 (0 2) 0 0 1 7 2 - 3

1. Introduction

Currently, there are two techniques available for functional magnetic resonance imaging (fMRI): blood oxygenation level dependent (BOLD) imaging and perfusion weighted imaging (PWI). Perfusion weighted imaging (PWI) detects the reactive increase in cerebral blood flow (CBV) while the BOLD effect reflects a convolution of the secondary changes of CBF, cerebral blood volume (CBF) and oxygenation [1]. The aim of our study was to measure the increased metabolic activity and, in consequence, to get one step closer to the true activation, i.e., the increased neuronal activity. For this purpose, we developed a completely MRI-based, non-invasive method, which allows the estimate the changes of cerebral oxygen metabolism ($\Delta CMRO_2$) with reasonable spatio-temporal resolution. Activation upon electrical forepaw stimulation was studied in α-chloralose anesthetized rats and $\Delta CMRO_2$ was determined by measuring the changes in the BOLD signal intensity (ΔSI_{BOLD}), SI_{PWI} and CBV.

We then used this technique to accurately localize the $CMRO_2$ changes by a center-of-mass analysis and compared this localization with the ones found for the BOLD, PWI and CBV changes during activation.

2. Materials and methods

2.1. Theory for $\Delta CMRO_2$ estimation

A detailed description of the method is presented elsewhere, therefore, the approach is only briefly summarized here [2]. Currently accepted models of the blood oxygenation level dependent (BOLD) contrast, express relative changes of SI_{BOLD} as a result of the changes in CBF, CBV and $CMRO_2$ [1]. Hence, changes of $CMRO_2$ can be calculated when changes of the BOLD, CBF and CBV are determined experimentally.

Using the assumption that all oxygen, which is extracted from the blood, will be rapidly metabolized, $CMRO_2$ can be calculated from the arterio-venous difference

$$OE = CMRO_2 \propto CBF(Ya - Yv) \qquad (1)$$

where Ya is the oxygenation of the arterial and Yv is the oxygenation of venous blood [1]. Then $\Delta CMRO_2$ can be calculated as

$$\frac{\Delta CMRO_2}{CMRO_{2rest}} = \left(1 + \frac{\Delta CBF}{CBF_{rest}}\right)\left(1 - \frac{\Delta Yv}{1 - Yv_{rest}}\right) - 1 \qquad (2)$$

where Δ indicates the difference between the stimulated and the resting state of the respective parameter, e.g. $\Delta CMRO_2 = CMRO_{2stim} - CMRO_{2rest}$.

Calculation of $\Delta CMRO_2$ thus requires determination of $\Delta CBF/CBF_{rest}$ and $\Delta Yv/(1 - Yv_{rest})$. According to Ogawa's relation between cerebral venous blood oxygenation and the BOLD signal [1], changes in $CMRO_2$ can be estimated by

$$\frac{\Delta CMRO_2}{CMRO_{2rest}} = \left(1 + \frac{\Delta CBF}{CBF_{rest}}\right)\left(1 - \left(\frac{\Delta SI_{BOLD}}{SI_{BOLD\ rest}}\right.\right.$$
$$\left.\left. \times \frac{1.32}{2\pi B_0 TE(1 - Yv_{rest})CBV_{rest}\Delta\chi} + \frac{\Delta CBV}{CBV_{rest}}\right)\right) - 1 \qquad (3)$$

2.2. Animal model

Five male Sprague–Dawley rats (300–400 g b.w.) were anesthetized with 1.5% halothane in a 7:3 N_2O/O_2 mixture. A femoral artery and vein were catheterized. The animals were artificially ventilated after tracheotomy and paralyzed with pancuronium bromide (0.4 mg kg^{-1} h^{-1}). For the functional activation studies, subcutaneous needle electrodes were inserted in both forepaws for electrical stimulation, and anesthesia was switched to α-chloralose (80 mg kg^{-1} i.v. supplemented by 40 mg kg^{-1} h^{-1}, N_2O replaced by N_2 [3]). Continuous monitoring included body temperature (37±0.5 °C), arterial blood pressure and arterial blood gas analyses at 30-min intervals.

2.3. Experimental and stimulation protocol

Experiments were carried out in two parts: in the first part we determined SI_{BOLD} and SI_{PWI} changes. A second part for measuring ΔCBV required the administration of an intravascular contrast agent.

We used a block design for stimulation consisting of seven blocks of 90 s OFF vs. 90 s ON stimulation. Stimulation parameters were as follows: 1 mA stimulation current, 0.3 ms pulse width and the stimulation frequency was varied from 3 Hz (three blocks) to 4.5 and 1.5 Hz (two blocks each, respectively) in order to get graded activation intensities [4].

The MRI experiments were carried out on a 7-T Bruker Biospec DBX system with actively shielded gradient coils (200 mT/m) and a bore size of 30 cm. The homebuilt rf-equipment consisted of a Helmholtz coil (12 cm diameter) for spin excitation and a passively decoupled surface coil (2.4 cm diameter) for signal detection.

2.3.1. BOLD and PWI

In the first part of the experiments, the BOLD and perfusion-weighted images were acquired with an arterial spin labeling technique [5], with an EPI readout module. The applied sequence allowed the simultaneous observation of both, perfusion and SI_{BOLD} changes [6] by using the untagged control images to extract the stimulation induced T_2^* changes. A single coronal slice of 2 mm thickness was acquired, 4.5 mm posterior of the rhinal fissure to cover the forepaw area: matrix size 64×32 (read×phase direction), field of view 2.56×1.28 cm^2, TE=27 ms, TR=3045 ms, gradient strength for labeling 10 mT/m. SI_{PWI} was calculated according to Detre et al. [7]

$$SI_{PWI} = \frac{\lambda}{T_{1app}} \frac{M_b^{cont} - M_b^{label}}{2\alpha M_b^{cont}} \tag{4}$$

where α is the efficiency of spin inversion, T_{1app} is the longitudinal relaxation time of the brain tissue, M_b^{cont} and M_b^{label} are the signal intensities in the control and the labeled image, respectively, and λ is the blood–brain partition coefficient of water. α was measured in the image plane, hereby accounting for relaxation due to arterial transfer from the labeling plane to the imaging plane. When λ, T_{1app} and α do not change during functional activation, SI_{PWI} reflects CBF and $\Delta CMRO_2$ can be calculated according to Eq. (3).

2.3.2. CBV

Cerebral blood volume (CBV) changes were measured according to Mandeville et al. [8]. Acquisition of the baseline signal intensity, $S_{CBV\ pre}$, was followed by i.v. administration of an intravascular paramagnetic contrast agent (SINEREM, Guerbet, France, 20 mg Fe kg^{-1} b.w.). Imaging parameters for the CBV investigations (same slice position and thickness as for the BOLD/PWI) were as follows: matrix size 64×32 (read $\times$ phase direction), field of view 2.56×1.28 cm^2, TE=27 ms, TR=500 ms.

2.4. Statistical parametric mapping, $\Delta CMRO_2$ calculation and center-of-mass analysis

Activated voxels were determined for all the acquired imaging modalities, i.e., ΔSI_{PWI}, ΔSI_{BOLD} and ΔCBV by statistical parametric mapping. A Student's t-test at a 95% confidence level was applied using the STIMULATE software package [9,10]. Changes in $CMRO_2$ were then calculated voxelwise from the measured changes in SI_{PWI}, CBV and SI_{BOLD} according to theory (see 2.1).

We used a center-of-mass analysis to compare the localization of the estimated $CMRO_2$ changes to the other modalities.

3. Results

3.1. Physiological parameters

The physiological parameters, i.e., blood pressure, heart rate, body temperature and blood gases were kept in the physiologic range throughout the experiments; there was no significant difference for any parameter between the two parts of the experiments. Furthermore, stimulation did not cause any transient blood pressure increases.

3.2. Measured changes of SI_{PWI}, BOLD and CBV and calculated $CMRO_2$ changes

Forepaw stimulation led to robust activations in the forepaw area of the somatosensory cortex for all three imaging modalities. Representative activation maps are shown in Fig.

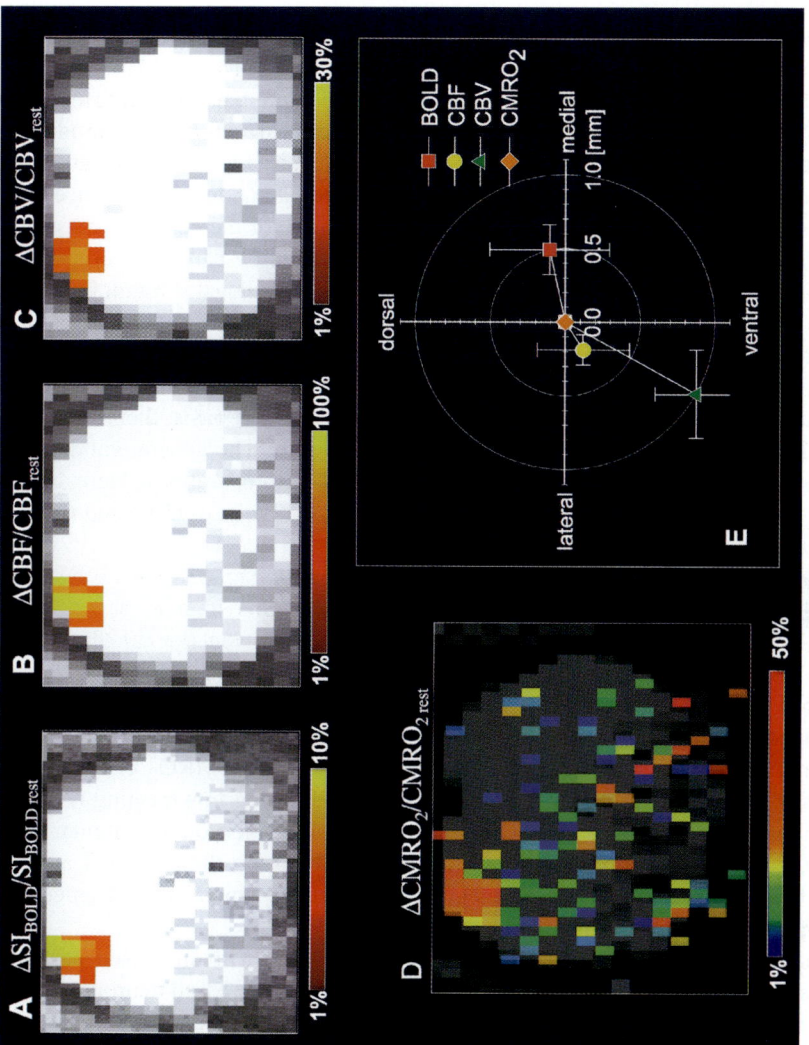

Fig. 1. Representative coronal activation maps for (A) ΔSI_{BOLD} (color bar from red <1% to yellow > 10%), (B) ΔSI_{PWI} (<1% to >100%) and (C) ΔCBV (<1% to >30%) after electrical forepaw stimulation. In (D), a $\Delta CMRO_2$ map calculated voxelwise according to theory is shown. (E) shows the averaged centers of gravity ±SEM for measured ΔSI_{BOLD}, ΔSI_{PWI} and ΔCBV, which are referenced to the calculated center-of-mass of the $CMRO_2$ changes. The largest mismatch is seen for CBV and SI_{BOLD} changes, while SI_{PWI} changes come closest to the $\Delta CMRO_2$.

1A–C. The most pronounced were the elicited changes in SI_{PWI} (66%), followed by changes in the CBV (23%) and SI_{BOLD} (5.2%). The responses decreased with increasing the stimulation frequency.

The measured values were then used to calculate $\Delta CMRO_2$ maps as described above. A representative example of such a map (1.5 Hz) is shown in Fig. 1D.

3.3. Localization and mismatch between BOLD, CBF, CBV and CMRO_2

As it can already be anticipated from the exemplary activation maps shown in Fig. 1A–C, the centers of activation did not co-localize for the three measured imaging modalities. This was clearly shown by means of a center-of-mass analysis: Fig. 1E shows the mean deviations of the centers of activation for the three measured parameters in reference to the center of mass of the $CMRO_2$ changes. The largest deviations for the center of mass were found for ΔCBV and ΔSI_{BOLD}, while $\Delta CMRO_2$ were matched best by ΔSI_{PWI}.

4. Discussion

Our approach allows mapping of $\Delta CMRO_2$ on a voxel by voxel basis; therefore spatial resolution is, in principle, only limited by hardware capabilities. The general validation of our technique will be published elsewhere (Burke et al., in preparation). Here, it may suffice to say that the magnitudes of all the changes in SI_{PWI}, SI_{BOLD}, CBV and $CMRO_2$ are in line with the literature [11–13].

4.1. Localization of activation

Our study has shown that the center of activation as detected by the different imaging modalities does not necessarily reflect the center of estimated $CMRO_2$ changes. The $CMRO_2$ changes were nicely matched by the SI_{PWI} changes, while the CBV and SI_{BOLD} changes were spatially different from the center of mass of the $CMRO_2$ changes. This observation is in line with work from Kim et al., presented during this meeting (Abstract No. 4), showing that the CBF response can resolve brain activation on a columnar level, whereas the (late) BOLD response cannot. A mismatch between the activated areas as detected by BOLD-fMRI and transcranial magnetic stimulation, which stimulates neuronal activity, was recently shown in human subjects [14].

An explanation for our finding could be as follows: tissue with increased perfusion encloses areas with and without increased neuronal activity. As increased neuronal activity leads to higher oxygen extraction, in these areas the concentration of paramagnetic deoxyhemoglobin will be higher than in those with an increased perfusion, however, without higher neuronal activity, resulting in a smaller BOLD-dependent signal increase in the area with neuronal activity. At this point, it should be mentioned that contributions from intrinsic susceptibility changes within the rat cerebral cortex, as described recently by M. Grüne et al. [15], to this spatial mismatch of the BOLD from the other parameters, cannot be fully excluded. However, against this speaks the fact that the CBV changes, also strongly dependent on susceptibility changes, shift in a direction almost opposite to that of the BOLD. Future studies using quantitative T_2* instead of T_2*-weighted BOLD imaging [15] should help to clarify this point.

We conclude that the BOLD-based fMRI may give misleading results for the exact localization of areas with increased neuronal activity. The activated area found with perfusion-weighted images better represents true activation.

2.1.4.6. On-Site Discussion

*2.1.4.6.1. **Question: (Bandettini)** A shortcoming of the technique for localization is that you do not know where you are measuring blood volume from: what vascular component.

Answer: (Schwindt) According to the Windkessel model of Mandeville et al. CBV changes first occur in the arterioles, thus allowing pressure and volume changes in downstream compartments. As these late changes were used to measure CBV changes, the signal presumably mainly comes from capillaries and veins.

References

[1] S. Ogawa, T.M. Lee, B. Barrere, The sensitivity of magnetic resonance image signals of a rat brain to changes in the cerebral venous blood oxygenation, Magnetic Resonance in Medicine 29 (2) (1993) 205–210.

[2] M. Burke, Die Bestimmung der Änderung des Sauerstoffverbrauchs unter funktioneller Aktivierung mittels Kernspintomographie. PhD thesis. Aachen: RWTH Aachen, http://sylvester.bth.rwth-aachen.de/dissertationen/2000/63/00_63.pdf, 2000.

[3] M. Ueki, F. Linn, K.A. Hossmann, Functional activation of cerebral blood flow and metabolism before and after global ischemia of rat brain, Journal of Cerebral Blood Flow and Metabolism 8 (4) (1988) 486–494.

[4] G. Brinker, C. Bock, E. Busch, H. Krep, K.A. Hossmann, M. Hoehn-Berlage, Simultaneous recording of evoked potentials and T*(2)-weighted MR images during somatosensory stimulation of rat, Magnetic Resonance in Medicine 41 (3) (1999) 469–473.

[5] D.S. Williams, J.A. Detre, J.S. Leigh, A.P. Koretsky, Magnetic resonance imaging of perfusion using spin inversion of arterial water, Proceedings of the National Academy of Sciences of the United States of America 89 (1) (1992) 212–216 [published erratum appears in Proc. Natl. Acad. Sci. U. S. A. 89 (9) (1992 May 1) 4220].

[6] A.C. Silva, S.P. Lee, G. Yang, C. Iadecola, S.G. Kim, Simultaneous blood oxygenation level-dependent and cerebral blood flow functional magnetic resonance imaging during forepaw stimulation in the rat, Journal of Cerebral Blood Flow and Metabolism 19 (8) (1999) 871–879.

[7] J.A. Detre, W. Zhang, D.A. Roberts, A.C. Silva, D.S. Williams, D.J. Grandis, et al., Tissue specific perfusion imaging using arterial spin labeling, NMR in Biomedicine 7 (1–2) (1994) 75–82.

[8] J.B. Mandeville, J.J. Marota, B.E. Kosofsky, J.R. Keltner, R. Weissleder, B.R. Rosen, et al., Dynamic functional imaging of relative cerebral blood volume during rat forepaw stimulation, Magnetic Resonance in Medicine 39 (4) (1998) 615–624.

[9] J.P. Strupp, Stimulate, Neuroimage 3 (3) (1996) S607.

[10] M. Burke, W. Schwindt, U. Ludwig, J. Hennig, M. Hoehn, Facilitation of electric forepaw stimulation-induced somatosensory activation in rats by additional acoustic stimulation: an fMRI investigation, Magnetic Resonance in Medicine 44 (2) (2000) 317–321.

[11] J.B. Mandeville, J.J.A. Marota, C. Ayata, M.A. Moskowitz, R.M. Weisskoff, B.R. Rosen, MRI measurement of the temporal evolution of relative $CMRO_2$ during rat forepaw stimulation, Magnetic Resonance in Medicine 42 (5) (1999) 944–951.

[12] S.G. Kim, E. Rostrup, H.B.W. Larsson, S. Ogawa, O.B. Paulson, Determination of relative $CMRO_2$ from CBF and BOLD changes: significant increase of oxygen consumption rate during visual stimulation, Magnetic Resonance in Medicine 41 (6) (1999) 1152–1161.

[13] M.S. Vafaee, E. Meyer, S. Marrett, T. Paus, A.C. Evans, A. Gjedde, Frequency-dependent changes in cerebral metabolic rate of oxygen during activation of human visual cortex, Journal of Cerebral Blood Flow and Metabolism 19 (3) (1999) 272–277.

[14] A. Wunderlich, U. Herwig, C. Schönfeld-Lecuona, H. Walter, R.J.P. Tomczak, M. Spitzer, et al., Functional MRI for validating neuronavigation of transcranial magnetic stimulation, Proceedings of the International Society for Magnetic Resonance in Medicine, Glasgow, UK, (2001) 666.

[15] M. Grüne, F. Pillekamp, W. Schwindt, M. Hoehn, Gradient echo time dependence and quantitative parameter maps for somatosensory activation in rats at 7 T, Magnetic Resonance in Medicine 42 (1) (1999) 118–126.

Linearity to neuronal activity

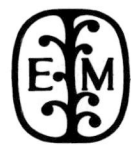

International Congress Series 1235 (2002) 57–71

Quantitative fMRI of rat brain by multi-modal MRI and MRS measurements

Fahmeed Hyder [a,b,c,*], Ikuhiro Kida [b], Arien J. Smith [b], Hal Blumenfeld [d,e], Robert G. Shulman [b,f], Douglas L. Rothman [a,b,c]

[a]*Department of Biomedical Engineering, Magnetic Resonance Center for Research in Metabolism and Physiology, Yale University, New Haven, CT, USA*
[b]*Department of Diagnostic Radiology, Magnetic Resonance Center for Research in Metabolism and Physiology, Yale University, New Haven, CT, USA*
[c]*Section of Bioimaging Sciences, Magnetic Resonance Center for Research in Metabolism and Physiology, Yale University, New Haven, CT, USA*
[d]*Department of Neurology, Magnetic Resonance Center for Research in Metabolism and Physiology, Yale University, New Haven, CT, USA*
[e]*Department of Neurobiology, Magnetic Resonance Center for Research in Metabolism and Physiology, Yale University, New Haven, CT, USA*
[f]*Department of Molecular Biophysics and Biochemistry, Magnetic Resonance Center for Research in Metabolism and Physiology, Yale University, New Haven, CT, USA*

Abstract

Quantitative magnetic resonance imaging (MRI) and spectroscopy (MRS) measurements of energy metabolism (i.e., cerebral metabolic rate of oxygen consumption (CMR_{O_2})), blood circulation (i.e., cerebral blood flow (CBF) and volume (CBV)), and functional MRI (fMRI) signal over a wide range of neuronal activity were used to interpret the energetic and physiologic basis of blood oxygenation level dependent (BOLD) image-contrast at 7 T in the rat brain. Since each parameter that can influence the BOLD image-contrast is measured quantitatively and separately, multi-modal measurements of changes in CMR_{O_2}, CBF, CBV, BOLD fMRI signal allow the calibration and validation of the BOLD image-contrast in glutamatergic neurons of the rat cerebral cortex. Good

Abbreviations: BOLD, blood-oxygenation level dependent; CBF, cerebral blood flow; CBV, cerebral blood volume; CMR_{O_2}, cerebral metabolic rate for oxygen consumption; EPI, echo planar imaging; fMRI, functional MRI; MRI, magnetic resonance imaging; MRS, magnetic resonance spectroscopy; PET, positron emission tomography; POCE, ^{1}H observed ^{13}C editing; R_1, longitudinal relaxation rate of tissue water; R_2^*, apparent tissue water relaxation rate; R_2, absolute tissue water relaxation rate; TE, echo time; TIR, inversion recovery time.
* Corresponding author. 126 MRC, 330 Cedar Street, Yale University, New Haven, CT 06510, USA.
Tel.: +1-203-785-6205; fax: +1-203-785-6643.
E-mail address: fahmeed.hyder@yale.edu (F. Hyder).

agreement between changes in CMR_{O_2} *calculated* from the BOLD theory and *measured* by ^{13}C MRS reveals that BOLD fMRI signal-changes at 7 T are closely linked with alterations in the neuronal glucose oxidation. Comparisons of CMR_{O_2} and CBF over a wide dynamic range of neuronal activity provide insight into the regulation of energy metabolism and oxygen delivery in the cerebral cortex. Consequences of these results from rat brain for similar calibrated BOLD fMRI studies in the human brain are discussed. The current results revealed the energetic and physiologic components of the BOLD fMRI signal and indicated the required steps towards mapping the neuronal activity quantitatively by fMRI at steady state. © 2002 Elsevier Science B.V. All rights reserved.

Keywords: Oxygen; Glucose; Lactate; Glutamate; Glycogen; Neurotransmitter; Energy; Blood flow; Metabolism; Neuron; Astrocyte; Glutamatergic synapse; Cerebral cortex; Electrical activity

1. Introduction

Functional imaging of the brain with magnetic resonance imaging (MRI) has become a popular modality in neurobiology [1], but the exact relationship between the measured blood-oxygenation level dependent (BOLD) signal and the underlying physiology remains unclear. The BOLD functional MRI (fMRI) method allows the detection of changes in the blood oxygenation during a physiological perturbation with the gradient-echo and spin-echo MRI sequences [2]. The image-contrast relies on physiologically induced changes in the magnetic properties of blood (oxyhemoglobin is diamagnetic and deoxyhemoglobin is paramagnetic), where an increase in the fractional BOLD fMRI signal-change ($\Delta S/S > 0$) is consistent with a drop in the venous deoxyhemoglobin concentration [1–5]. At steady state, $\Delta S/S$ is related to the underlying changes in several physiological parameters [3–5]

$$\Delta S/S = \acute{A}((\Delta CBF/CBF - \Delta CMR_{O_2}/CMR_{O_2})/(1 + \Delta CBF/CBF)$$

$$- \Delta CBV/CBV) \tag{1}$$

where $\acute{A}$ is a measurable constant which is dependent on the baseline physiology and the static magnetic field strength, and $\Delta CMR_{O_2}/CMR_{O_2}$, $\Delta CBF/CBF$, and $\Delta CBV/CBV$ are the changes in the cerebral metabolic rate of oxygen consumption, cerebral blood flow, and cerebral blood volume, respectively. Of these physiological parameters, $\Delta CMR_{O_2}/CMR_{O_2}$ is the most relevant for studying the brain function [2,6], because it is proportional to the change in energy consumption associated with the changes in neuronal activity induced by the stimulation.

Several studies have attempted to calibrate the BOLD signal to estimate $\Delta CMR_{O_2}/CMR_{O_2}$ from the MRI measurements [1,2]. The term calibration usually means that by the standardization of $\Delta S/S$ over a wide range of neuronal activity, $\Delta CMR_{O_2}/CMR_{O_2}$ can be predicted with a certain confidence level from the multi-modal MRI data. In this paper, we present the multi-modal measurements of changes in CMR_{O_2}, CBF, CBV, and BOLD signal in the rat cerebral cortex at 7 T over a wide range of neuronal activity. This approach differs from others in the field [7–9] because each parameter in Eq. (1) that influences the image-contrast is measured independently. Furthermore, this current approach allows the validation of BOLD image-contrast because the *predicted* changes in CMR_{O_2} based on the BOLD theory (Eq. (1) rearranged) can be compared with the independently *measured* changes in CMR_{O_2} from in vivo ^{13}C magnetic resonance spectroscopy (MRS) detection of ^{13}C label flow from glucose to glutamate, which provide the metabolic fluxes of the brain energy metabolism [10]. We explored the neuroenergetic basis of the BOLD signal at 7 T in glutamatergic neurons of the rat cerebral cortex and the relevance of these multi-modal measurements for mapping the neuronal activity by fMRI at steady state.

2. Material and methods

2.1. Animal preparation

Adult, male, Sprague–Dawley rats (fasted >16 h) were tracheotomized under halothane (~ 1%) anesthesia and artificially ventilated (70% N_2O/30% O_2). A femoral artery was cannulated for the continuous mean arterial blood pressure monitoring and periodic sampling for the measurement of blood gases, pH, pressure, and glucose. Femoral veins were cannulated for intravenous (i.v.) infusions of nicotine hydrogen tartrate and iron oxide contrast agent (AMI-227; Advanced Magnetics, Cambridge, MA), or D-[1-^{13}C] or [1,6-^{13}C]glucose (99 at.%; Cambridge Isotopes, Andover, MA). Intraperitoneal (i.p.) lines were inserted for the administration of anesthetic, paralyzing agent, and/or pharmaco-logical agent. The scalp was retracted and a layer of Saran Wrap was placed over the skull. The rat was placed prone in a cradle and covered with a water blanket to maintain body temperature (~ 37 °C). Halothane anesthesia was discontinued after the positioning and anesthesia was maintained throughout with either morphine sulfate or α-chloralose and paralyzed with D-tubocurarine chloride (initial 0.5 mg/kg; supplemental 0.25 mg/kg/0.5 h; i.p.). The head was secured in a frameless stereotaxic device and tightly fixed by foam cushions to minimize head movements. The center of the radio-frequency surface-coil was placed above the bregma.

2.2. Experimental protocols

Multi-modal measurements were divided into five treatment groups. The rats in Group α ("control I") were anesthetized with morphine sulfate (initial dose of 50 mg/kg; supplemental doses 30 mg/kg/0.5 h; i.p.), where the rats in Groups β and γ received, in addition, sodium pentobarbital (initial dose of 45 mg/kg initial; supplemental doses of 10 mg/kg/0.5 h; i.p.) and nicotine hydrogen tartrate (dose of 4 mg/kg; rate of 16.7 µl/min; i.v.), respectively [11–14]. The rats in Group δ ("control II") were anesthetized with α-chloralose (initial dose of 40–80 mg/kg; supplemental dose of 20 mg/kg/0.5 h; i.p.), where the rats in Group ε received electrical stimulation (2–3 V square pulses of 0.3 ms duration at 3 Hz; Harvard Apparatus Limited, Kent, MA) of the forepaw [11,12]. Prior to the start of each MRI and MRS protocol, delays alternating with nutations for tailored excitation (DANTE) method was used (see below) for the estimation of the static magnetic field distortions, ΔB_o [13,14]. Values of BOLD fMRI signal (both gradient-echo and spin-echo), CBF, and CBV were obtained (by averaging) from the same region of interest (48 or 8 µl) as the CMR_{O_2} measurements were made from [11–14]. All data were acquired under steady-state conditions.

2.3. MRI and MRS measurements

All in vivo MRI and MRS data were obtained on a modified 7 T Bruker Biospec or AVANCE horizontal-bore spectrometer (Bruker Instruments, Billerica, MA) operating at 300.6 and 75.5 MHz for ^1H and ^{13}C, respectively, using a ^1H resonator transmit (8 cm diameter) for the homogeneous radio-frequency transmission with a ^1H surface-coil receiver (10 mm in diameter) for local radio-frequency reception and a concentric ^{13}C radio-frequency surface-coil (20 mm in diameter) for the transmission and decoupling in the ^1H observed ^{13}C editing (POCE) experiments for the absolute CMR_{O_2} measurements (see below). High resolution, multi-slice, coronally oriented gradient-echo MRI data were acquired to provide coordinates for the placement of a $7.5 \times 1.6 \times 4.0$-mm^3 region of interest for the POCE experiments in the sensorimotor region of the rat brain. The static magnetic field homogeneity of that region of interest was optimized. All multi-modal MRI data (see below) were acquired with sequentially sampled echo planar imaging (EPI) data [15] with spatial resolution of $430 \times 430 \times 1000$ μm^3, using a sinc pulse for the slice excitation and an adiabatic fast passage hyperbolic secant pulse for the slice refocusing or inversion (see below).

Absolute values of CMR_{O_2} were obtained either from 48 μl voxels using the POCE method [16,17] or 8 μl with a method which combines the speed of EPI with $^{13}C-^1H$ J-editing and semi-selective water suppression [18]. Time courses of brain C4-glutamate labeling from each rat were normalized to the ^{13}C fractional enrichment of plasma C1- or C1,6-glucose [16,17]. A set of coupled differential equations was used to describe the model [19,20] and an iterative method was used to fit the model to the C4-glutamate turnover data to yield absolute values of CMR_{O_2}. The modeling parameters which have secondary effects on CMR_{O_2} have been described and discussed previously [10,16–20]. For rats in Group ϵ only, partial-volume corrected CMR_{O_2} values were obtained for the forepaw stimulation data as previously described [17] using the relationship of ω(activa-(activated)=$[\omega$(observed) $- (1 - f) \times \omega$(rest)$]/f$, where f represents the fraction of activated tissue in the compartment (e.g., 0.7 ± 0.2 from Ref. [11]) using the activated CBF threshold maps at the resting CBF value, and ω represents CMR_{O_2}.

The multi-modal MRI measurements were made with a new EPI sequence [21] that allows the measurement of changes in CBF and CBV in a rapid manner ($\sim$ 1 min). The method allows interleaved measurements of both transverse (apparent tissue water relaxation rate (R_2) and absolute tissue water relaxation rate (R_2^*)) and longitudinal (R_1) relaxation rates of tissue water in conjunction with the pulsed arterial spin labeling. The image-contrasts are intrinsically oxygenation and flow weighted but each contrast is made quantitative by two echo time (TE) and inversion recovery time (TIR) acquisitions with EPI. This method has been validated in the rat brain by comparison of the multi-modal maps obtained by using the two-point and multi-point fitting approaches during varied levels of activity [21]. By the use of an MRI contrast agent and repeated measurements of changes in R_2 and R_2^* with stimulation (in the same subject), the CBV changes can be determined with the same method [12–14].

A single-exponential fit of the gradient-echo and spin-echo data was used to obtain $R_2^*(\text{obs})$ and $R_2(\text{obs})$ maps, respectively. We used the following relaxation rate term to describe the BOLD fMRI signal

$$R_2'(Y) = R_2^*(\text{obs}) - R_2(\text{obs}) - R_2^*(\Delta B_o) \qquad (2)$$

where $R_2^*(\Delta B_o)$ is the relaxation component of the tissue water relaxation rate attributed to the macroscopic distortions of the static magnetic field (ΔB_o), and $R_2'(Y)$ is the reversible relaxation component tissue water relaxation rate due to the blood oxygenation effects. The $R_2^*(\Delta B_o)$ component within the region of interest was estimated ($6 \pm 1 \text{ s}^{-1}$) by an MRI sequence [22] with a double spin tagging sequence using DANTE pulses as described previously [13,14]. The BOLD fMRI signal-change at steady state in Eq. (1) is also given by

$$\Delta S/S = \exp(-\Delta R_2'(Y) \times \text{TE}) - 1 \qquad (3)$$

where TE is 25 ms and $\Delta R_2'(Y)$ is the change in the relaxation rate term described in Eq. (2). The advantage of this definition for the BOLD signal is that the common (and unknown) terms between $R_2^*(\text{obs})$ and $R_2(\text{obs})$ are subtracted away [4] leaving only the pure oxygenation term, which can be described as [1–5]

$$R_2'(Y) = Cv_{\max}(1 - Y)b\text{Hct} \qquad (4)$$

where C is a BOLD fMRI signal proportionality constant, $v_{\max}$ is the magnetic field dependent deoxyhemoglobin susceptibility frequency shift, b is the blood volume fraction, $(1 - Y)$ is the blood deoxygenation, and Hct is the blood hematocrit.

The relative changes in CBV from the baseline to lower or higher conditions were measured by the administration of a high susceptibility MRI contrast agent to enhance the blood volume induced changes in $R_2(\text{obs})$ or $R_2^*(\text{obs})$. The blood volume susceptibility was raised through serial injections (2 mg/kg/0.9 ml bolus) of an iron oxide contrast agent AMI-227 which remains in the intravascular space for several hours [23]. The relative changes in CBV were calculated by $\Delta\text{CBV}/\text{CBV} = (\Delta R^w - \Delta R^{w/o})/(R^w - R^{w/o})$, where R^w and $R^{w/o}$ are the rates at the reference conditions with and without agents, respectively, and ΔR^w and $\Delta R^{w/o}$ are the rate differences as a consequence of transition from the baseline to lower or higher conditions with and without agents, respectively. Details of relative CBV measurement and experimental errors have been described earlier [23,24].

The absolute CBF maps were obtained using the spin-echo slice selective and non-slice selective inversion-recovery weighted EPI data [21]. A single-exponential recovery fit to the TIR data was used to create R_1 maps for the slice selective (R_{1s}) and non-slice selective (R_{1n}) images. The longitudinal relaxation rate of the arterial blood water (R_{1b}) was determined ($0.50 \pm 0.03 \text{ s}^{-1}$) from the high resolution CBF data [11,21] and the brain–blood partition coefficient for water (λ) was assumed to be 0.95 ml/g [25]. Absolute perfusion was calculated by $\text{CBF} = 60\lambda(R_{1\text{app}} - R_{1b})$, where $R_{1\text{app}}$ is the apparent relaxation rate given by $\{R_{1b} + (R_{1s} - R_{1n})/(1 + v)\}$ and v is a small correction factor, given by $3/4(1 - R_{1b}/R_{1n})$, which accounts for the difference between the longitudinal relaxation rates of the tissue water and arterial blood water [25]. Details of the absolute CBF measurement and associated experimental errors have been described previously [21,26].

2.4. Calibration and validation of the BOLD fMRI signal

To compare the values of $\Delta S/S$ over a wide range of neuronal activity in a meaningful manner requires standardization because the change in the BOLD fMRI signal (measured by MRI) is dependent on the relative differences of fractional changes in three parameters (Eq. (1)). We have measured each parameter separately and quantitatively, namely, $\Delta CBF/CBF$ (measured by MRI), $\Delta CBV/CBV$ (measured by MRI), and $\Delta CMR_{O_2}/CMR_{O_2}$ (measured by MRS). The normalization of the BOLD fMRI signal can be obtained by dividing both sides of Eq. (1) by $\Delta CBF/CBF$ and rearranging to result in

$$\acute{A} = \theta/((1 - \Psi)/(1 + \Delta CBF/CBF) - \Lambda) \tag{5}$$

where $\theta = (\Delta S/S)/(\Delta CBF/CBF)$, $\Psi = (\Delta CMR_{O_2}/CMR_{O_2})/(\Delta CBF/CBF)$, and $\Lambda = (\Delta CBV/CBV)/(\Delta CBF/CBF)$. Since each term in Eqs. (1) and (5) was measured over a wide range of neuronal activity at 7 T in the rat cortex, the parameter $\acute{A}$ was completely determined from the experimental data. The normalized approach for the determination of $\acute{A}$ (Eq. (5)) avoids biases towards arbitrary values of $\Delta S/S$, which has potential to be affected by the resting baseline values [27]. The value of $\Delta CMR_{O_2}/CMR_{O_2}$ is calculated by the rearrangement of Eq. (1)

$$\Delta CMR_{O_2}/CMR_{O_2} = \Delta CBF/CBF - \{(\Delta S/S)/\acute{A} + \Delta CBV/CBV\}$$
$$\times (1 + \Delta CBF/CBF) \tag{6}$$

which can be further simplified by the relationship between CBV and CBF [28]

$$\Delta CBV/CBV = (1 + \Delta CBF/CBF)^\phi - 1 \tag{7}$$

to allow the calculation of $\Delta CMR_{O_2}/CMR_{O_2}$ only from the BOLD and CBF measurements (by MRI only)

$$\Delta CMR_{O_2}/CMR_{O_2} = \Delta CBF/CBF - \{(\Delta S/S)/\acute{A} + (1 + \Delta CBF/CBF)^\phi - 1\}$$
$$\times (1 + \Delta CBF/CBF). \tag{8}$$

The value of ϕ used in Eq. (8) can be determined experimentally from the CBV and CBF data (Eq. (7)) over a wide dynamic range of conditions [12–14]. Although the relationship expressed in Eq. (8) is similar to others [7–9], we have sought to measure each parameter on the right-hand side of Eq. (8) to predict $\Delta CMR_{O_2}/CMR_{O_2}$ [12–14]. Comparison of predicted (in Eq. (8) using the MRI data) and measured (by POCE using the MRS data) values of $\Delta CMR_{O_2}/CMR_{O_2}$ can allow the validation of this method

$$[\Delta CMR_{O_2}/CMR_{O_2} \text{ (predicted by Eq. (8))}]$$
$$= m[\Delta CMR_{O_2}/CMR_{O_2} \text{ (measured by POCE)}] \tag{9}$$

where m approaches identity if the *predicted* and *measured* values $\Delta CMR_{O_2}/CMR_{O_2}$ are in agreement.

3. Results

The changes in CBV (measured by MRI) and CMR_{O_2} (measured by MRS) are compared with the changes in CBF (measured by MRI) in Fig. 1A. The relative changes in CBV for the global perturbations (Groups β and γ) were small, ranging from 2% to 7% with respect to the control condition I (Group α), whereas the localized changes in the CBV measured during the forepaw stimulation (Group ϵ) were slightly larger, ranging from 7% to 21% with respect to the control condition II (Group δ). The relationship between CBV and CBF (Eq. (7)) shows that although the relative magnitudes in CBV changes for the two control conditions (Groups α and δ) were different (i.e., $5 \pm 3\%$ vs. $14 \pm 9\%$, respectively), the value of ϕ determined from Eq. (7) were of the same magnitude (i.e., 0.10 ± 0.06) for all perturbations. Therefore, the relative changes in CBV in relation to the absolute changes in CBF could be scaled to the awake resting CBF value for the nonanesthetized resting awake condition and used in Eq. (8) for the calibration.

In Fig. 1A, the comparison of relative changes in CBV (measured by MRI) and CMR_{O_2} (measured by MRS) shows that $\Delta CMR_{O_2}/CMR_{O_2} \gg \Delta CBV/CBV$ over the same range of changes in CBF (measured by MRI). Because the measured $\Delta CMR_{O_2}/CMR_{O_2}$ values above the nonanesthetized resting awake condition (Group ϵ; top right quadrant) were partial-volume corrected, a nonlinear fit over the whole dynamic range is a better representative for the relationship between CMR_{O_2} and CBF (see below and Fig. 3A). Fig. 1B shows the summary of all multi-modal MRI and MRS data which have been used to standardize the BOLD fMRI signal-changes over a wide range of neuronal activity (Groups α–ϵ). The average values of Ψ, Λ, and θ in Eq. (5) were determined to be 0.75 ± 0.16, 0.12 ± 0.07, and 0.10 ± 0.06, respectively, to provide a standardized value of 0.36 ± 0.09 for $\acute{A}$ representing the nonanesthetized resting awake condition.

Fig. 2A shows the comparison of the *predicted* $\Delta CMR_{O_2}/CMR_{O_2}$ (in Eq. (8)) and *measured* $\Delta CMR_{O_2}/CMR_{O_2}$ (by POCE). Because most of the data points representing the MRI-predicted and MRS-measured values of $\Delta CMR_{O_2}/CMR_{O_2}$ lie close to the line of identity over a wide dynamic range of neuronal activity (Groups α–ϵ), there is high confidence ($m = 0.9 \pm 0.1$; Eq. (9)) of the BOLD fMRI signal calibration at 7 T in the rat cortex ($n = 28$). Fig. 2B shows the mapping of localized changes in CBF, CBV, and BOLD signal (using R_2' (Y) as in Eq. (3)) during the forepaw stimulation in a lightly anesthetized rat. The magnitudes of localized changes in CBF, CBV, and BOLD signal were 1.22 ± 0.45, 0.08 ± 0.05, and 0.06 ± 0.02, respectively ($n = 4$). Comparison of the localized changes in CBV and CBF shows that the value of ϕ for the functional data (~ 0.1) in this lightly anesthetized condition is in agreement with the other conditions measured in Fig. 1 (see above). Therefore, Eq. (8) could be used with the high confidence of the linear regression in Fig. 2A ($R^2 = 0.95$) to predict the regional alterations in CMR_{O_2} from the localized changes in CBF and BOLD signal and the experimentally determined values of $\acute{A}$ (Eq. (5)) and ϕ (Eq. (7)). The regional alterations in CMR_{O_2} was estimated to be 0.97 ± 0.36 using Eq. (8) for the lightly anesthetized condition ($n = 4$). Alternatively, using Eq. (6) with the fractional changes in CBF, CBV, and BOLD signal yielded statistically insignificantly different predictions of $\Delta CMR_{O_2}/CMR_{O_2}$ (0.97 ± 0.36 vs. 0.93 ± 0.40; $p > 0.3$). While magnitudes of changes in CBF and CMR_{O_2} were smaller than

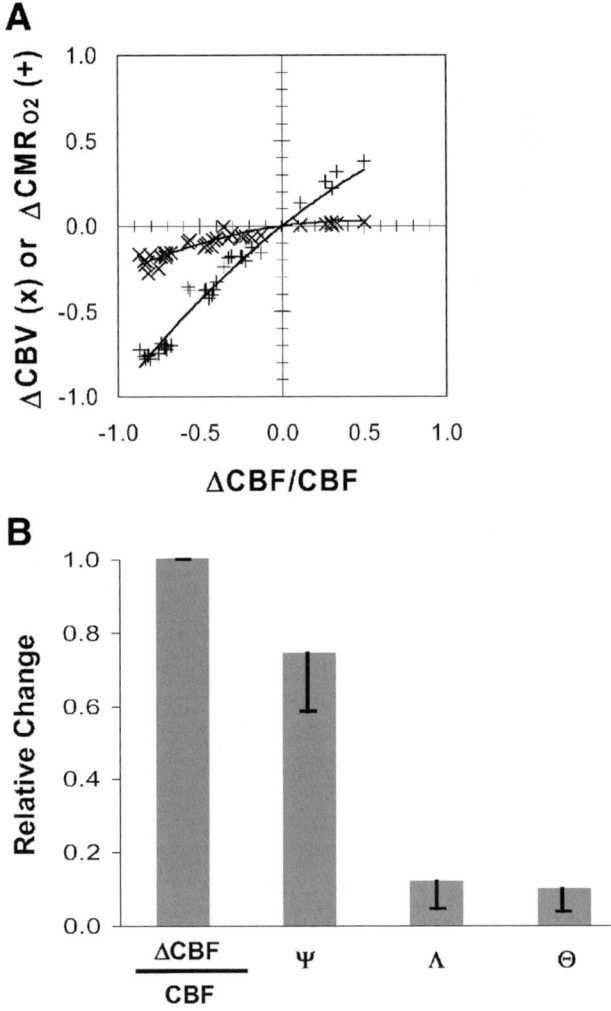

Fig. 1. (A) Comparisons of $\Delta CBV/CBV$ ($\times$) and $\Delta CMR_{O_2}/CMR_{O_2}$ (+) vs. $\Delta CBF/CBF$ for the different conditions (Groups $\alpha-\epsilon$). The ratios of ($\Delta CMR_{O_2}/CMR_{O_2})/(\Delta CBF/CBF)$ and ($\Delta CBV/CBV)/(\Delta CBF/CBF)$, given by Ψ and Λ, respectively in Eq. (5), are significantly different (slopes through origin are $\sim$ 0.8 and $\sim$ 0.1, respectively). The origin represents the resting awake state for the rat cerebral cortex [11,12]. Modified from Hyder et al. [11,12] and Kida et al. [13,14]. (B) Summary of quantitative MRI and MRS measurements of relative changes in CBF, CMR_{O_2}, CBV, and BOLD signal, over a wide range of neuronal activity (Groups $\alpha-\epsilon$). For each condition, the changes in CBF, CMR_{O_2}, CBV, and BOLD signal were normalized by changes in CBF which resulted in ratios of 1, Ψ, Λ, and θ, respectively (Eq. (5)). This normalization procedure provides a comparison of relative changes in each parameter during the changes in neuronal activity. These findings show that CBF and CMR_{O_2} play a more dominant role in the modulation of BOLD image-contrast at 7 T in glutamatergic neurons of rat brain. The average values of Ψ, Λ, and θ in Eq. (5) were 0.75 ± 0.16, 0.12 ± 0.07, and 0.10 ± 0.06, respectively, to provide a standardized value of 0.36 ± 0.09 for $\acute{A}$ ($n=28$) representing the nonanesthetized resting awake condition. The error bars represent the standard deviation from the mean. Modified from Hyder et al. [12].

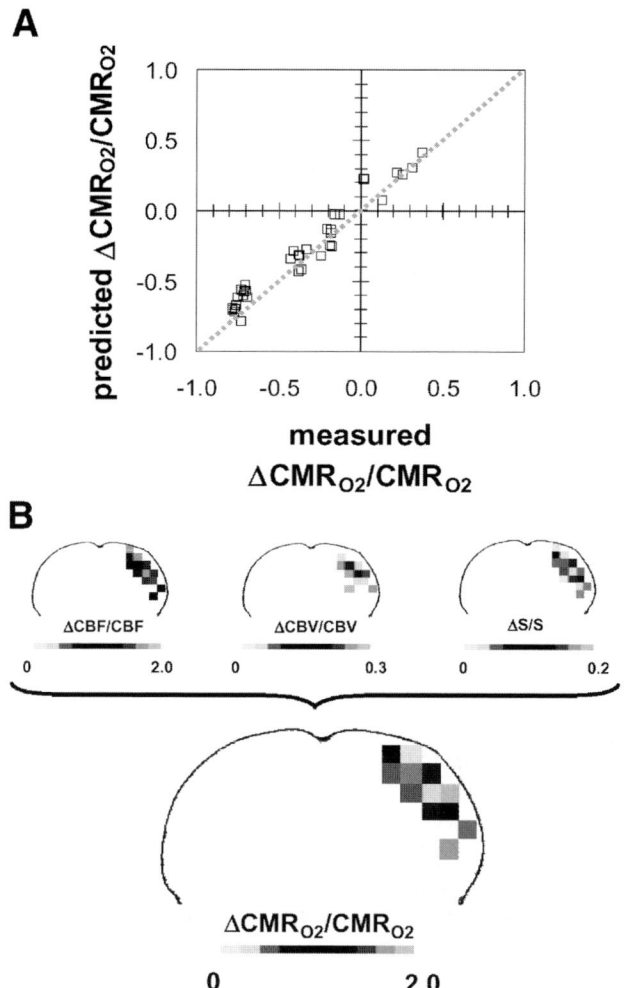

Fig. 2. (A) The *predicted* $\Delta CMR_{O_2}/CMR_{O_2}$ (by Eq. (8)) and *measured* $\Delta CMR_{O_2}/CMR_{O_2}$ (by POCE) values are compared to provide validation of BOLD calibration at 7 T in the rat cerebral cortex. The dotted line represents the line of identity and a linear regression analysis of the data provides a value of $m = 0.9 \pm 0.1$ (Eq. (9)) with $R^2 = 0.95$. These results indicate that at very high static magnetic fields strengths deoxygenation effects in blood dominate the relaxation effects in tissue which can be accentuated by combining the gradient-echo and spin-echo data (Eq. (2)). Since the validation of BOLD calibration relies on standard errors of independent measures for the relaxation rate, blood flow, and volume, by comparing the *calculated* and *measured* $\Delta CMR_{O_2}/CMR_{O_2}$, it can be calculated that the validation accuracy for high resolution CMR_{O_2} mapping by multi-modal MRI at 7 T in the rat cortex is at least 80% [12]. Modified from Hyder et al. [12] and Kida et al. [14]. (B) Multi-modal maps of localized changes in CBF, CBV, and BOLD signal obtained during the forepaw stimulation in an α-chloralose anesthetized rat which were used to calculate a relative CMR_{O_2} map using Eq. (8). The rats in this group ($n = 4$) received an initial α-chloralose dose of 40 mg/kg (i.p.). The magnitudes of changes in CBF, CBV, and BOLD signal were 1.17 ± 0.41, 0.07 ± 0.04, and 0.06 ± 0.02, respectively, and the localized change in CMR_{O_2} was 0.93 ± 0.33 (for this rat only). Each map is scaled differently. The regional correlation observed between changes in CMR_{O_2} and CBF is very similar to the regional correlation between the changes in glucose metabolism and perfusion for the same rat model [29]. Modified from Hyder et al. [12].

the previous values for the forepaw stimulation [11], the value of Ψ (Eq. (5)) which is given by the ratio of $(\Delta CMR_{O_2}/CMR_{O_2})/(\Delta CBF/CBF)$ for the lightly anesthetized condition in the current study (0.7 ± 0.3) is in good agreement with the previous observations [11] under deeper anesthesia (0.8 ± 0.2).

4. Discussion

The approach we employed to calibrate the BOLD image-contrast [12–14] differs from the previous animal studies which used the nonphysiological challenges (e.g., hypoxia or hypercapnia) to perturb CBF [7,30]. In these previous studies, the changes in CBV were assumed to follow the dependence proposed in Eq. (7) for hypercapnic challenges in primates [28] and changes in CMR_{O_2} and CBV were not measured. The value of ϕ in Eq. (7) was determined to be ~ 0.4 by Grubb et al. [28] in a positron emission tomography (PET) study, whereas the value of ϕ determined in the current MRI study was ~ 0.1 for a wide range of activity in the rat brain (Fig. 1B). This discrepancy could be partially attributed to the different tracers used in the MRI and PET methods for CBV measurements. Because the distribution spaces and half-lives of PET and MRI tracers are different, the changes in tracer kinetics of each label reflect changes in different compartments of blood (e.g., plasma vs. hemoglobin). Alternatively, hypoxia and hypercapnia induce some level of uncoupling between the oxygen delivery and consumption, and alterations in blood pH and/or hematocrit [31], which may lead to a different coupling between CBF and CBV than with physiological stimulation.

The BOLD calibration was tested by the comparison of $\Delta CMR_{O_2}/CMR_{O_2}$ predicted (in Eq. (8)) and measured (by POCE). The accuracy of the BOLD calibration in Fig. 2A ($m = 0.9 \pm 0.1$) is consistent over a wide range of neural activity, from the deeply anesthetized condition (bottom left quadrant) to highly activated condition (top right quadrant). The highest levels of activity are above the nonanesthetized resting awake condition (origin). Although the confidence limit of calibration of the BOLD signal is quite high (Fig. 2A), there are limitations to the calibration. One potential source of uncertainty in comparing the MRI-predicted CMR_{O_2} (in Eq. (8)) with the MRS-measured CMR_{O_2} (by POCE) is the heterogeneity in metabolism within larger MRS voxels in comparison to the $\Delta CBF/CBF$, $\Delta CBV/CBV$, and $\Delta S/S$ measurements which all have substantially superior spatial resolution. The CMR_{O_2} measured (by POCE) in the region of interest is equivalent to the average of CMR_{O_2} predicted (in Eq. (8)) from all MRI subvoxels. If the theory is correct, by calculating $\Delta CMR_{O_2}/CMR_{O_2}$ in each voxel from the MRI data and then, summing them up, the average value determined from the BOLD calibration should agree with the MRS measurement. The finding of good experimental agreement between these independent measures (Fig. 2A) strongly supports the combined use of the BOLD signal, CBF, and CBV measurements to map CMR_{O_2} at 7 T (see below; Fig. 2B). A detailed discussion of the biophysical consequences of these results has been described earlier [12,14]. In summary, the results indicate that the strongest modulator of the BOLD fMRI signal is the $R_2'(Y)$ component (Eq. (2)), utilized here by the difference of $R_2^*(\text{obs})$ and $R_2(\text{obs})$ after the removal of the $R_2^*7(\Delta B_o)$ term, which is associated with the extravascular compartment at a high static magnetic field strength [1–5].

We expect the accuracy of the BOLD calibration at 7 T in the rat cortex to be high over a wide range of neuronal activity (Fig. 2A) because of the linear relationship observed between CBF and CMR_{O_2} over the same range. Fig. 3A indicates that CBF (measured by MRI) and CMR_{O_2} (measured by MRS) change proportionately in the rat somatosensory

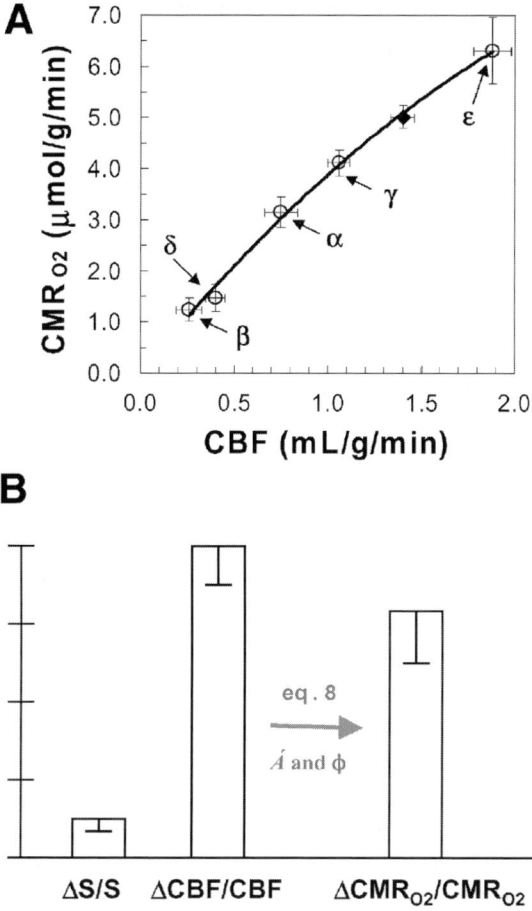

Fig. 3. (A) Comparison of CMR_{O_2} (measured by MRS) vs. CBF (measured by MRI) for the different conditions (Groups α–ϵ). For the observed relationship between CBF and CMR_{O_2}, the tissue pO_2 has to remain significantly lower than the vessel pO_2 values [11,32,33], which supports a situation in which the effective mass transfer coefficient for oxygen (D) must change. Since the ratio of $(\Delta D/D)/(\Delta CBF/CBF)$ expressed as a constant Ω was determined to be 0.8 ± 0.2, it is suggested that the efficiency of oxygen delivery plays an important role for the regulation of oxygen delivery in vivo. The filled symbol represents the resting awake state for the rat cerebral cortex [11,12]. The error bars represent the standard deviation from the mean. Modified from Hyder et al. [11,12]. (B) A schematic for using the multi-modal measurements of changes in BOLD signal and CBF during a functional study to calculate the changes in CMR_{O_2} using Eq. (8). This approach may be particularly useful for human studies where previously determined values of $\acute{A}$ and ϕ (using Eqs. (5) and (7), respectively) can be used in conjunction with the measured changes in BOLD signal and CBF to predict the changes in CMR_{O_2} (as in Fig. 2B). The error bars represent the standard deviation from the mean.

cortex over a wide dynamic range [11,12]. Since the normalization of the BOLD signal described above is valid for the same range of activity (Fig. 2A), Eq. (6) can be used in conjunction with the multi-modal measurements of BOLD signal, CBF, and CBV to calculate changes in CMR_{O_2}. While the use of the long half-life superparamagnetic MRI contrast agent for the CBV measurements [23,24] provides valuable data in these experiments, the use of these agents for human experiments is not yet approved. Alternatively, BOLD and CBF data can be used in conjunction with the experimentally derived values of $\acute{A}$ and ϕ to calculate changes in CMR_{O_2} (Eq. (8); see Fig. 2B) as shown graphically in Fig. 3B. Recent BOLD fMRI experiments in the awake human visual cortex [34,35] and in the anesthetized rat sensorimotor cortex [12,21,36] have shown that $\Delta S/S$ and $\Delta CBF/CBF$ are linearly correlated. These observations, in conjunction with Eq. (6), indicate that the relationship between $\Delta CBF/CBF$ and $\Delta CMR_{O_2}/CMR_{O_2}$ would also be linear with the functional activation [11] as we have observed experimentally in the rat cortex (Fig. 3A).

Since the linear relationship between CBF and CMR_{O_2} has been observed in the rat and human cortex under a variety of conditions [32,33], this BOLD calibration approach may be applied to human studies. Recent fMRI studies by Hoge et al. [8] and Kim et al. [9] in the human visual cortex also suggest a linear relationship between CBF (measured by MRI) and CMR_{O_2} (predicted by MRI), where the predicted value of Ψ (Eq. (5)) given by the ratio of $(\Delta CMR_{O_2}/CMR_{O_2})/(\Delta CBF/CBF)$ ranged from 0.5 to 0.7 which is in good agreement with the value of Ψ in the current rat studies (0.7 ± 0.3). The slight difference in the relationship between CBF vs. CMR_{O_2} for rats and humans may be due to an actual species difference in the mechanisms of the cerebral oxygen delivery. However, experimentally measured values of $\acute{A}$ and ϕ along with some validation experiments in human brain studies may improve the agreement between the rat and human data.

In summary, the BOLD image-contrast in the rat cerebral cortex at 7 T has been calibrated by multi-modal measurements and the neuroenergetic weighting of the fMRI signal has been validated with the ^{13}C MRS measurements of CMR_{O_2}. Regional correlation was observed for the changes in CMR_{O_2} and CBF with functional activation over a wide range of neuronal activity. Although the exact cellular processes that underlie the BOLD phenomenon are yet to be revealed [37], the current results reveal the energetic and physiologic ingredients of the BOLD fMRI signal and indicate the necessary steps towards mapping the neuronal activity quantitatively by fMRI at steady state [38,39].

2.2.1.7. On-Site Discussion

2.2.1.7.1. *Question: (Lauritzen)* Just to comment that the interpretation of the increased field potential amplitude is not necessary an indicator of increased neuronal firing, most likely it indicates the increased synaptic action by, probably, in postsynaptic cellular elements.

Answer: (Hyder) Exactly. These field potential measurements are reflective of synaptic activity.

2.2.1.7.2. **Question: (Bandettini)** Transit time artifact in MRI perfusion measurement may vary depending on the CO_2 stimulation as neuronal activation. This depends on the MRI technique.

Answer: (Hyder) These were all steady-state measurements using arterial spin labeling techniques with appropriate (slow) methods to minimize the transit-time related artifacts.

2.2.1.7.3. **Question: (Kim)** CBV in the BOLD model is venous, not total CBV. However, MRI CBV technique measures the total CBV change. Based on our MR and video-microscopic measurements, the venous CBV change is small compared to the arterial CBV change.

Answer: (Hyder) Yes, I am aware of the work. While your ^{19}F work shows differential extent of change in the arterial and venous (+capillary) compartments, I think the assumption of arterial volume being the dominant fraction in the cerebral vasculature is questionable.

2.2.1.7.4. **Question: (Kanno)** We measured the fractional change of arterial blood in PET. It was 30% of the total CBV.

Answer: (Hyder) Yes, I know. With MRI, we measure about 10% change in CBV in relation to the 100% change in CBF. This difference between the two methods may be due to the tracer in PET and MRI being markers of hemoglobin and plasma, respectively.

2.2.1.7.5. **Question: (Buxton)** Is the picture presented for the rat different from the picture we have for human? Specifically, our data shows nearly matched changes in CBF and CMR_{O_2}, which would not change the blood oxygen saturation. So, how does the BOLD effect arise?

Answer: (Hyder) The BOLD effect is well intact and in effect in the rat data as well. The ratio of $(\Delta CMR_{O_2}/CMR_{O_2})/(\Delta CBF/CBF)$ is about 0.6 to 0.8 in the rat data which is about what is being measured in the human experiments.

Acknowledgements

The authors thank Drs. Kevin L. Behar and Richard P. Kennan for their helpful discussions. The authors also thank engineers T. Nixon, P. Brown, and S. McIntyre for the maintenance of the spectrometer and for the radio-frequency probe designs, and B. Wang for the technical support. Supported by the National Institutes of Health grants NS-32126 (DLR), DK-27121 (RGS), and NS-37203 (FH); National Science Foundation grant DBI-9730892 (FH), and DBI-0095173; and Pfizer (HB) and Howard Hughes (AJS) fellowships.

References

[1] S. Ogawa, R.S. Menon, S.G. Kim, K. Ugurbil, On the characteristics of functional magnetic resonance imaging of the brain, Annu. Rev. Biophys. Biomol. Struct. 27 (1998) 447–474.
[2] K. Ugurbil, G. Adriany, P. Andersen, C. Wei, R. Gruetter, X. Hu, H. Merkle, D.S. Kim, S.G. Kim, J. Strupp,

X. Hong, S. Ogawa, Magnetic resonance studies of brain function and neurochemistry, Annu. Rev. Biomed. Eng. 2 (2000) 633–660.

[3] S. Ogawa, T.M. Lee, B. Barrere, The sensitive of magnetic resonance image signals of rat brain to changes in the cerebral venous blood oxygenation, Magn. Reson. Med. 29 (1993) 205–210.

[4] R.P. Kennan, J. Zhong, J.C. Gore, Intravascular susceptibility contrast mechanisms in tissue, Magn. Reson. Med. 31 (1994) 9–21.

[5] R.M. Weisskoff, C.S. Zuo, J.L. Boxerman, B.R. Rosen, Microscopic susceptibility variation and transverse relaxation: theory and experiment, Magn. Reson. Med. 31 (1994) 601–610.

[6] R.G. Shulman, D.L. Rothman, Interpreting functional imaging studies in terms of neurotransmitter cycling, Proc. Natl. Acad. Sci. U. S. A. 95 (1998) 11993–11998.

[7] P.C.M. van Zijl, S.M. Efefe, J.A. Ulatowski, J.M.E. Oja, A.M. Ulug, R.J. Traystman, R.A. Kauppinen, Quantitative assessment of blood flow, blood volume and blood oxygenation effects in functional magnetic resonance imaging, Nat. Med. 4 (1998) 159–167.

[8] R.D. Hoge, J. Atkinson, B. Gill, G.R. Crelier, S. Marrett, G.B. Pike, Linear coupling between cerebral blood flow and oxygen consumption in activated human cortex, Proc. Natl. Acad. Sci. U. S. A. 96 (1999) 9403–9408.

[9] S.G. Kim, E. Rostrup, H.B. Larsson, S. Ogawa, O.B. Paulson, Determination of relative CMR_{O_2} from CBF and BOLD changes: significant increase of oxygen consumption rate during visual stimulation, Magn. Reson. Med. 41 (1999) 1152–1161.

[10] D.L. Rothman, N.R. Sibson, F. Hyder, J. Shen, K.L. Behar, R.G. Shulman, In vivo nuclear magnetic resonance spectroscopy studies of the relationship between the glutamate–glutamine neurotransmitter cycle and functional neuroenergetics, Philos. Trans. R. Soc. London, Ser. B 354 (1999) 1165–1177.

[11] F. Hyder, R.P. Kennan, I. Kida, G.F. Mason, K.L. Behar, D.L. Rothman, Dependence of oxygen delivery on blood flow in rat brain: a 7 Tesla nuclear magnetic resonance study, J. Cereb. Blood Flow Metab. 20 (2000) 485–498.

[12] F. Hyder, I. Kida, K.L. Behar, R.P. Kennan, P.K. Maciejewski, D.L. Rothman, Quantitative functional imaging of the brain: towards mapping neuronal activity by BOLD fMRI, NMR Biomed. 14 (2001) 413–431.

[13] I. Kida, F. Hyder, R.P. Kennan, K.L. Behar, Towards absolute quantitation of BOLD functional MRI, Adv. Exp. Med. Biol. 471 (1999) 681–689.

[14] I. Kida, R.P. Kennan, D.L. Rothman, K.L. Behar, F. Hyder, High-resolution CMR_{O_2} mapping in rat cortex: a multi-parametric approach to calibration of BOLD image contrast at 7 Tesla, J. Cereb. Blood Flow Metab. 20 (2000) 847–860.

[15] F. Hyder, D.L. Rothman, A.M. Blamire, Image reconstruction of sequentially sampled echo-planar data, Magn. Reson. Imaging 13 (1995) 97–103.

[16] F. Hyder, J.R. Chase, K.L. Behar, G.F. Mason, M. Siddeek, D.L. Rothman, R.G. Shulman, Increased tri-carboxylic acid cycle flux in rat brain during forepaw stimulation detected with $^1H–[^{13}C]$ NMR, Proc. Natl. Acad. Sci. U. S. A. 93 (1996) 7612–7617.

[17] F. Hyder, D.L. Rothman, G.F. Mason, A. Rangarajan, K.L. Behar, R.G. Shulman, Oxidative glucose metabolism in rat brain during single forepaw stimulation: a spatially localized $^1H[^{13}C]$NMR study, J. Cereb. Blood Flow Metab. 17 (1997) 1040–1047.

[18] F. Hyder, R. Renken, D.L. Rothman, In vivo carbon-edited detection with proton echo-planar spectroscopic imaging (ICED PEPSI): [3,4-$^{13}CH_2$]glutamate/glutamine tomography in rat brain, Magn. Reson. Med. 42 (1999) 997–1003.

[19] G.F. Mason, D.L. Rothman, K.L. Behar, R.G. Shulman, NMR determination of the TCA cycle rate and α-ketoglutarate/glutamate exchange rate in rat brain, J. Cereb. Blood Flow Metab. 12 (1992) 434–447.

[20] G.F. Mason, R. Gruetter, D.L. Rothman, K.L. Behar, R.G. Shulman, E.J. Novotny, Simultaneous determination of the rates of the TCA cycle, glucose utilization, α-ketoglutarate/glutamate exchange, and glutamine synthesis in human brain by NMR, J. Cereb. Blood Flow Metab. 15 (1995) 12–25.

[21] F. Hyder, R. Renken, R.P. Kennan, D.L. Rothman, Quantitative multi-modal functional MRI with blood oxygenation level dependent exponential decays adjusted for flow attenuated inversion recovery (BOLDED AFFAIR), Magn. Reson. Imaging 18 (2000) 227–235.

[22] T.J. Mosher, M.B. Smith, Mapping the static magnetic field using a double-DANTE tagging sequence, J. Magn. Reson. 93 (1991) 624–629.

[23] R.P. Kennan, B.E. Scanley, R.B. Innis, J.C. Gore, Physiological basis for BOLD MR signal changes due to neuronal stimulation: Separation of blood volume and magnetic susceptibility effects, Magn. Reson. Med. 40 (1998) 840–846.

[24] J.B. Mandeville, J.J.A. Marota, B.E. Kosofsky, J.R. Keltner, R. Weissleder, B.R. Rosen, R.M. Weisskoff, Dynamic functional imaging of relative cerebral blood volume during rat forepaw stimulation, Magn. Reson. Med. 39 (1998) 615–624.

[25] C. Schwarzbauer, S.P. Morrissey, A. Haase, Quantitative magnetic resonance imaging of perfusion using magnetic labeling of water proton spins within the detection slice, Magn. Reson. Med. 35 (1996) 540–546.

[26] F. Calamante, Dl. Thomas, G.S. Pell, J. Wiersma, R. Turner, Measuring cerebral blood flow using magnetic resonance imaging techniques, J. Cereb. Blood Flow Metab. 19 (1999) 701–735.

[27] R.G. Shulman, D.L. Rothman, F. Hyder, Stimulated changes in localized cerebral energy consumption under anesthesia, Proc. Natl. Acad. Sci. U. S. A. 96 (1999) 3245–3250.

[28] R.L. Grubb, M.E. Raichle, J.O. Eichling, M.M. Ter Pogosian, The effects of changes in pCO$_2$ on cerebral blood volume, blood flow, and vascular mean transit time, Stroke 5 (1974) 630–639.

[29] M. Ueki, F. Linn, K.A. Hossman, Functional activation of cerebral blood flow and metabolism and after global ischemia of rat brain, J. Cereb. Blood Flow Metab. 8 (1988) 486–494.

[30] S. Ogawa, T.M. Lee, B. Barrere, The sensitive of magnetic resonance image signals of rat brain to changes in the cerebral venous blood oxygenation, Magn. Reson. Med. 29 (1993) 205–210.

[31] B.K. Siesjo, Brain Energy Metabolism, Wiley, New York, NY, 1978.

[32] T.L. Davis, K.K. Kwong, R.M. Weisskoff, B.R. Rosen, Calibrated functional MRI: mapping the dynamics of oxidative metabolism, Proc. Natl. Acad. Sci. U. S. A. 95 (1998) 1834–1839.

[33] X.H. Zhu, S.G. Kim, P. Andersen, S. Ogawa, K. Ugurbil, W. Chen, Simultaneous oxygenation and perfusion imaging study of functional activity in primary visual cortex at different visual stimulation frequency: quantitative correlation between BOLD and CBF changes, Magn. Reson. Med. 40 (1998) 703–711.

[34] A.C. Silva, S.P. Lee, G. Yang, C. Iadecola, S.G. Kim, Simultaneous BOLD and CBF functional MRI during forepaw stimulation in rat, J. Cereb. Blood Flow Metab. 19 (1999) 871–879.

[35] F. Hyder, R.G. Shulman, D.L. Rothman, A model for the regulation of cerebral oxygen delivery, J. Appl. Physiol. 85 (1998) 554–564.

[36] F. Hyder, R.G. Shulman, D.L. Rothman, Regulation of cerebral oxygen delivery, Adv. Exp. Med. Biol. 471 (1999) 99–109.

[37] I. Kida, F. Hyder, K.L. Behar, Inhibition of voltage-dependent sodium channels suppresses the functional MRI response to forepaw somatosensory activation in the rodent, J. Cereb. Blood Flow Metab. 21 (2001) 585–591.

[38] R.G. Shulman, F. Hyder, D.L. Rothman, Cerebral energetics and the glycogen shunt: neurochemical basis of functional imaging, Proc. Natl. Acad. Sci. U. S. A. 98 (2001) 6417–6422.

[39] L. Pellerin, N.R. Sibson, N. Hadjikhani, F. Hyder, What you see is what you think—or is it? Trends Neurosci. 24 (2001) 71–72.

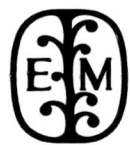

International Congress Series 1235 (2002) 73–85

Dynamic nonlinearities in BOLD contrast: neuronal or hemodynamic?

Peter A. Bandettini*, Rasmus M. Birn, Dan Kelley, Ziad S. Saad

Laboratory of Brain and Cognition, Unit on Functional Imaging Methods, National Institute of Mental Health, NIH, Bldg. 10, Rm. 1D80, 10 Center Dr., Bethesda, MD 20892-1366, USA

Abstract

A primary goal of the functional MRI (fMRI) methods development is to characterize the relationship between the blood oxygenation level-dependent (BOLD) signal changes and neuronal activation. Recent studies of blood oxygenation level-dependent (BOLD) signal responses have demonstrated nonlinear behavior with respect to stimulus duration. Specifically, shorter duration stimuli produce larger signal changes than expected from a linear system. The precise reasons for this nonlinearity are not clearly understood. The goal of this study is to further clarify the origin of dynamic BOLD contrast nonlinearities—either neuronal or hemodynamic or both, by a combined approach of task timing modulation, spatial mapping, and modeling/fitting of the BOLD response using the "Balloon model." In this study, we found that (1) in agreement with the literature, the dynamic BOLD "on" response is nonlinear and has significant spatial heterogeneity. Spatial maps of nonlinearity, while highly reproducible, do not correlate with maps of the BOLD response magnitude or latency, but do show some correlation with functional segregation; (2) the dynamic BOLD "off" response is sublinear; and (3) while data fitted with Balloon model hemodynamic parameters, assuming linear neuronal input, generally create nonlinear dynamic BOLD responses, the Balloon model was not able to fit all BOLD contrast response task timing modulations simultaneously. These findings suggest that the dynamic BOLD response may be a linear function of the neuronal input function and that the neuronal input function is not a simple "on/off" boxcar function, but rather a nonlinear function that has an initial overshoot that lasts for approximately 4 s until reaching a steady state. © 2002 Elsevier Science B.V. All rights reserved.

Keywords: BOLD fMRI; Linearity; Stimulus duration; Visual; Motor; Balloon model

* Corresponding author. Tel.: +1-301-402-1333; fax: +1-301-402-1370.
E-mail address: bandettini@nih.gov (P.A. Bandettini).

0531-5131/02 © 2002 Elsevier Science B.V. All rights reserved.
PII: S0531-5131(02)00174-7

1. Introduction

An increase in neuronal activity leads to a localized increase in the neuronal firing rate, metabolism, blood flow, blood volume, and blood oxygenation, resulting in changes in the local amount of deoxyhemoglobin in each voxel, to which MRI is sensitive. The utility of the functional MRI (fMRI) is directly related to the degree to which neuronal activation can be implied through these hemodynamic changes and the resulting effects on the MRI contrast, most importantly, blood oxygenation level-dependent (BOLD) contrast. An important step in characterizing the relationship between the neuronal firing and measured fMRI signal is by the assessment of the linearity of the measured BOLD signal in response to neural stimulation. While recent studies have suggested that, at steady state (i.e., activation lasting longer than 10 s), the BOLD response shows proportionality to the neuronal firing rate [1] or implied measures of task intensity [2–5], the dynamic BOLD response. Meaning, the magnitude of response as a function of task durations less than 5 s has been shown to have highly nonlinear behavior. The BOLD response does not obey the superposition for certain stimuli [6–8]. While longer duration stimuli behave in an approximately linear fashion, short duration stimuli produce responses larger than the predicted from a linear model.

The purpose of the present work is to examine more closely these nonlinearities and to determine if the source of the nonlinearity is neuronal, hemodynamic, or both. Specifically, we approach this question with three studies. In the first study, we systematically vary the stimulus duration in the motor and visual cortexes and calculate, on a voxel-wise basis, the degree that the response deviates from a linear system. We then compare these "non-linearity" maps with simultaneously derived maps of latency and magnitude (dominated by hemodynamic response variables). If a spatial correlation were found between the linearity maps and the other maps, it would imply that the nonlinearities were of a hemodynamic origin. In the second study, instead of modulating the "on" response, we modulated the "off" response timing and performed a linearity assessment. The assump-

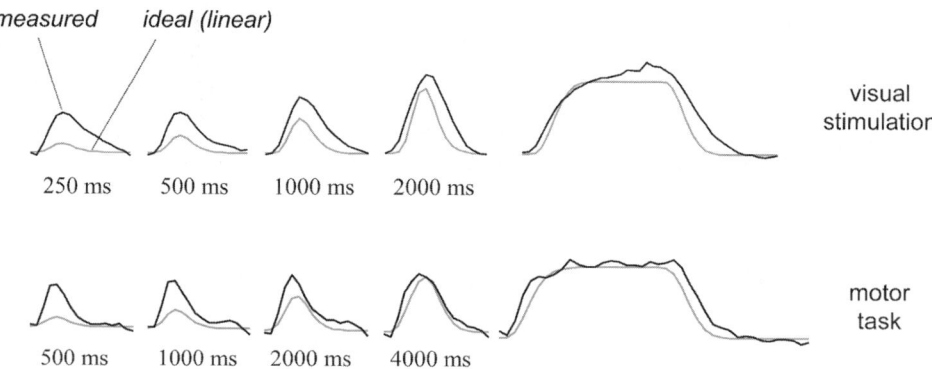

Fig. 1. Top: measured and ideal linear BOLD responses after visual stimulation of 250-, 500-, 1000-, 2000-ms, and 20-s duration. Bottom: measured and ideal responses after finger tapping of 500-, 1000-, 2000-, and 4000-ms, and 20-s duration. Measured and ideal linear responses are also shown superimposed. Short duration stimuli are larger than predicted from a linear system.

Nonlinearity

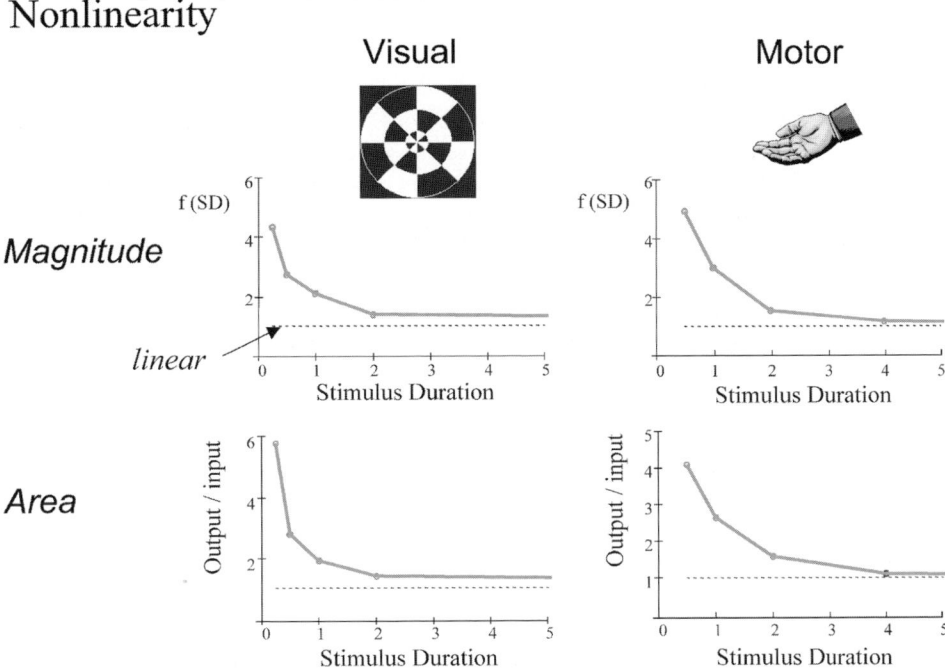

Fig. 2. The amount by which the amplitude (top) and the area (bottom) of the responses are larger at each stimulus duration than the response from a linear system, determined by a linear extrapolation of the responses at the blocked design. In this figure, the nonlinearity curves are averaged over all activated voxels. Left: nonlinearity in the visual cortex; right: nonlinearity in the motor cortex.

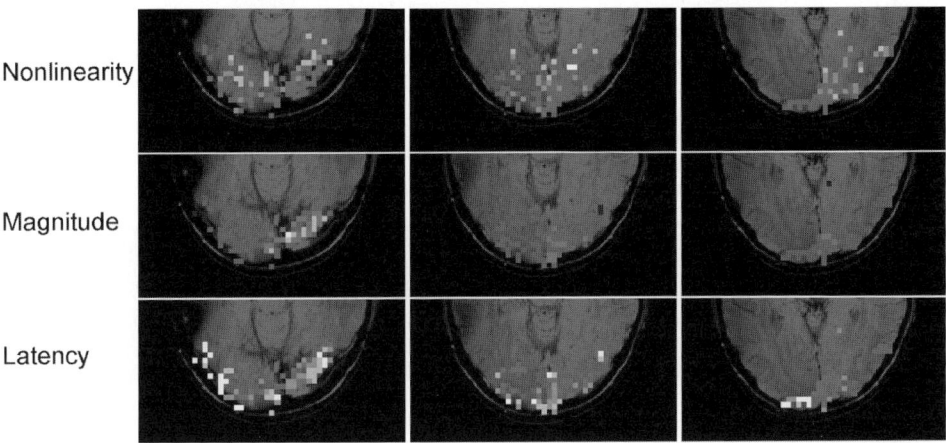

Fig. 3. The nonlinearity (top), activation amplitude (middle), and latency (bottom) for three slices in the visual cortex assessed with a contrast reversing the checkerboard stimulus. Nonlinearity was assessed from the activation amplitude relative to a linear prediction. Spatial variation in the nonlinearity is evident, but does not appear to be correlated with either magnitude or latency.

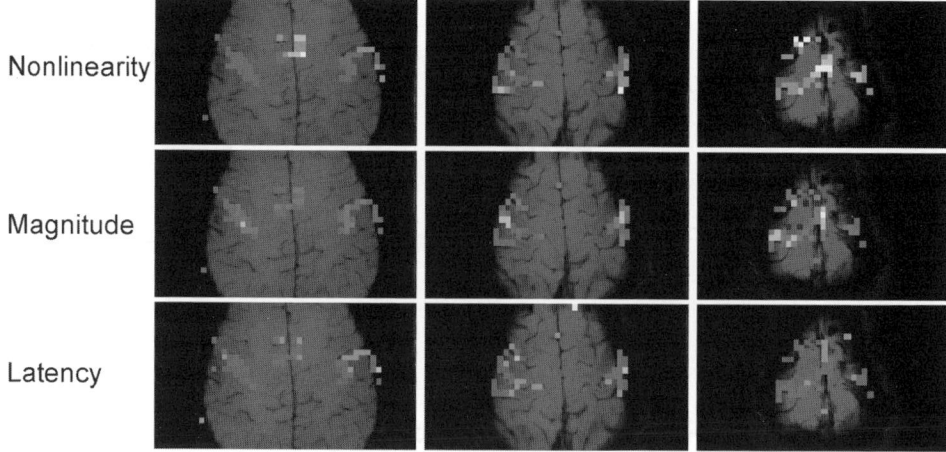

Fig. 4. The nonlinearity (top), activation amplitude (middle), and latency (bottom) for three slices in the motor cortex assessed with a contrast reversing the checkerboard stimulus. Nonlinearity was assessed from the activation amplitude relative to a linear prediction. Spatial variation in the nonlinearity is evident, however, does not appear to be correlated with either magnitude or latency. It appears that the supplementary motor cortex shows greater nonlinearity than the primary motor cortex.

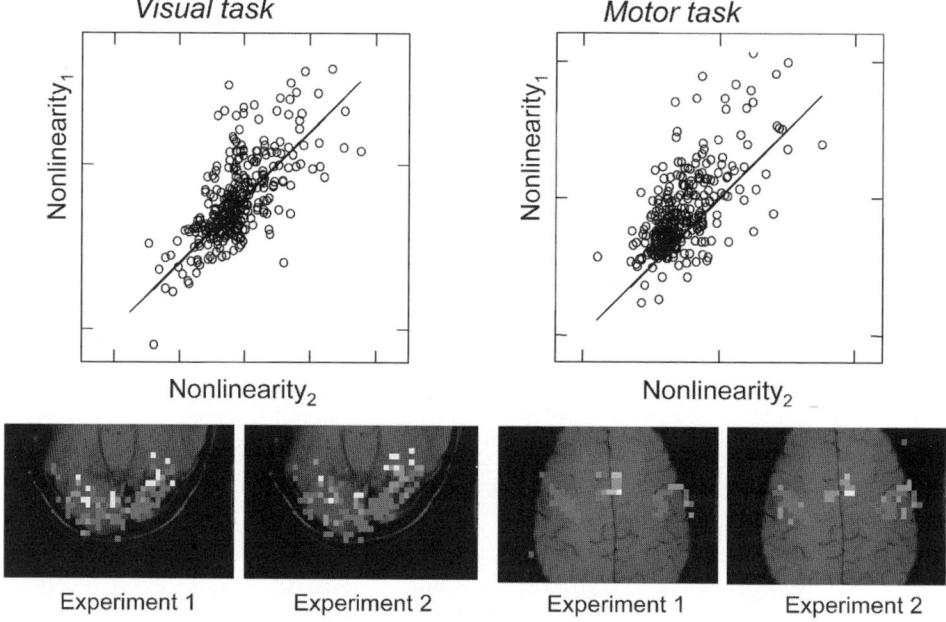

Fig. 5. Computed nonlinearity (as measured by the amplitude of the response compared to a linear model) in two separate runs in the same subject for the visual stimulation experiment (left) and the motor task (right). The line indicates the ideal case of identical nonlinearity values for both runs. The measure of nonlinearity is consistent and reproducible for both tasks. Using the area of the average response instead of the magnitude was equally reproducible.

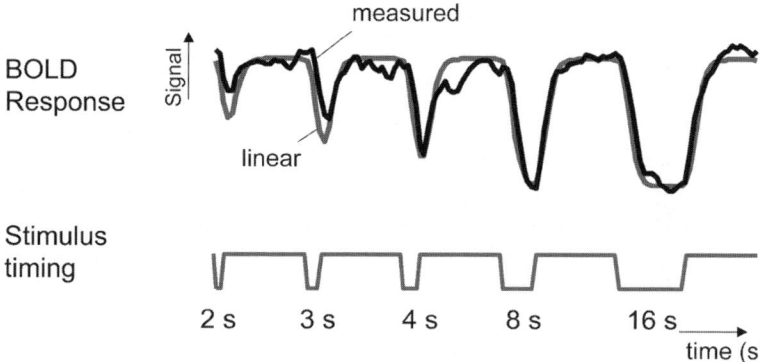

Fig. 6. Measured and ideal linear BOLD responses for "off" durations for 2-, 3-, 4-, 8-, and 16-s durations. Measured and ideal linear responses are also shown superimposed. Short duration "off" is smaller than the predicted from a linear system.

tion here is based on an understanding that the "on" and "off" responses differ neuronally. In the third study, we attempted to fit the BOLD response to a single-time series of different task timings, ranging from 250 ms to 20 s, to the Balloon model, assuming a boxcar neuronal input function.

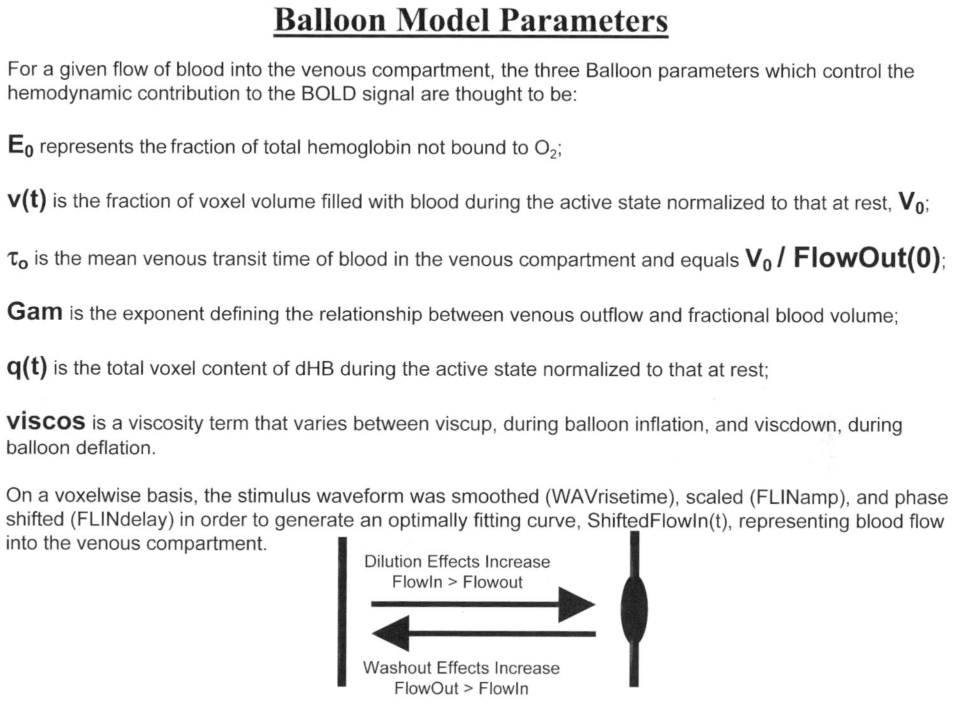

Balloon Model Parameters

For a given flow of blood into the venous compartment, the three Balloon parameters which control the hemodynamic contribution to the BOLD signal are thought to be:

E_0 represents the fraction of total hemoglobin not bound to O_2;

v(t) is the fraction of voxel volume filled with blood during the active state normalized to that at rest, **V_0**;

τ_o is the mean venous transit time of blood in the venous compartment and equals **V_0 / FlowOut(0)**;

Gam is the exponent defining the relationship between venous outflow and fractional blood volume;

q(t) is the total voxel content of dHB during the active state normalized to that at rest;

viscos is a viscosity term that varies between viscup, during balloon inflation, and viscdown, during balloon deflation.

On a voxelwise basis, the stimulus waveform was smoothed (WAVrisetime), scaled (FLINamp), and phase shifted (FLINdelay) in order to generate an optimally fitting curve, ShiftedFlowIn(t), representing blood flow into the venous compartment.

Dilution Effects Increase
FlowIn > Flowout

Washout Effects Increase
FlowOut > FlowIn

Fig. 7. Balloon model parameters used in the fitting routine in this study.

2. Study 1: spatial heterogeneity assessment

Results of this study are published in Birn et al. [9]. The linearity of the response with respect to the stimulus duration (the "on" period) was assessed in two tasks—a motor task consisting of bilateral finger tapping and a visual task where the subject viewed an 8-Hz contrast reversing checkerboard. In the motor task, the subject performed finger tapping during the presentation of a visual cue. Both tasks were performed at four different stimulus durations. The visual stimuli were presented at durations of 250, 500, 1000, and 2000 ms; and the finger tapping was performed at durations of 500, 1000, 2000, and 4000 ms, respectively. During each scan run, 20 repetitions of each stimulus were presented once every 16 s. Images were also acquired in a blocked trial paradigm, alternating eight

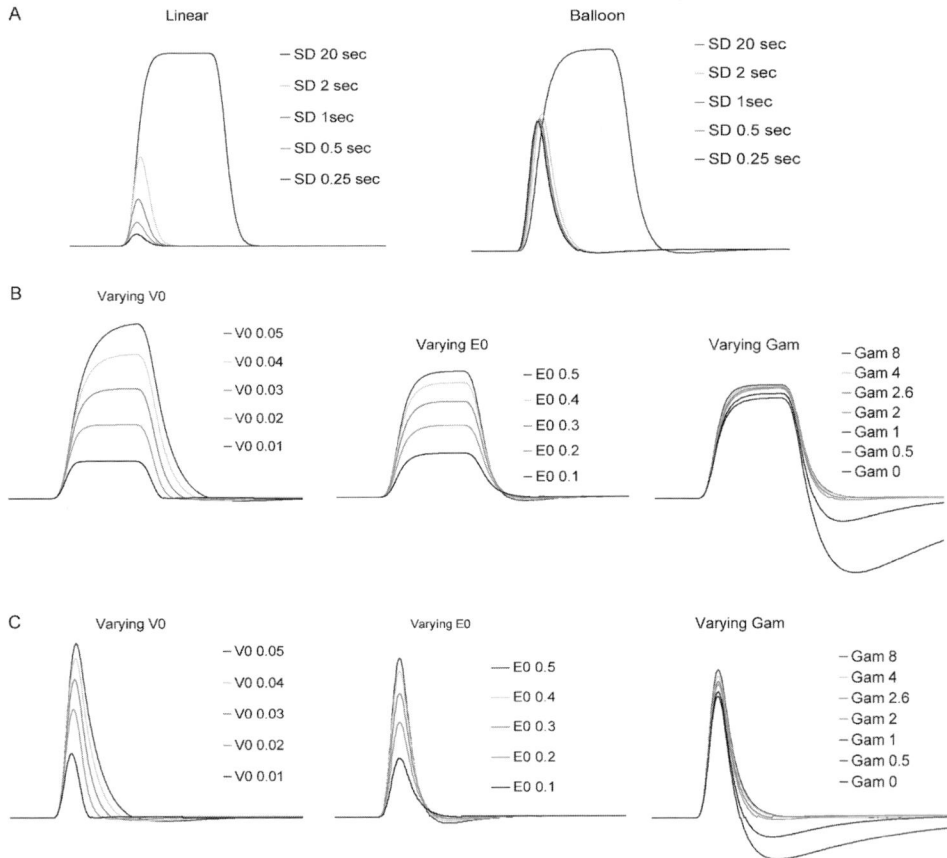

Fig. 8. Simulated BOLD curves: (A) linear and nonlinear "Balloon" BOLD curves for stimulus durations of 20, 2, 1, 0.5, 0.25 s. (B) Stimulus duration=20 s: one parameter is varied at a time. When they are not varied they are set equal to V_0=0.03, E_0=0.3, and Gam=2.6. (C) Stimulus duration=2 s: one parameter is varied at a time. When they are not varied, they are set equal to V_0=0.03, E_0=0.3, and Gam=2.6.

20-s periods of stimulation with eight 20-s periods of rest for a total duration of 320 s. Three subjects were studied for each task using an approved protocol.

During these tasks, a series of 320 echo-planar images (EPI) were acquired on a 3T GE Signa (Waukesha, WI, USA) magnet, equipped with a local birdcage RF coil (Medical Advances, Milwaukee, WI, USA). Eight axial slices with a 24-cm field of view and 5-mm slice thickness were used to cover the visual cortex during the visual task, and the motor cortex during the finger-tapping task (TR: 1000 ms, TE: 30 ms, matrix size: 64×64). The entire experiment, consisting of five 320-s runs, was performed twice in one scanning session to assess the repeatability of the nonlinearity measurements.

In a linear system, the area of the input (the stimulus) is directly proportional to the stimulus duration. Therefore, the area for the average response for the duration of each stimulus was divided by the stimulus duration to produce a measure of linearity—the output of the system for a given level of input. For each voxel, the area of the response as the function of stimulus duration was determined and normalized by the area or amplitude of the fMRI response to a blocked design, respectively. To map the nonlinearity across space, these curves were reduced to one number by computation of the area under the nonlinearity curve. To determine both the magnitude and the latency of the response on a voxel-wise basis, multiple reference functions with varying delays (increments of 100 ms) were generated.

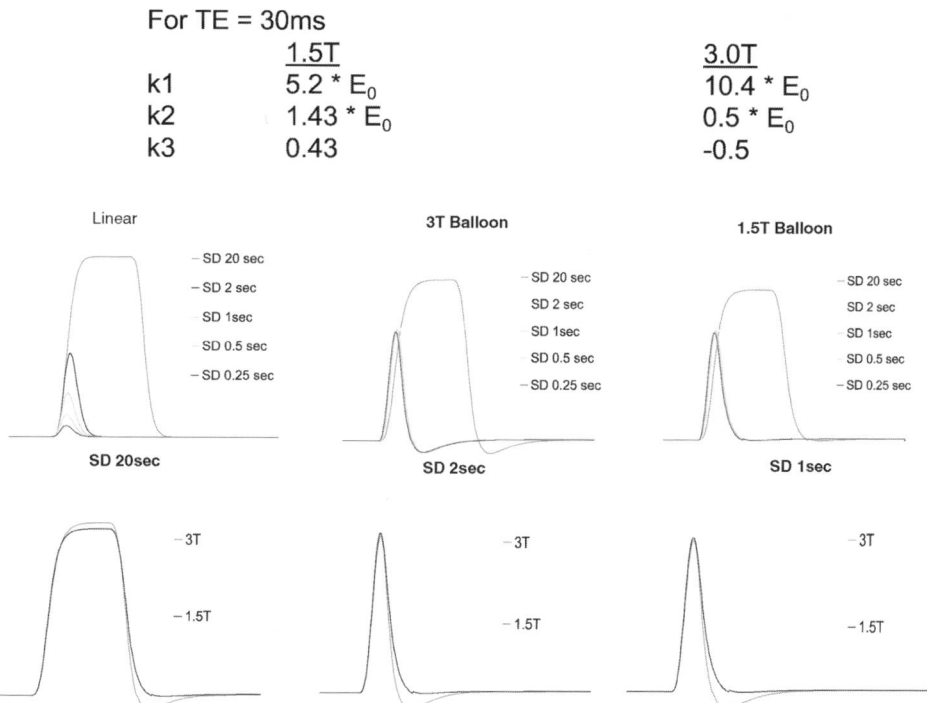

Fig. 9. Balloon model simulations at different field strengths, S.D.=20 s. V_0=0.03, E_0=0.3, and Gam=2.6.

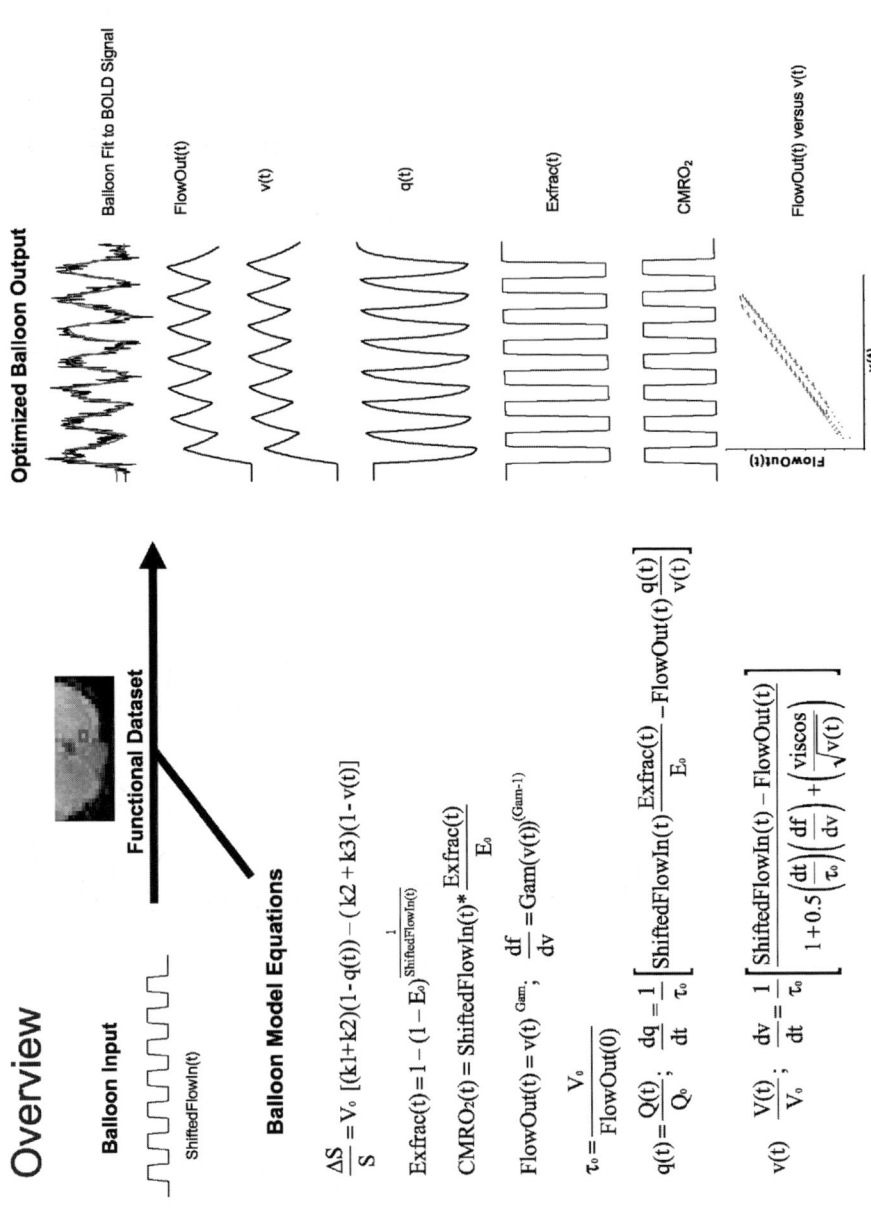

Fig. 10. Overview of the Balloon model fitting routine and resulting output curves of each neurovascular coupling/hemodynamic component that can be obtained. This was performed on a voxel-wise basis.

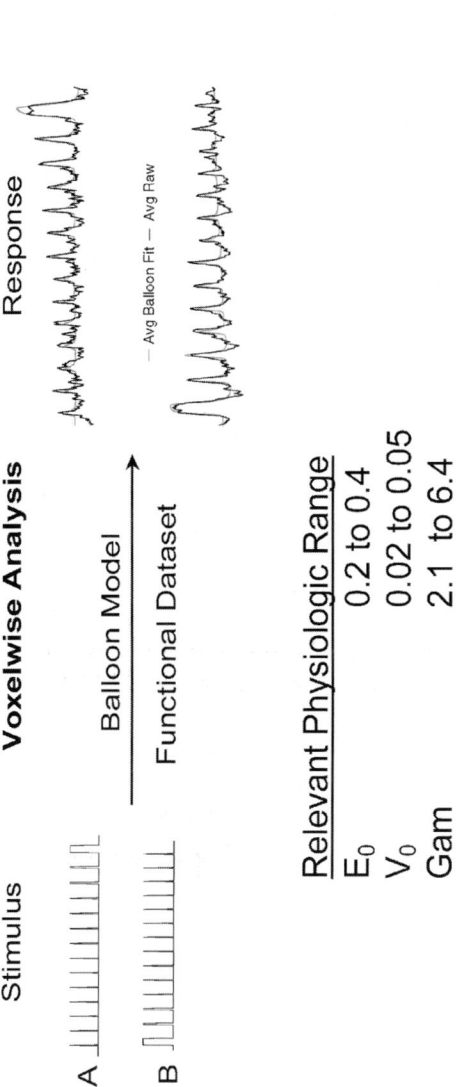

Balloon Model Parameter Estimation

	A1	A2	Mean	StdDev	%StDev/Mean	B1	B2	Mean	StdDev	%StDev/Mean
constant	726.422	719.873	723.148	4.631	0.640	687.650	695.451	691.551	5.516	0.798
linear	-0.008	0.029	0.011	0.026	241.779	0.023	0.005	0.014	0.013	94.457
FLINamp	0.598	0.491	0.545	0.076	13.938	0.582	0.603	0.592	0.015	2.498
FLINdelay	-0.794	-0.808	-0.801	0.010	-1.227	0.662	0.545	0.604	0.083	13.748
Vo	0.051	0.049	0.050	0.002	3.825	0.034	0.041	0.037	0.004	12.007
Eo	0.330	0.295	0.312	0.025	7.982	0.436	0.393	0.415	0.030	7.288
Gam	4.151	3.723	3.937	0.303	7.687	3.742	3.495	3.618	0.175	4.830
WAVrisetime	2.572	2.788	2.680	0.153	5.706	2.431	2.625	2.528	0.138	5.445
viscup	3.780	3.206	3.493	0.406	11.620	8.529	7.115	7.822	1.000	12.782
viscdown	8.870	11.086	9.978	1.567	15.704	9.945	10.250	10.098	0.215	2.133

Stimulus

Voxelwise Analysis

Response

— Avg Balloon Fit — Avg Raw

A

B

Balloon Model

Functional Dataset

Relevant Physiologic Range

E_0 0.2 to 0.4

V_0 0.02 to 0.05

Gam   2.1 to 6.4

Fig. 11. Summary of the results from an ROI in the visual cortex showing that, if the fitting parameters are allowed to vary within a physiologically reasonable range, the curves fit best the BOLD responses to the longer duration stimuli.

In agreement with previous studies, the BOLD response was found to be nonlinear for stimuli under a 5-s duration, with activation amplitudes larger than the predicted from a linear model at shorter stimulus durations. This is illustrated in Fig. 1, which shows the BOLD response averaged over all stimulation epochs and activated voxels for stimulus duration and the responses predicted from a linear system. The amount by which the area and the magnitude of the responses at stimulus duration are larger than expected from a linear model is shown in Fig. 2 for both the visual and motor tasks.

Maps of nonlinearity, latency, and magnitude are shown in Figs. 3 and 4. While the degree of nonlinearity is spatially heterogeneous, there appears to be distinct differences between the degree of nonlinearity in the primary and supplementary motor areas. While responses in both areas are nonlinear, the manifestations of the nonlinearity are different. The responses in the supplementary motor cortex are almost the same amplitude regardless of the stimulus duration.

The response latency and percentage signal change have been thought to discriminate between signals from large veins (with a large percentage signal change and long latency) and small vessels (with a small percentage signal change and short latency) [10]. The nonlinearity is not significantly correlated with either response amplitude or latency at a p-value of 0.01.

The high correlation between repeated voxel-wise measurements of nonlinearity (significant at a p-value of 0.001), which are shown in Fig. 5, demonstrate that the variability of the nonlinearity is not an artifact of noise.

3. Study 2: response to varying "off" durations

To assess the linearity of the visual system BOLD "off" response, the visual stimulus paradigm was performed in which the baseline was activated and the durations of blank fixation were varied from 2 to 16 s. The MRI and visual stimulus characteristics were identical to those in Study 1: spatial heterogeneity assessment. Fig. 6 shows the basic results. The BOLD response behaves in a sublinear manner for the "off" response.

4. Study 3: Balloon model studies

Using a physiologically based model for the BOLD contrast dynamics known as the "Balloon model" [11,12], we intend to address how details of the hemodynamic effects can be extracted from the BOLD response in humans. The observed dynamic non-linearities may be due to neuronal or hemodynamic effects or a combination of both. In this study, we varied the stimulus durations within a run and forced the Balloon model to fit all stimulus durations within a voxel with the same balloon parameters. A precise fit for all stimulus durations would imply that the nonlinearities could be accounted for by

Fig. 12. Breakdown of the results for each stimulus duration, indicating that the short duration BOLD signal changes are consistently underestimated by the Balloon model fit when the same parameters are applied to all durations simultaneously.

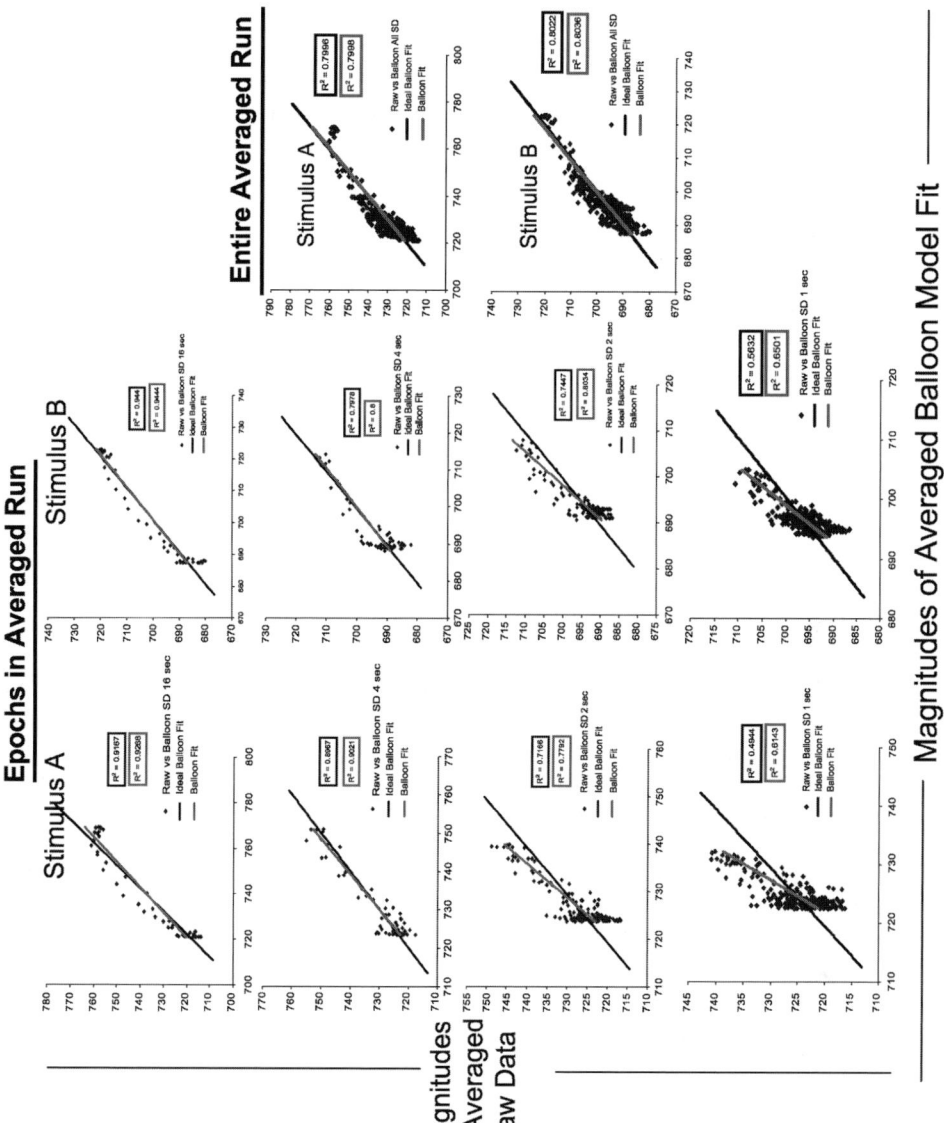

hemodynamic factors alone. A breakdown of the fit would imply that the neuronal input function for the model (a simple on–off boxcar function) is inaccurate.

4.1. Balloon model

Summaries of the Balloon model parameters, some examples of the effects of varying the Balloon model parameters and the model fitting procedure are given in Figs. 7–12, respectively. For a given flow of blood into the venous compartment, the three balloon parameters which control the hemodynamic contribution to the BOLD signal are thought to be E_0, V_0, and Gam[2]. E_0 represents the fraction of total hemoglobin not bound to O_2; $v(t)$ is the fraction of voxel volume filled with blood during the active state normalized to that at rest, V_0; Gam is the exponent defining the relationship between venous outflow and fractional blood volume; τ_o is the mean venous transit time of blood in the venous compartment; $q(t)$ is the total voxel content of dHB during the active state normalized to that at rest; viscos is a viscosity term that varies between viscup, during balloon inflation, and viscdown, during balloon deflation. The stimulus waveform was smoothed (WAVrisetime), scaled (FLINamp), and phase shifted (FLINdelay) on a voxel-wise basis to generate an optimal curve (ShiftedFlowIn(t)) representing the blood flow into the venous compartment.

The stationary of the model parameters across the stimulus timing was assessed using a visual task consisting of an 8-Hz flashing checkerboard. The visual stimuli were presented at durations of 1000, 2000, and 4000 ms, and 16 s. Standard deviations of each stimulus duration epoch were matched to prevent biasing our fitting routine.

During these tasks, a series of axial 510 echo-planar images (EPI) of the visual cortex were acquired on a 3T GE Signa magnet, with a 24-cm field of view, 5-mm slice thickness, and 64×64 matrix size (TR: 1000 ms, TE: 30 ms). Each run was performed twice to assess the reliability of the fitted parameters. To achieve the best least squares fit to the BOLD signal on a voxel-wise basis, the Balloon model parameters were varied independently by using a balloon signal model, inflater, as a plug in for the nonlinear simplex fitting routine, 3dNLfim, packaged with AFNI [13]. A linear noise model, with a constant and linear term, was incorporated into the fitting procedure. Data from two subjects were acquired, showing similar results.

In this study, shown in Figs. 11 and 12, we found that the Balloon model hemodynamics do not fully account for the human BOLD signal nonlinearities. Within a run, the Balloon model better characterizes epochs of longer stimulus duration than the shorter stimulus durations.

5. Conclusion

For brief stimulus "on" periods, signal increases are larger than expected. These nonlinearities show considerable yet reproducible spatial heterogeneity that does not correlate with the hemodynamic latency or magnitude maps. For brief stimulus "off" periods, signal decreases are smaller than expected from a linear system. We also found that the Balloon model hemodynamics do not fully account for the human BOLD signal dynamic nonlinearities. Within a run for a given stimulus, the Balloon model is better at characterizing epochs of longer stimulus duration than shorter stimulus duration.

In general, these studies imply that the BOLD response nonlinearities may be explained by a combination of a nonlinear neuronal input and nonlinearities in the hemodynamic response. A recent publication by Logothetis et al. [14] demonstrates that, in nonhuman primates, integrated postsynaptic potential measures can almost fully explain the simultaneously measured dynamic BOLD response magnitude. More studies involving carefully constructed stimuli in combination with more measures of hemodynamic variables will shed further light on these issues. In general, all the results seem to indicate that the BOLD response is more sensitive to subtleties of neuronal activity than previously thought.

2.2.2.7. On-Site Discussion

2.2.2.7.1. *Comment: (Harder)* There is an integrating cell type or "function" between neural activity and blood flow.

References

[1] G. Rees, K. Friston, C. Koch, A direct quantitative relationship between the functional properties of human and macaque V5, Nat. Neurosci. 3 (7) (2000) 716–723.
[2] J.R. Binder, et al., Syllable rate determines functional MRI response magnitude during a speech discrimination task, Proc., SMR, 2nd Annual Meeting, San Francisco, 1994.
[3] S.M. Rao, et al., Relationship between finger movement rate and functional magnetic resonance signal change in human primary motor cortex, J. Cereb. Blood Flow Metab. 16 (1996) 1250–1254.
[4] K.K. Kwong, et al., Dynamic magnetic resonance imaging of human brain activity during primary sensory stimulation, Proc. Natl. Acad. Sci. U. S. A. 89 (1992) 5675–5679.
[5] G. Rees, et al., Characterizing the relationship between BOLD contrast and regional cerebral blood flow measurements by varying the stimulus presentation rate, Neuroimage 6 (4) (1997) 270–278.
[6] K.J. Friston, et al., Nonlinear event-related responses in fMRI, Magn. Reson. Med. 39 (1998) 41–52.
[7] A.L. Vazquez, D.C. Noll, Nonlinear aspects of the BOLD response in functional MRI, Neuroimage 7 (2) (1998) 108–118.
[8] G.M. Boynton, et al., Linear systems analysis of functional magnetic resonance imaging in human V1, J. Neurosci. 16 (1996) 4207–4221.
[9] R.M. Birn, Z.S. Saad, P. Bandettini, Spatial heterogeneity of the nonlinear dynamics in the fMRI BOLD response, Neuroimage, in press.
[10] A.T. Lee, G.H. Glover, C.H. Meyer, Discrimination of large venous vessels in time-course spiral blood–oxygen-level-dependent magnetic-resonance functional neuroimaging, Magn. Reson. Med. 33 (6) (1995) 745–754.
[11] R.B. Buxton, E.C. Wong, L.R. Frank, Dynamics of blood flow and oxygenation changes during brain activation: the balloon model, Magn. Reson. Med. 39 (1998) 855–864.
[12] R.B. Buxton, E.C. Wong, L.R. Frank, A biomechanical interpretation of the BOLD signal time course: the balloon model, Proc., ISMRM 5th Annual Meeting, Vancouver, 1997.
[13] R.W. Cox, AFNI: software for analysis and visualization of functional magnetic resonance neuroimages, Comput. Biomed. Res. 29 (3) (1996) 162–173.
[14] N. Logothetis, et al., Neurophysiological investigation of the basis of the fMRI signal, Nature 412 (2001) 150–157.

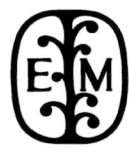

International Congress Series 1235 (2002) 87–97

Oxygen delivery to the brain during behavioral activation at acute normobaric hypoxemia

Ian Law [a,b,*], Robert C. Roach [c,d], Niels V. Olsen [e], Søren Holm [b], Markus Nowak [b], Thomas F. Hornbein [f], Olaf B. Paulson [a]

[a] The Neurobiology Research Unit, N 9201, Copenhagen University Hospital,
Rigshospitalet, Copenhagen, Denmark
[b] The PET and Cyclotron Unit, KF 3982, Department of Clinical Physiology and Nuclear Medicine,
Copenhagen University Hospital, Rigshospitalet, Copenhagen, Denmark
[c] The Copenhagen Muscle Research Center, Copenhagen University Hospital,
Rigshospitalet, Copenhagen, Denmark
[d] Cardiopulmonary Research Laboratory, New Mexico Highlands University, Las Vegas, NM, USA
[e] The Department of Neuroanesthesiology, Copenhagen University Hospital,
Rigshospitalet, Copenhagen, Denmark
[f] The University of Washington School of Medicine, Seattle, WA, USA

Abstract

In order to examine the hypothesis that the regional cerebral blood flow (rCBF) is fully regulated to maintain regional cerebral oxygen delivery (rO_2-delivery), we reanalyzed quantified positron emission tomography (PET) CBF data obtained in eight healthy subjects. The regional CBF to the hand area was sampled during rest or finger movements, during normoxemia (20%) or acute hypoxemia (8% or 10%), and when acclimatized either to sea level or high altitude (5260 m). Hypoxemia significantly increased the global CBF (gCBF) and rCBF, and decreased the global cerebral oxygen delivery (gO_2-delivery), thus the O_2-delivery does not entirely regulate CBF. The reduction in rO_2-delivery by hypoxemia was significantly larger during high altitude acclimatization than during sea level acclimatization. Acclimatization to high altitude did not significantly change the gCBF or rCBF, while gO_2-delivery and rO_2-delivery were both significantly increased, however, only during normoxemia. Finger movements significantly increased the rCBF and rO_2-delivery to the hand area, while the corresponding global values were unchanged. There were no differences in the rCBF and rO_2-delivery increases during finger movements by hypoxemia or acclimatization

* Corresponding author. The Neurobiology Research Unit, N 9201, Copenhagen University Hospital, Rigshospitalet, 9 Blegdamsvej, 2100 Copenhagen, Denmark. Tel.: +45-35456712; fax: +45-35456713.
  E-mail address: ilaw@pet.rh.dk (I. Law).

altitude. This study shows that CBF is not perfectly regulated to maintain O_2-delivery in every situation. © 2002 Elsevier Science B.V. All rights reserved.

Keywords: Hypoxemia/brain; High altitude; Positron emission tomography; Activation; Regional cerebral blood flow

1. Introduction

The regional cerebral blood flow (rCBF) increase during neuronal activation is unproportionally large, relative to the regional metabolic rate of oxygen (rCMRO$_2$) known as uncoupling. It has been hypothesized that the rCBF and the rCMRO$_2$ have in fact preserved coupling, but nonlinearly, with a pronounced neural activation induced rCBF increase intended to sustain adequate tissue oxygenation by overpowering the diffusion, and solubility limitations of oxygen in the brain tissue [1].

The relationship between CMRO$_2$ and CBF can be defined using Fick's principle as:

$$CMRO_2 = CBF \cdot (C_a - C_v)O_2 = C_aO_2 \cdot CBF \cdot OEF = O_2\text{-delivery} \cdot OEF$$

Thus, when the arterial oxygen content (C_aO_2) is reduced during hypoxemia, CMRO$_2$ can be sustained either by increasing CBF or the oxygen extraction fraction (OEF), and a decrease in O_2-delivery can only be met by an increase in OEF. If the rCBF is regulated to maintain O_2-delivery, a decrease in C_aO_2 must be counteracted by a proportional increase in the rCBF. Conversely, if the rCBF is not regulated to maintain O_2-delivery, the rCBF is not sufficiently increased to compensate for a C_aO_2 decrease. Furthermore, data have been presented to suggest the latter relationship. Visual stimulation during normoxemia and acute hypoxemia by inhalation of gas with a fractional inspired oxygen content (F_IO_2) of 12% provided the same relative rCBF activation responses (32%) in the visual cortex, thus resulting in a net decrease in the change of O_2-delivery during hypoxemia [2].

We have recently collected positron emission tomography (PET) rCBF data with the purpose of examining the consequences of various behavioral conditions in acute and chronic hypoxemia. These data have been reanalyzed in order to address the above relationship between the rCBF and O_2-delivery.

2. Methods

2.1. Subjects

Eight healthy volunteers (four males; four females; median age: 25 years; range 22–27 years), from a cohort of sixteen, were acclimatized to chronic hypoxemia during a 12-week sojourn in Chacaltaya in the Andes, Bolivia. The altitude was 5260 m above sea level, corresponding to a F_IO_2 of 11%. After breathing room air during a plane trip to Copenhagen, Denmark, the subjects spent the night in a pressure chamber at oxygen tensions, simulating an altitude of 6000 m in order to conserve acclimatization as much as possible.

2.2. PET scanning

A total of 20 PET scans was acquired per subject with quantification of the rCBF using standard $H_2^{15}O$ autoradiographic techniques [3] with appropriate corrections of the arterial input function [4]. A dose of 230 MBq (6.2 mCi) $H_2^{15}O$ was administered per scan and the acquisition time was 90 s in 3D mode [5] using the Advance-GE PET scanner. A total of 10 scans were sampled within 24 h of return from high altitude and the remaining 10 scans after an acclimatization period of 5–7 months at sea level. In addition, the arterial blood gas values were measured.

2.3. Experimental design

2.3.1. Behavioral conditions

The 10 scans at each acclimatization level were divided into four behavioral conditions: rest; repetitive (1 Hz) finger-to-thumb opposition movements with the right hand; leg exercise; and visual stimulation (see Table 1).

2.3.2. The fractional inhaled oxygen content

Apart from the behavioral differences between scans, F_1O_2 was also manipulated toobserve responses at acute hypoxemia at a given altitude of acclimatization. Hence, the PET scans were acquired at normoxemia ($F_1O_2 = 20\%$) and acute hypoxemia with a F_1O_2 of 8% (simulating an ascend to approximately 7500 m) at high altitude acclimatization or 10% at sea level acclimatization.

2.4. Analysis

Image analysis was performed using standard SPM99 techniques (http://www.fil.io-n.ucl.ac.uk/spm), except that the global CBF (gCBF) or P_aCO_2 were not removed as confounders. The gCBF values were sampled using an identical region of interest in all subjects and scans covering predominantly cortical, cerebellar and subcortical gray matter.

Table 1
The experimental design with the distribution of measurements among conditions at acclimatization to high altitude and at sea level and different F_1O_2s

Level of Acclimatization	Normoxia ($F_1O_2 = 20\%$)				Acute Hypoxia ($F_1O_2 = 8/10\%$)			
	Rest	Hand	Leg	Visual	Rest	Hand	Leg	Visual
High Altitude	1	1	0	0	2	2	2	2
Sea Level	2	2	2	2	1	1	0	0

Only data within the broken line box are presented.

Only data from the finger movement vs. rest comparison will be presented, as this is the only comparison in which independent data were sampled in all treatments (Table 1). Quantitative rCBF values were sampled from a 20-mm diameter spherical volume of interest placed on the peak activation in the left hemisphere hand area. The corresponding O_2-delivery values for rCBF and gCBF were calculated based on corresponding values of hemoglobin concentrations and O_2-saturation. We also performed analysis after normalization by the gCBF values. Statistical analyses of the blood gas data, absolute and relative CBF values, and O_2-delivery values were performed using repeated measures, ANOVA with F_IO_2, with condition and acclimatization level as treatments. A one-sampled t-test was used for comparison of the hemoglobin concentrations. The significance threshold was found to be $p < 0.05$.

3. Results

3.1. Blood gasses and hemoglobin

As expected, decreasing F_IO_2 significantly decreased P_aO_2 ($F_{1,7} = 1782$; $p < 0.0001$) from values of 100 to 33 mm Hg, while the O_2-saturation decreased from 97% to 68%

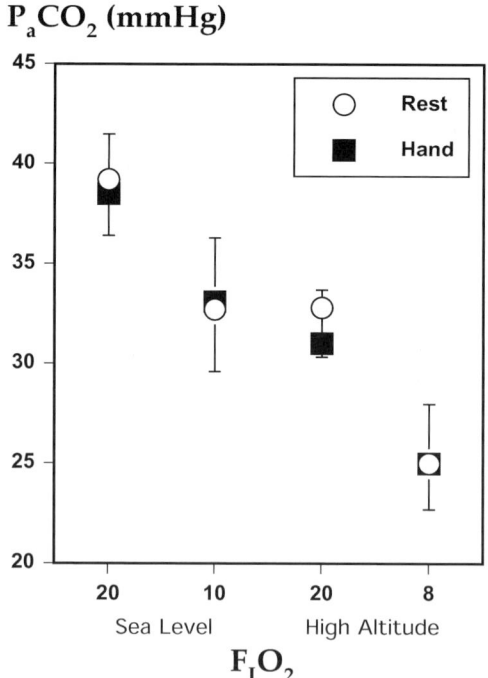

Fig. 1. The arterial carbon dioxide tension during room air, and hypoxemia at acclimatization to sea level and high altitude.

($F_{1,7} = 1153$; $p < 0.0001$). Although we used two different F_IO_2 levels, the P_aO_2 and O_2-saturation values were reduced to similar values. The hypoxemic ventilatory response induced significant hypocapnia ($F_{1,7} = 164.9$; $p < 0.0001$), but hypocapnia was also more significantly pronounced during the acclimatization to high altitude as an independent and additive effect ($F_{1,7} = 37.1$; $p < 0.0005$) (Fig. 1). In addition, finger movements did not produce hypocapnia. The hemoglobin concentration at high altitude and sea level was 14.4 ± 1.8(SD) g/dl and 13.4 ± 1.2(SD) g/dl, respectively ($t = 3.22$, $df = 7$, $p < 0.05$), and hypoxemia increased the average arterial pH from 7.400 ± 0.026(SD) to 7.466 ± 0.023(SD) ($F_{1,6} = 185$; $p < 0.0001$).

3.2. Cerebral blood flow

Hypoxemia significantly increased gCBF ($F_{1,7} = 14.4$; $p < 0.01$). There were no significant effects of acclimatization to the altitude, condition or interaction effects (Fig. 2). Although the observed average change by hypoxemia was larger at acclimatization to sea level compared to that at high altitude, this was not significantly different ($F_{1,7} = 2.2$; $p = 0.18$).

The pattern of regional activation revealed the expected configuration with significant increases in the left pre- and post-central gyrus (Talairach coordinates $(x, y, z) = (-42, -20,$

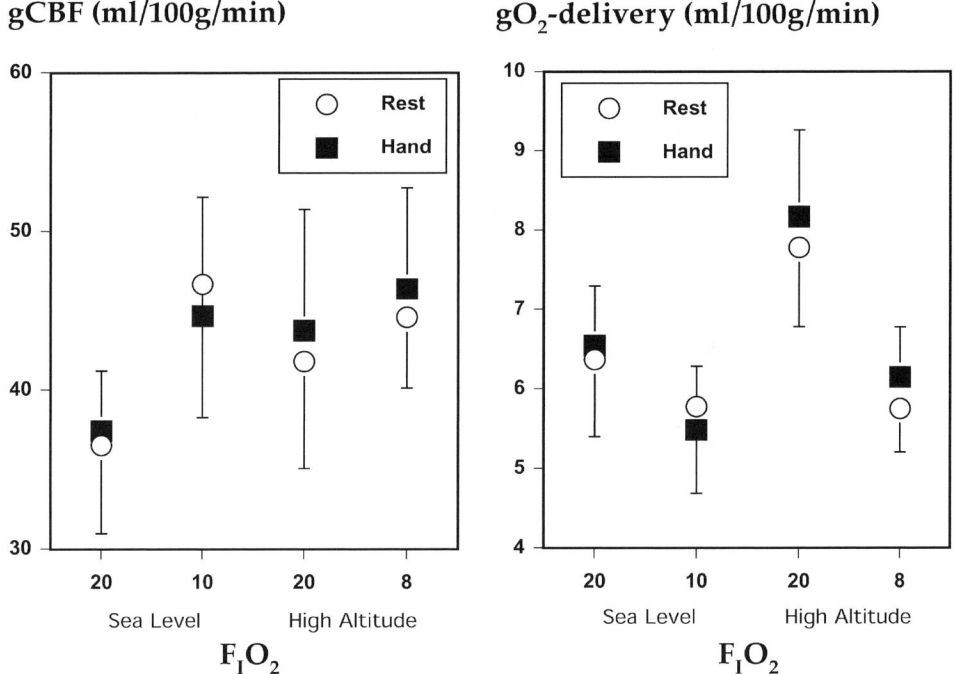

Fig. 2. The global blood flow and the global oxygen delivery to the brain during room air and hypoxemia at acclimatization to sea level and high altitude.

64); SPM$\{T_{140}\}$ =6.8, $p<0.0001$ corrected for multiple independent comparisons), the left medial frontal gyrus, the cerebellar hemispheres, the thalami and the right pre-central gyrus (Fig. 3). Post hoc ANOVAs from the putative hand area showed significantly increased rCBF as a result of both conditions ($F_{1,7}$=51.7; $p<0.0005$) and F_1O_2 ($F_{1,7}$=8.1; $p<0.05$). There were no significant interaction effects or acclimatization effects (Fig. 4); thus, the observed average rCBF changes with finger movements did not change significantly.

3.3. Oxygen delivery

The global cerebral oxygen delivery (gO$_2$-delivery) was significantly larger during acclimatization to high altitude ($F_{1,7}$=12.7; $p<0.01$) and significantly lower during

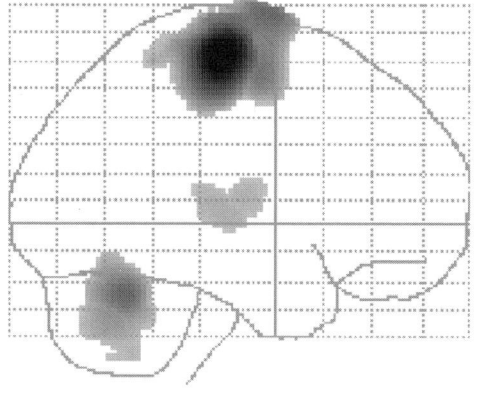
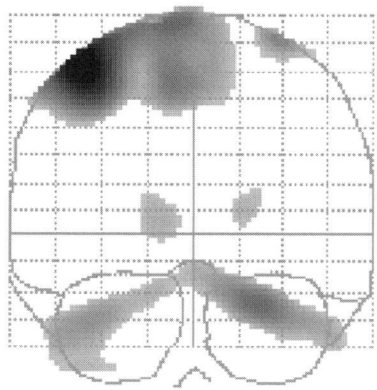
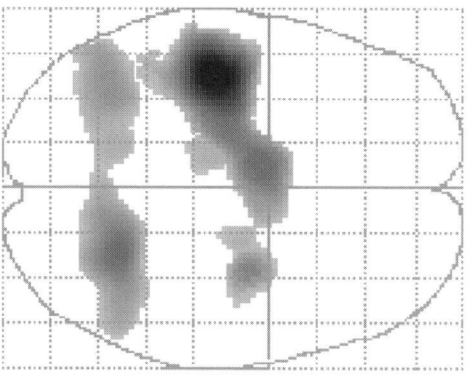

Fig. 3. The rCBF activation pattern, SPM$\{T_{140}\}$, of right-handed finger movements vs. rest. The data are presented in orthogonal sagittal, coronal, and axial projections through a transparent brain. For display purposes, the image is thresholded at $p<0.001$, uncorrected.

rCBF (ml/100g/min)   **rO$_2$-delivery (ml/100g/min)**

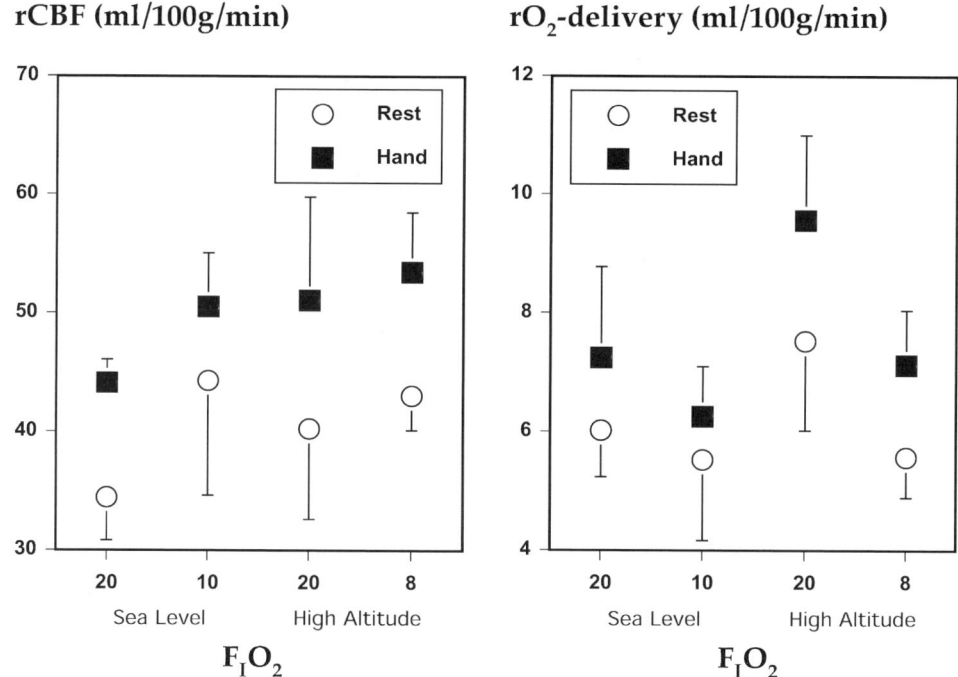

Fig. 4. The regional cerebral blood flow and regional cerebral oxygen delivery to the hand area in the left hemisphere during room air, and hypoxemia at acclimatization to sea level and high altitude.

hypoxemia ($F_{1,7}=59.1; p<0.0001$). Furthermore, the response to hypoxemia depended on the acclimatization altitude. Separate ANOVA analyses revealed that hypoxemia significantly lowered the gO$_2$-delivery both at acclimatization to sea level ($F_{1,7}=11.4; p<0.05$) and high altitude ($F_{1,7}=36.3; p<0.0005$), although the magnitude of decrease was significantly greater in the latter ($F_{1,7}=6.9; p<0.05$). As the O$_2$-saturation reached approximately the same normoxemic and hypoxemic levels at both acclimatization altitudes, this effect can be attributed to the relative polycythemia increasing gO$_2$-delivery in normoxemia (Fig. 2).

The regional cerebral oxygen delivery (rO$_2$-delivery) calculated in the hand area (Fig. 4) was significantly larger overall when acclimatized to high altitude ($F_{1,7}=28.0; p<0.005$), significantly decreased by hypoxemia ($F_{1,7}=15.5; p<0.01$), and increased by finger movements ($F_{1,7}=29.2; p<0.001$). As for the global effects, the decrease in rO$_2$-delivery was significantly larger during hypoxemia at high altitude acclimatization compared to that at sea level acclimatization ($F_{1,7}=7.1; p<0.05$). Analyzing the sea level and high altitude conditions separately revealed only a significant decrease by hypoxemia during acclimatization to high altitude ($F_{1,7}=38.6; p<0.0005$). Although the change in rO$_2$-delivery during finger movements at sea level acclimatization was less pronounced during hypoxemia, this was not significant ($F_{1,7}=4.2; p=0.08$).

Normalized rCBF & rO$_2$ (%)

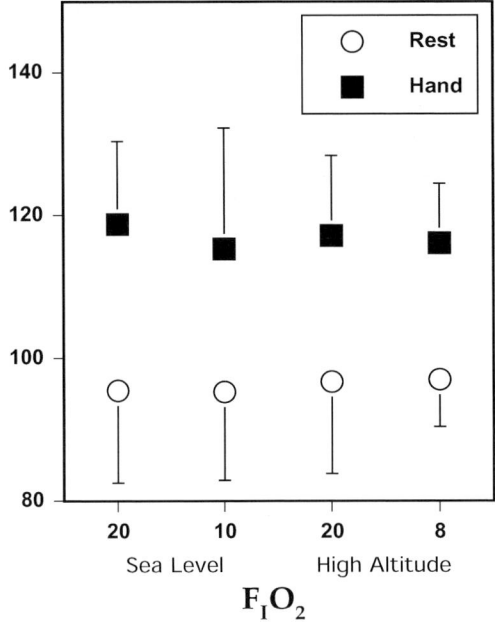

Fig. 5. The regional cerebral blood flow to the hand area normalized by global cerebral blood flow during room air and hypoxemia at acclimatization to sea level and high altitude.

3.4. Relative rCBF and rO$_2$-delivery

The rCBF and consequently, rO$_2$-delivery relative to the global values were strikingly similar regardless of F$_I$O$_2$ or the acclimatization altitude (Fig. 5). The only significant effect was an increase in the hand area due to finger movements ($F_{1,7} = 59.1$; $p < 0.0001$).

4. Discussion

Kety and Schmidt [6] already described the increased gCBF in response to hypoxemia in a normal man in 1948 using a F$_I$O$_2$ of 10%. The release of several substances including adenosine, prostaglandins, vasopressin, opioids and nitric oxide [7–9] has subsequently been shown to mediate the hypoxemia-induced vasodilation. One mechanism of action is through activation of calcium sensitive potassium channels in vascular smooth muscle [10]. However, hypoxemia is by no means a neutral paradigm for general cerebrovascular vasodilatation, which is an important limitation of the hypoxemia paradigm. As shown in Fig. 1, hypoxemia has profound effects on a number of important physiological blood parameters, which could influence the rCBF with varying regional sensitivities [11]. Moreover, hypoxemia is a potent stimulator of counter-regulatory mechanisms to minimize development of tissue hypoxia and organ dysfunction revolving around autonomic nervous adjustments. Acutely, the cardiovascular responses are dominated by increases in ventilatory drive, heart rate and sympathetic vasoconstrictor tone, without large changes in blood pressure, cardiac output or peripheral blood flow [12,13]. Chronic intermittent hypoxemia in rats, a model for the obstructive sleep apnea syndrome, evokes the expression of c-*fos*, an immediate early gene, in a number of primarily limbic cortical and subcortical regions related to the activation of circuits that adaptively regulate sympathetic and cardiovascular activities [14,15]. The cerebral correlates of autonomic cardiovascular arousal have previously been demonstrated in man [16]. Thus, hypoxemia has a regional activation pattern representing an ill-defined conglomerate of cerebrovascular responses to physiological blood parameters and the ongoing generation, maintenance or representation of different states of autonomic arousal and possibly related conditioned responses, all of which could interact with the magnitude of an rCBF activation response. During hypoxemia, we found particularly significant rCBF responses bilaterally in the sensorimotor strip, insulae, visual cortex, cingulate cortex and thalami (data not shown).

In the present study, hypoxemia significantly increased gCBF and hand area rCBF by an overall average of 6.6 ml/100 g/min (14%) and 5.3 ml/100 g/min (12%), respectively. The gCBF was not sufficiently increased during acute hypoxemia, nor sufficiently decreased during normoxemia and the relative polycythemia at acclimatization to high altitude, to perfectly regulate gO_2-delivery. We cannot, with certainty, ascertain whether the findings during acclimatization to high altitude were particular to this state or would also generalize to sea level polycythemia. A further difficulty in interpreting the high altitude data relates to $gCMRO_2$. Some species have the ability to decrease $CMRO_2$ during long-term hypoxemia, presumably as a neuroprotective strategy [17]. Short-term changes, however, are unlikely. Acute hypoxia at sea level ($F_1O_2 = 10\%$) does not change $gCMRO_2$ significantly [6]. Furthermore, the gCBF and $gCMRO_2$ were measured using Kety–Schmidt in nine of the subjects from the Bolivia expedition, three of which also provided data in the present study, at high altitude and 6 months after at sea level, at room air [18]. No significant differences were found in either. Thus, $gCMRO_2$ can be assumed constant in our study.

The rCBF increase to the hand area during hypoxemia at sea level acclimatization was sufficiently high to compensate for the reduction in arterial oxygen content, maintaining rO_2-delivery unaltered. This was not the case for rO_2-delivery during the high altitude acclimatization, which was significantly reduced by hypoxemia. Thus, we can demonstrate one, possibly abnormal physiological condition, where the rCBF was not regulated adequately to maintain a constant rO_2-delivery.

Finger movements significantly increased rO_2-delivery to the hand area. This was at an unchanged magnitude of increase, unaffected by hypoxemia ($p = 0.08$) or acclimatization altitude, and within an rCBF activation increase, that did not change significantly. Finally, the changes in gCBF did not influence the observed rCBF change, whether measured by an absolute or a relative scale.

Thus, there is ample evidence in human and animal studies showing that factors that determine oxygen content, such as hemoglobin concentration and O_2-saturation, have profound regulatory effects on CBF. This study shows that this regulation does not perfectly maintain O_2-delivery in every situation.

2.2.3.7. On-Site Discussion

2.2.3.7.1. *Question: (Pearce)* Isn't it true that the preservation of regional blood flow responsiveness in the altitude-acclimatized subjects actually represents successful adaptation to chronic hypoxemia? Animal studies suggest that many cerebrovascular characteristics involved in signaling are dramatically different in normoxic and chronically hypoxemic animals. To what extent have you considered, or examined, the possibility that aspects of neurohumoral reactivity may be changed by hypoxemic acclimatization, whereas regional responsiveness to neuronal activation, is not?

Answer: (Law) Correct! In this particular study, our experimental design was connected to a hypothesis of compromised rCBF activation response during cerebral hypoxia, so the neurohumoral responses were not measured simultaneously in the PET scanner. However, the subjects participating in the Bolivia expedition participated in more than 30 separate physiological experiments, one of which showed persistently increased microneural activity even 3 weeks after descent from high altitude (Hansen et al., personal communication).

Acknowledgements

This work was supported by a grant from the Danish medical research council. The John and Birthe Meyer Foundation is gratefully acknowledged for the donation of the Cyclotron and PET scanner.

References

[1] R.B. Buxton, L.R. Frank, A model for the coupling between cerebral blood flow and oxygen metabolism during neural stimulation, J. Cereb. Blood Flow Metab. 17 (1) (1997) 64–72.

[2] M.A. Mintun, G.L. Shulman, A.V. Snyder, M.E. Raichle, Cerebral blood flow during regional activation is not regulated to maintain oxygen delivery (abstract), J. Neurosci. 26 (2000) 645.11.

[3] I. Kanno, H. Iida, S. Miura, M. Murakami, K. Takahashi, H. Sasaki, et al, A system for cerebral blood flow measurement using an $H_2{}^{15}O$ autoradiographic method and positron emission tomography, J. Cereb. Blood Flow Metab. 7 (143) (1987) 143–153.

[4] H. Iida, S. Higano, N. Tomura, F. Shishido, I. Kanno, S. Miura, et al, Evaluation of regional differences of tracer appearance time in cerebral tissues using water and dynamic positron emission tomography, J. Cereb. Blood Flow Metab. 8 (285) (1988) 285–288.

[5] I. Law, H. Iida, S. Holm, S. Nour, E. Rostrup, C. Svarer, et al, Quantitation of regional cerebral blood flow corrected for partial volume effect using O-15 water and PET II. Normal values and gray matter blood flow response to visual activation, J. Cereb. Blood Flow Metab. 20 (8) (2000) 1252–1263.

[6] S.S. Kety, C.F. Schmidt, The effects of altered arterial tensions of carbon dioxide and oxygen on cerebral blood flow and cerebral oxygen consumption of normal young men, J. Clin. Invest. 27 (1948) 484–492.

[7] W.M. Armstead, Opioids and nitric oxide contribute to hypoxia-induced pial arterial vasodilation in newborn pigs, Am. J. Physiol. 268 (1 Pt. 2) (1995) H226–H232.

[8] D.A. Pelligrino, Q. Wang, H.M. Koenig, R.F. Albrecht, Role of nitric oxide, adenosine, N-methyl-D-aspartate receptors, and neuronal activation in hypoxia-induced pial arteriolar dilation in rats, Brain Res. 704 (1) (1995) 61–70.

[9] M.G. Coyle, W. Oh, B.S. Stonestreet, Effects of indomethacin on brain blood flow and cerebral metabolism in hypoxic newborn piglets, Am. J. Physiol. 264 (1 Pt. 2) (1993) H141–H149.

[10] G. Ben-Haim, W.M. Armstead, Stimulus duration-dependent contribution of k(ca) channel activation and cAMP to hypoxic cerebrovasodilation, Brain Res. 853 (2) (2000) 330–337.

[11] H. Ito, I. Yokoyama, H. Iida, T. Kinoshita, J. Hatazawa, E. Shimosegawa, et al, Regional differences in cerebral vascular response to P_aCO_2 changes in humans measured by positron emission tomography, J. Cereb. Blood Flow Metab. 20 (8) (2000) 1264–1270.

[12] K.P. Davy, P.P. Jones, D.R. Seals, Influence of age on the sympathetic neural adjustments to alterations in systemic oxygen levels in humans, Am. J. Physiol. 273 (2 Pt. 2) (1997) R690–R695.

[13] S.D. Lucy, R.L. Hughson, J.M. Kowalchuk, D.H. Paterson, D.A. Cunningham, Body position and cardiac dynamic and chronotropic responses to steady-state isocapnic hypoxemia in humans, Exp. Physiol. 85 (2) (2000) 227–237.

[14] A.L. Sica, H.E. Greenberg, S.M. Scharf, D.A. Ruggiero, Chronic-intermittent hypoxia induces immediate early gene expression in the midline thalamus and epithalamus, Brain Res. 883 (2) (2000) 224–228.

[15] A.L. Sica, H.E. Greenberg, S.M. Scharf, D.A. Ruggiero, Immediate-early gene expression in cerebral cortex following exposure to chronic-intermittent hypoxia, Brain Res. 870 (2000) 204–210.

[16] H.D. Critchley, D.R. Corfield, M.P. Chandler, C.J. Mathias, R.J. Dolan, Cerebral correlates of autonomic cardiovascular arousal: a functional neuroimaging investigation in humans, J. Physiol. 523 (Pt. 1) (2000) 259–270.

[17] J.M. Mulvey, G.M. Renshaw, Neuronal oxidative hypometabolism in the brainstem of the epaulette shark (*Hemiscyllium ocellatum*) in response to hypoxic pre-conditioning, Neurosci. Lett. 290 (1) (2000) 1–4.

[18] K. Moller, O.B. Paulson, T.F. Hornbein, W.N. Colier, A.S. Paulson, R.C. Roach, et al, Unchanged cerebral blood flow and oxidative metabolism after acclimatization to high altitude, J. Cereb. Blood Flow Metab. 22 (1) (2002) 118–126.

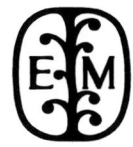

International Congress Series 1235 (2002) 99–106

Quantitative aspects of changes in cerebral blood flow induced by neuronal activation

Iwao Kanno*, Tetsuya Matsuura, Hiroshi Ito

*Department of Radiology and Nuclear Medicine, Akita Research Institute of Brain and Blood Vessels,
6-10 Senshu-Kubota-Machi, Akita, Akita 010-0874, Japan*

Abstract

We examined the quantitative aspects of neurovascular coupling by revisiting and reanalyzing published cerebral blood flow (CBF) data, measured by positron emission tomography (PET) and laser Doppler flowmetry (LDF). The proportional increase of absolute CBF with the baseline CBF even under constant stimulation suggests that the CBF increase is independent of the nutritional demand induced by neuronal activity. In contrast, the linearity of the normalized CBF relative to the baseline CBF in PET and the linearity of the relative CBF to the frequency of electrical stimulation in LDF, both suggest that relative CBF change is beautifully regulated by the strength of neuronal activity. In addition, we will discuss the features of the two CBF regulation factors, $PaCO_2$ and neuronal activity. © 2002 Elsevier Science B.V. All rights reserved.

Keywords: Cerebral blood flow; Baseline CBF; Activation CBF; $PaCO_2$; Neuronal activity

1. Introduction

It has been naively believed that the magnitude of the signals from neurovascular coupling [1], such as CBF change, BOLD contrast, or the optical image signal, is basically linear with the strength of neuronal activity. Brain-imaging methods, mapping the brain function in man and animals, have relied on this robust characteristic of

Abbreviations: CBF, cerebral blood flow; CeBF, cerebellar blood blow; LDF, laser Doppler flowmetry; PET, positron emission tomography; CCD, crossed cerebellar diaschisis; MDLT, modified random digit learning test; CBV, cerebral blood volume.
* Corresponding author. Fax: +81-18-833-2104.
E-mail address: kanno@akita-noken.go.jp (I. Kanno).

neurovascular coupling. However, quantitative aspects of the magnitude of hemodynamic change in relation to the strength of neuronal activation have not yet been established [2]. We have revisited quantitative data obtained in studies carried out on man and rats, to elucidate the physiological mechanisms that quantitatively govern the magnitude of CBF response during neuronal stimulation. Our goal is to answer questions about the quantitative relationship between the magnitude of CBF changes and the strength of neuronal activity.

2. CBF response in absolute and relative scales

In order to establish a quantitative relationship between activation CBF and baseline CBF, we used PET to measure the activation of the CBF induced in the visual cortex by an 8-Hz flicker stimulus during hypocapnia, normocapnia and hypercapnia. It was found that increases in CBF in the visual cortex, caused by this stimulation, were proportional to the baseline CBF ($n=12$) (Fig. 1) [3]. This finding suggests that the baseline CBF level, that is $PaCO_2$, modifies the increase in CBF. We also observed with PET that under forced hyperventilation, the absolute CBF change in the motor area associated with the diaphragm was lower than that under normal ventilation. However, the relative CBF (i.e., CBF normalized by the global average CBF) showed a clear positive value in the same area ($n=14$) (Fig. 2) [4]. This also implies that the $PaCO_2$ level modulates the neuronal activity, and in this case, regulation by neuronal activity is overridden by $PaCO_2$ regulation.

Both of these findings clearly demonstrate that absolute CBF in the absolute scale does not reflect the strength of the neuronal activity, while the relative CBF is relevant to the neuronal activity rather than the absolute CBF. In addition, it is clearly confirmed that the

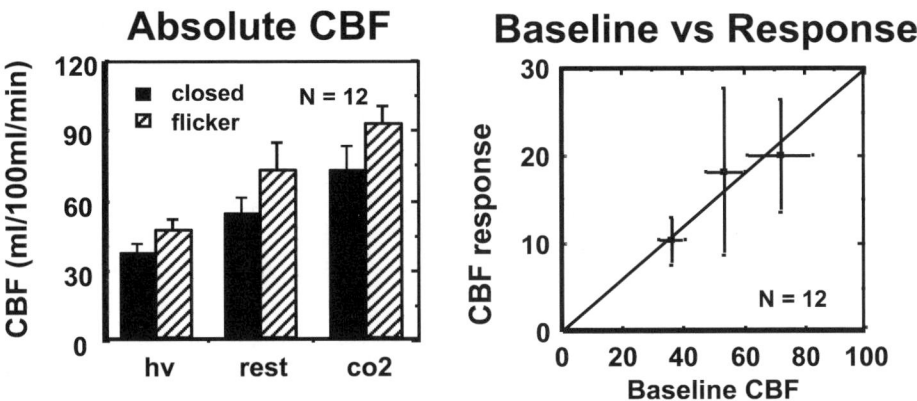

Fig. 1. The CBF in the visual cortex measured during eye-closed and 8 Hz flicker stimulation for each $PaCO_2$ level (left), and their difference as a function of baseline CBF (right). All CBF values plotted in either graph were the absolute value. The CBF response was revealed to be proportional to the baseline CBF.

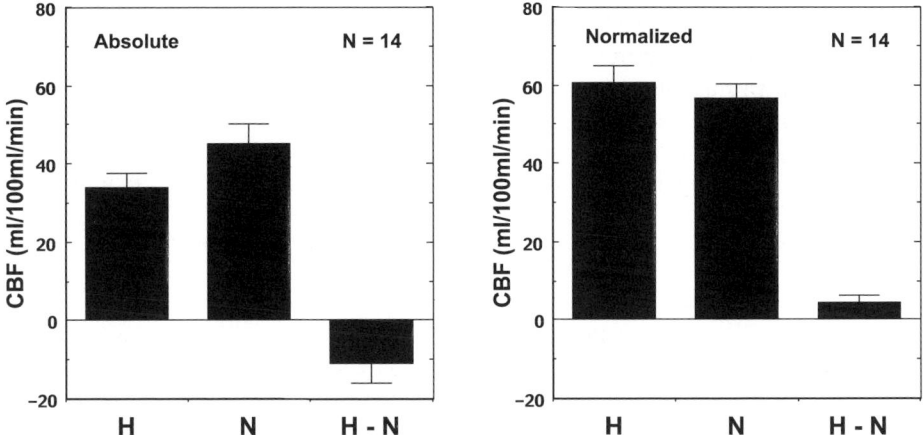

Fig. 2. The CBF in the motor cortex corresponding to the diaphragm during normal breathing, hyperventilation and their difference were plotted using absolute CBF (left graph), and using relative CBF (whole brain CBF normalized to be 50 ml/100 g/min) (right graph). Absolute CBF in the diaphragm motor area during hyperventilation was lower than that during normal breathing. This relationship became the opposite in the relative CBF, and the relative CBF in the diaphragm function was positive. This normalization is a conventional process in mapping brain function.

driving force to elevate CBF during stimulation is independent of the demand for nutrition during energy metabolism.

3. Linearity in the coupling of relative CBF to neuronal activity

The next question is the quantitative relationship between the magnitude of the CBF response and the strength of the neuronal activity. We analyzed PET CBF data obtained from a psychological task; the modified random digit learning test (MDLT) was carried out in a relatively large population (n=20). The CBF in the midbrain was plotted as a function of the behavior score from the MDLT. The CBF in the absolute scale did not show any correlation with the behavior score, whereas the CBF in the relative scale showed a significant correlation with the behavior score (Fig. 3). This implies that behavior, or neuronal activity, is tightly coupled with the relative CBF but not with the absolute CBF.

The quantitative relationship between the strength of neuronal activity and the relative CBF change was also confirmed by experiments using LDF and an α-chloralosed rat. In these experiments, we manipulated the strength of neuronal activity by changing the frequency of electrical stimulation at the hind paw. The stimulus duration was fixed at 5 s. The LDF probe was placed at the same location as the electrode used to measure the field potential in the somatosensory cortex. Assuming that the strength of neuronal activity was determined by the integral of the field potential, we found that CBF was clearly proportional to the strength of neuronal activity (Fig. 4) [5]. As CBF determined by LDF is always on a relative scale with respect to the baseline level, it is clear that the relative CBF was once again tightly bound to the strength of neuronal activity.

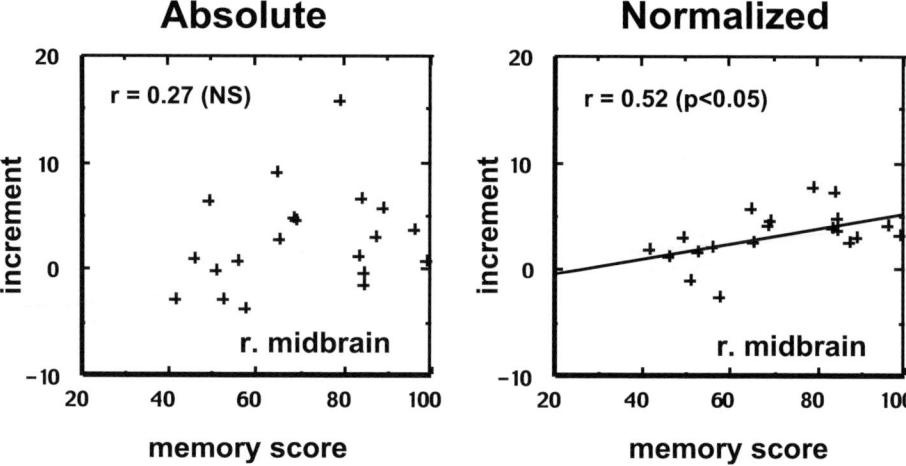

Fig. 3. The CBF in the midbrain during the modified digit learning test (MDLT) was plotted as a function of MDLT behavior score. Again the absolute CBF (on the left) and relative CBF (on the right) were plotted in each graph. It was clear that there was little correlation between absolute CBF and the behavior score, but a high correlation was revealed for the relative CBF.

The quantitative aspects of neurovascular coupling were first established through the slow process of PET, which provides the mean CBF average over a few minutes. Then, we tested and confirmed it in a fast process using LDF, which follows the almost instantaneous CBF and needs, at the longest, a few seconds for quantification. Thus, the servomechanism adjusting the magnitude of CBF response to the strength of neuronal activity performs its function not only in the slow steady-state process, but also in faster

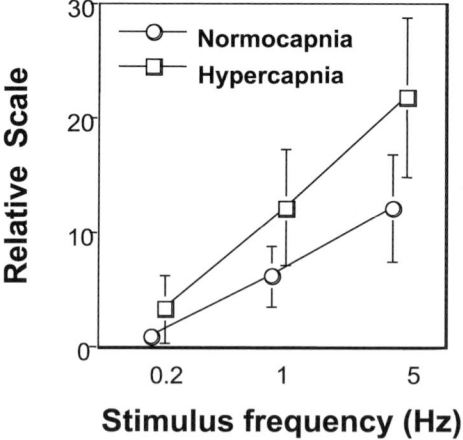

Fig. 4. The CBF obtained by LDF in a rat with hind paw stimulation was increased as its frequency increased from 0.2 to 5 Hz. In hypercapnia, the relationship between the CBF increase and the frequency became steeper than that in normocapnia. The effect of $PaCO_2$ was modulated by the strength of neuronal activity.

processes. The practical realization of the servomechanism remains to be clarified, including the investigation of factors for feedback and feed forward.

4. Symmetrical feature of neuronal activity with PaCO2 in CBF regulation

Two control factors, $PaCO_2$ and neuronal activity, are found to "symmetrically" affect the CBF regulation. As shown in Fig. 1, increases in the absolute CBF were revealed to be proportional to the $PaCO_2$ level when the stimulus was kept constant, so that neuronal activity was approximately the same at all times [3]. Similarly, with neuronal deactivation associated with the crossed cerebellar diaschisis (CCD) of a minor stroke, it was found that the difference in cerebellar blood flow of the contralateral cerebellum (deactivated neuronal activity) from that of the ispilateral cerebellum (normal neuronal activity) was proportional to the $PaCO_2$ ($n=17$) (Fig. 5) [6]. These data, demonstrated by an increase or decrease in CBF induced by neuronal activation or deactivation, is modified by the $PaCO_2$ level in a way that is proportional to the baseline CBF [7]. On the other hand, LDF experiments with a graded strength of neuronal activity and a fixed $PaCO_2$ level, demonstrated that the $PaCO_2$ affected the increase in CBF [8]. Thus, the two factors of neuronal activity and $PaCO_2$ behave in a "symmetrical" fashion in the regulation of CBF.

Now because the level of microcirculatory $PaCO_2$ is uniform across the whole of the brain, $PaCO_2$ can be considered a global factor in the regulation of CBF. In addition, the neuronal activity is a local factor because it only affects a small area corresponding to specific neuronal regions of the brain. Based on these presuppositions, the twin schematic relationships between CBF and local (i.e., neuronal activity) and global (i.e., $PaCO_2$) regulation factors have been sketched in Fig. 6.

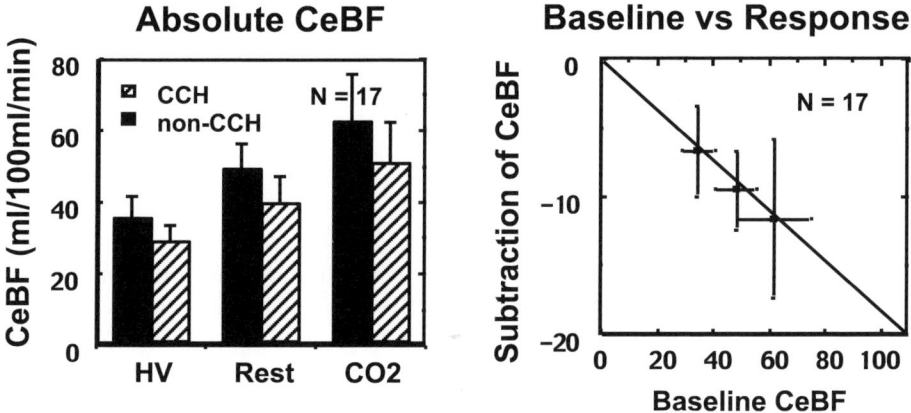

Fig. 5. Cerebellar blood flow (CeBF) of the contralateral (deactivate) (solid bar) and ipsilateral (control) (hatched bar) cerebellar hemispheres in minor stroke patients with hemispheric cerebral vascular disease during hypocapnia, normocapnia and hypercapnia (left graph). The decrease in CBF was again proportional to the baseline CBF level. The subtraction from the contraleteral side of the ipsilateral side, plotted as a function of the ipsilateral side, revealed a clear negative relationship (right graph).

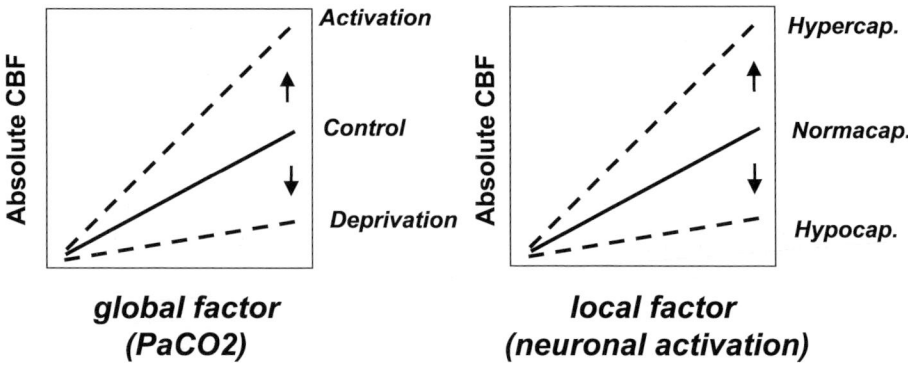

Fig. 6. Schematic relationships between the local CBF for different levels of a global factor (PaCO$_2$) (left), and between global CBF as a function of the control global CBF for different levels of local factor (neuronal activity). Furthermore, the global and local factors interact symmetrically with each other.

Recently, we found that the relationship between CBF and the cerebral blood volume (CBV) during neuronal stimulation, was almost the same as that obtained by Grubb et al. [9] and Ito et al. [10] during PaCO$_2$ regulation. This supports the similarity of the affects that either PaCO$_2$ or neuronal activity has on microcirculation when the other factor is held constant. Both components probably interact at the same site of the microvascular structure.

5. Closing remarks

These results imply that only the relative CBF response was closely linked to the strength of neuronal activity. They also imply that only the relative CBF was closely linked to the neuronal activation and that its magnitude was linearly related to the intensity of neuronal activity change. Regulation of CBF by the neuronal activity was found to be similar to that produced by PaCO$_2$.

2.2.4.8. On-Site Discussion

2.2.4.8.1. *Question: (Dirnagl)* Your data in which you show that neuronally evoked responses in CBF are increased when baseline CBF is increased are at variance with data shown in several presentations this morning. Do you have any explanations for this discrepancy?

Answer: (Kanno) As I showed in my talk, magnitudes of response are a function of baseline level. Therefore, if response was varied, it would be due to different baseline as well as difference magnitude of stimulation.

2.2.4.8.2. *Question: (Heiss)* Your results that responses at a low resting flow rate are less pronounced than at a higher resting flow are surprising. I wonder if the "resting state" during a more complex situation — active background — would not rather have a modulating effect on the stimulus-related response. For example, if you are aroused and expecting a stimulus — your background "resting" flow would be high, but the response to the stimulus might be relative small. Do you have any results concerning this influence of absolute flow on the extent of response to a stimulus?

Answer: (Kanno) What I showed was absolute CBF increase from the baseline level to activation level of neuronal activity. Thus, the "active background" is no more "resting-state" in my talk, therefore, I have not had such data. However, I suppose the additive stimulation might cause a proportional increase based on an "arousal" baseline.

2.2.4.8.3. *Question: (Bandettini)* It seems that if hypercapnia causes enhanced blood flow responses with activation then this relationship would break down at some high level of flow. Flow increases cannot continue without bound. Where do you think this breaks down?

Answer: (Kanno) I do not have such threshold for the breakdown, but I believe, it must be within physiological range, say 50 mm Hg at maximum.

2.2.4.8.4. *Question: (Hoge)* How wide is the range of perturbation of $PaCO_2$?

Answer: (Kanno) It was minus 10 mm Hg for hypocapnia, and plus 5 mm Hg for hypercapnia. Since normocapnia level was 40 mm Hg in average, range was from 30 to 45 mm Hg. We measured $PaCO_2$ by arterial blood sampling.

2.2.4.8.5. *Question: (Nemoto)* Hypercapnia produces a significant catecholamine responses and increases in arterial blood pressure. Did you measure arterial pressure and was it unchanged with hypercapnia.

Answer: (Kanno) We monitored blood pressure by hand finger in all cases, and found no systematic change of mean blood pressure in either hypocapnia or hypercapnia.

Acknowledgements

This work was partially supported by the Japan Science and Technology Corporation grant on "Measurement and Mechanism of the Secondary Signal Induced by Neuronal Activation" (1996–2000).

References

[1] C.S. Roy, C.S. Sherrington, On the regulation of the blood-supply of the brain, J. Physiol. 11 (1890) 85–108.

[2] N.A. Lassen, I. Kanno, The metabolic and hemodynamic events secondary to functional activation — notes from a workshop held in Akita, Japan, Magn. Reson. Med. 38 (1997) 521–523.

[3] E. Shimosegawa, I. Kanno, J. Hatazawa, H. Fujita, H. Iida, S. Miura, M. Murakami, A. Inugami, H. Itoh, T. Okudera, K. Uemura, Photic stimulation study of changing the arterial partial pressure level of carbon dioxide, J. Cereb. Blood Flow Metab. 15 (1995) 111–114.

[4] I. Kanno, E. Shimosegawa, H. Fujita, J. Hatazawa, Uncoupling of absolute CBF to neural activity, Adv. Exp. Med. Biol. 413 (1997) 209–214.

[5] R. Bakalova, T. Matsuura, I. Kanno, Frequency dependence of local cerebral blood flow induced by somatosensory hind paw stimulation in rat under normo- and hypercapnia, Jpn. J. Physiol. 51 (2001) 201–208.

[6] K. Ishii, I. Kanno, K. Uemura, J. Hatazawa, T. Okudera, A. Inugami, T. Ogawa, H. Fujita, E. Shimosegawa, Comparison of carbon dioxide responsiveness of cerebellar blood flow between affected and unaffected sides with crossed cerebellar diaschisis, Stroke 25 (1994) 826–830.

[7] I. Kanno, J. Hatazawa, E. Shimosegawa, K. Ishii, H. Fujita, Proportionality of reaction CBF to baseline CBF with neural activation and deactivation, in: R. Myers, V. Cunninghan, D. Bailey, T. Jones (Eds.), Quantification of Brain Function Using PET, Academic Press, Oxford, 1996, pp. 362–364.

[8] T. Matsuura, H. Fujita, K. Kashikura, I. Kanno, Modulation of evoked cerebral blood flow under excessive blood supply and hyperoxic conditions, Jpn. J. Physiol. 50 (2000) 115–123.

[9] R.L. Grubb Jr., M.E. Raichle, J.O. Eichling, M.M. Ter-Pogossian, The effects of changes in $PaCO_2$ on cerebral blood volume, blood flow, and vascular mean transit time, Stroke 5 (1974) 630–639.

[10] H. Ito, K. Takahashi, J. Hatazawa, S.G. Kim, I. Kanno, Changes in human regional cerebral blood flow and cerebral blood volume during visual stimulation measured by positron emission tomography, J. Cereb. Blood Flow Metab. 21 (2001) 608–612.

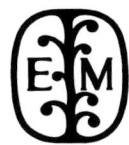
International Congress Series 1235 (2002) 107–113

Evoked cerebral blood flow is linear to neuronal activation but independent of metabolic oxygen demand

Tetsuya Matsuura*, Iwao Kanno

Department of Radiology and Nuclear Medicine, Akita Research Institute of Brain and Blood Vessels, 6-10 Senshu-kubota machi, Akita 010-0874, Japan

Abstract

The purpose of this study was to test the hypothesis that the degree of evoked local cerebral blood flow (LCBF) is dependent on neuronal activity, but not on oxygen consumption. We measured the field potential and evoked LCBF using laser-Doppler flowmetry in alpha-chloralose anesthetized rats during activation of the somatosensory cortex. The findings of this study are: (1) change in response magnitude of evoked LCBF reflects the change in the integrated amplitude of field potentials; (2) hyperoxia enhances the evoked LCBF; and (3) the evoked LCBF is proportional to the baseline flow. These suggest that the evoked LCBF is not directed toward supplying oxygen and some substrates for oxidative metabolism, but it could be modified by mechanisms operating on the blood vessels, which are proportional to neuronal activity. © 2002 Elsevier Science B.V. All rights reserved.

Keywords: Cerebral blood flow; Hyperoxia; Hypercapnia; Laser-Doppler flowmetry; Neuronal activity

1. Introduction

Since the coupling between cerebral blood flow (CBF) and neuronal activity was first proposed by Roy and Sherrington [1], a number of researchers have demonstrated the relationship between neuronal activity and change in local CBF (evoked LCBF). One important role of the evoked LCBF is to supply oxygen to the brain tissue. However, Fox and Raichle [2] demonstrated a lack of coupling between LCBF and oxygen metabolism. This suggests that the degree of increase in LCBF is dependent on neuronal activity, but not on oxygen consumption. The purpose of this study was to test the hypothesis that the

---

* Corresponding author. Department of Biology and Earth Sciences, Faculty of Science, Ehime University, Bunkyo-cho 3, Matsuyama, 790-8577, Japan. Tel./fax: +81-89-927-8928.

E-mail address: matsuurat@sci.ehime-u.ac.jp (T. Matsuura).

evoked LCBF is not directed toward supplying oxygen for oxidative metabolism by measuring the evoked LCBF under hyperoxia, hypocapnia and hypercapnia using laser-Doppler flowmetry (LDF).

Another objective of this study was to determine the quantitative relationship between neuronal activity and the changes in evoked LCBF using both electrophysiological and LDF techniques. There are few reports which have evaluated the relationship between neuronal activity and evoked LCBF [3–7]. These observations indicate the existence of a discrepancy between the evoked LCBF and electrical signal, when the selected signal which is used to evaluate the neuronal activity is different, i.e., number of spikes, amplitude of evoked potential, or product of amplitude of evoked potential and stimulus frequency. In the present study, we recorded the field potential of a local area using an electrode inserted into the cortex, and evaluated the relationship between this recording and evoked LCBF.

2. Materials and methods

Sprague–Dawley rats (320–460 g) were anesthetized with halothane (4% for induction and 1.5% during surgery) in 30% oxygen and 70% nitrous oxide. The tail artery and the left femoral vein were cannulated for blood pressure monitoring, blood gas sampling, and intravenous drug administration. Following tracheotomy, alpha-chloralose (75 mg/kg, i.v.) was administered, and halothane and nitrous oxide administrations were discontinued. The rat was immobilized with pancuronium bromide (0.7 mg/kg, i.v.), and ventilated with a respirator (SN-480-7, Shinano, Japan) using room air and supplemental oxygen throughout the experimental period. Anesthesia was maintained with alpha-chloralose (45 mg/kg/h, i.v.), and muscle relaxation, with pancuronium bromide (0.8 mg/kg/hr, i.v.). The body temperature was maintained at approximately 37.0°C using a heating pad (ATC-101, Unique Medical, Japan). The rat was fixed in a stereotactic frame, and the parietal bone was thinned to translucency at the left somatosensory area. The $PaCO_2$ and PaO_2 levels were maintained in the range of 32–40 and 90–120 mm Hg, respectively, by regulating the stroke volume of ventilation and the fractional concentration of oxygen in the gas inspired.

LCBF was measured with an LDF (Periflux 4001 Master, Perimed, Sweden) equipped with an LDF probe with a tip diameter of 0.46 mm (Probe 411, Perimed, Sweden). The LDF probe was placed in the somatosensory area of the hind paw, perpendicular to the brain surface. It was attached to the thinned parietal bone, avoiding areas with large blood vessels. To ensure a stable condition of the animal, measurements were performed 2–3 h after the preparation of the parietal bone. Activation of the cortex was carried out by electrical stimulation of the hind paw with 0.1-ms rectangular pulses through a pair of small needle electrodes inserted under the skin of the right hind paw. In the experiments for the analysis of frequency dependency, we used 12 rats, and varied the frequency (0.2, 1, 5 and 10 Hz) of the electrical stimuli applied for a 5-s duration at an intensity of 1.5 mA. This stimulus intensity did not cause any change in the systemic arterial blood pressure during stimulation [5,8]. The order of the stimulus frequencies was selected randomly; at each stimulus frequency, 30 successive stimuli were applied at 60-s intervals. The field potentials of the somatosensory cortex were recorded in another set of 12 rats. A tungsten microelectrode (12 MΩ) was inserted into the somatosensory cortex of the hind paw area through the thinned portion of the skull, and fixed using dental cement. The tip of the electrode was set at a depth of approximately 0.5 mm from the surface of the cortex. An Ag–AgCl indifferent electrode was placed between the skull bone and the scalp [9].

In the hyperoxia experiment ($n = 22$), we first examined the responses of LCBF at 5- or 10-Hz electrical stimulation under normoxia, followed by those under hyperoxia after 20 min of 100% oxygen ventilation ($n = 13$ at 5 Hz, $n = 9$ at 10 Hz). For the experiments under hypocapnia and hypercapnia, we used 20 rats (hypocapnia, $n = 10$; hypercapnia, $n = 10$), and first examined the LCBF responses to normocapnia, followed by those to hypocapnia after 20 min of hypocapnic ventilation (hyperventilation) or hypercapnia after 20 min of hypercapnic ventilation. For hypercapnic ventilation, approximately 2.5% carbon dioxide was mixed with the gas administered under the normal gas condition.

The LDF signal and recording of field potential of 30–50 successive measurements were accumulated in order to reduce the noise level of the signal using the MacLab data-acquisition software (AD Instruments, Australia). The response magnitude for 5-s stimulation was calculated as the integral of the response curve from the rise time to the termination time, and was considered to reflect the total amount of increase in blood flow [5]. Parameters among each stimulus frequency were statistically analyzed by ANOVA (repeated measurements) and multiple comparisons (Bonferroni) or the t-test. Values are presented as means $\pm$ S.D.

3. Results

3.1. Relationship between evoked LCBF and neuronal activity

The response of evoked LCBF during the 5-s stimulation period increased with increasing stimulus frequency up to 5 Hz, and decreased at 10 Hz. The pattern of change in the response magnitude of evoked LCBF correlated with that in the integrated amplitude of field potentials (total amplitude: product of the number of spikes and mean amplitude of field potential) during 5-s stimulation ($r = 0.992$, $p < 0.01$) (Fig. 1A), but not with those in the number of spikes and mean amplitude of field potentials (Fig. 1B). The number of spikes during the 5-s stimulation nearly corresponded to the pulse of hind-paw stimuli up to a frequency of 5 Hz, but that during 10-Hz stimulation decreased. The mean amplitude of field potentials declined with increasing stimulus frequency ($p < 0.05$), although there was no significant difference in the mean amplitude between 0.2 and 1 Hz.

3.2. Effect of hyperoxia on evoked LCBF

Physiological variables were within the normal range throughout the experiments, except for PaO_2 under hyperoxia ($PaO_2 = 106.4 \pm 8.4$ mm Hg during normoxia, $PaO_2 = 513.5 \pm 48.4$ mm Hg during hyperoxia). There was no significant difference in the $PaCO_2$ and MABP levels between normoxia and hyperoxia.

The baseline level of LCBF under hyperoxia was $5.6 \pm 3.3\%$ lower than that under normoxia ($p < 0.01$), suggesting mild vasoconstriction at rest under hyperoxia. The normalized response magnitudes of evoked LCBF, which was calculated by dividing

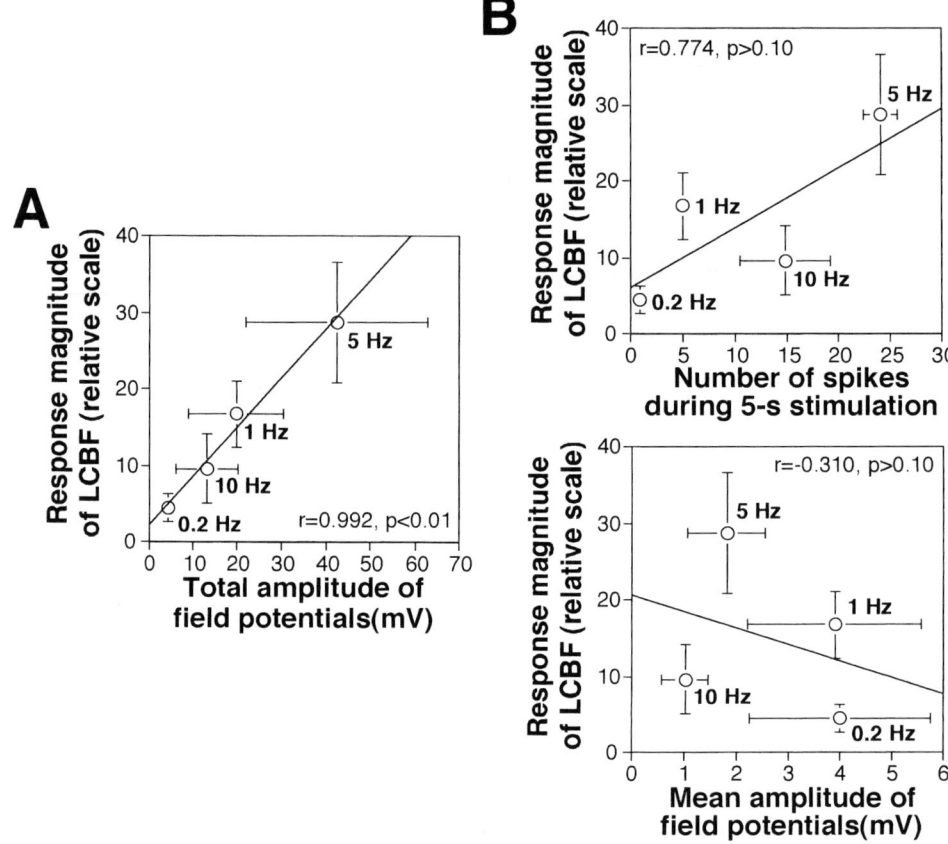

Fig. 1. Correlation between parameters of neuronal activity (number of spikes, mean amplitude and integrated amplitude of field potentials) and response magnitude of evoked LCBF. (A) Significant correlation between integrated amplitude of field potentials and evoked LCBF. (B) Lack of correlation between the number of spikes and evoked LCBF, and the mean amplitude and evoked LCBF. The mean values at each stimulus frequency were used for statistical analysis. Error bars indicate ±S.D. ($n = 12$).

the raw data by each baseline value, at 5- and 10-Hz stimulation under hyperoxia were, respectively, 68.2±48.0% and 44.6±32.0% greater than those under normoxia ($p<0.05$) (Fig. 2). The absolute response magnitudes of evoked LCBF under hyperoxia were also greater than those under normoxia [10].

3.3. Changes in evoked LCBF under hypocapnia and hypercapnia

Under hypocapnia and hypercapnia, physiological variables were within the normal range throughout the experiments, except for the $PaCO_2$ level under hypocapnia ($PaCO_2 = 26.4±1.1$ mm Hg) and hypercapnia ($PaCO_2 = 73.4±13.3$ mm Hg).

The baseline levels of LCBF under hypocapnia and hypercapnia were, respectively, 10.0±0.04% lower and 47.0±22.0% higher than those under normocapnia ($p<0.01$)

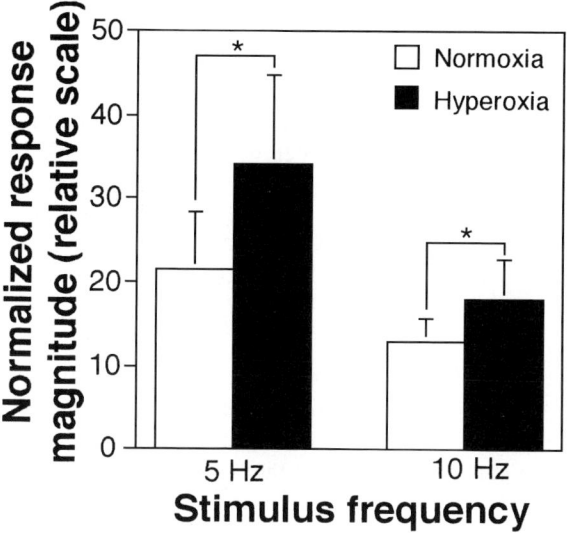

Fig. 2. Comparison of normalized response magnitudes of evoked LCBF. Note that normalized response magnitudes under hyperoxia at 5 and 10 Hz were greater than those under normoxia (*$p < 0.01$). Error bars indicate S.D. (5 Hz, $n = 13$; 10 Hz, $n = 9$).

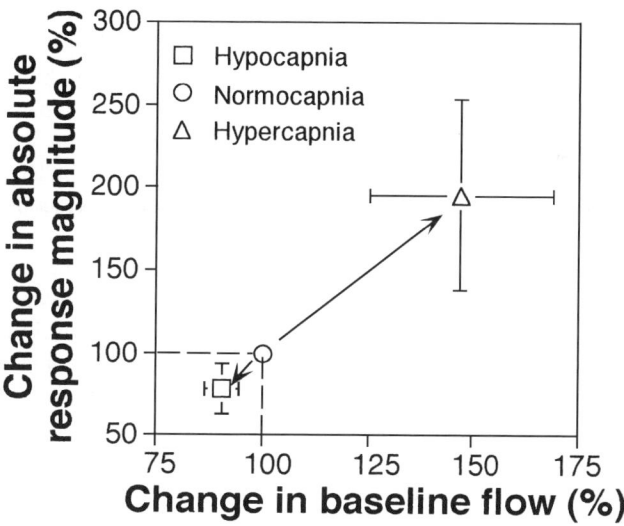

Fig. 3. Changes in baseline levels and response magnitudes of evoked LCBF; values of the parameters obtained under normocapnia were considered as 100%. Note that the response magnitude of evoked LCBF proportionally changed with baseline levels. Data were normalized with respect to those under normocapnia after statistical analysis. Error bars indicate ±S.D. (hypocapnia, $n = 10$; hypercapnia, $n = 10$).

(Fig. 3). The absolute response magnitudes of evoked LCBF to 5-Hz stimulation under hypocapnia and hypercapnia were, respectively, $21.8 \pm 14.9\%$ lower and $95.5 \pm 57.4\%$ higher than those under normocapnia ($p < 0.05$) (Fig. 3). However, after normalization with respect to each baseline level, there was no significant difference in the normalized response magnitude of evoked LCBF either between hypocapnia and normocapnia or between hypercapnia and normocapnia [11]. This indicates that the evoked LCBF is proportional to the baseline flow, which is consistent with previous reports [12,13].

4. Discussion

In this study, we have determined the relationship between the field potential and evoked LCBF in response to electrical stimulation of the rat hind paw. Changes in field potential and evoked LCBF were detected using an electrode inserted into the cortex and LDF, respectively. The pattern of change in the response magnitude of the evoked LCBF to various stimulus frequencies during the 5-s stimulation correlated with that in the integrated amplitude of field potentials during the stimulation period, but not with those in the number of spikes and mean amplitude of field potentials (Fig. 1). This indicates that the response magnitude of the evoked LCBF, which reflects the total amount of blood flow supplied during stimulation, reflects the integrated neuronal activity [9], and supports the concept of the coupling between the evoked LCBF and the neuronal activity. Previous studies on the neurovascular response assumed that the response of evoked LCBF to neuronal activity is linked by the integrated neuronal response to successive stimulations [7,14]. This was confirmed in our present study.

The brain has a high rate of aerobic metabolism. During cortical activation, the brain tissue exhibits an increased demand for oxygen supply and the supply of other substrates (e.g., glucose) as an energy source of neuronal spiking. The PO_2 level in the cerebral cortex has been reported to be 20% higher under hyperoxia (500 mm Hg) than under normoxia (100 mm Hg) [15]. The baseline level of LCBF under hypercapnia was approximately 47.0% higher than that under normocapnia (Fig. 3). If the evoked LCBF response was to increase the supply of oxygen and any substrates for oxidative metabolism, the response magnitude of evoked LCBF under hypercapnia or hyperoxia would be lower than that under the normal gas condition. Nevertheless, hyperoxia enhanced the response of evoked LCBF (Fig. 2), and the evoked LCBF proportionally changed with the baseline flow which is caused by the change in the $PaCO_2$ level (Fig. 3). It has been confirmed that the field potentials detected during stimulation under hyperoxia and hypercapnia were not significantly different from those under the normal gas condition [8,16], indicating that neuronal activity was not affected by hypercapnia and hyperoxia in our experiments. In the present study, we also indicated the linear correlation between evoked LCBF and neuronal activity. These suggest that the increase in LCBF is not directed toward supplying oxygen and some substrates for oxidative metabolism [8,10,11], and it could be modified by mechanisms operating on the blood vessels, which are proportional to neuronal activity.

The mechanisms of the enhancement of evoked LCBF under hyperoxia remain to be elucidated. Some vasodilator products, e.g., potassium, nitric oxide, hydrogen ion and adenosine, have been reported as mediators of evoked LCBF [17]. One possible mechanism underlying the enhancement of evoked LCBF is the interference of hyperoxia by these mediators of neuronal activation. A direct oxygen action, as a mediator of evoked LCBF regulation, is also a possible mechanism underlying the enhancement of evoked LCBF. We speculate that the combined action of mediators and oxygen may be involved in the enhancement of evoked LCBF under hyperoxia [8,10].

Acknowledgements

Part of this study was supported by Japan Science and Technology Corporation (JST).

References

[1] C.S. Roy, C.S. Sherrington, On the regulation of the blood supply of the brain, J. Physiol. 11 (1890) 85–108.

[2] P.T. Fox, M.E. Raichle, Focal physiological uncoupling of cerebral blood flow and oxidative metabolism during somatosensory stimulation in human subjects, Proc. Natl. Acad. Sci. U. S. A. 83 (1986) 1140–1144.

[3] E. Leniger-Follert, K.A. Hossmann, Simultaneous measurements of microflow and evoked potentials in the somatosensory cortex of the cat brain during specific sensory activation, Pflügers Arch. 380 (1979) 85–89.

[4] V. Ibáñez, M.P. Deiber, N. Sadato, C. Toro, J. Grissom, R.P. Woods, J.C. Mazziotta, M. Hallett, Effects of stimulus rate on regional cerebral blood flow after median nerve stimulation, Brain 118 (1995) 1339–1351.

[5] T. Matsuura, H. Fujita, C. Seki, K. Kashikura, K. Yamada, I. Kanno, CBF change evoked by somatosensory activation measured by laser-Doppler flowmetry: independent evaluation of RBC velocity and RBC concentration, Jpn. J. Physiol. 49 (1999) 289–296.

[6] T. Matsuura, H. Fujita, C. Seki, K. Kashikura, I. Kanno, Hemodynamics evoked by microelectrical direct stimulation in rat somatosensory cortex, Comp. Biochem. Physiol. A 124 (1999) 47–52.

[7] A.C. Ngai, M.A. Jolley, R. D'Ambrosio, J.R. Meno, H.R. Winn, Frequency-dependent changes in cerebral blood flow and evoked potentials during somatosensory stimulation in the rat, Brain Res. 837 (1999) 221–228.

[8] T. Matsuura, H. Fujita, K. Kashikura, I. Kanno, Modulation of evoked cerebral blood flow under excessive blood supply and hyperoxic conditions, Jpn. J. Physiol. 50 (2000) 115–123.

[9] T. Matsuura, I. Kanno, Quantitative and temporal relationship between local cerebral blood flow and neuronal activation induced by somatosensory stimulation in rats, Neurosci. Res. 40 (2001) 281–290.

[10] T. Matsuura, K. Kashikura, I. Kanno, Hemodynamics of local cerebral blood flow induced by somatosensory stimulation under normoxia and hyperoxia in rats, Comp. Biochem. Physiol. A 129 (2001) 363–372.

[11] T. Matsuura, H. Fujita, K. Kashikura, I. Kanno, Evoked local cerebral blood flow induced by somatosensory stimulation is proportional to the baseline flow, Neurosci. Res. 38 (2000) 341–348.

[12] I. Kanno, E. Shimosegawa, H. Fujita, J. Hatazawa, Uncoupling of absolute CBF to neuronal activity, Adv. Exp. Med. Biol. 413 (1997) 209–214.

[13] E. Shimosegawa, I. Kanno, J. Hatazawa, H. Fujita, H. Iida, S. Miura, M. Murakami, A. Inugami, T. Ogawa, H. Itoh, T. Okudera, K. Uemura, Photic stimulation study of changing the arterial partial pressure level of carbon dioxide, J. Cereb. Blood Flow Metab. 15 (1995) 111–114.

[14] P.T. Fox, M.E. Raichle, Stimulus rate dependence of regional cerebral blood flow in human striate cortex, demonstrated by positron emission tomography, J. Neurophysiol. 51 (1984) 1109–1120.

[15] T. Shinozuka, E.M. Nemoto, P.M. Winter, Mechanisms of cerebrovascular O_2 sensitivity from hyperoxia to moderate hypoxia in the rat, J. Cereb. Blood Flow Metab. 9 (1989) 187–195.

[16] R. Bakalova, T. Matsuura, I. Kanno, The frequency dependence of evoked local CBF induced by somatosensory stimulation in rat under normo- and hypercapnia, Jpn. J. Physiol. 51 (2001) 201–208.

[17] A. Villringer, U. Dirnagl, Coupling of brain activity and cerebral blood flow: basis of functional neuroimaging, Cerebrovasc. Brain Metab. Rev. 7 (1995) 240–276.

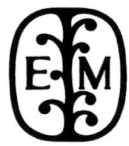

International Congress Series 1235 (2002) 115–122

Cortical blood flow through individual capillaries in rat vibrissa S1 cortex: stimulus-induced changes in flow are comparable to the underlying fluctuations in flow

David Kleinfeld*

*Department of Physics and Graduate Program in Neurosciences 0319, University of California,
9500 Gilman Drive, La Jolla, San Diego, CA 92093, USA*

Abstract

Cortical blood flow was probed via the motion of red blood cells (RBCs) in individual capillaries that lay as much as 600 μm below the pia matter of primary somatosensory cortex in rat. The flow was quite variable, with a speed of 0.8 ± 0.5 mm/s (mean $\pm$ S.D.) and a flux of 60 ± 40 RBC/s, averaged over all capillaries and over time. The fluctuations in the flow were dominated by a spectral band near 0.1 Hz. This band coincides with the spectral band of fluctuations previously seen across whole capillary beds with optical [Neuroimage 4 (1996) 183] and ƒMRI [Mag. Reson. Med. 37 (1997) 511] imaging techniques. Time-locked increases in the flow of red blood cells (RBCs) within individual capillaries were observed in response to stimulation of multiple vibrissae at natural levels of deflection. The magnitude of the stimulus-evoked change in speed was, at most, equal to 20% of the basal speed. This change is comparable to the level of the fluctuations in speed seen in single capillaries. Thus, changes in flow evoked by natural stimuli are largely masked by basal fluctuations. In toto, the results of our study suggest that fluctuations at the level of the microvasculature limit the sensitivity of brain imaging techniques, at least at low frequencies. © 2002 Elsevier Science B.V. All rights reserved.

Brain homeostasis depends on adequate levels of blood flow to insure the delivery of nutrients and to facilitate the removal of metabolites and heat. The exchange of material between constituents in the blood and neurons and glia occurs at the level of individual capillaries. Further, sensory stimulation, or even ideation, may lead to an increase in the

---

* Tel.: +1-858-822-0342; fax: +1-858-534-7697.
E-mail address: dk@physics.ucsd.edu (D. Kleinfeld).

0531-5131/02 © 2002 Elsevier Science B.V. All rights reserved.
PII: S 0 5 3 1 - 5 1 3 1 (0 2) 0 0 1 7 8 - 4

electrical activity within populations of neurons that subsequently results in a shift in blood flow between activated and quiescent regions [1]. These shifts are of sufficient duration and magnitude to form the basis of imaging techniques in which neuronal activity is inferred from changes in blood flow and blood oxygenation [2,3]. However, such changes are only observed with extensive averaging over time and/or trials.

What is the noise source that limits the sensitivity of brain imaging techniques? An elegant anatomical study performed by Morri et al. [4] provides graphic illustration that the capillary bed is tortuous, with a high degree of connectivity in the form of "T" junctions and closed loops that bridge between arterioles and venules (Fig. 1). Other studies provide evidence for local sphincters in the arterioles, which suggests that blood flow is controlled at the level of only a few capillaries [5]. In light of analogies between the geometry of the microvasculature and that of models for transport in weakly connected networks [6], one may conjecture that the basal flow through capillaries may support a multitude of stable flow patterns. Further, the flow may be highly variable if small changes in the microvasculature result in a shift among such patterns. The present physiological relevance of such variability is that it may set a baseline level for meaningful changes in blood flow that occur as a result of changes in brain electrical activity and/or metabolism.

Here, we address the issue of determining the magnitude of the basal fluctuations in red blood cell (RBC) flow in individual capillaries in comparison with the change in flow in response to natural stimuli. We used two-photon laser scanning microscopy as a means to study flow deep to the pia matter with diffraction limited optical resolution [7,8]. Flow was imaged at depths up to 600 μm [9], which corresponds to the level of layer 4. This layer is the primary locus of afferent input and, consistent with a large density of presynaptic terminals and their concomitant metabolic needs, contains the highest density of vasculature throughout the neocortex [10].

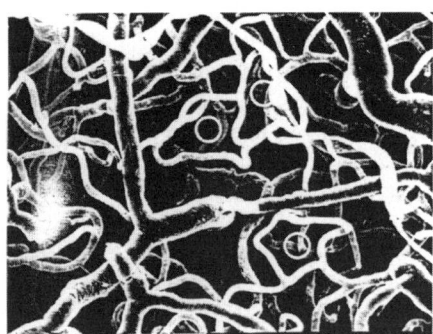
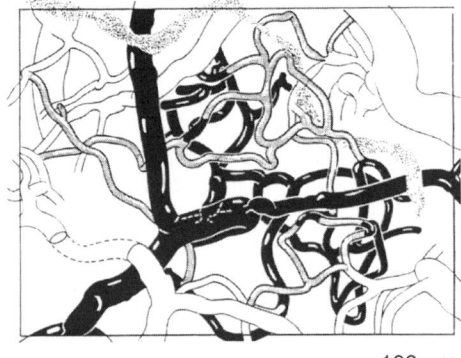

━━━ 100 μm

Fig. 1. Reconstruction of the capillary bed in rat cortex. The vasculature was filled with a casting material. After curing, the soft tissue was removed by corrosion in KOH and the casting was coated with gold and observed in the scanning electron microscope (SEM). The image on the left is the SEM data and the image on the right is the interpretation of the SEM image, with arterioles drawn in black, venules drawn in white, and capillaries shaded as gray. Note the closed loops and "T" junctions in the capillary bed. Data extracted from Fig. 9 in the work of Motti et al. [4].

Adult Sprague–Dawley rats that were anesthetized with urethane served as our preparation. We report on results for 8 animals and 42 capillaries. Contrast was supplied by labeling the blood serum was fluorescein isothiocynate-dextran (77 kDa) in physiological saline; the concentration of dye in the serum was estimated to be 300 μM. The RBCs appeared as dark objects on a fluorescent background [11]. Natural stimulation was performed by tapping a group of approximately 15 vibrissa that encompassed the straddlers and rostral vibrissae of rows B through E. Sinusoidal motion, typically 2° in amplitude, was delivered at 10 Hz for a period of 1 s, in concurrence with the rate at which rats palpate objects with their vibrissae [12]. The extent of cortical activation by the stimulus was inferred from an electrocorticogram (ECoG).

We readily imaged single microvessels and the surrounding vasculature at submicron resolution (Fig. 2a and b). Successive, rapidly acquired planar images of such microvessels revealed a train of dark objects that moved across a sea of fluorescently labeled serum (Fig. 2c). The dark spots are red blood cells. The change in position of the spots between successive images is proportional to the speed (arrows; Fig. 2c).

In general, we had insufficient temporal resolution to characterize the motion of RBCs from planar images of the entire vessel. Thus, we acquired repetitive line scans along the central axis of a capillary. The data comprise a matrix with one spatial (x) and one temporal (t) dimension. In this mode, the motion of RBCs leads to dark bands in the data set (Fig. 2d). The average time between bands at a fixed position, denoted Δt, is inversely proportional to the flux, the average distance between bands at a fixed time, denoted Δx, is inversely proportional to the linear density of RBCs, and the average slope of the band, $\Delta t/\Delta x$, is inversely proportional to the speed of the RBCs (Fig. 2c). These three quantities are related by flux = linear density × speed. The average flux of RBCs was determined by manually counting the number of bands in successive, 0.5-s intervals. The average speed of RBCs in either 0.05- or 0.1-s intervals was determined by an automatic procedure.

The passage of RBCs appeared to occur at irregular intervals (Fig. 3a–c). The spectral composition of this variability was not uniform; in essentially all cases the speed exhibited a spectral peak between 0.1 and 0.2 Hz (Fig. 3d). The time-averaged properties of the blood flow through each vessel were examined in terms of the values of the speed and flux averaged over a 20-s interval. We observed that the speed and flux vary over a range of values mainly between 0 and 1 mm/s, and 0 and 100 RBC/s, respectively, and that they linearly track each other at low values of flux (Fig. 3e). At high values of flux, the speed has a tendency to plateau (Fig. 3e).

We observed frequent instances of highly irregular flow in which the speed and flux changed suddenly (Fig. 3f) or in which individual RBCs stalled for extended periods of time (Fig. 3g). The most extensive irregularities occurred at the confluence of three vessels that formed a "T" junction. We simultaneously scanned the two collinear arms and often observed stalls in one arm, as well as sustained reversals in the direction of flow in one or both arms (Fig. 3h).

To examine the effect of stimulation on the flux and linear density of the RBCs, as well as explore the issue of single-trial variability, we consider the analysis of records that were free of stalls or other large irregularities over an entire 128 s period of acquisition. For the example of Fig. 4a, we observed considerable trial-to-trial variability in the value of the stimulus-induced change in the speed of RBCs (top line; Fig. 4a), as well as in the change in flux (second line). An examination of the averaged quantities for this trial reveals that the flux as well as the speed transiently increase upon stimulation (Fig. 4b). Nonetheless, the spectral composition of the speed indicates that the magnitude of the peak at the repetition rate of the stimulus (0.05 Hz; ♦ in Fig. 4c) is similar to the magnitude for peak

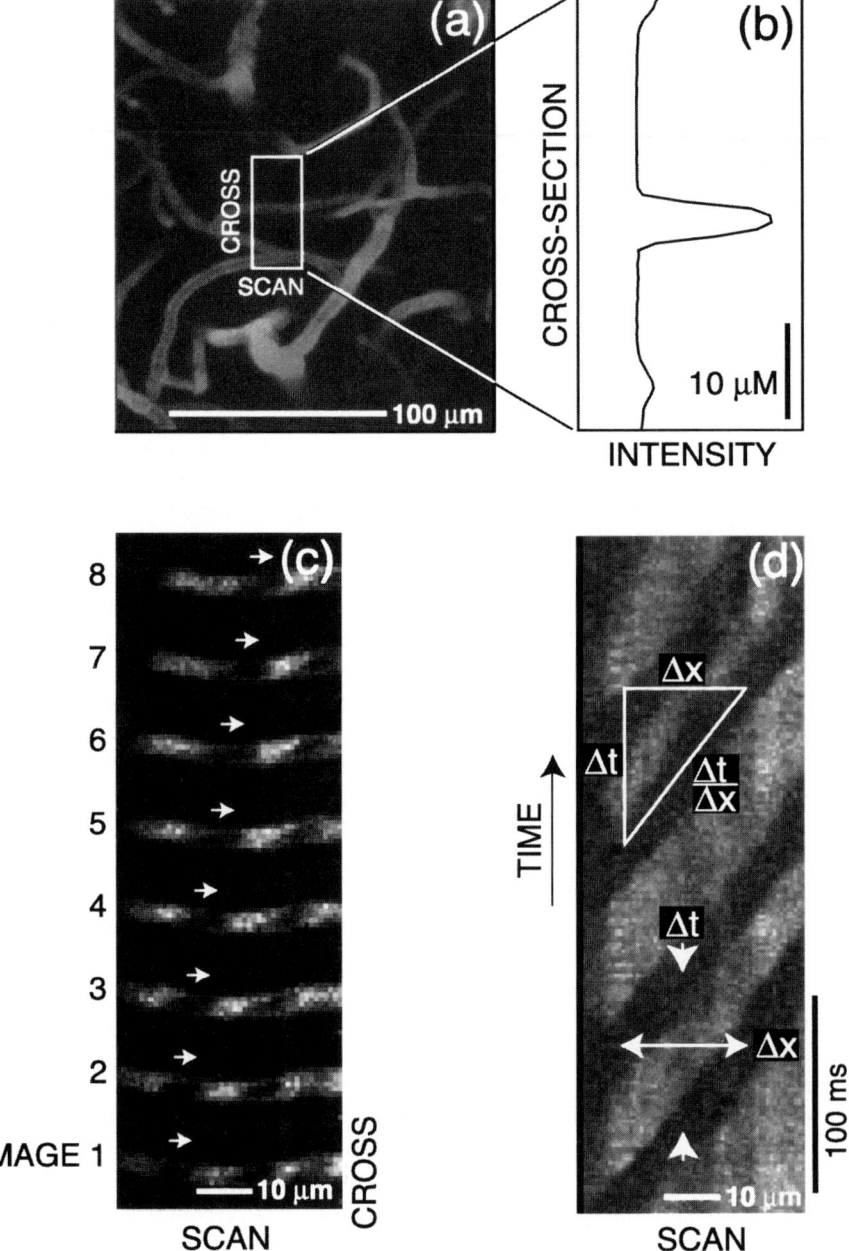

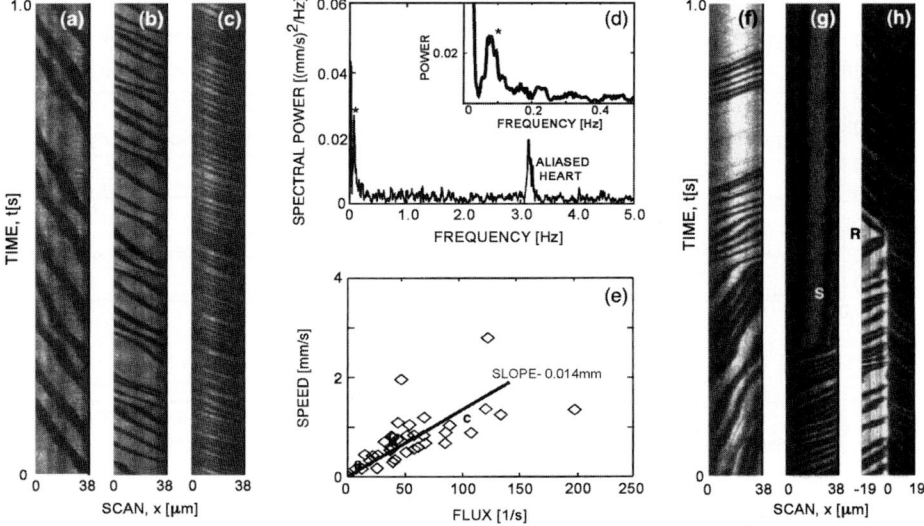

Fig. 3. Characterization of the basal motion of RBCs in capillaries. The vessels were scanned at 2 ms/line, except for one vessel with very fast flow that was scanned at 1 ms/line. (a–c) Selected 1-s segments of the line-scan data for flow in three different vessels. Note the increase in speed and flux in the progression (a) → (b) → (c). (d) Representative plot of the spectral power in a 128-s record of speed versus time; we used multi-taper estimation techniques [22] with a half-bandwidth of 0.02 Hz. Note the peak near 0.1 Hz (*); the peak at 3.2 Hz is the aliased heart rate of 6.8 Hz. (e) Plot of the speed versus flux for flow in 38 vessels. The solid line is a best fit to points in the data set. (h) A 1-s segment of the line-scan data through a straight section of capillary in which the speed changes from relatively slow (large slope) to fast (small slope). (i) A 1-s segment of data at the onset of a transient stall in flow (S). Note that the RBCs remain stuck in the vessel. (j) A 1-s segment of data that shows the flow in two collinear arms of a junction. Note the reversal in the direction of flow in the arm on the left (R).

that corresponds to low frequency oscillations (0.1 Hz; * in Fig. 4c). The latter peak is present independent of stimulation (Fig. 4c).

A final point concerns the possibility that the capillary flow was largely unresponsive to stimulation in our preparations. As a control experiment, we measured the change in flow of RBCs in response to mild electrical shock to the tail. We collected data from both vibrissa S1 cortex as well as more medial parts of S1 cortex, which respond to stimulation of the trunk and lower limbs. In all cases, we observed changes in flow that were 50–

Fig. 2. Characterization of individual capillaries and flow in the capillaries. (a) Tangential projection in the vicinity of a single capillary that is reconstructed from a set of 100 planar scans acquired every 1 μm between 310 and 410 μm. (b) The intensity profile along the cross-section for the scan that passed through the central axis of the capillary in question ($z = 360$ μm). The caliber is defined by the number of pixels whose intensity is above the background level, as noted. (c) Successive planar images through a small vessel, acquired every 60 ms. The change in position of a particular unstained object, interpreted as a RBC, is indicated by the series of arrows (→); the velocity of the RBC is +0.18 mm/s. Depth = 450 μm. (d) Succession of line-scans (2 ms/line) through the axis of a capillary, shown solely to illustrate the characterization of RBC flow.

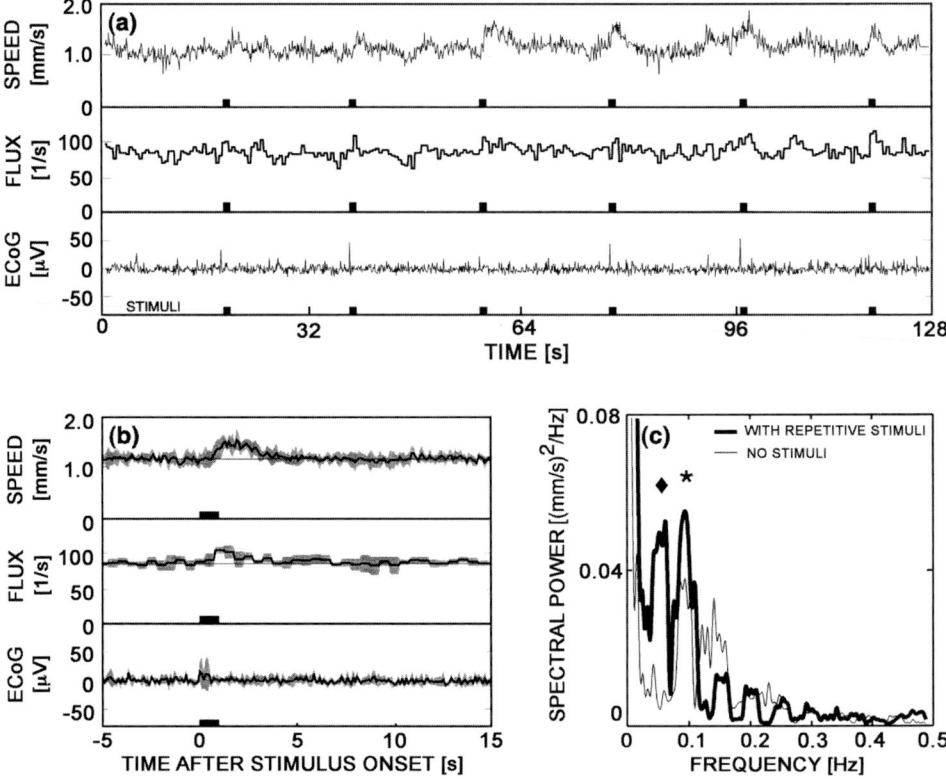

Fig. 4. The nature of the single-trial response of red blood cell flow to vibrissa stimulation in a capillary in vibrissa primary S1 cortex. (a) A complete 128-s time-series with six separate stimuli, spaced 20 s apart. Shown are the speed, the flux, and the ECoG recorded from a site 2 mm lateral to the optical measurement. Depth = 255 μm. (b) Trial-average of the quantities shown in part (a). The dark line is the average over all 6 trials, the gray band is the standard deviation of the trial average, and the thin straight line is drawn through the prestimulus portion of the data. (c) Spectral power for the speed shown in part (a) (thick line) along with the power for a record taken immediately after that in part (a) but in the absence of simulation (thin line). The '♦' corresponds to variation in the speed at the 0.05 Hz repetition frequency of the stimulation and the '*' corresponds to a peak at 0.1 Hz associated with vasomotor oscillations. The half-bandwidth of the spectral estimation was 0.016 Hz.

100% of the basal level, as typified by the data of Fig. 5 and consistent with past work using electrical stimulation [13]. This implies that the level of response we observe with natural vibrissa stimulation is not an artifact of compromised physiology.

To summarize, we observe low frequency fluctuations in the speed of RBC flow. The frequency of these oscillations are similar to those reported for the speed of RBCs imaged in capillaries close to at the cortical surface by wide-field techniques [14] and inferred from laser-Doppler measurements [15]. Further, oscillations with a similar spectral character are observed with intrinsic optical imaging of cortical function in rat [16] and result in changes in blood flow that are coherent over distances of 1 mm or more across cortex [17]. These oscillations are generally termed "vasomotion" and, consistent with their extended correlations, are believed to result from oscillations in the arterial supply

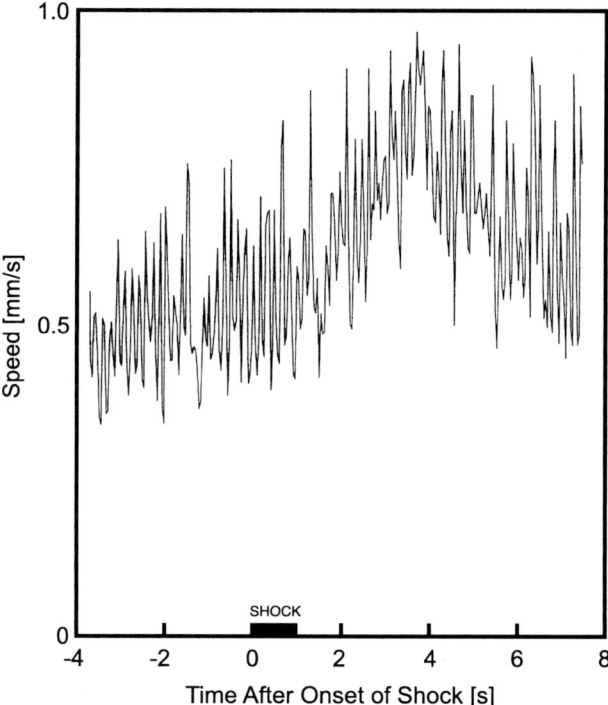

Fig. 5. The single-trial time series of the speed of red blood cell flow during an epoch that includes mild electrical shock to the tail (1-s train of 3-ms pulses delivered at 20 Hz). The oscillations in the speed corresponds to 6.5-Hz modulation from cardiac pulsations. Note that the increase in flow in response to simulation peaks at 65% above the basal level, as opposed to the much smaller change seen in response to natural vibrissa stimulation (Fig. 4a).

[18,19]. From the perspective of functional imaging of nervous activity, these oscillations appear as a physiological noise source that are likely to limit the sensitivity of optical or magnetic resonance imaging techniques [16,20] in which the contrast mechanism is related to changes in blood flow [21].

Acknowledgements

I thank my past and present collaborators, Winfried Denk, Fritjof Helmchen, Partha P. Mitra, Nozomi Nishimuri, and Philbert S. Tsai, for their efforts. This work was sponsored by the NINDS.

References

[1] T.A. Woolsey, C.M. Rovainen, S.B. Cox, M.H. Henger, G.E. Liange, D. Liu, Y.E. Moskalenko, J. Sui, L. Wei, Neuronal units linked to microvascular modules in cerebral cortex: response elements for imaging the brain, Cereb. Cortex 6 (1996) 647–660.

[2] M.E. Raichle, Circulatory and metabolic correlates of brain function in normal humans, in: V.B. Mountcastle, F. Plum, S.R. Geiger (Eds.), Handbook of Physiology. Section I. The Nervous System, American Physiological Society, Bethesda, 1987, pp. 643–674.

[3] S. Ogawa, R.S. Menon, S.-G. Kim, K. Ugurbil, On the characteristics of functional magnetic resonance imaging of the brain, Annu. Rev. Biophys. Biomol. Struct. 27 (1998) 447–474.

[4] E.D.F. Motti, H.-G. Imhof, M.G. Yasargil, The terminal vasculature bed in the superficial cortex of the rat: an SEM study of corrosion casts, J. Neurosurg. 65 (1986) 834–846.

[5] K. Nakai, H. Imai, I. Kamei, T. Itakura, N. Komari, H. Kimura, T. Nagai, T. Maeda, Microangioarchitecture of rat parietal cortex with special reference to vascular "sphincters": scanning electron microscopic and dark field microscopic study, Stroke 12 (1981) 653–659.

[6] B.D. Hughes, Random Walks and Random Environments, Random Environments, vol. 2, Oxford Press, New York, 1996.

[7] D. Kleinfeld, P.P. Mitra, F. Helmchen, W. Denk, Fluctuations and stimulus-induced changes in blood flow observed in individual capillaries in layers 2 through 4 of rat neocortex, Proc. Natl. Acad. Sci. U. S. A. 95 (1998) 15741–15746.

[8] P.S. Tsai, N. Nishimura, E.J. Yoder, E.M. Dolnick, G.A. White, D. Kleinfeld, Principles, design, and construction of a two photon laser scanning microscope for in vitro and in vivo brain imaging, in: R.D. Frostig (Ed.), Vivo Optical Imaging of Brain Function, CRC Press, 2001.

[9] D. Kleinfeld, W. Denk, Two-photon imaging of neocortical microcirculation, in: R. Yuste, F. Lanni, A. Konnerth (Eds.), Imaging Neurons: A Laboratory Manual, Cold Spring Harbor Laboratory Press, Cold Spring Harbor, 2000, pp. 23.1–23.15.

[10] U. Patel, Non-random distribution of blood vessels in the posterior region of the rat somatosensory cortex, Brain Res. 289 (1983) 65–70.

[11] U. Dirnagl, A. Villringer, K.M. Einhaupl, In-vivo confocal scanning laser microscopy of the cerebral microcirculation, J. Microsc. 165 (1992) 147–157.

[12] G.E. Carvell, D.J. Simons, Biometric analyses of vibrissal tactile discrimination in the rat, J. Neurosci. 10 (1990) 2638–2648.

[13] A.C. Ngai, J.R. Meno, H.R. Winn, Simultaneous measurements of pial arteriolar diameter and laser-Doppler flow during somatosensory stimulation, J. Cereb. Blood Flow Metab. 15 (1995) 124–127.

[14] B.B. Biswal, A.G. Hudetz, Synchronous oscillations in cerebrocortical capillary red blood flow after nitric oxide synthase inhibition, Microvasc. Res. 52 (1996) 1–12.

[15] E.V. Golanov, S. Yamamoto, D.J. Reis, Spontaneous waves of cerebral blood flow associated with a pattern of electrocortical activity, Am. J. Physiol. 266 (1994) R204–R214.

[16] J.E.W. Mayhew, S. Askew, Y. Zeng, J. Porrill, G.W.M. Westby, P. Redgrave, D.M. Rector, R.M. Harper, Cerebral vasomotion: 0.1 Hz oscillation in reflectance imaging of neural activity, Neuroimage 4 (1996) 183–193.

[17] P.P. Mitra, B. Pesaran, S. Ogawa, D. Kleinfeld, K. Ugerbil, Characterization and removal of respiratory, cardiac and vasomotor oscillations in dynamic brain images, Society for Neuroscience Annual Meeting, San Diego, CA, 1995.

[18] M. Tomita, F. Gotoh, T. Sato, N. Tanahashi, K. Tanaka, 4–6 cycle per minute fluctuation in cerebral blood volume of feline cortical tissue in situ, J. Cereb. Blood Flow Metab. 1 (1981) S443–S444 (abstract).

[19] A. Colantuoni, S. Bertuglia, M. Intaglietta, Microvascular vasomotion: origin of laser Doppler flux motion, Int. J. Microcirc. 14 (1994) 151–158.

[20] P.P. Mitra, S. Ogawa, X. Hu, K. Ugurbil, The nature of spatiotemporal changes in cerebral hemodynamics as manifested in functional magnetic resonance imaging, Magn. Reson. Med. 37 (1997) 511–518.

[21] D. Malonek, U. Dirnagl, U. Lindauer, K. Yamada, I. Kanno, A. Grinvald, Vascular imprints of neuronal activity: relationships between the dynamics of cortical blood flow, oxygenation, and volume changes following sensory stimulation, Proc. Nat. Acad. Sci. U. S. A. 94 (1997) 14826–14831.

[22] D.J. Thomson, Spectral estimation and harmonic analysis, Proc. IEEE 70 (1982) 1055–1096.

Oxygen delivery and microcirculation

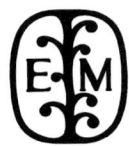

International Congress Series 1235 (2002) 123–135

Model of oxygen delivery to brain tissue in vivo explains beneficial effect of hypothermia in ischemia

Albert Gjedde*, Sean Marrett, Masaharu Sakoh, Manouchehr Vafaee

Pathophysiology and Experimental Tomography Center, Aarhus University Hospital, Aarhus University, Norrebrogade 44, Aarhus, Denmark

Knowledge of the relationship between neuronal activity and energy metabolism in brain tissue is essential to the understanding of how the brain functions. The relationship is complex and likely to involve several interrelated factors [1]. These include the cell types involved in brain activity, the mechanisms that link cellular activity to energy production and consumption, and the mechanisms that relate nutrient supply to energy production in the brain.

Two theories have been proposed to account for the distribution of energy production and use among the different cell types in the brain. The sodium conductance theory proposes that changes of electrochemical gradients across the postsynaptic membranes of neurons impose the bulk of the energy demand of the working brain [2,3]. The glutamate–glutamine neurotransmitter cycling theory forms the alternative hypothesis [4]. According to this second theory, energy is consumed by both astrocytes and neurons in proportion to the release of excitatory neurotransmitters, and there is compartmentalization of the glycolytic and oxidative components of glucose metabolism between these two cell types. In astrocytes, metabolism of glucose produces two molecules of lactate for each molecule of glutamate imported from the extracellular space, and the energy gained by this metabolism is stored in two molecules of ATP. The lactate is transferred to neurons where it is converted to pyruvate. The energy released by the oxidative metabolism of pyruvate in neuronal mitochondria is stored in as many as 36 molecules of ATP [5]. Thus, according to this latter theory, the total glucose consumption in the brain (total CMR_{glc}) is the sum of a glycolytic (astrocytic) component, which generates only two molecules of ATP per glucose molecule, and an oxidative (neuronal) component, which generates 36 molecules of ATP per glucose molecule.

The studies outlined here used PET to investigate the break up of energy use between astrocytes and neurons [6–8], and the changes of energy use in ischemia accompanied by hypothermia. By comparing experimental data with modelling studies, it is suggested that the lactate generation in neurons and astrocytes at different stages of activation are

---

* Corresponding author.

0531-5131/02 © 2002 Elsevier Science B.V. All rights reserved.
PII: S0531-5131(02)00179-6

influenced by the different subtypes of lactate dehydrogenase (LDH) that are present in these two cell types. In neurons, the lactate generation from pyruvate is catalysed by another subtype of the enzyme than the one used by pyruvate in astrocytes. The comparison indicates that pyruvate and lactate of neuronal origin are the primary substrates for oxidative phosphorylation in neurons [9]. Although the identification of the neuronal source of neuronal pyruvate may not definitively establish the validity of one theory over the other, the evidence presented here as well as the absence of evidence either of net transfer of lactate from astrocytes to neurons, or of privileged access of glucose to astrocytes, raise the need for a synthesis of the key elements of both theories into a single concept with important consequences for the interpretation of functional brain images.

1. Brain energetics

The claim that cerebral blood flow (CBF) is closely regulated to meet the local metabolic requirements of oxygen as well as glucose has been inferred from early studies [10]. Under normal physiological conditions, it is known that the majority of energy required for the ATP generation by mitochondria in the adult mammalian brain is supplied almost exclusively via complete oxidative metabolism of glucose in the TCA cycle [11]. Thus, the steady-state glucose and oxygen requirements of different areas of the brain change constantly depending on their activity. As the complete oxidation of glucose is described by the equation $C_6H_{12}O_6+6O_2=6CO_2+6H_2O$, the oxygen–glucose ratio index (OGI), or molar ratio, calculated from the theoretical values of the total oxygen and glucose requirements in situations in which glucose metabolism is fully oxidative, is 6. However, on theoretical grounds, judging from the pyruvate and lactate exchange, as well as from the presence of lactate transporters in the brain endothelium, a 5–10% lower OGI of close to 5.5 is predicted and confirmed in most studies in vivo. This lower ratio indicates that there is a small glycolytic contribution to energy production, under steady-state circumstances, which lowers the gain of ATP to 34–36 mol per mol of glucose consumed. As evidenced by a transient increase in lactate concentration within the brain when activity increases [11,12], the OGI may drop further when the brain metabolism changes. The mechanism responsible for this decline is poorly understood.

Although not all studies report an OGI value of 5.5 in the living brain (for reviews, see Refs. [1,5], the time courses of glycolytic and oxidative changes could be different and the OGI value in non-steady states would then depend on the time at which the measurements were made [7]. Another consideration is that the transport mechanisms for oxygen and glucose across the blood–brain barrier are different [13]. Thus, while cerebral perfusion and oxygen diffusivity play integral roles in oxygen delivery [8,14–16], glucose delivery is less dependent on the blood supply than oxygen is.

Allowing for these factors, we combined data from previously published studies in conscious humans and showed that the responses of brain metabolism to somatosensory and simple visual stimulation, on one hand, and complex visual stimulation and motor activity, on the other, appear to fall into two distinct categories [13]. One category includes simple ('primary') somatosensory stimuli with little information content and the other complex ('secondary') somatosensory stimuli and motor activity (Fig. 1), based on a qualitative

Stimulus	Duration [min]	ΔCBF	Supply ΔJ_{glc} [%]	ΔJ_{O_2}	Products ΔJ_{ATP} [μmol g^{-1} min^{-1}]	ΔJ_{lact}
Primary						
Somatosensory	1[a]	28	[17]	9*	0.96*	0.05
	1[b]	31	[18]	13*	1.35*	0.03
	1[c]	18	[8]	0	0.04	0.04
	20[d]	18	8	[0]	0.04	0.04
	20[e]	18	[8]	0	0.04	0.04
	45[e]	27	17	[0]	0.10	0.10
Visual (Photic)	30[f]	43	27	0	0.15	0.15
	45[g]	49	51	5*	0.76*	0.26
Mean		29	19	3.4	0.43	0.089
Secondary and Motor						
Visual (Checkerboard)	5[h]	25	[28]	28	3.17	0
	10[h]	26	[29]	29	3.29	0
	4[i] (1Hz)	32	[32]	10	1.27	0.133
	4[i] (4Hz)	38	[38]	16	1.96	0.133
	4[i] (8Hz)	42	[42]	6	0.90	0.217
Thalamic Stimulation	8[j]	88	[88]	47	5.60	0.247
Internal Visualization	1[k]	31	[37]	37	4.18	0
Tactile Learning	1[l]	23	[23]	-	-	-
Hand Grip	8[m]	30	[40]	40	4.50	0
Sequential Finger Touching	4.5[n] (1.5Hz, M1)	22	[22]	8	1.00	0.084
Mean		36	38	25	2.89	0.090

From [a] Fox & Raichle (1986), [b] Seitz & Roland (1992), [c] Fujita et al. (1993a), [d] Kuwabara et al. (1992), [e] Ginsberg et al. (1988), [f] Ribeiro et al. (1993), [g] Fox et al. (1988), [h] Marrett & Gjedde (1997); [i] Vafaee & Gjedde (2000); [j] Katayama (1986); [k] Roland et al. (1987); [l] Roland et al. (1989); [m] Raichle (1976); [n] Iida et al. (1993); values in brackets are estimates; *J_{O_2} increase not significant.

Fig. 1. Table of studies carried out in humans comparing changes of the CBF (ΔCBF) and CMRO$_2$ (ΔJ_{O2}), as summarized by Ref. [13]. In addition, table lists changes of glucose consumption (ΔJ_{glc}), and ATP (ΔJ_{ATP}) and lactate (ΔJ_{lact}) turnover. In humans, the relative increases in CMRO$_2$ following simple somatosensory stimuli are less than that following complex somatosensory or motor stimulation [13]. Also see Seitz and Roland [18], Fujita et al. [19], Kuwabara et al. [20], Ginsberg et al. [21], Ribeiro et al. [22], Fox et al. [17], Marrett and Gjedde [23], Vafaee and Gjedde [8], Katayama et al. [24], Roland et al. [25], Raichle et al. [26], Iida et al. [27].

evaluation of the information content of the stimuli. Complex visual stimuli (e.g., looking at a rapidly reversing blue–yellow radial checkerboard for 4 min) increases both blood flow and O$_2$ consumption, leading to an OGI of approximately 5 [9]. Stimulation with a photic flash (e.g., from white-light-emitting goggles) produces a smaller increase in O$_2$ consumption and gives rise to an OGI of approximately 0.5 [17].

We suggest that the marked differences in the OGI values is an indirect measure of differences in the transient generation of lactate during stimulation [13], related to the degree of information processing which these stimuli give rise to. This suggestion leads to the hypothesis that simple stimulation is unaccompanied by a significant increase in oxidative metabolism because of the limited postsynaptic depolarization, despite substantial presynaptic impulse activity. An important prediction arising from this hypothesis is the claim that the glycolytic and oxidative responses are additive, the glycolytic response reflecting the work of astrocytes importing glutamate, and the oxidative response reflecting the degree of

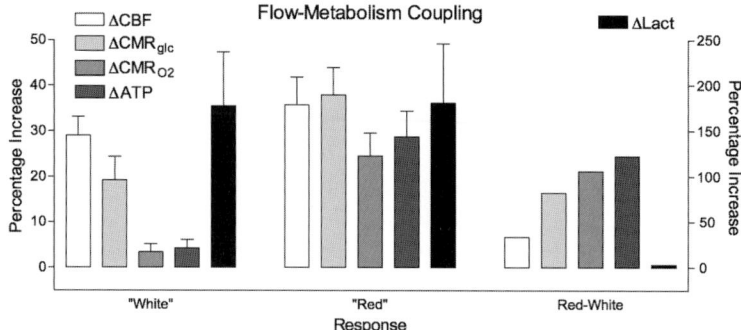

Fig. 2. Comparison of "red" and "white" metabolic reactivity in the two groups of data shown in Fig. 1, and subtraction of the "white" from the "red", yielding a third, "red-white" group. Data are mean±S.E.M., pooled from several PET studies as listed in Fig. 1 (from Ref. [28]).

postsynaptic neuronal depolarization and the consequent activation of neuronal mitochondria concentrated in the dendrites.

In analogy to the reactivity of muscle tissue, the two responses may be called "white" for the simple response in which the oxidative component and ATP gain are low and much lactate is being generated, for example by astrocytes, and "red" for the complex response in which there is the same amount of lactate being generated, but also much ATP (Fig. 2). If the two responses were additive and independent, the oxidative response would not be expected to reduce the amount of lactate produced in the tissue. The absence of a diminished lactate accumulation would, in turn, be evidence against any neuronal metabolism of lactate generated in the astrocytes. Subtracting the 'complex' or 'red' response from the 'simple or white' activation can test this prediction of the additive responses. The subtraction shown in Fig. 2 reveals a state in which oxygen consumption and ATP generation rise; however, there is no further change in blood flow or lactate concentration. The subtraction confirms that the lactate accumulation is not attenuated by more oxidative metabolism.

2. Cellular compartmentalization

Astrocytic processes possess glutamate transporters that remove glutamate released into the synaptic cleft from presynaptic nerve terminals [5]. Within astrocytes, glutamine synthetase converts glutamate to glutamine, which, in turn, is released from astrocytes, taken up by neurons and converted back to glutamate by glutaminase, a neuronal enzyme. Thus, the localization of key transporters and enzymes leads to compartmentalization of glutamate and glutamine between neurons and astrocytes.

In contrast, we suggest that the locations of the transporters and enzymes of the glycolytic and oxidative pathways indicate that there is little potential for further segregation of the metabolic processes between neurons and astrocytes. Glucose transporters on astrocyte and neuronal membranes allow glucose in the bloodstream to diffuse across the blood–brain barrier and cell membranes into all cells (Fig. 3), and permit equilibration of glucose concentrations in the extra- and intracellular spaces. Hexokinase, a cytosolic enzyme, converts each molecule of glucose into two molecules of pyruvate, a monocarboxylic acid (two molecules of ATP are also generated by this reaction). Theoretically, pyruvate has several potential fates, which may differ in neurons and astrocytes: First, it enters mitochondria via the mitochondrial monocarboxylic transporter (mMCT) where it forms a substrate for pyruvate dehydrogenase. Second, pyruvate within the cytoplasm also converts to lactate in a reversible reaction that is catalysed by LDH. Third, pyruvate is a substrate for transport out of the cells and out of the brain by the monocarboxylate transporters. The abundance of monocarboxylic acid transporters that transport both lactate and pyruvate, and the near-equilibrium between pyruvate and lactate pools, ensure rapid and reversible exchange between intra- and extracellular pools of pyruvate and lactate. For this reason, it is unlikely that major concentration differences can exist among different pools of pyruvate, or among different pools of lactate. Thermodynamically, it is probable that all pyruvate and lactate in the brain tissue outside of the mitochondria form a single substrate pool.

Although it has been hypothesized that lactate is synthesized preferentially in glial and equally preferentially oxidized in the neurons [4], it is unclear how this selectivity might be achieved with a single pool of pyruvate and lactate as described above (Fig. 3). Recently,

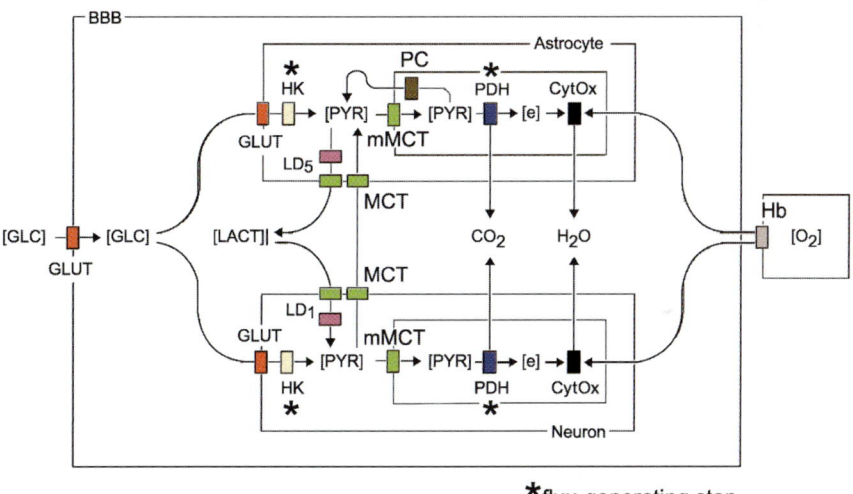

*flux-generating step

Fig. 3. A model relating to the metabolism of lactate and pyruvate in the astrocytes and neurons, with glucose metabolism. Glucose (GLC) and O_2 are the main energy-forming substrates in the brain. Glucose is actively transported across the blood–brain barrier and enters astrocytes and neurons by specific glucose transporters (GLUT). Oxygen passively diffuses throughout the brain. The breakdown of glucose to pyruvate (PYR) involves a flux-generating step (*) mediated by hexokinase (HK). In addition, pyruvate carboxylase (PC) activity in the cytosol of astrocytes indicates that some TCA cycle intermediates could also form pyruvate in this cell type. A near-equilibrium concentration ratio between pyruvate and lactate is established by lactate dehydrogenase. LD_5, the astrocyte-specific subtype of this enzyme, catalyses a low ratio between pyruvate and lactate, whereas LD_1, the neuron-specific subtype, catalyses a high ratio. This forms the basis of the use of the ratio between pyruvate and lactate to determine whether neurons or astrocytes are the origin of pyruvate in a given functional state.

however, different subtypes of LDH have been identified, each with a distinct localization and activity: LD_1, the oxidative subtype with a low ratio of lactate to pyruvate in vitro, is present in neurons; and LD_5, the glycolytic subtype with a high ratio of lactate to pyruvate in vitro, is located in glial cells [29,30]. As it is difficult to understand how these differences translate into compartmentalization in vivo, we suggest that different lactate-to-pyruvate ratios mediated by these LDH subtypes predominate in different situations and at different times, rather than at different places in the tissue. In turn, these temporal variations establish different changes in the concentrations of pyruvate and lactate generated in the neurons and astrocytes, under different conditions of activation.

We have taken advantage of this prediction of temporally selective distribution of LDH activity to test the hypothesis that during stimulation, the speed with which lactate is generated depends on the enzyme responsible for the generation, either LD_1, the oxidative subtype in neurons, or LD_5, the glycolytic subtype found only in astrocytes.

Thus, a higher lactate-to-pyruvate ratio, which occurs for the approach of the LD_5-catalysed reaction towards a new near equilibrium, must commensurately delay the onset of the increase in cerebral metabolic rate of oxygen consumption ($CMRO_2$), if this increase depends on the transfer of lactate from astrocytes to neurons. In addition, this transfer determines the relative contribution of the two cell types to the total pyruvate concentration. The hypothesis predicts that the time course of the lactate generation is an important index of the relative amount of pyruvate contributed by each type of cell.

Using this hypothesis as the basis for a model, we derived differential equations for the changes in pyruvate and lactate concentrations, for the consequent change in $CMRO_2$ with time, as well as for the resulting OGI,

$$\Delta M_{pyr}(t) = 2.0\Delta CMR_{glc}(t)[1 - \exp(-kt)]/(1+\lambda)k \text{ and } \Delta CMRO_2(t) = 3.0\Delta M_{pyr}(t)$$

where ΔCMR_{glc}=the change in CMR_{glc}, $\Delta CMRO_2$=the change in $CMRO_2$, t=time, λ=[lactate]/[pyruvate], k_{pyr}=rate of pyruvate clearance from the cytosol, k_{lact}=rate of lactate clearance from the cytosol, $k = (k_{pyr}+\lambda k_{lact})/(1+\lambda)$, and ΔM_{pyr} the changing pyruvate concentration. The oxygen–glucose index (OGI) is the steady-state plateau approached by the term,

$$\Delta CMRO_2(t)/\Delta CMR_{glc}(t) = 6(1 - \exp(-kt))/(1 + r\lambda)$$

where $r=k_{lact}/k_{pyr}$. By using the known values of the affinity of LDH subtypes for lactate and pyruvate in these equations, we have simulated the rate of change of pyruvate concentration $[\Delta M_{pyr}(t)]$ and the rate of change of $CMRO_2$ $[\Delta CMRO_2(t)]$ that would be expected if pyruvate were generated either in the neurons or from lactate generated in the astrocytes (Fig. 4, left panel). In one kinetic profile we used λ=16.7, which corresponds to the value for the oxidative LH_1 subtype in the neurons; in the other λ=200 [9], which corresponds to the value for the glycolytic LD_5 subtype in the astrocytes. In the unstimulated state CMR_{glc} is 0.26 µmol g^{-1} min^{-1} and $CMRO_2$ is 1.40 µmol g^{-1} min^{-1}, which correspond to a basal OGI of 5.4. Assuming that $\Delta CMR_{glc}(t)$ requires ~ 15 min to reach steady-state levels, the simulated values of $\Delta M_{pyr}(t)$ and $\Delta CMRO_2(t)$ result in an OGI value of 5.3 for the LD_1 subtype and 2.5 for the LD_5. In each case, $\Delta CMRO_2(t)$ is quantitatively reflected by $\Delta M_{pyr}(t)$, where a greater change in $CMRO_2$ is proportional to a larger

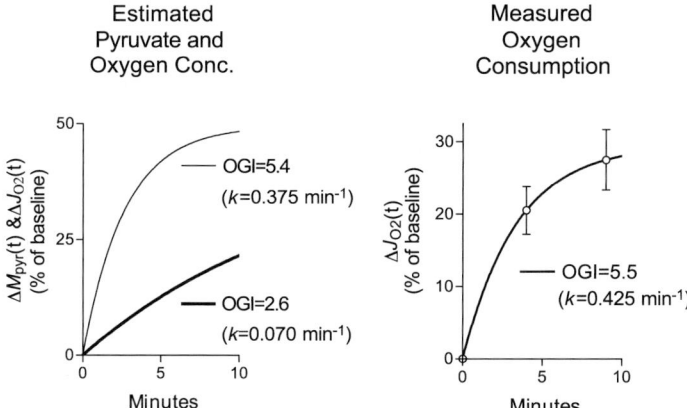

Fig. 4. Consumption of pyruvate and O_2 increases with increasing duration of stimulation. (a) Simulation of the rate of change in M_{pyr} [$\Delta M_{pyr}(t)$] and $CMRO_2$ [$\Delta CMRO_2(t)$, shown as $J_{O2}(t)$] as a function of increased stimulus duration. Data was calculated using the equations in the text, with λ([lactate]/[pyruvate]) of 16.7 for LD_1 and 200 for LD_5. All simulations were obtained using $r=0.0067$, which corresponds to a k_{lact} of 0.04 min^{-1} and k_{pyr} of 6 min^{-1}, respectively. (b) Values of $\Delta CMRO_2(t)$ measured by PET during visual stimulation are plotted. The best fit of the model to the data gives λ of 14.5 (adapted from Ref. [9]).

pyruvate pool. At rest, i.e., when no external stimuli are applied, values of CMR_{glc} and $CMRO_2$ measured experimentally correspond to an OGI of 5.4.

Thus, calculations on the basis of biochemical data from the neuronal LD_1 isoform, results in an OGI value that is similar to that observed experimentally at rest. This finding is consistent with the claim that the pyruvate used by the neurons at rest is generated in the neurons without first being converted from lactate generated in the astrocytes by the LD_5 enzyme.

3. Oxidative vs. nonoxidative metabolism

We used the model to investigate the metabolic consequences of visual stimulation in humans, using PET to measure the rate of change in $CMRO_2$ during stimulation. The stimulus consisted of exposure to a semiannular checkerboard in the area to the left of the midline, while the right eye was occluded. The baseline condition was fixation on a cross-hair. Experimental recordings were made for 3 min, starting at 3 or 8 min after the stimulus was presented. The average increase in $CMRO_2$ measured during the 3-min stimulation was 20.5% and during the 8-min stimulation 27.5%. We investigated whether the increased energy production that accompanies neuronal activation comes from oxidative (neuronal) or glycolytic (astrocytic) metabolism by comparing the values measured experimentally with the theoretical predictions for each LDH isoform [8,9]. Furthermore, varying the length of stimulation also allowed us to examine whether there is a shift in the metabolic preferences as the duration of stimulation increases.

The average increase in $CMRO_2$ evoked by visual stimulation was used to produce a best fit of the model presented above (Fig. 4, right panel). The experimental data is similar to the

OGI observed at rest, and consistent with an OGI of 5.5. These results indicate that neuronal work (i.e., an LD_1 subtype reaction) was elevated during sustained stimulation, and with prolonged stimulation there was an ever-increasing oxidative contribution to the work. The data suggests that the neuronal metabolism is fully oxidative, albeit waiting for a rise of pyruvate to sustain the increased demand for oxygen. The data also shows that during stimulation, lactate is not generated by a switch of substrate from LD_1 in the neurons to LD_5 in the astrocytes, but rather by increased exposure of LD_1 to pyruvate generated in the neurons.

4. Inverse flow-metabolism coupling

Fig. 2 raises the possibility that three fundamentally different levels of focal activity exist in the brain, one characterized by baseline values of blood flow and oxygen metabolism, a second level characterized by increased blood flow, but little increase of oxygen consumption, because of collateral inhibition of postsynaptic depolarization, a condition best described as "stand-by"; and a third level characterized by increased blood flow and increased oxygen consumption because of significant postsynaptic depolarization and efferent impulse traffic. A model of the cellular relationships suggested by this possibility is shown in Fig. 5. The stand-by condition has efferent activity and, hence, causes the release of excitatory neurotransmitters, however, the postsynaptic depolarization is prevented by collateral inhibition. The excitatory neurotransmitters are removed by adjacent astrocytes, which undergo a limited activation of glial metabolism. The oxidative response is low because the mitochondria that are located preferentially in the dendrites are not stimulated. Only when the collateral inhibition is lifted will postsynaptic depolarization ensue and significant oxygen consumption commence. The switch from a stand-by condition to the fully activated situation would depend on a top-down-directed selection of

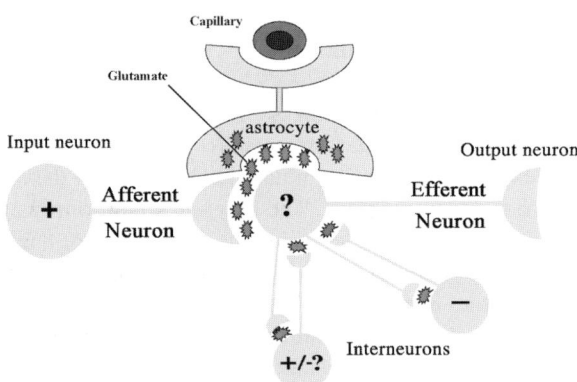

Fig. 5. Model of neuronal and glial relationships hypothetically explaining the three levels of functional brain activity suggested by observations summarized in Fig. 2. Depending on the degree of positive and/or negative feedback, output or projection neuron may be more or less depolarised.

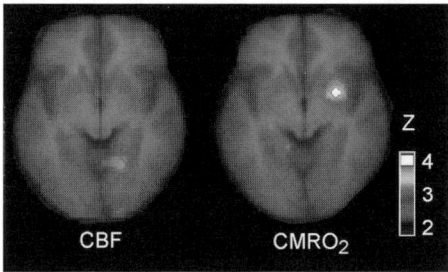

Fig. 6. Result of functional PET measurements of changes in blood flow and oxygen consumption in putamen of 14 volunteers performing right-hand fingers-to-thumb apposition taps at a frequency of 3/s (3 Hz). The figure illustrates a subset of studies involving frequencies ranging from 0 (baseline) to 4 Hz. Note the significant increase of oxygen consumption but the absence of a significant increase in the blood flow. Calculated from the *t*-statistic, the increase of oxygen consumption exceeded the increase in blood flow by 3.3-fold.

the appropriate functional responsiveness to the incoming efferent impulse traffic. Incoming traffic with a low informational content, as in primary or simple stimulation, presumably would not lead to a fully activated condition and, therefore, would not cause a major change in oxygen consumption.

Interestingly, Figs. 2 and 5 predict that activations can occur as a transition from the stand-by condition to the fully activation situation in which oxygen consumption would rise significantly, however, there would be little change in the blood flow. Thus, if stimulation happened to activate a region in which the baseline state were on stand by, no blood flow increase would be registered, but a significant increase of oxygen consumption would be measured. Such a condition is shown in Fig. 6.

5. Oxygen metabolism in hypothermic ischemia

The functional role of the hypothetical "stand-by" condition is unclear. It has been claimed, as outlined in Fig. 3, that the oxygen reserve in mitochondria is so low that the brain regions with a consistently fluctuating oxygen demand depend on a flow-limited supply of oxygen, driven by the average oxygen tension of the brain's capillaries. This claim predicts that reduction of the brain metabolism as seen in hypothermia ($Q10 \sim 2-3$, i.e., metabolism declines by 50–67% for each 10° of temperature reduction) must be accompanied by a commensurate reduction of flow. We observed such a reduction of flow in the brain cortex of anaesthetised pigs by means of positron emission tomography, as shown in Fig. 7.

The change in hypothermia is consistent with a concept of flow regulation according to which the blood flow level established in the stand-by condition is regulated to supply the necessary additional oxygen for a fully activated condition, should a negative feedback be replaced by a positive feedback. According to this concept, ischemic hypoxia must impair the supply of oxygen by reducing the mean capillary oxygen tension to a level incompatible with the supply of oxygen to the tissues, in which the mitochondrial oxygen ten-

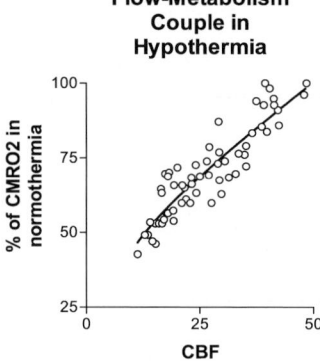

Fig. 7. Flow metabolism coupling in hypothermia. The figure shows preserved cerebral flow metabolism in hypothermia in pigs. Flow and oxygen consumption were measured in the cerebral cortex of anaesthetised pigs by positron emission tomography adapted from [31].

sion is effectively close to zero. The available supply of oxygen would be exhausted by the neurons closest to the source of oxygen, as shown in Fig. 9.

This explanation is the basis for a hypothesis of the mechanism underlying the beneficial effect of hypothermia in ischemic hypoxia. The hypothesis was tested as shown in Fig. 8: Pigs were subjected to experimental brain ischemia with and without hypothermia. The portions of the tissue served at the prevailing oxygen consumption were calculated as the ratio between the ischemic and the nonischemic oxygen consumption for normo- as well as hypothermia. The results show that hypothermia of 32 °C can stretch the

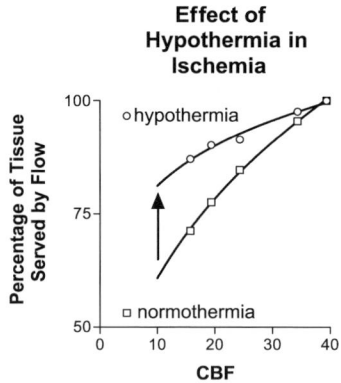

Fig. 8. Change of blood flow and oxygen consumption in the focal ischemia of a pig brain, established by surgical middle cerebral artery occlusion. Brain venous temperature was lowered to 32 °C exposure of the pig to air cooled by dry ice. Abscissa is blood flow to ischemic core. Ordinate is the percentage of tissue served at prevailing flow, calculated from the fraction of oxygen consumption in the non-ischemic control state covered in ischemic condition (adapted from Ref. [31]).

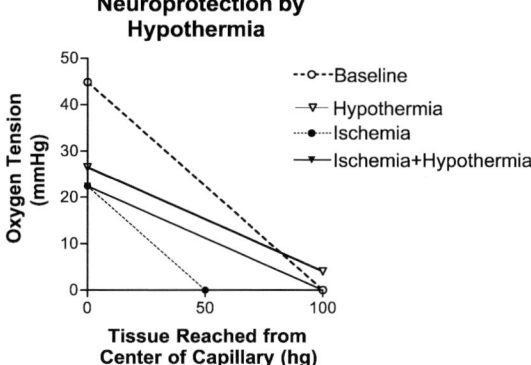

Fig. 9. Model of oxygen supply to brain tissue explaining beneficial effect of hypothermia in ischemic hypoxia: Ischemia lowers oxygen tension in brain capillaries (by increasing the extraction fraction), depriving distant sections of the region of oxygen because the existing oxygen is exhausted by normally metabolising regions closer to the source. Hypothermia distributes the existing oxygen to greater portions of the tissue by lowering metabolism of all cells, including those close to the remaining sources of oxygen.

oxygen supply to 80% or more of the tissue, compared to 50% served at normothermic ischemia, as shown in Fig. 9.

6. Conclusion

The observations summarized in this chapter allow a distinction to be made between a presynaptic phase and a postsynaptic phase of functional activation. The presynaptic phase involves the presynaptic terminals and astrocytes, while the postsynaptic phase involves the dendrites and cell bodies of projections neurons and interneurons. The changes of metabolism occurring in each phase appear to be additive and to rule out significant transfer of lactate from astrocytes to neurons. In addition to the release of neuro-transmitters from the presynaptic terminals and the import of the neurotransmitter into astrocytes, the function of the presynaptic phase appears to be the establishment of a blood flow level sufficient to support the projected metabolic rate. The effect of hypothermia in ischemia underscores the effect the disruption of this adjustment causes. However, the variable metabolic rate of the postsynaptic phase makes it difficult to draw firm conclusions about the functional state from changes of blood flow alone. In fact, it is possible that the most dramatic examples of uncoupling of flow from oxidative metab-olism reflect the situations in which the postsynaptic activation is minimal. In this sense, it is possible that changes of flow and glycolysis, which are dissociated from changes in oxygen consumption, could signify states of inhibition of functional activity.

2.3.1.9. On-Site Discussion

2.3.1.9.1. *Comment: (Lauritzen)* A comment related to the quote of Bob Shulman with respect to Creutzfeldt's calculation of the neural basis of brain energy consumption.

Creutzfeldt's point was that spiking activity alone explained only a very little fraction of energy consumption. The remaining—all important—part was explained by restorations of function following synaptic activity in the dendritic tree. This notion has a strong support for considerations of ion fluxes during synaptic activity and the dendritic localization of mitochondria. The point of Creutzfeldt, concluding from the earliest work of Hodgkin and Huxley, was the low energy requirement of axonal action potential activity (AC potentials) compared to the high energy requirements of dendutic membrane potential changes (DC potentials).

2.3.1.9.2. **Question: (Villringer)** I am interested in the pronounced dissociation which you describe between changes in CBF and $CMRO_2$. This should be reflected in very significant differences between PET-based vs. fMR1-based activation studies, from which testable hypotheses can be derived. Do you have any evidence for that?

Answer: (Gjedde) The conclusions emphasize the possibility of great variations in the relationship between blood flow and $CMRO_2$, depending on the nature of the baseline. I am struck by the great variability of BOLD responses, except for the most primary stimuli. Most reports are anecdotal (for obvious reasons), pinpointing the need for more detailed reporting of aberrant fMR1 BOLD responses.

2.3.1.9.3. **Question: (Nemoto)** Historically, one of the problems of asserting the protection effect of hypothermia to a single reduction in $CMRO_2$ is that barbiturates, which reduce $CMRO_2$ even more, do not offer as much protection against ischemic brain damage.

Answer: (Gjedde) Almost all drugs tested have failed to improve the outcome after ischemia, except when they also depress body and/or brain temperature. The reason for this feature is not understood, but may be related to a feature to depress all cellular processes equally. It is possible that only hypothermia has such a global effect.

References

[1] A. Gjedde, The relation between brain function and cerebral blood flow and metabolism, in: H.H. Batjer (Ed.), Cerebrovascular Disease, Lippincott-Raven, Philadelphia, 1997, pp. 23–40.
[2] A. Gjedde, The energy cost of neuronal depolarization, in: B. Gulyas, D. Ottoson, P.E. Roland (Eds.), Functional Organization of the Human Visual Cortex, Pergamon, Oxford, 1993, pp. 291–306.
[3] S.B. Laughlin, R.R. de Ruyter van Steveninck, J.C. Anderson, The metabolic cost of neural information, Nat. Neurosci. 1 (1998) 36–41.
[4] P.J. Magistretti, L. Pellerin, D.L. Rothman, R.G. Shulman, Energy on demand, Science 283 (1999) 496–497.
[5] R.G. Shulman, D.L. Rothman, Interpreting functional imaging studies in terms of neurotransmitter cycling, Proc. Natl. Acad. Sci. U. S. A. 95 (1998) 11993–11998.
[6] M.S. Vafaee, S. Marrett, E. Meyer, A.C. Evans, A. Gjedde, Increased oxygen consumption in human visual cortex response: to visual stimulation, Acta Neurol. Scand. 98 (1998) 85–89.
[7] M.S. Vafaee, E. Meyer, S. Marrett, T. Paus, A.C. Evans, A. Gjedde, Frequency-dependent changes in cerebral metabolic rate of oxygen during activation of human visual cortex, J. Cereb. Blood Flow Metab. 19 (1999) 272–277.
[8] M.S. Vafaee, A. Gjedde, Model of blood–brain transfer of oxygen explains non-linear flow-metabolism coupling during stimulation of visual cortex, J. Cereb. Blood Flow Metab. 20 (2000) 747–754.
[9] A. Gjedde, S. Marrett, Glycolysis in neurons, not astrocytes, delays oxidative metabolism of human visual

cortex during sustained checkerboard stimulation in vivo, J. Cereb. Blood Flow Metab., submitted for publication.

[10] C.S. Roy, C.S. Sherrington, On the regulation of the blood supply of the rat brain, J. Physiol. (London) 11 (1890) 85–108.

[11] L. Sokoloff, Energetics of functional activation in neural tissues, Neurochem. Res. 24 (1999) 321–329.

[12] J. Prichard, D. Rothman, E. Novotny, O. Petroff, T. Kuwabara, M. Avison, A. Howseman, C. Hanstock, R. Shulman, Lactate rise detected by NMR in human visual cortex during physiologic stimulation, Proc. Natl. Acad. Sci. U. S. A. 88 (1991) 5829–5831.

[13] A. Gjedde, Brain energy metabolism and the physiological basis of the hemodynamic response, in: P. Jezzard, P.M. Matthews, S. Smith (Eds.), Functional Magnetic Resonance Imaging: Methods for Neuroscience, Oxford Univ. Press, Oxford, 2001, In press.

[14] A. Gjedde, S. Ohta, H. Kuwabara, E. Meyer, Is oxygen diffusion limiting for blood–brain transfer of oxygen? In: N.A. Lassen, D.H. Ingvar, M.E. Raichle, L. Friberg (Eds.), Brain Work and Mental Activity, Alfred Benzon Symp., vol. 31. Munksgaard, Copenhagen, 1991, pp. 177–184.

[15] F. Hyder, R.G. Shulman, D.L. Rothman, A model for the regulation of cerebral oxygen delivery, J. Appl. Physiol. 85 (1998) 554–564.

[16] A. Gjedde, P. Høst Poulsen, L. Østergaard, On the oxygenation of hemoglobin in the human brain, Adv. Exp. Biol. Med. 471 (1999) 67–81.

[17] P.T. Fox, M.E. Raichle, M.A. Mintun, C. Dence, Nonoxidative glucose consumption during focal physiologic neural activity, Science 241 (1988) 462–464.

[18] R.J. Seitz, P.E. Roland, Vibratory stimulation increases and decreases the regional cerebral blood flow and oxidative metabolism a positron emission tomography (PET) study, Acta Neurol. Scand. 86 (1992) 6067.

[19] H. Fujita, H. Kuwabara, D.C. Reutens, A. Gjedde, Oxygen consumption of cerebral cortex fails to increase during continued vibrotactile stimulation, J. Cereb. Blood Flow Metab. 19 (1999) 266–271.

[20] H. Kuwabara, S. Ohta, P. Brust, E. Meyer, A. Gjedde, Density of perfused capillaries in living human brain during functional activation, Prog. Brain Res. 91 (1992) 209–215.

[21] M.D. Ginsberg, J.Y. Chang, R.E. Kelley, F. Yoshii, W.W. Barker, G. Ingenito, T.E. Boothe, Increases in both cerebral glucose utilization and blood flow during execution of a somatosensory task, Ann. Neurol. 23 (1988) 152–160.

[22] L. Ribeiro, H. Kuwabara, E. Meyer, H. Fujita, S. Marrett, A. Evans, A. Gjedde, Cerebral blood flow and metabolism during non-specific bilateral visual stimulation in normal subjects, in: K. Uemura, N.A. Lassen, T. Jones, I. Kanno (Eds.), Quantification of Brain Function. Tracer Kinetics and image Analysis in Brain PET, Elsevier, Amsterdam, 1993, pp. 217–224.

[23] S. Marrett, A. Gjedde, Changes of blood flow and oxygen consumption in visual cortex of living humans, Adv. Exp. Med. Biol. 413 (1997) 205–208.

[24] Y. Katayama, T. Tsubokawa, T. Hirayama, G. Kido, T. Tsukiyama, M. Iio, Response of regional cerebral blood flow and oxygen metabolism to thalamic stimulation in humans as revealed by positron emission tomography, J. Cereb. Blood Flow Metab. 6 (1986) 637–641.

[25] P.E. Roland, L. Eriksson, S. Atone-Elander, L. Widen, Does mental activity change the oxidative metabolism of the brain? J. Neurosci. 7 (1987) 2373–2389.

[26] M.E. Raichle, R.L. Grubb, M.H. Gado, J.O. Eichling, M.M. Ter-Pogossian, Correlation between regional cerebral blood flow and oxidative metabolism, Arch. Neurol. 33 (1976) 523–526.

[27] H. Iida, T. Jones, S. Miura, Modeling approach to eliminate the need to separate arterial plasma in oxygen-15 inhalation positron emission tomography, J. Nucl. Med. 34 (1993) 1333–1340.

[28] M.S. Vafaee, A. Gjedde (2001).

[29] G. Tholey, B.F. Roth-Schechter, P. Mandel, Activity and isoenzyme pattern of lactate dehydrogenase in neurons and astroblasts cultured from brains of chick embryos, J. Neurochem. 36 (1981) 77–81.

[30] P.G. Bittar, Y. Charnay, L. Pellerin, C. Bouras, P.J. Magistretti, Selective distribution of lactate dehydrogenase isoenzymes in neurons and astrocytes of human brain, J. Cereb. Blood Flow Metab. 16 (1996) 1079–1089.

[31] M. Sakoh, L. Østergaard, A. Gjedde, Comparison of multitracer PET and functional MRI in a pig MCAO model for acute ischemic stroke, in: Y. Fukuuchi, M. Tomita, A. Koto (Eds.), Ischemic Blood Flow in the Brain, Springer Verlag, Tokyo, 2001, pp. 226–231.

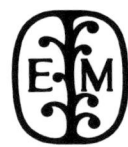

International Congress Series 1235 (2002) 137–144

Neuronal activation induced changes in microcirculatory haemoglobin oxygenation: to dip or not to dip

Ute Lindauer [a,*], Georg Royl [a], Christoph Leithner [a], Marc Kühl [a], Jörn Gethmann [a], Matthias Kohl-Bareis [b], Arno Villringer [b], Ulrich Dirnagl [a]

[a]*Department of Experimental Neurology, Charité Hospital, Humboldt University, Berlin 10098, Germany*
[b]*Department of Neurology, Charité Hospital, Humboldt University, Berlin 10098, Germany*

Abstract

A tight temporal and spatial relationship exists between neuronal activity, metabolism, and blood flow in the brain, and different temporal and spatial kinetics of oxygen consumption and blood flow lead to complex changes in regional cerebral haemoglobin oxygenation. Until now, it remains unclear whether neuronal activation leads to an early deoxygenation termed 'initial dip' preceding the rCBF response accompanied by hyperoxygenation. Although several studies have reported the 'initial dip', other studies did not confirm these findings, regardless of the species used. In an extensive series of experiments in anesthetized rats, we did not robustly find the dip using various modes of cortical O_2-measurements. Our findings for the first time demonstrate that the appearance of an initial dip and its amplitude may be correlated to the kinetics of the rCBF response. In addition, we show that the mode of analysis of spectroscopic data critically affects results. In our experiments, the finding of an initial dip was sensitive to the mode of spectroscopic analysis. Advanced models of spectroscopic analysis, including differential pathlength correction, should become standard in optical imaging spectroscopy studies. We conclude that in the rodent the initial dip is not a robust phenomenon, the occurrence of which may depend on the level of baseline CBF and thus mean transit time. © 2002 Elsevier Science B.V. All rights reserved.

Keywords: Early deoxygenation; Functional activation; Neurovascular coupling; Oxygen metabolism; Whisker stimulation

* Corresponding author. Tel.: +49-30-450-560198; fax: +49-30-450-560915.
E-mail address: ute.lindauer@charite.de (U. Lindauer).

0531-5131/02 © 2002 Elsevier Science B.V. All rights reserved.
PII: S 0 5 3 1 - 5 1 3 1 (0 2) 0 0 1 8 0 - 2

1. To dip or not to dip: the controversy

A tight temporal and spatial relationship exists between neuronal activity, metabolism, and blood flow in the brain. Changes in neuronal activity induce localized changes in metabolism and regional cerebral blood flow (rCBF), a phenomenon termed 'neurometabolic and neurovascular coupling' [1]. Consequently, consumption and delivery of oxygen and glucose, the metabolic substrates that fuel the brain, change at the same time.

Using modern functional brain imaging techniques such as positron emission tomography (PET), functional magnetic resonance imaging (fMRI), near infrared spectroscopy (NIRS), and optical imaging spectroscopy (OIS), the human or animal brain can be visualized at work due to neurometabolic and neurovascular coupling. These techniques do not directly measure neuronal and glial activity, however, the associated changes in regional blood flow, blood oxygenation or glucose/energy metabolism. Whereas the rCBF and the metabolic rate of glucose increase approximately to the same extent, the fractional change in oxygen metabolism during neuronal activation is much smaller. This discrepancy between the cerebral metabolic rate of oxygen ($CMRO_2$) on the one hand, and glucose metabolism and blood flow on the other, was first discovered by Fox et al. [2,3] in a PET study. Furthermore, different temporal and spatial kinetics of oxygen consumption and blood flow lead to complex changes in regional cerebral haemoglobin oxygenation. Deoxygenised haemoglobin (deoxy-Hb) has paramagnetic properties; changes in the functional activity of the brain can therefore indirectly be mapped using the blood oxygenation level dependent (BOLD)-fMRI. This signal results from the complex interaction of stimulation-induced changes in $CMRO_2$ and oxygen delivery via changes in rCBF. During increases in neuronal activity BOLD-fMRI detects robust decreases in deoxy-Hb (=increase in the BOLD-fMRI signal), which result from a disproportionate increase of rCBF in relation to the increase in $CMRO_2$. The deoxy-Hb decreases because it is washed out by arteriolarized (i.e. high in oxygenated haemoglobin, oxy-Hb) blood. This well-characterized hyperoxygenation, which sets in $1-2$ s after stimulation onset and peaks with higher amplitude, does not necessarily mean an 'uncoupling' of rCBF and oxygen metabolism. Large changes in CBF may be necessary to sustain small changes in oxygen metabolism, as explained by the oxygen limitation model [4–6], in which a linear coupling exists between rCBF and oxygen metabolism [7].

Despite our knowledge on the hyperoxygenation phase of the vascular response to functional activation, it remains unclear whether neuronal activation leads to early (<2 s after stimulation onset) deoxygenation, preceding the rCBF response accompanied by hyperoxygenation. This phenomenon has been termed 'initial dip' since it is detected as a decrease in the MR signal induced by the paramagnetic deoxy-Hb.

Optical imaging studies in cats, rats, and monkeys have provided evidence for an initial increase in deoxy-Hb following the onset of neuronal stimulation [8–13]. This early increase has been interpreted as the consequence of oxygen extraction at a time point when vascular mechanisms have not yet increased rCBF. Furthermore, it has been postulated that this deoxygenation might be the critical signal initiating and possibly maintaining the increase in blood flow in functionally active brain areas [14,15]. Concerning the issue of functional brain mapping, it has been proposed that this early activity-dependent increase in deoxy-Hb concentration is more tightly co localized with electrical activity than the delayed increase in oxy-Hb, which is associated with the later increase in blood flow. However, recently it has been shown that the columnar structure of the cat visual cortex can be equally mapped by CBF-fMRI (arterial spin labelling technique) compared to BOLD-fMRI [16].

Over the last years, several fMRI studies in man or animals have reported an early BOLD signal decrease, which has been interpreted as evidence for early deoxygenation [12,17–20]. However, other studies did not confirm this finding [21–24] and the 'initial dip' detected in monkeys [12] was reported to be not of acceptable consistency to reveal cortical micro architecture in a later communication of the same group [25]. A comparable lack of robustness has recently been reported for BOLD-fMRI measurements of early deoxygenation in cats (K. Ugurbil, personal communication).

To summarize, although several studies have reported the 'initial dip' in optical imaging and BOLD-fMRI studies, scepticism remains because of the unpublished negative findings by a number of groups. In the cat and in the monkey the data seems to be unequivocally pointing towards the existence of early deoxygenation, although with variable robustness, while in man the issue remains controversial. The existence of early deoxygenation also remains controversial for rats. As mentioned above, several optical imaging studies have detected the 'initial dip' [10,11], while fMRI studies [22,24] were unable to detect it even at high field strength [24].

2. The initial dip in rats: contribution of different algorithms of spectral analysis

In order to try to solve some of the controversies in the field, we have evaluated the time course of oxygen delivery and consumption in SI cortex in rats in response to a physiological stimulus (whisker deflection) using independent methodological approaches (optical imaging spectroscopy, microfibre spectroscopy, oxygen-dependent phosphorescence quenching), as shown in our recent publication [26]. Spectroscopic data were evaluated using different algorithms including constant pathlength in comparison to differential pathlength correction. The experiments were performed in α-chloralose/ urethane anesthetized rats under full physiological control. Optical imaging was followed either by imaging spectroscopy performed over a slit (imaging in one dimension, time resolution ~ 500 ms, wavelength range 480–680 nm) above the whisker barrel cortex, or by micro fiber spectroscopy (no imaging, light guide 0.2 mm diameter, time resolution ~ 330 ms, wavelength range 480–920 nm). We applied two different algorithms based on the Lambert–Beer law. For constant pathlength analysis, we used the Lambert–Beer law without the inclusion of a wavelength dependent pathlength term [9]. We then compared the results of this algorithm to an algorithm that employed a differential pathlength factor (total hemoglobin concentration 20 μM, saturation 60%), since the extinction spectra are distorted in tissue due to light scattering, and the photon pathlength within scattering tissue is wavelength dependent. Using the pathlength corrected algorithm, the description of the attenuation spectra was significantly improved, as revealed by a decrease in the residues. The activity-dependent oxygen tension changes during whisker stimulation were measured using oxygen-dependent phosphorescence quenching. Further details of the methods and data analysis used are provided in our recent publications in 'Physics in Medicine and Biology' and in 'NeuroImage' [26,27].

Using optical imaging as well as micro fibre spectroscopy, we consistently found monophasic hyperoxygenation during whisker stimulation. While fitting with differential pathlength corrected extinction spectra, the oxygenated haemoglobin in the microcirculatory region (centre of the activated barrel) started to increase ≤1 s after stimulation onset, and reached its maximum at 3–4 s (peak of the response) and decreased below the baseline for the rest of the data acquisition period (sustained oxy-Hb undershoot). The deoxy-Hb concentration did not change during the first 1.5 s of stimulation, and started to decrease at the end of the 2-s stimulation period. The maximum decrease was reached 4 s after stimulation onset, and the deoxy-Hb concentration returned to the baseline followed by a transient deoxy-Hb overshoot. Using constant pathlength analysis, the time course of oxy-Hb concentration changes during and after stimulation did not qualitatively differ from those achieved by differential pathlength correction analysis. In contrast, however, the deoxy-Hb concentration started to increase at the same time as the oxy-Hb, reached its maximum at the end of the stimulation period (2 s), decreased during the following 2–3 s, and returned to a higher level than the pre-stimulation baseline. Using the constant pathlength analysis, significant parts of the measured attenuation spectra were not explained, leading to high values of residues of the fitting curves. The maximum residue changes, using the constant pathlength analysis, was 1.5 times larger than in the differential pathlength correction analysis, representing inferior quality of the constant pathlength fitting procedure.

The phosphorescence decay time minimally increased 1 s after stimulation onset, however, no statistically significant early deoxygenation was found in the averaged data from the experiments. In only one animal was statistically significant early deoxygenation found, the amplitude of the oxygen tension decrease amounted to approx 10% of the following hyperoxygenation. In all of the animals, the phosphorescence decay time significantly decreased to a maximum 4 s after stimulation onset, representing a significant increase in microvascular oxygen tension due to whisker deflection, which was followed by small poststimulation undershoot.

In summary, according to our data using optical imaging spectroscopy, no early deoxygenation occurs during functional activation in the SI cortex of the rat. In addition, we have shown that constant pathlength analysis of spectroscopic data may lead to the erroneous detection of early deoxygenation.

3. Robustness of the dip: implications for 'dip-imaging'

The 'dip' controversy has recently been heated up by the publication of our study [26] together with spectroscopic data from the rat whisker system by Jones et al. [28] in the same issue of NeuroImage, accompanied by commentaries by Buxton [29] and Vanzetta and Grinvald [30].

Two important issues have been discussed by the two commentaries, which may be related to each other. (1) The high variability of the dip in rise time and amplitude in optical imaging studies in cats and monkeys [30], also recently discussed for fMRI data in monkeys [25] and cats (K. Ugurbil, personal communication). (2) The influence of rise time of rCBF and of baseline hemoglobin saturation in correlation to oxygen metabolism as a possible explanation for the variability of the initial dip [29,30].

Vanzetta and Grinvald pointed to different criteria for accepting or rejecting experiments before subjecting the data to statistical analysis in our study, compared to that of the Mayhew group. In our study, the only criteria for rejecting experiments were (1) microscopically visible damage to the brain surface due to cranial window preparation and (2) lack of optical imaging maps at 570 and 605 nm during whisker deflection preceding imaging spectroscopy. Therefore, no bias towards special deoxy-Hb features is to be expected.

In an extended series of experiments of whole whisker pad stimulations using micro fiber spectroscopy subjected to differential pathlength analysis with an improved time resolution (160 ms), we now evaluated a correlation of the occurrence of an early increase in deoxy-Hb with amplitude and rise time of the oxy-Hb signal in our experimental setup. Oxy- and deoxy-Hb time courses of different animals are shown in the figure. Fig. 1A demonstrates the most common feature, occurring in ~ 60% of the experiments, which also corresponds to the averaged data shown in Fig. 5B in Ref. [26]. No early increase in deoxy-Hb was detectable. The increase of oxy-Hb started at ~ 0.5 s. As shown in Fig. 1C, in ~ 10% of our experiments, an initial dip occurred (Fig. 1C; despite pathlength correction of the spectroscopic analysis). In these experiments, oxy-Hb started to increase approximately 1–1.5 s later than in the experiments in which no dip appeared. In the remaining ~ 30% of experiments, a very small and inconsistent deoxy-Hb increase was observed (Fig. 1B), and the oxy-Hb started to increase > 0.5–1.5 s after stimulation onset. These hemoglobin oxygenation responses implicate a dynamic range between 'no occurrence of the dip' and 'significant occurrence of the dip'. Commonly, in experiments in which the dip occurred, and the onset of oxy-Hb increase was delayed, the amplitude of the peak response in oxy-Hb was small compared to responses without dip. However, as shown in Fig. 1D, in animals with small oxy-Hb peak amplitudes the initial dip did not necessarily occur. These data provide preliminary evidence for a correlation of the occurrence of the dip and the temporal onset of the rCBF response (which very much parallels the oxy-Hb increase), as postulated by Buxton [29]. Hypothetically, a lower baseline CBF and thus higher mean transit time of red blood cells through the cerebral microvasculature may favor a condition in which oxygen delivery lags behind oxygen extraction. In their comment, Vanzetta and Grinvald [30] stated that the well-known variability of amplitude and rise time of the dip in experiments in cats and monkeys depend on the anesthesia depth and on the anesthetic. One of the main differences of Mayhew's experiments and our experiments is indeed the issue of anesthesia. However, until now we do not know which anesthetic regime resembles most the conditions of the conscious state.

To summarize the results of our recently published data and the extended study shown here, we did not robustly find a dip in the anesthetized rat using various modes of cortical O_2-measurements. The mode of analysis for spectroscopic data critically affects findings. We postulate that advanced models of spectroscopic analysis, such as the one used by us including the differential pathlength correction, should become standard in optical imaging spectroscopy studies.

The inconsistency of the early increase of deoxy-Hb makes it unlikely to be the initial signal for the blood flow response to occur. However, future studies are required to understand which factors affect the elusiveness of the dip. Resolving the 'dip enigma' will further our understanding of neurovascular coupling, while at the same time advance our

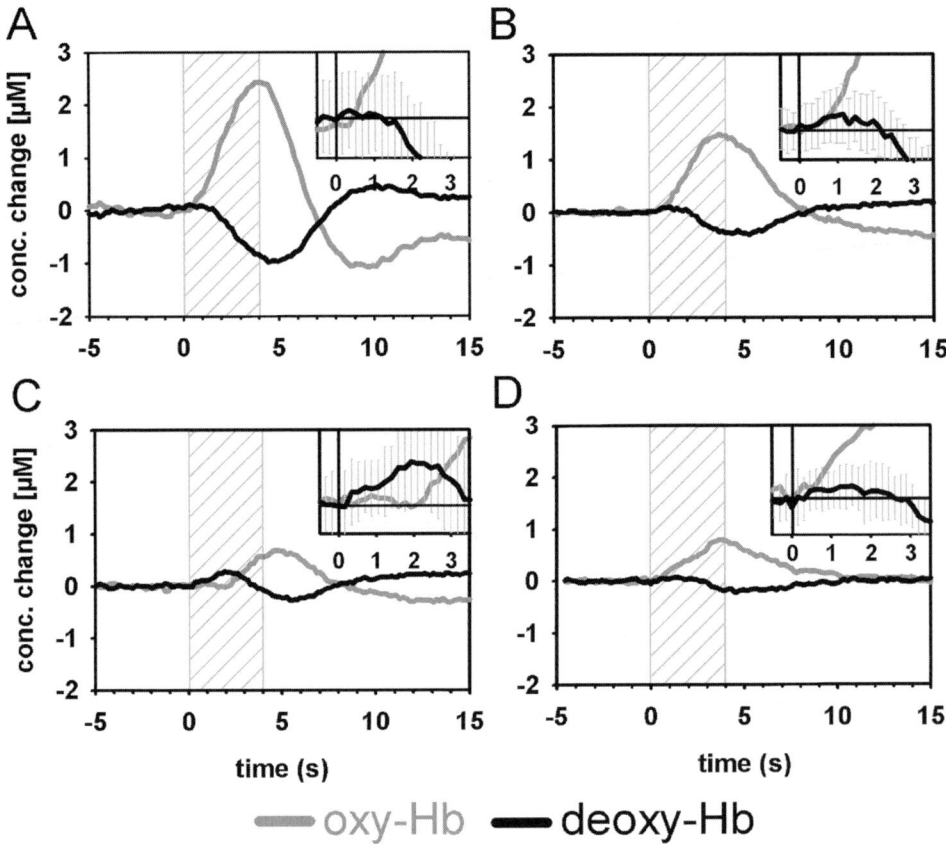

Fig. 1. Oxy- and deoxy-Hb time courses of different experiments during whisker stimulation in anesthetized rats: no early increase in deoxy-Hb is detectable in ~ 60% of the experiments (A). In ~ 30% of the experiments, a very small and inconsistent deoxy-Hb increase occurs (B), and in 10% of our experiments, an initial dip can be detected (C). Please note that in the experiments in which the dip occurs, the onset of oxy-Hb increase is delayed, and the amplitude of the peak response in oxy-Hb is small compared to the responses without a dip. However, in animals with small oxy-Hb peak amplitudes, the initial dip does not necessarily occur (D).

knowledge on the strengths and weaknesses of techniques such as BOLD-fMRI, imaging and near infrared spectroscopy, as well as phosphorescence lifetime quenching.

2.3.2.6. On-Site Discussion

2.3.2.6.1. *Question: (Busija)* You presented data on variability among animals. What happens in animals that show the "dip" with repeated interventions?

Answer: (Dirnagl) Intra animal variability is smaller than inter animal variability, but it exists.

2.3.2.6.2. **Question: (Gjedde)** Does the absence of a "dip" mean that EO_2 cannot rise under normal physiological circumstances?

Answer: (Dirnag) Not necessarily. If there is an oxygen "buffer" like in the Buxton model, the extra amount of O_2 needed before the flow response starts could be extracted from the buffer.

2.3.2.6.3. **Question: (Kim)** Dynamics of BOLD response in cat visual cortex is dependent on basal PCO_2 level. Thus, the magnitude of the dip can be modulated by changing PCO_2 level.

Answer: (Dirnagl) This is a very interesting observation. It agrees with an observation of a relationship between a delay of the flow response and the appearance of early deoxygenation.

2.3.2.6.4. **Question: (Nemoto)** The presence or absence of the dip may be simply reflected to collateral circulation heterogeneity relating to a "steal" phenomenon.

Answer: (Dirnagl) I do not believe so, since this could not explain inter-animal variability in one species.

Acknowledgements

Supported by the German Israel Science Foundation, the Hermann and Lilly Schilling Stiftung, and the DFG.

References

[1] A. Villringer, U. Dirnagl, Coupling of brain activity and cerebral blood flow: basis for functional neuro-imaging, Cerebrovasc. Brain Metab. Rev. 7 (1995) 240–276.

[2] P.T. Fox, M.E. Raichle, Focal physiological uncoupling of cerebral blood flow and oxidative metabolism during somatosensory stimulation in human subjects, Proc. Natl. Acad. Sci. 83 (1986) 1140–1144.

[3] P.T. Fox, M.E. Raichle, M.A. Mintun, C. Dence, Nonoxidative glucose consumption during focal physiologic neural activity, Science 241 (1988) 462–464.

[4] A. Gjedde, S. Ohta, H. Kubawara, et al., Is oxygen diffusion limiting for blood–brain transfer of oxygen? in: N.A. Lassen, D.H. Ingvar, M.E. Raichle, L. Friberg (Eds.), Brain Work and Mental Activity. Alfred Benzon Symposium, vol. 31. Munskgaard, Copenhagen, 1991, pp. 177–184.

[5] R.B. Buxton, L.R. Frank, A model for the coupling between cerebral blood flow and oxygen metabolism during neural stimulation, J. Cereb. Blood Flow Metab. 17 (1) (1997) 64–72.

[6] F. Hyder, R.G. Shulman, D.L. Rothman, A model for the regulation of cerebral oxygen delivery, J. Appl. Physiol. 85 (2) (1998) 554–564.

[7] R.D. Hoge, J. Atkinson, B. Gill, G.R. Crelier, S. Marrett, G.B. Pike, Linear coupling between cerebral blood flow and oxygen consumption in activated human cortex, Proc. Natl. Acad. Sci. U. S. A. 96 (16) (1999) 9403–9408.

[8] D. Malonek, A. Grinvald, Interactions between electrical activity and cortical microcirculation revealed by imaging spectroscopy: implications for functional brain mapping, Science 272 (1996) 551–554.

[9] D. Malonek, U. Dirnagl, U. Lindauer, K. Yamada, I. Kanno, A. Grinvald, Vascular imprints of neuronal activity: relationships between the dynamics of cortical blood flow, oxygenation, and volume changes following sensory stimulation, Proc. Natl. Acad. Sci. U. S. A. 94 (26) (1997) 14826–14831.

[10] M. Nemoto, Y. Nomura, C. Sato, M. Tamura, K. Houkin, I. Koyanagi, H. Abe, Analysis of optical signals evoked by peripheral nerve stimulation in rat somatosensory cortex: dynamic changes in hemoglobin concentration and oxygenation, J. Cereb. Blood Flow Metab. 19 (3) (1999) 246–259.

[11] J. Mayhew, D. Johnston, J. Berwick, M. Jones, P. Coffey, Y. Zheng, Spectroscopic analysis of neural activity in brain: increased oxygen consumption following activation of barrel cortex, NeuroImage 12 (6) (2000) 664–675.

[12] N.K. Logothetis, H. Guggenberger, S. Peled, J. Pauls, Functional imaging of the monkey brain, Nat. Neurosci. 2 (6) (1999) 555–562.

[13] E. Shtoyerman, A. Arieli, H. Slovin, I. Vanzetta, A. Grinvald, Long-term optical imaging and spectroscopy reveal mechanisms underlying the intrinsic signal and stability of cortical maps in V1 of behaving monkeys, J. Neurosci. 20 (21) (2000) 8111–8121.

[14] J.S. Stamler, L. Jia, J.P. Eu, T.J. McMahon, I.T. Demchenko, J. Bonaventura, K. Gernert, C.A. Piantadosi, Blood flow regulation by S-nitrosohemoglobin in the physiological oxygen gradient, Science 276 (5321) (1997) 2034–2037.

[15] H.H. Dietrich, M.L. Ellsworth, R.S. Sprague, R.G.J. Dacey, Red blood cell regulation of microvascular tone through adenosine triphosphate, Am. J. Physiol.: Heart Circ. Physiol. 278 (4) (2000) H1294–H1298.

[16] T.Q. Duong, D.S. Kim, S.G. Kim, Simultaneous CBF and BOLD fMRI of the cat visual cortex: comparison of spatial specificity at sub-millimeter resolution, Proc. Int. Soc. Mag. Reson. Med. 8 (2000) 980.

[17] T. Ernst, J. Hennig, Observation of a fast response in functional MR, Magn. Reson. Med. 32 (1) (1994) 146–149.

[18] R.S. Menon, S. Ogawa, X. Hu, J.P. Strupp, P. Anderson, K. Ugurbil, BOLD based functional MRI at 4 Tesla includes a capillary bed contribution: echo-planar imaging correlates with previous optical imaging using intrinsic signals, Magn. Reson. Med. 33 (3) (1995) 453–459.

[19] X. Hu, T.H. Le, K. Ugurbil, Evaluation of the early response in fMRI in individual subjects using short stimulus duration, Magn. Reson. Med. 37 (6) (1997) 877–884.

[20] D.S. Kim, T.Q. Duong, S.G. Kim, High-resolution mapping of iso-orientation columns by fMRI, Nat. Neurosci. 3 (2) (2000) 164–169.

[21] P. Fransson, G. Kruger, K.D. Merboldt, J. Frahm, Temporal characteristics of oxygenation-sensitive MRI responses to visual activation in humans, Magn. Reson. Med. 39 (6) (1998) 912–919.

[22] J.B. Mandeville, J.J. Marota, C. Ayata, M.A. Moskowitz, R.M. Weisskoff, B.R. Rosen, MRI measurement of the temporal evolution of relative CMRO (2) during rat forepaw stimulation, Magn. Reson. Med. 42 (5) (1999) 944–951.

[23] J.J. Marota, C. Ayata, M.A. Moskowitz, R.M. Weisskoff, B.R. Rosen, J.B. Mandeville, Investigation of the early response to rat forepaw stimulation, Magn. Reson. Med. 41 (2) (1999) 247–252.

[24] A.C. Silva, S.P. Lee, C. Iadecola, S.G. Kim, Early temporal characteristics of cerebral blood flow and deoxyhemoglobin changes during somatosensory stimulation, J. Cereb. Blood Flow. Metab. 20 (1) (2000) 201–206.

[25] N.K. Logothetis, Can current fMRI techniques reveal the microarchitecture of cortex? Nat. Neurosci. 3 (5) (2000) 413–414.

[26] U. Lindauer, G. Royl, C. Leithner, M. Kuhl, L. Gold, J. Gethmann, M. Kohl-Bareis, A. Villringer, U. Dirnagl, No evidence for early decrease in blood oxygenation in rat whisker cortex in response to functional activation, NeuroImage 13 (6) (2001) 988–1001.

[27] M. Kohl, U. Lindauer, G. Royl, M. Kühl, L. Gold, A. Villringer, U. Dirnagl, Physical model for the spectroscopic analysis of cortical intrinsic optical signals, Phys. Med. Biol. 45 (2000) 3749–3764.

[28] M. Jones, J. Berwick, D. Johnston, J. Mayhew, Concurrent optical imaging spectroscopy and Laser–Doppler flowmetry: the relationship between blood flow, oxygenation, and volume in rodent barrel cortex, NeuroImage 13 (6) (2001) 1002–1015.

[29] R.B. Buxton, The elusive initial dip, NeuroImage 13 (6) (2001) 953–958.

[30] I. Vanzetta, A. Grinvald, Evidence and lack of evidence for the initial dip in the anesthetized rat: implications for human functional brain imaging, NeuroImage 13 (6) (2001) 959–967.

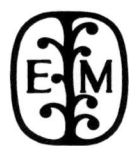

International Congress Series 1235 (2002) 145–153

Spatio-temporal characteristics of neurovascular coupling in the anesthetized cat and the awake monkey

Ivo Vanzetta, Hamutal Slovin, Amiram Grinvald*

The Department of Neurobiology and the Grodetsky Center for the Studies of Higher Brain Functions, Weizmann Institute of Science, Rehovot 76100, Israel

Abstract

Understanding of the spatio-temporal characteristics of the sensory-evoked cortical blood-volume and oxygenation changes is important from the physiological perspective as well as for the interpretation of results obtained by various neuroimaging techniques, such as optical imaging, PET and f-MRI, and for their improvement. The detailed picture, however, has remained elusive for more than a century. We investigated the blood-volume and oxygenation changes in anesthetized cats and awake monkeys using intrinsic imaging at isosbestic and other wavelengths, laser Doppler, imaging spectroscopy, phosphorescence quenching and fluorescence imaging of activity-dependent responses of intravenously injected extrinsic probes. We found that the onset of blood-volume changes was delayed (>300 ms) with respect to a fast decrease in blood oxygenation. Thus, the blood-volume effects cannot merely explain the "initial dip". 570-nm measurements and high-resolution imaging (80 ms, 7 μm) of a fluorescent tracer injected into the blood circulation facilitated the resolution of the responses of different microvascular compartments. Preliminary results show that the arterioles led the blood volume increase, rapidly spreading towards the other microvascular compartments. Veins lagged behind. Functional maps of stimulus vs. blank (single condition maps) in a conscious macaque and an anesthetized cat were obtained only during the early deoxygenation phase at 605 nm. At later times or at 570 nm, the vessel artifacts dominated. These results indicated a stronger co-localization of oxygen consumption and electrical activity as compared to the subsequent volume and flow increase, which are not well regulated at the cortical column level. © 2002 Elsevier Science B.V. All rights reserved.

Keywords: Oxygenation; CBV; Microvasculature; Hemodynamics; Functional brain mapping; Optical imaging; f-MRI

* Corresponding author.

E-mail addresses: ivo.vanzetta@weizmann.ac.il (I. Vanzetta), hamutal.slovin@weizmann.ac.il (H. Slovin), amiram.grinvald@weizmann.ac.il (A. Grinvald).

0531-5131/02 © 2002 Elsevier Science B.V. All rights reserved.
PII: S0531-5131(02)00181-4

About 15 years ago, Fox and Raichle "shocked the Neuroscience world" [1] by reporting results from PET measurements implying a large mismatch (50% vs. 5%) between a big activity-dependent increase in the local cerebral glucose metabolic rate, and only a small increase in the cerebral metabolic rate for oxygen [2,3]. Since then, opinions have been divided on whether, in the living brain, neuronal activation causes a significative increase in oxidative metabolism, or if the increased energy demands are met by other, anaerobic mechanisms or by both [4–17].

Evidence in favor of activity-dependent oxygen consumption has been provided by the detection of the "initial dip," an early increase in the concentration of deoxyhemoglobin (Hbr) following neuronal activation, observed by Malonek and Grinvald [18] in the anesthetized cat using imaging spectroscopy. With this technique, the initial dip was also seen in the anesthetized rat [19] and in the conscious monkey [20]. Objections have, however, been raised with respect to the quantitative and qualitative accuracy of deoxyhemoglobin and oxyhemoglobin concentration ([Hbr] and [HbO$_2$], respectively) time courses, obtained with simplified spectroscopic models as used by Malonek and Grinvald [18] and Nemoto et al. [19]. In fact, their simplified model ignored the well-known photons' path length dependency on wavelength. Intense modeling efforts have been made [21–23] and application on imaging spectroscopy data has been set forth by several groups [24–26], however, unambiguous interpretation of imaging spectroscopy data still remains a challenge, as shown by the opposite conclusions reached with respect to the initial dip in the rat by different groups [13,14,24,27,28].

The initial dip was also seen with high field BOLD-fMRI in humans, monkeys and cats [29–33]. With some exceptions, however [34], at low field strength it was not detected [35,36]. It was suggested that the weight of the capillaries' contribution to the BOLD signal grows with field strength [34], but altogether the exact sources of the different BOLD-fMRI signals are still to be determined (e.g., [29]). It has also been debated whether a detected increase in [Hbr] necessarily implies blood deoxygenation due to increased oxygen consumption, or if the detected initial dip rather results from blood volume increase, e.g., by an accumulation of deoxygenated blood in the venular/venous compartment of the microcirculation [13–15,28,37–41].

To address the outlined questions, we measured [9,28] activity-evoked oxygen tension changes in the cortical microvasculature together with blood volume changes, using phosphorescence quenching [42] together with optical imaging of intrinsic signals upon illumination at the isosbestic wavelength of 570 nm (Fig. 1).

The results showed a very fast (beginning 100 ms from stimulus onset), activity-evoked, increase in the phosphorescence decay time, beginning at least 300 ms before the onset of blood volume (and thus flow) changes, thus proving a drop in the blood oxygenation level following visual stimulation. This time lag in fact, drastically simplifies the interpretation of the multi-exponential phosphorescence decay curves, which, in the general case, present a number of pitfalls that must be carefully taken into account [9,27]. Furthermore, since the detected deoxygenation precedes blood volume changes, it cannot merely be an effect of the accumulating Hbr due to the increased blood volume, as hypothesized by the Balloon Model in its restrictive interpretation. The results actually indicate an increase in neuronal or glial oxygen consumption. These results are in line with previous laser Doppler studies in the cat [43], which detected a delay in the onset of blood

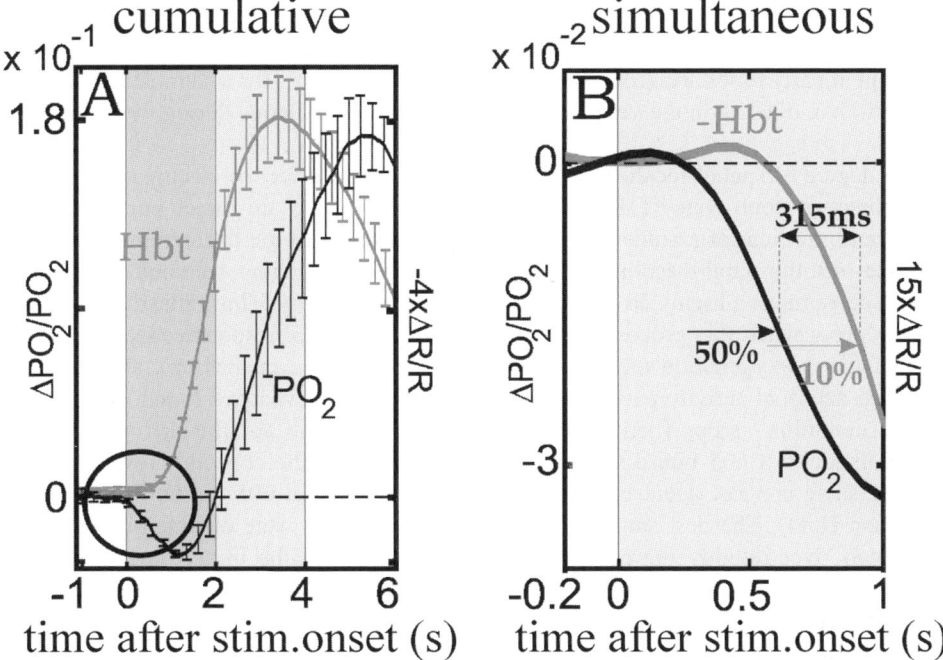

Fig. 1. PO₂ and Hbt measurements in the anesthetized cat area 18. PO₂ (black) was derived from the phosphorescence decay-time measurements, whereas Hbt (red) changes (equivalent to CBV) were measured by recording the reflected light upon illumination at 570 nm. (**A**) Grand average of separate phosphorescence quenching and reflection measurements. (**B**) Time-zoom into the first 1 s of an experiment where the two methods were employed simultaneously on the same patch of cortex. Note that when the initial deoxygenation has reached 50% of its maximum, the blood volume increase has hardly started; it reaches 10% of its peak only 315 ms later (black and red arrows). To facilitate timing comparisons, the Hbt curve in (B) is displayed upside down. The shaded areas mark the stimulus (durations of 2 and 4 s were averaged together). Modified from Ref. [28].

flow increase as compared to the increase in [Hbr], as derived from concomitant imaging spectroscopy measurements (1.5 and 0.5 s after stimulus onset, respectively). An inflating venous/venular compartment would in fact pre-suppose increased inflow, and if the detected deoxygenation was due to such Balloon-like effects, the corresponding flow increase, as measured by the laser Doppler should precede it rather than lag behind it. Similar results, albeit a smaller delay (0.2 s), were obtained in recent studies on the rat [13]. Different capillary-transit times between the two species might be responsible for this reduced delay.

Obviously, increased oxygen consumption and the mismatch between in- and outflow from the veins and venules as predicted by the Balloon scenario do not exclude each other, and both processes may contribute to the initial increase in [Hbr]. Indeed, the [Hbr] peak measured by imaging spectroscopy [18,20] or BOLD-fMRI [32,33] is delayed by 0.5–1 s, with respect to the time of minimum oxygen tension measured by phosphorescence quenching [9]. With the caveats of possible timing inaccuracies introduced by the approximations used in the applied spectroscopic models or by the interpretation of

BOLD-fMRI data, this delay supports the hypothesis of two separate processes which contribute, with different timings, to the initial dip: (a) increased oxygen consumption, dominant at early times and (b) a somewhat delayed, transient, Hbr accumulation, due to a larger in- than outflow in the veins, venules and perhaps capillaries during their expansion phase.

The degree of spatial localization of the initial dip to the loci of electrical activity has been object of controversy [18,32,33,44–46]. Clearly, there are direct implications for functional brain imaging, since the spatial regulation scales of the different hemodynamic processes set the upper resolution limit of the different imaging techniques. Increased oxygen consumption highly co-localizes with electrical activity. Thus, Hbr maps obtained at early times when this process dominates (at 1.5 s from the response onset, i.e., at the peak of the deoxygenation measured from phosphorescence quenching), should reflect increased neuronal activity particularly well. Indeed, this is what we found by analyzing "single condition" maps (i.e., maps of stimulated vs. blank conditions) obtained with optical imaging at 605 nm, a wavelength that emphasizes the concentration changes of Hbr, the same contrast agent used by BOLD-fMRI, which at 605 nm absorbs six times more than HbO_2. The best single condition functional maps were obtained by averaging the signals over roughly the period of somewhat less than the initial dip (first 2–3 s, compare also (B) to (D) in Fig. 2). These data were obtained from anesthetized cats and conscious monkeys [28,45] with stimulus durations of 2, 4 and 6 s, and may be similar to the results obtained with high field BOLD-fMRI by Kim et al. [33]. However, because optical imaging and fMRI do not measure the same phenomena, one would like to see an independent confirmation of Kim et al.'s results. In this important context, a recent paper by Cannestra et al. [47] employing both optical imaging and fMRI, lend support for our earlier prediction from optical imaging and the fMRI results of Kim et al. [33].

The "quality" of such single condition maps increases up to 1.5 s from the onset of the response. Afterwards, the maps deteriorate due to blood-vessel artifacts, up to the point that after 5 s from the stimulus onset the functional architecture is essentially unrecogniz-able (Fig. 2). In fact, blood-volume and flow also influence the [Hbr] distribution, but the brain microcirculation's active response appears to have a relatively diffuse character [18,20,48], in line with the low spatial resolution of the late, positive BOLD-fMRI signal [33]. To better characterize the microcirculation's response, we performed experiments on the anesthetized cat, in which sensory-evoked blood volume changes were imaged at a high spatio-temporal resolution (7 μm, 80 ms), by optical imaging of a fluorescent tracer injected into the blood circulation. Preliminary results indicate that the vasodilatation begins at the arteriolar level, spreading rapidly towards the other vascular compartments; veins lag somewhat behind. The arteriolar and arterial signal were also largest in amplitude. A simple geometrical consideration points to an important conclusion: Arteries and arterioles, as well as venules and veins run preferentially parallel to the cortical sheet, thereby crossing several functional domains. Furthermore, their density is rather low compared to that of the capillaries' density. Thus, it appears that only the capillaries can contribute to the stimulus specific high-resolution mapping component of the volume/flow signal change. Consistently with this purely anatomical consideration, we indeed found that the blood volume signals are inadequate for obtaining single condition maps of the functional architecture, as shown in Fig. 3A–D, which compares single condition ocular

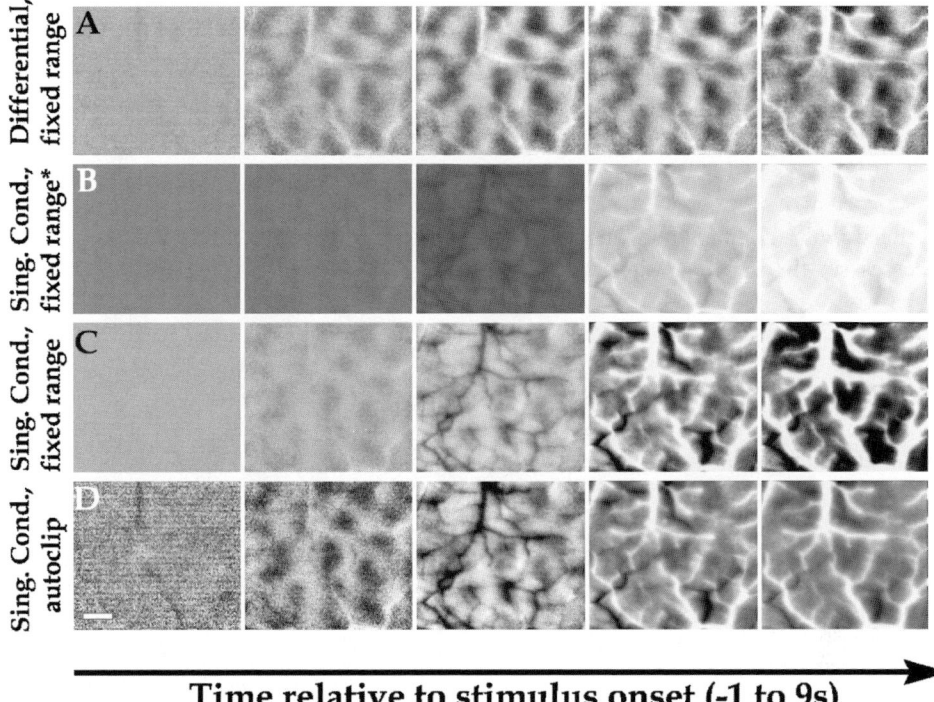

Time relative to stimulus onset (-1 to 9s)

Fig. 2. Single condition and differential maps of ocular dominance columns in the behaving monkey obtained by optical imaging. The exposed cortex was illuminated at a wavelength of 605 nm to emphasize small concentration changes in deoxyhemoglobin. (**A**) A series of differential images taken 2 s apart, obtained by subtracting the cortical images taken during contralateral eye stimulation from the corresponding images taken when the ipsilateral eye was stimulated. To show the time development of the differential map all the frames were clipped at the same range. (**B**) The corresponding single condition maps, obtained by normalizing the cortical image to the overall illumination intensity pattern without any additional processing, when the contralateral eye viewed the stimulus. The same grayscale-mean and -range was used in all frames to emphasize the large global changes. (**C**) Same as in (B), however, to emphasize the mapping signal, the grayscale's mean was matched to the mean intensity of each individual frame. (**D**) Same as in (C), but here the grayscale range is proportional to the intensity variance of each individual frame, in order to maximize the dynamic range of each image. Stimulus duration was 2 s. Scale bar: 1 mm. Modified from Ref. [45].

dominance maps recorded with optical imaging of intrinsic signals in the behaving monkey upon illumination at 605 and 570 nm. In the latter case, the images are dominated by a stimulus unspecific response, showing up as large vascular artifacts.

In most cases, when using differential techniques this large global component cancels out leaving only the stimulus specific part of the signal. Thus, also blood volume-based signals can be advantageously used for functional mapping as shown in the behaving monkey in Fig. 3E–F, provided that "orthogonal" stimuli are available and differential imaging is warranted. For the BOLD-fMRI experiments, this allows to significantly increase the S/N ratio by acquiring long data series [49–51], as compared to the short time of the initial negative signal. In the general case, however, single condition imaging is

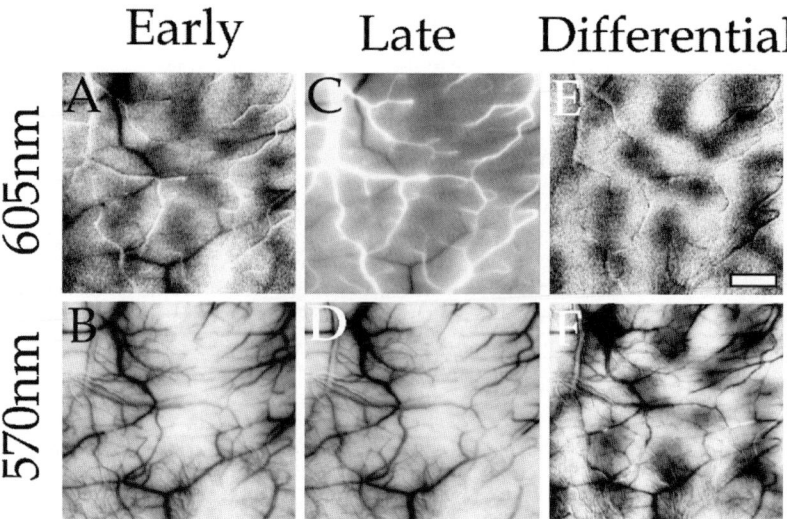

Fig. 3. A comparison of orientation maps derived from oximetry and blood volume changes. (**A**) and (**B**) Early single condition maps of the contralateral eye, imaged at 605 and 570 nm, respectively, obtained by averaging from 1 until 4 s after the stimulus onset. (**C**) and (**D**) Same as in (A) and (B), but late (averaging from 6 until 9 s) maps. Note that functional patches are visible only upon illumination at 605 nm, at early times. (**E**) Differential ocular dominance map (contralateral vs. ipsilateral eye open) obtained at 605 nm, averaging from 1 until 9 s. (**F**) Same as in (E), but with a 570-nm illumination. Range of maps in (A)–(F) 0.08%, 0.9%, 0.8%, 2.06%, 0.13%, 0.5%. Scale bar: 1 mm.

required. In this case, our results suggest that the time window used for data acquisition is critical [9,33,45]: it should be restricted to the early part of the response, when the increase in [Hbr] is prevalently due to increased oxygen consumption by the active neurons or the surrounding glia, avoiding contributions by the less localized blood volume and flow changes.

Acknowledgements

This study was supported by grants from GIF, the Grodetsky Center and the Goldsmith Foundation to A.G.

References

[1] Research News, What makes brain neurons run? Science 276 (1997) 196–198.
[2] P.T. Fox, M.E. Raichle, Focal physiological uncoupling of cerebral blood flow and oxidative metabolism during somatosensory stimulation in human subjects, Proc. Natl. Acad. Sci. U. S. A. 83 (1986) 1140–1144.
[3] P.T. Fox, M.E. Raichle, M.A. Mintun, C. Dence, Nonoxidative glucose consumption during focal physio-logic neural activity, Science 241 (1988) 462–464.
[4] M.E. Raichle, Circulatory and metabolic correlates of brain function in normal humans, in: V.B. Mountcastle,

F. Plum, S.R. Geiger (Eds.), Handbook of Physiology: The Nervous System 1(V), Am. Physiol. Soc., Bethesda, MD, 1987, pp. 643–674.

[5] M.E. Raichle, Behind the scenes of functional brain imaging: a historical and physiological perspective, Proc. Natl. Acad. Sci. U. S. A. 95 (1998) 765–772.

[6] P.E. Roland, L. Eriksson, S. Stone-Elander, L. Widen, Does mental activity change the oxidative metabolism of the brain? J. Neurosci. 7 (1987) 2373–2389.

[7] T. Davis, K.K. Kwong, R.M. Weisskoff, B.R. Rosen, Calibrated functional MRI: mapping the dynamics of oxidative metabolism, Proc. Natl. Acad. Sci. U. S. A. 95 (1998) 1834–1839.

[8] H. Fujita, H. Kuwabara, D.C. Reutens, A. Gjedde, Oxygen consumption of cerebral cortex fails to increase during continued vibrotactile stimulation, J. Cereb. Blood Flow Metab. 19 (1999) 266–271.

[9] I. Vanzetta, A. Grinvald, Increased cortical oxidative metabolism due to sensory stimulation: implications for functional brain imaging, Science 286 (1999) 1555–1558.

[10] J.B. Mandeville, J.J. Marota, C. Ayata, M.A. Moskowitz, R.M. Weisskoff, B.R. Rosen, MRI measurement of the temporal evolution of relative $CMRO_2$ during rat forepaw stimulation, Magn. Reson. Med. 42 (1999) 944–951.

[11] S.G. Kim, E. Rostrup, H.B.W. Larrson, S. Ogawa, O.B. Paulson, Determination of relative $CMRO_2$ from CBF and BOLD changes: significant increase in oxygen consumption rate during visual stimulation, Magn. Reson. Med. 41 (1999) 1152–1161.

[12] M.S. Vafaee, A. Gjedde, Model of blood–brain transfer of oxygen explains nonlinear flow-metabolism coupling during stimulation of visual cortex, J. Cereb. Blood Flow Metab. 20 (2000) 747–754.

[13] M. Jones, J. Berwick, D. Johnston, J. Mayhew, Concurrent optical imaging spectroscopy and laser-Doppler flowmetry: the relationship between blood flow, oxygenation and volume in rodent barrel cortex, Neuroimage 13 (2001) 1002–1015.

[14] J. Mayhew, D. Johnston, J. Berwick, M. Jones, P. Coffey, Y. Zheng, Spectroscopic analysis of neural activity in brain: increased oxygen consumption following activation of barrel cortex, Neuroimage 12 (2000) 664–675.

[15] J. Mayhew, M. Jones, J. Berwick, D. Johnston, Y. Zheng, Increased oxygen consumption following activation of brain: theoretical footnotes using spectroscopic data from barrel cortex, Neuroimage 13 (2001) 975–987.

[16] R.G. Shulman, F.L. Hyder, D.L. Rothman, Cerebral energetics and the glycogen shunt: neurochemical basis of functional imaging, Proc. Natl. Acad. Sci. U. S. A. 98 (2001) 6417–6422.

[17] B.M. Ances, D.F. Wilson, J.H. Greenberg, J.A. Detre, Dynamic changes in cerebral blood flow, O_2 tension, and calculated cerebral metabolic rate of O_2 during functional activation using oxygen phosphorescence quenching, J. Cereb. Blood Flow Metab. 21 (2001) 511–516.

[18] D. Malonek, A. Grinvald, Interactions between electrical activity and cortical microcirculation revealed by imaging spectroscopy: implications for functional brain mapping, Science 272 (1996) 551–554.

[19] M. Nemoto, Y. Nomura, C. Sato, M. Tamura, K. Houkin, I. Koyanagi, H. Abe, Analysis of optical signals evoked by peripheral nerve stimulation in rat somatosensory cortex: dynamic changes in hemoglobin concentration and oxygenation, J. Cereb. Blood Flow Metab. 19 (1999) 246–259.

[20] E. Shtoyerman, A. Arieli, H. Slovin, I. Vanzetta, A. Grinvald, Long-term optical imaging and spectroscopy reveal mechanisms underlying the intrinsic signal and stability of cortical maps in V1 of behaving monkeys, J. Neurosci. 20 (2000) 8111–8121.

[21] S.R. Arridge, M. Cope, D.T. Delpy, The theoretical basis for the determination of optical pathlengths in tissue: temporal and frequency analysis, Phys. Med. Biol. 37 (1992) 1531–1560.

[22] E. Gratton, S. Fantini, M.A. Franceschini, G. Gratton, M. Fabiani, Measurements of scattering and absorption changes in muscle and brain, Philos. Trans. R. Soc. London, Ser. B 352 (1997) 727–735.

[23] S.J. Matcher, M. Cope, D.T. Delpy, In vivo measurements of the wavelength-dependence of tissue scattering coefficients between 760 and 900 nm measured with time-resolved spectroscopy, Appl. Opt. 36 (1997) 386–396.

[24] J. Mayhew, Y. Zheng, Y. Hou, B. Vuksanovic, J. Berwick, S. Askew, P. Coffey, Spectroscopic analysis of changes in remitted illumination: the response to increased neural activity in brain, Neuroimage 10 (1999) 304–326.

[25] M. Kohl, U. Lindauer, G. Royl, M. Kühl, L. Gold, A. Villringer, U. Dirnagl, Physical model for the spectroscopic analysis of cortical intrinsic optical signals, Phys. Med. Biol. 45 (2000) 3749–3764.

[26] C. Sato, M. Nemoto, M. Tamura, Reassessment of activity-related optical signals by an algorithm including wavelength-dependent path length. Submitted, 2001.

[27] U. Lindauer, G. Royl, C. Leithner, M. Kühl, L. Gold, J. Gethmann, M. Kohl-Bareis, A. Villringer, U. Dirnagl, No evidence for early decrease in blood oxygenation in rat whisker cortex in response to functional activation, Neuroimage 13 (2001) 988–1001.

[28] I. Vanzetta, A. Grinvald, Evidence and no evidence for the initial dip in the anesthetized rat; implications for human functional brain imaging, Neuroimage 13 (2001) 959–967.

[29] T. Ernst, J. Hennig, Observation of a fast response in functional MR, Magn. Reson. Med. 32 (1994) 146–149.

[30] R.S. Menon, S. Ogawa, X. Hu, J.P. Strupp, P. Anderson, K. Ugurbil, BOLD based functional MRI at 4 Tesla includes a capillary bed contribution: echo-planar imaging correlates with previous optical imaging using intrinsic signals, Magn. Reson. Med. 33 (1985) 453–459.

[31] X. Hu, T.H. Le, K. Ugurbil, Evaluation of the early response in fMRI in individual subjects using short stimulus duration, Magn. Reson. Med. 37 (1997) 877–884.

[32] N.K. Logothetis, H. Guggenberger, S. Peled, J. Pauls, Functional imaging of the monkey brain, Nat. Neurosci. 2 (1999) 555–562.

[33] D.S. Kim, T.Q. Doung, S.G. Kim, High-resolution mapping of iso-orientation columns by fMRI, Nat. Neurosci. 3 (2000) 164–199.

[34] E. Yacoub, X. Hu, Detection of the early negative response in f-MRI at 1.5 Tesla, Magn. Reson. Med. 41 (1999) 1088–1092.

[35] J. Frahm, H. Bruhn, K.D. Merboldt, W. Haenicke, Dynamic MRI of human brain oxygenation during rest and photic stimulation, J. Magn. Reson. Imaging 2 (1992) 501–505.

[36] P. Fransson, G. Kruger, K.D. Merboldt, J. Frahm, Temporal characteristics of oxygenation-sensitive MRI responses to visual activation in humans, Magn. Reson. Med. 39 (1998) 912–919.

[37] R.B. Buxton, L.R. Frank, A model for the coupling between cerebral blood flow and oxygen metabolism during neural stimulation, J. Cereb. Blood Flow Metab. 17 (1997) 64–72.

[38] R.B. Buxton, E.C. Wong, L.R. Frank, Dynamics of blood flow and oxygenation changes during brain activation: the balloon model, Magn. Reson. Med. 39 (1998) 855–864.

[39] F. Hyder, R.G. Shulman, D.L. Rothman, A model for the regulation of cerebral oxygen delivery, J. Appl. Physiol. 85 (1998) 554–564.

[40] J.B. Mandeville, J.J. Marota, C. Ayata, G. Zaharchuk, M.A. Moskowitz, B.R. Rosen, R.M. Weisskoff, Evidence for a cerebrovascular postarteriolar windkessel with delayed compliance, J. Cereb. Blood Flow Metab. 19 (1999) 679–689.

[41] K.J. Friston, A. Mechelli, R. Turner, C.J. Price, Nonlinear responses in fMRI: the Balloon model, Volterra kernels, and other hemodynamics, Neuroimage 12 (2000) 466–477.

[42] M. Pawlowski, D.F. Wilson, Monitoring of the oxygen pressure in the blood of live animals using the oxygen dependent quenching of phosphorescence, Adv. Exp. Med. Biol. 316 (1992) 179–185.

[43] D. Malonek, U. Dirnagl, U. Lindauer, K. Yamada, I. Kanno, A. Grinvald, Vascular imprints of neuronal activity: relationships between the dynamics of cortical blood flow, oxygenation, and volume changes following sensory stimulation, Proc. Natl. Acad. Sci. U. S. A. 94 (1997) 14826–14831.

[44] D.S. Kim, Can current fMRI techniques reveal the micro-architecture of cortex, Nat. Neurosci. 3 (2000) 414.

[45] A. Grinvald, H. Slovin, I. Vanzetta, Non-invasive visualization of Cortical Columns by f-MRI, Nat. Neurosci. 3 (2000) 105–107.

[46] N.K. Logothetis, Can current fMRI techniques reveal the micro-architecture of cortex, Nat. Neurosci. 3 (2000) 413.

[47] F.C. Cannestra, N. Pouratian, S.Y. Bookheimer, N.A. Martin, D.P. Becker, A.W. Toga, Temporal spatial differences observed by functional MRI and human intraoperative optical imaging, Cereb. Cortex. 11 (2001) 773–782.

[48] R.D. Frostig, E.E. Lieke, D.Y. Ts'o, A. Grinvald, Cortical functional architecture and local coupling between neuronal activity and the microcirculation revealed by in vivo high-resolution optical imaging of intrinsic signals, Proc. Natl. Acad. Sci. U. S. A. 87 (1990) 6082–6086.

[49] R.S. Menon, S. Ogawa, J.P. Strupp, K. Ugurbil, Ocular dominance in human V1 demonstrated by functional magnetic resonance imaging, J. Neurophysiol. 77 (1997) 2780–2787.

[50] R.S. Menon, B.G. Goodyear, Submillimeter functional localization in human striate cortex using BOLD contrast at 4 Tesla: implications for the vascular point-spread function, Magn. Reson. Med. 4 (1999) 230–235.

[51] K. Cheng, R.A. Waggoner, K. Tanaka, Patterns of ocular dominance columns as revealed by high-field (4T) functional magnetic resonance imaging (fMRI), Soc. Neurosci. Abstr. 25 (1999) 572.3 (Abstract).

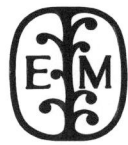

International Congress Series 1235 (2002) 155–163

Simultaneous measurements of brain tissue pO_2 and cerebral blood flow during functional stimulation[☆]

Beau M. Ances [a,*], Donald G. Buerk [b], Joel H. Greenberg [a,c], John A. Detre [a,c]

[a]*Department of Neurology, University of Pennsylvania School of Medicine, 3400 Spruce Street, Philadelphia, PA 19104, USA*
[b]*Department of Physiology and Bioengineering, University of Pennsylvania School of Medicine, 3400 Spruce Street, Philadelphia, PA 19104, USA*
[c]*Cerebrovascular Research Center, University of Pennsylvania School of Medicine, 3400 Spruce Street, Philadelphia, PA 19104, USA*

Abstract

Simultaneous partial pressure of tissue oxygen (pO_2) and laser Doppler (LD) flowmetry measurements of cerebral blood flow (CBF) were obtained from the rat somatosensory cortex during periodic electrical forepaw stimulation of either 1-min or 4-s duration. For both stimulus durations, a transient significant decrease or "initial dip" in tissue pO_2 preceded blood flow changes, followed by a peak in blood flow and an overshoot in tissue pO_2. A sustained poststimulus undershoot in tissue pO_2 was observed only for the 1-min stimulus. The magnitude of this poststimulus tissue pO_2 decrease was significantly greater than the "initial dip" observed after stimulus onset, suggesting that relative tissue hypoxia alone does not mediate blood flow changes observed with functional stimulation. Our results suggest a complex dynamic relationship between oxygen utilization and blood flow exists during functional stimulation. © 2002 Elsevier Science B.V. All rights reserved.

Keywords: Tissue oxygen electrode; Cerebral blood flow; Laser Doppler flowmetry

1. Introduction

The coupling between functional stimulation and regional changes in cerebral blood flow (CBF) and cerebral metabolism has been recognized for over a century, although the

Abbreviations: CBF, cerebral blood flow; CMRO$_2$, cerebral metabolic rate of oxygen; LD, laser Doppler.
☆ Adapted from Ances et al., Temporal Dynamics of Brain Tissue pO_2 During Functional Stimulation, *Neuroscience Letters 306 (2001) 106–110.*
* Corresponding author. Tel.: +1-215-662-7341; fax: +1-215-614-1927.
E-mail address: bances@mail.med.upenn.edu (B.M. Ances).

specific mediators and modulators involved have not been elucidated [21]. Controversy exists concerning the relative extents of the increases in CBF and cerebral metabolic rate of oxygen ($CMRO_2$) during functional activation. Protracted functional activation paradigms in both humans and animals have demonstrated small or no task-induced increases in $CMRO_2$ [7], or comparable CBF and $CMRO_2$ changes [16,19].

With the advent of functional magnetic resonance imaging (fMRI), the blood oxygenation level dependent (BOLD) contrast technique has heightened interest in better defining the temporal dynamics of CBF and $CMRO_2$ changes for the purpose of modeling the expected BOLD contrast responses. Early investigations of the temporal dynamics of the blood flow response were performed in the cat visual cortex using near-infrared optical spectroscopy and spectroscopic imaging techniques [8,14]. These optical imaging techniques, which are primarily sensitive to changes in the concentrations of intravascular oxyhemoglobin and deoxyhemoglobin, demonstrated an early decrease in oxyhemoglobin, an "initial dip", followed by a later less localized washout increase in oxyhemoglobin due to flow increases. This "initial dip" has subsequently been confirmed using oxygen-dependent phosphorescence quenching [20] that is sensitive to the partial pressure of intravascular oxygen. However, the extent to which intravascular oxygen changes accurately reflect tissue changes and the applicability of these observations to other brain regions and species remains uncertain as some groups using BOLD-fMRI have not observed this "initial dip" [15,18].

The partial pressure of tissue oxygen (pO_2) can be measured using O_2 microelectrodes, which have relatively rapid response times (ms) that are accurate to low microvascular oxygen pressures (<0.1 Torr), and can be used in vivo [4]. Laser Doppler flowmetry (LD) and an O_2 microelectrode previously were used simultaneously to monitor blood flow and tissue pO_2 changes in the cat optic nerve during photic stimulation [3]. We have characterized the magnitude and localization of functional activation induced blood flow changes in the somatosensory cortex using a rat forepaw stimulation model [1]. To further characterize the changes in tissue O_2 and blood flow during functional activation, we used an O_2 microelectrode in conjunction with LD over the somatosensory cortex of rats during electrical forepaw stimulation.

2. Methods and materials

Under 1–2% halothane anesthesia, adult Sprague–Dawley rats ($n=6$) were tracheostomized and mechanically ventilated. A tail artery catheter was placed, the scalp retracted, and the skull thinned. A small amount of thinned skull and underlying dura was removed from an area 5-mm lateral to bregma. Anesthesia was maintained using 60 mg/kg of α-chloralose i.p., followed by hourly supplemental doses of 30 mg/kg. Electrical forepaw stimulation was performed using two subdermal needle electrodes inserted into the dorsal forepaw. A function generator was used to control the stimulus frequency with frequency fixed at 5 Hz while the stimulus amplitude was maintained at 2.0 mA using a constant current dense stimulus isolation device.

Recessed gold microsensors [22] were fabricated from glass micropipettes with tip dimensions ~ 3–7 μm and recesses ~ 20–50 μm deep. An O_2 microelectrode was inserted into the brain and the LD probe was positioned adjacent to the microelectrode. The O_2 microelectrode was inserted at various levels (200–400 μm deep) into the somatosensory cortex. Simultaneous flow and tissue pO_2 measurements were made for repetitive periodic stimulation trials of either 1 min of stimulation and 1-min interstimulus interval or 4 s of stimulation with a 20-s interstimulus interval. All data were recorded on a virtual instrument using an analog to digital converter. A single trial consisted of 10 iterations with at least two trials performed for each electrode depth. Signal averaging was performed across multiple periodic trials to increase the signal to noise. The signal averaged flow and tissue pO_2 data were converted to percent changes from baseline by dividing the average baseline value obtained over the 2 s prior to stimulation. Overall averages for both blood flow and tissue pO_2 for all rats were determined along with intersubject standard errors.

3. Results

Physiological variables measured during the stimulation paradigm were (mean±S.E.M), pH=7.39±0.02, P_aCO_2=39.0±0.6 mm Hg, P_aO_2=123±2 mm Hg. The overall signal averaged time courses of changes in tissue pO_2 and relative blood flow in the somato-sensory cortex during 1-min forepaw stimulation with a 1-min interstimulus interval are

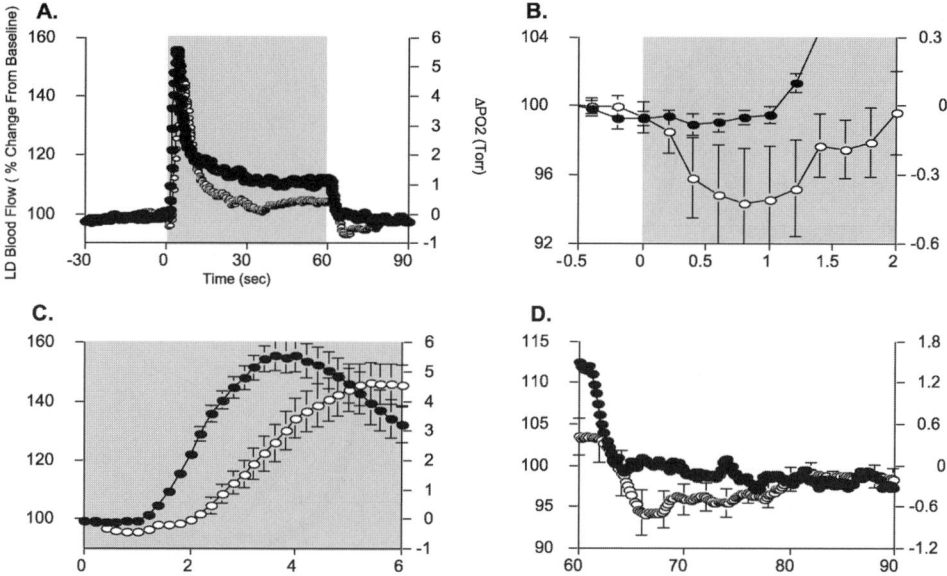

Fig. 1. (A) Overall time course of the signal averaged changes in cerebral blood flow (CBF) (●) and partial pressure of tissue oxygen (pO_2) (○) during 1 min of forepaw stimulation with a 1-min interstimulus interval. (B) The initial 2 s after the onset of forepaw stimulation for CBF and tissue pO_2. (C) The peak responses for both CBF and tissue pO_2. (D) The poststimulus time period for both CBF and tissue pO_2. For all figures, the shaded area represents the 1-min stimulation period. Error bars indicate standard error for all figures (From Ances et al., *Neuroscience Letters, in press*).

shown in Fig. 1A. Functional stimulation led to a rapid peak in flow and tissue pO_2 followed by a much lower magnitude plateau for both measurements over the final 30 s of the stimulus. Fig. 1B shows the early temporal responses of flow and tissue pO_2 changes during the first 2 s of stimulation. Shortly after the stimulus onset, tissue pO_2 decreased from baseline prior to blood flow changes. As shown in Fig. 1C, the maximum flow response of 155.8±5.9% of baseline blood flow was at 4.0±0.3 s, and is comparable to previous results [2]. This increase in flow was accompanied by a delayed increase in tissue pO_2 with the maximum change (4.6±0.7 Torr) occurring 5.6±0.2 s after stimulus onset. A mismatch between flow changes and tissue oxygen utilization occurs during the first few seconds of stimulation. The peak increase in tissue pO_2 was ~11-fold larger than the "initial dip" in tissue pO_2. At the end of protracted stimulation, tissue pO_2 remained only slightly above the prestimulus baseline, while blood flow was maintained at 10±2% of baseline (Fig. 1D). These results suggest that during steady-state stimulation, blood flow increases are reasonably well matched to increases in tissue oxygen utilization. The relatively greater increase in blood flow versus tissue pO_2 may be attributable to a decrease in oxygen extraction fraction [5,6]. During the poststimulus period, blood flow rapidly returned to baseline while a prominent undershoot was observed in tissue pO_2, and presumably reflects an increase in tissue oxygen metabolism required to compensate for a metabolic debt incurred with protracted stimulation [9,12]. The magnitude of this

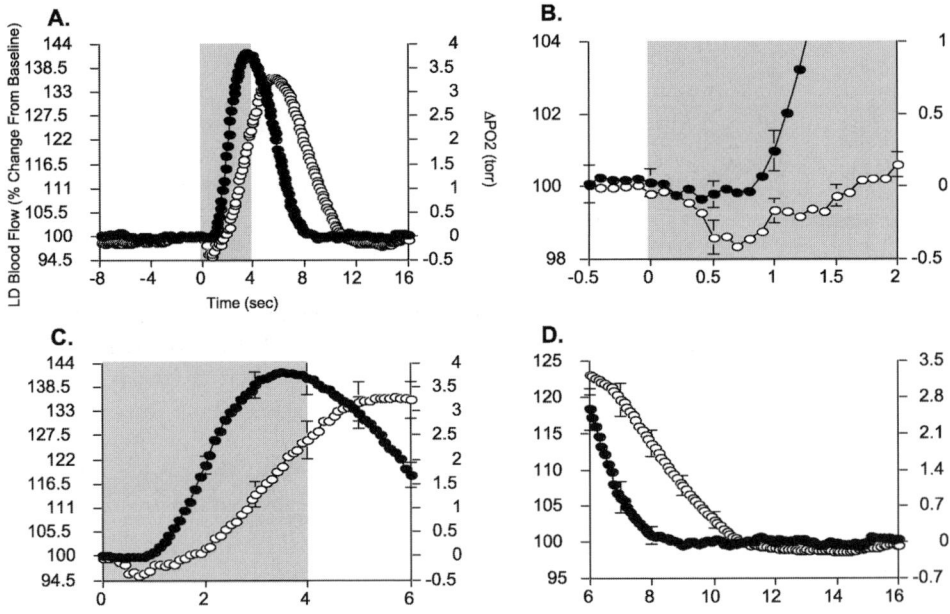

Fig. 2. (A) Overall time course of CBF (●) and tissue pO_2 (○) (relative to a baseline) for 4 s of forepaw stimulation with a 20-s interstimulus interval. For both responses, a peak was observed. (B) The initial 2 s after the onset of forepaw stimulation for CBF and tissue pO_2. (C) The peak responses for both CBF and tissue pO_2. (D) The poststimulus time period for CBF and tissue pO_2. The shaded area represents the 4-s stimulation period and error bars indicate standard error for all figures (From Ances et al., Neuroscience Letters, in press).

poststimulus tissue pO_2 decrease (-0.71 ± 0.31 Torr at 66.4 s) was significantly greater than the initial decrease (-0.42 ± 0.24 Torr) observed after the stimulus onset and was not accompanied by changes in blood flow, suggesting that relative tissue hypoxia alone does not mediate flow changes observed with functional stimulation.

Fig. 2A shows the overall signal averaged flow and tissue pO_2 results for a shorter stimulus paradigm consisting of 4 s of stimulation with a 20-s interstimulus interval. Peaks in blood flow expressed as a percent of the baseline and changes in tissue pO_2 resemble those seen for the longer stimulus. The early temporal sequence of blood flow and tissue pO_2 for the 4-s stimulus was also similar to longer stimulus results, with a decrease in tissue pO_2 occurring prior to flow changes (Fig. 2B). As seen in Fig. 2C, a large flow response again preceded the tissue pO_2 overshoot. A lag of 1.9 ± 0.2 s between the peak in flow and tissue pO_2 could reflect the capillary transit time required for O_2 to diffuse out of the blood into the tissue. For the 4-s stimulus, a prominent poststimulus undershoot was not observed in tissue pO_2 (Fig. 2D). Our data suggest that the metabolic debt incurred for the 4-s stimulus may be less than that for the 1-min stimulus, and is comparable to our previous study in which both the flow response and neural activity, as measured by somatosensory evoked potentials, were shown not to be refractory for a periodic 4-s stimulus with a 20-s interstimulus interval [1].

4. Conclusion

These simultaneous measurements of blood flow and tissue pO_2 during functional stimulation confirm the presence of an early decrease, or "initial dip", in tissue pO_2 in rat somatosensory cortex, indicating an early rise in $CMRO_2$. For both stimulus durations tested, the temporal dynamics of the changes in tissue pO_2 were similar to the results obtained using intravascular tracers in the cat visual cortex [8,14,20]. Our results suggest that the "initial dip" in tissue pO_2 is generalizable to other brain regions besides the primary visual cortex, and that intravascular measures accurately reflect tissue pO_2 changes. The failure to reliably observe an "initial dip" using BOLD-fMRI or optical imaging outside of the cat visual cortex may be attributable to richer vascularization in the visual cortex [23] and/or the increased metabolic demands of the visual cortex [17] as compared to other cortical regions.

The initial decrease in tissue pO_2 as measured by O_2 microelectrode occurred faster than those previous measurements obtained from optical imaging and oxygen phosphorescence quenching. The maximum decrease in tissue pO_2 occurred ~ 0.7 s after the onset of stimulation compared to ~ 1.5 s for optical imaging and oxygen phosphorescence studies [13,14,20]. This latency between the tissue and intravascular measurements is in agreement with previous results that have estimated the time required for oxygen to diffuse from the vasculature to the tissue [10]. In addition, our oxygen microelectrode measurements likely reflect local parenchymal changes at the site of increased neural activity [3,4], while optical imaging and oxygen phosphorescence measurements survey intravascular oxygen changes in vessels in as well as surrounding the activated region [8,20].

The initial increases in deoxyhemoglobin of the BOLD-fMRI may be a better localizer of neural activity as compared to the large delayed decrease in deoxyhemoglobin due to blood flow increases [11]. Our results suggest that the relationship between blood flow and oxygen metabolism varies considerably during functional activation. Thus, while transient changes in BOLD-fMRI may be used to improve the spatial and temporal resolution of functional neuroimaging, it may be difficult to interpret these changes quantitatively in terms of neural metabolism. However, with more protracted stimulation, blood flow changes appear to be well matched to tissue oxygen utilization.

2.3.4.7. On-Site Discussion

2.3.4.7.1. *Question: (Pelligrino)* (1) How did you measure NO? (2) Have you examined whether neuronal NOS inhibition affects the CBF response?

Answer: (Ances) (1) We measured changes in NO using a gold microsensor that was calibrated prior to experiments. Polarographic currents for the electrochemical reduction of O_2 (-650 mV relative to Ag/AgCl reference) typically ranged between 30 and 60 pA in room air equilibrated saline at 37 °C, with zero currents <1% of the room air calibration, and 90% response times <100 ms. This experimental set-up is similar to previous work by Buerk et al., Adv. Exp. Med. Biol. 1998; 454: 159) for measurement of tissue NO that was performed in the cat retina. (2) We have not attempted nNOS inhibition with these experiments of simultaneous measurements of NO and CBF using the NO electrode, and laser Doppler (LD). We do have previous data concerning the effect of nNOS inhibition on the CBF using the neuronal NOS inhibitor 7-Nitroindazole (7-NI). In these experiments, we have shown that 7-NI leads significantly reduced the CBF response while neuronal activity remained unaffected (Ances et al., J. Cereb. Blood Flow Metab. 2001; 21: P124). These results are also similar to work that has previously been performed using 7-NI (Lindauer et al., Am. J. Physiol. 1999; 277(2 Pt 2): H799).

2.3.4.7.2. *Question: (Harder)* The "Dip" is very small, for it to be relevant physiologically in needs to be amplified.

Answer: (Ances) The dip is quite small in our measurements with this initial dip approximately 1/10 in magnitude compared to later increases in tissue pO_2 as seen with an increases in CBF. Our results are different then those previously seen with oxygen phosphorescence quenching where 1/4 ratio was observed. As shown in the last scene of slides in this presentation, a potential mechanism that could relatively increase the magnitude of this initial dip would be stronger variations in the inter-stimulus interval (ISI). As we have previously shown with shorter ISIs, the relative magnitude of the initial dip increases (Ances et al., 2000; J. Cereb. Blood Flow Metab. 20: 290). Further pharmacological interventions using NOS inhibitors (as suggested in above question) will be investigated to magnify or minimize the dip.

2.3.4.7.3. *Question: (Pearce)* Did you measure and correct for differences in the time constants of measurements of both CBF and tissue pO_2? How confident are you that the relative registrations of the CBF and pO_2 signals were not out of phase?

Answer: (Ances) In these experiments, the temporal resolution of the experiments were limited by laser Doppler (LD) collection. If we had only obtained tissue pO_2 values with stimulation, we could have had a temporal resolution of milliseconds. However, since these experiments investigated the simultaneous measurements of CBF and tissue pO_2 we were limited by the temporal resolution of LD. We are quite confident that the CBF and pO_2 signals that we obtained were not out of phase.

2.3.4.7.4. *Question: (Gjedde)* In your conclusions, you mentioned that tissue pO_2 might serve as a buffer for increased $CMRO_2$ without affecting the mitochondrial pO_2. As stated in your conclusion, these results would be in agreement with calculations offered by Dr. Buxton in his opening presentation. It is of interest to know how the tissue pO_2 might be able to fall without affecting mitochondrial pO_2?

Answer: (Ances) Mitochondrial O_2 may remain elevated in the face of decreasing tissue pO_2 by a siphoning of tissue pO_2. An increase in neuronal activity will lead to an increase in metabolic requirements. In order to maintain mitochondrial O_2 that is required for metabolic processes, tissue pO_2 may decrease with O_2 flowing from the tissue into the mitochondria. Therefore, the initial dip in tissue pO_2 we observed may occur due to this siphoning of tissue pO_2 by the mitochondria. Once blood flow increases, a corresponding increase in tissue pO_2 will occur. These results are entirely consistent with the model proposed by Buxton at this meeting.

2.3.4.7.5. *Question: (Golanov)* (1) What are the reasons to choose the particular paradigm of stimulation used in experiments? Have you tried single pulse stimulation? (2) Did you try other anesthetics?

Answer: (Ances) (1) We used the paradigm of either 1-min stimulation and 1 min of interstimulus interval or 4 s of stimulation with a 20-s of interstimulus interval (ISI) as we have previous experience using these paradigm (Detre et al., Brain Research 1998; 726 (1–2): 91 and Ances et al., Neurosci. Lett. 1999; 257 (1): 25) Furthermore, we were interested at seeing if the initial dip could be seen for both short and long stimulus durations. Our paradigm allowed us to signal average our results and is similar to paradigms that we used in functional neuroimaging studies. We have not tried a single pulse experiment. However, even with one iteration (i.e. one stimulation of 4-s duration and a 20-s interstimulus interval) we were able to see thus initial dip. In the future, we plan to investigate the minimum stimulus duration required for producing the "initial dip". (2) In other experiments, we initially anesthetized the rat with halothane and then maintained anesthesia with α-chloralose. This anesthetic was chosen as α-chloralose has previously been shown to maintain the coupling of CBF and neuronal activity with functional stimulation (Ueki et al., J. Cereb. Blood Flow Metab. 1988; 8: 486). We have not attempted to use other anesthetic agents.

2.3.4.7.6. *Comment: (Bandettini)* Use of 4-s ISI is difficult to interpret. Even a predicted response is sensitive to what type of function you use as a model. So any difference between predicted and revealed may not have much meaning.

2.3.4.7.7. *Question: (Jones)* Was your data controlled for the initial brain tissue pO_2? My fear is that your results might be influenced by the wide variations possible in brain tissue. pO_2 have been noted previously by many workers (Wilson et al., J. Appl. Physiol. 1993; 74: 580; Kozniewska et al., J. Cereb. Blood Flow Metab. 1987; 7: 464; Silver. Med. Electron Biol. Eng. 1965; 3: 377; Smith et al., Microvasc. Res. 1977; 13: 233). Your dip results might be different if your probe was placed in a region with a brain pO_2 of 4 mm Hg vs. a region with a pO_2 of 40 mm Hg.

Answer: (Ances) We attempted to control for variations in the tissue pO_2 by sampling over a depth of a few microns. In these experiments we advanced the O_2 electrode from depths of 200–400 mm in order to ensure that we sampled from similar regions that were measured using the LD probe (1 mm^3). In our experiments, we did not see significant variations in the tissue pO_2 with advancement of the tissue pO_2 probe. Furthermore, tissue pO_2 values were also similar across all rats.

2.3.4.7.8. *Question: (Gaehtgens)* My question is related to the lack of synchrony between the signals for pO_2, NO and LDF. While the observations are very interesting, I think the interpretation depends on the measurements being made at identical locations in the tissue. (1) Therefore, do you have information about the precise location of your electrode, e.g. in relation to neighbouring blood vessels, etc.? (2) Since NO- and CBF-signals are clearly not "in phase" but CBF increase with a delay relative to NO, how can one conclude that NO is initiating the flow increase?

Answer: (Ances) (1) In these experiments, we placed the LD probe with a few microns of either the O_2 or NO microelectrode. Both prior to and after removal of the microelectrodes we obtained flow responses from the region from which the O_2 probe was inserted. We did not do post-mortem studies looking at the exact site of the microelectrode tip placement. We therefore cannot be sure that electrodes were not next to blood vessels. However, since we never recorded extremely elevated NO or pO_2 measurements, our results strongly suggest that we were within the tissue and not in blood vessels. (2) All of our tissue measurements had the same temporal resolution. In our results, we have shown that with stimulation there is an almost immediate increase in tissue NO after the stimulus onset. These results suggest that an increase in tissue NO occurs prior to the onset of CBF changes. With an increase in CBF, we observe a decrease in NO and our data show very similar shape curves with increases in CBF leading to decrease in NO due to a washout effect by CBF. However, the NO still remains above baseline until the end of stimulation. Once the stimulus is terminated NO decreases with an undershoot observed before returning to baseline during the understimulus interval. In the future, we plan to perform mathematical modeling concerning the relationship between the changes in NO and CBF.

Acknowledgements

This work was supported by MH12078, NS02079, NS337859, and EY09260.

References

[1] B.M. Ances, J.H. Greenberg, J.A. Detre, Effects of variations in interstimulus interval on activation-flow coupling response and somatosensory evoked potentials with forepaw stimulation in the rat, J. Cereb. Blood Flow Metab. 20 (2000) 290–297.

[2] B.M. Ances, D.F. Wilson, J.H. Greenberg, J.A. Detre, Dynamic changes in cerebral blood flow, O_2 tension,

and calculated cerebral metabolic rate of O_2 during functional activation using oxygen phosphorescence quenching, J. Cereb. Blood Flow Metab. 21 (5) (2001) 511–516.

[3] D.G. Buerk, D.N. Atochin, C.E. Riva, Simultaneous tissue pO_2, nitric oxide, and laser Doppler blood flow measurements during neuronal activation of optic nerve, Adv. Exp. Med. Biol. 454 (1998) 159–164.

[4] D.G. Buerk, P. Nair, PtiO$_2$ and CMRO$_2$ changes in cortex and hippocampus of aging gerbil brain, J. Appl. Physiol. 74 (1993) 1723–1728.

[5] R.B. Buxton, L.R. Frank, A model for the coupling between cerebral blood flow and oxygen metabolism during neural stimulation, J. Cereb. Blood Flow Metab. 17 (1997) 64–72.

[6] R.B. Buxton, E.C. Wong, L.R. Frank, Dynamics of blood flow and oxygenation changes during brain activation: the balloon model, Magn. Reson. Med. 39 (1998) 855–864.

[7] P.T. Fox, M.E. Raichle, Focal physiological uncoupling of cerebral blood flow and oxidative metabolism during somatosensory stimulation in human subjects, Proc. Natl. Acad. Sci. U. S. A. 83 (1986) 1140–1144.

[8] A. Grinvald, E. Leike, R.D. Frostig, C.D. Gilbert, T.N. Weisel, Functional architecture of the cortex revealed by optical imaging of intrinsic signals, Nature 324 (1986) 269–271.

[9] J. Hamer, K. Wiedemann, H. Berlet, F. Weinhardt, S. Hoyer, Cerebral glucose and energy metabolism, cerebral oxygen consumption, and blood flow in arterial hypoxaemia, Acta Neurochir. 44 (1978) 151–160.

[10] A.G. Hudetz, Mathematical model of oxygen transport in the cerebral cortex, Brain Res. 817 (1999) 75–83.

[11] D.S. Kim, T.Q. Duong, S.G. Kim, High-resolution mapping of iso-orientation columns by fMRI [see comments], Nat. Neurosci. 3 (2000) 164–169.

[12] D. Kintner, J.H. Fitzpatrick, J.A. Louie Jr., D.D. Gilboe, Cerebral oxygen and energy metabolism during and after 30 minutes of moderate hypoxia, Am. J. Physiol. 247 (1984) E475–E482.

[13] D. Malonek, U. Dirnagl, U. Lindauer, K. Yamada, I. Kanno, A. Grinvald, Vascular imprints of neuronal activity: relationships between the dynamics of cortical blood flow, oxygenation, and volume changes following sensory stimulation, Proc. Natl. Acad. Sci. U. S. A. 94 (1997) 14826–14831.

[14] D. Malonek, A. Grinvald, Interactions between electrical activity and cortical microcirculation revealed by imaging spectroscopy; implications for functional brain mapping, Science 272 (1996) 551–554.

[15] J.J. Marota, C. Ayata, M.A. Moskowitz, R.M. Weisskoff, B.R. Rosen, J.B. Mandeville, Investigation of the early response to rat forepaw stimulation, Magn. Reson. Med. 41 (1999) 247–252.

[16] S. Marrett, H. Fujita, E. Meyer, L. Ribeiro, A. Evans, H. Kuwabara, A. Gjedde, Stimulus specific increases of oxidative metabolism in human visual cortex, in: K. Uemura, N.A. Lassen, T. Jones, I. Kanno (Eds.), Quantification of Brain Function. Tracer Kinetics and Image Analysis in Brain PET, Elsevier, New York, 1993, pp. 217–228.

[17] T.M. Preuss, J.H. Kaas, Cytochrome oxidase 'blobs' and other characteristics of primary visual cortex in a lemuroid primate, *Cheirogaleus medius*, Brain Behav. Evol. 47 (1996) 103–112.

[18] A.C. Silva, S.P. Lee, C. Iadecola, S.G. Kim, Early temporal characteristics of cerebral blood flow and deoxyhemoglobin changes during somatosensory stimulation, J. Cereb. Blood Flow Metab. 20 (2000) 201–206.

[19] L. Sokoloff, R. Mangold, R.L. Wechsler, C. Kennedy, S. Kety, The effects of mental activation cerebral circulation and metabolism, J. Clin. Invest. 34 (1955) 1101–1108.

[20] I. Vanzetta, A. Grinvald, Increased cortical oxidative metabolism due to sensory stimulation: implications for functional brain imaging, Science 286 (1999) 1555–1558.

[21] A. Villringer, U. Dirnagl, Coupling of brain activity and cerebral blood flow: basis of functional neuro-imaging, Cereb. Brain Metab. Rev. 7 (1995) 240–276.

[22] W.J. Whalen, J. Riley, P. Nair, A microelectrode for measuring intracellular pO_2, J. Appl. Physiol. 23 (1967) 798–801.

[23] D. Zheng, A.S. LaMantia, D. Purves, Specialized vasculaturization of the primate visual cortex, J. Neurosci. 91 (1991) 2622–2629.

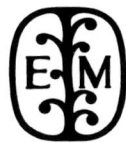

International Congress Series 1235 (2002) 165–171

Contribution of blood volume changes to intrinsic optical signals

Fukuda Mitsuhiro, Rajagopalan Uma Maheswari,
Homma Ryota, Tanifuji Manabu*

Laboratory for Integrative Neural Systems, Brain Science Institute, RIKEN, 2-1, Wako, Saitama 351-0198, Japan

Abstract

Hemodynamic responses evoked by neural activation are used to visualize active brain areas in various functional brain imaging techniques, such as PET, fMRI and intrinsic signal imaging. Though the major focus of these techniques is spatial localization of the active areas, the spatial precision of hemodynamic responses is not well understood. The purpose of this study was to investigate the spatial precision of hemodynamic responses by using intrinsic signal imaging. In particular, we focused on activity-dependent changes in the blood volume. We visualized sub-millimeter-scale functional structures such as orientation columns in the feline visual cortex using intrinsic signal imaging. To investigate the spatial precision of changes in the blood volume, we extracted the blood volume component from intrinsic signals using the Beer–Lambert equation, and directly visualized changes in the blood volume by observing absorption changes of an extrinsic dye infused into the bloodstream. In both cases, we succeeded in visualizing sub-millimeter-scale functional structures as changes in the blood volume. Taking into account that spatial separation of arteries is coarser than the spatial layout of sub-millimeter-scale functional structures, we believe these results suggest that there are supplementary control mechanisms of blood flow, probably in the capillary beds, in addition to arterial global control. © 2002 Elsevier Science B.V. All rights reserved.

Keywords: Hemodynamic responses; Capillary; Beer–Lambert law; Orientation column; Visual cortex

1. Introduction

Recent functional brain imaging techniques (PET, fMRI, intrinsic signal imaging) rely on hemodynamic responses induced by neural activities [1]. Researchers have debated whether the individual components of hemodynamic responses are precise enough to

---

* Corresponding author. Tel.: +81-48-462-1111; fax: +81-48-462-4696.
E-mail address: tanifuji@postman.riken.go.jp (T. Manabu).

allow the visualization of sub-millimeter-scale functional structures [2–4]. In this study, we examined the spatial precision of hemodynamic responses; in particular changes in blood volume, by using intrinsic signal imaging. First, we recorded intrinsic signals from the feline visual cortex at the following wavelengths 540, 570 and 620 nm simultaneously, and we then decomposed the signals into their components based on the Beer–Lambert equation. The analysis showed that spatial patterns of changes in the blood volume were almost identical to the sub-millimeter-scale functional structures revealed by the intrinsic signals. We also injected an absorption dye into the feline bloodstreams and visualized the spatial patterns of changes in the blood volume as dye-specific absorption changes. The contrast in images of the functional structures was enhanced under the presence of the absorption dye. These results suggest that the changes in blood volume have enough precision to allow the visualization of sub-millimeter-scale functional structures. Since the spatial separation of arteries is larger than 500 μm, we hypothesize that there are blood flow fine-control mechanisms in the capillaries, in addition to the global control of blood flow in the arteries.

2. Materials and methods

2.1. Measurement of intrinsic signals

We recorded intrinsic signals at the wavelengths of 540, 570 and 620 nm simultaneously, from anesthetized feline visual cortices. Orthogonal grating patterns were presented binocularly in the whole feline visual fields to induce intrinsic signals in the visual cortex. We analyzed the intrinsic signals as changes in light reflection ($\Delta R/R$), where ΔR is the difference between the intensity of reflected light after and before stimulus onset and R is the intensity of reflected light before stimulus onset.

In order to evaluate the spatial localization of the intrinsic signals and their components, we generated differential images by mutual subtraction of the two responses evoked by the orthogonal orientation stimuli. The differential images gave activity patches, which were specific for one of two orientations.

2.2. Spectroscopic analysis

We used the following equation to quantify the changes in the concentrations of oxyhemoglobin (oxyHb) and deoxyhemoglobin (deoxyHb).

$$\Delta OD_\lambda \approx \varepsilon_\lambda^{\text{oxyHb}} \cdot d \cdot \Delta[\text{oxyHb}] + \varepsilon_\lambda^{\text{deoxyHb}} \cdot d \cdot \Delta[\text{deoxyHb}] + \text{residual},$$

where d and ε_λ represent the path length and the absorption coefficients of each component at wavelength λ, respectively. In the equation, a change in light reflection is expressed by a change in optical density (OD). Changes in the blood volume were defined as changes in the total hemoglobin concentration, that is, the sum of oxyHb and deoxyHb concentration changes.

2.3. Measurement of changes in blood volume

In general, changes in the total hemoglobin concentration are associated with changes in the plasma volume [5]. To measure changes in the blood volume as changes in the plasma volume, we injected an absorption dye intravenously that has a broadband absorption spectrum (Nigrosin, water-soluble Acid Black 2, Sigma: 20–34 mg/kg). Then, we measured the changes in plasma volume as the dye-specific absorption changes. The absorption changes were recorded at 620 nm, where light absorption by hemoglobin was relatively small.

3. Results

3.1. Stimulus-specific and -non-specific parts of intrinsic signals

A typical example of intrinsic signals is shown in the gray-scale images in Fig. 1, where darkening indicates decreased reflection. Although, neurons selective to a particular orientation are localized in 500-μm patches, a grating pattern having horizontal orientation, evoked initial darkening of the entire cortex (Fig. 1b). Similar responses were also obtained by an orthogonal stimulus. However, if we look at the spatial profiles of the reflection

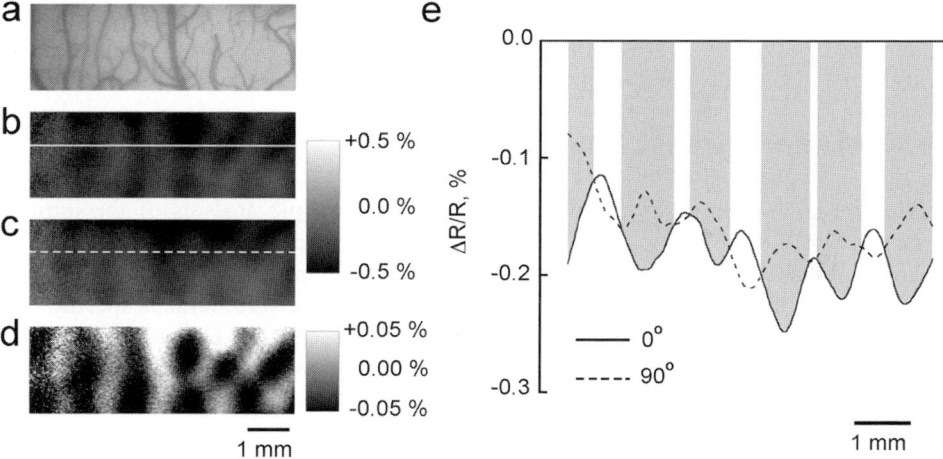

Fig. 1. Stimulus-specific and -non-specific parts of intrinsic signal. (a) The image of the cortical surface at 540 nm. (b and c) Non-specific parts of the intrinsic signals at 2.0 s after the stimulus onset recorded at 620 nm. The signals were induced by grating stimuli, which have orientations of horizontal (0°) and vertical (90°), respectively. (d) The stimulus-specific part of the intrinsic signal revealed by subtracting the image c from the image b. Black and white patches were regions selective to bars of 0° and 90° orientations, respectively. Dark gray (darkening) indicates a decrease of light reflection. (e) Spatial profiles of the intrinsic signals along solid and broken lines in the images of b and c, respectively. In the shaded regions, the stimulus having 0° orientation evoked more darkening than the orthogonal stimulus. The negative values in $\Delta R/R$ indicate a decrease of light reflection relative to reflected light intensity before the stimulus onset.

changes along solid and broken lines in Fig. 1b and c, we note stimulus-specific modulations (Fig. 1e). For example, in the shaded areas the grating pattern having horizontal
orientation evoked more darkening than the orthogonal grating pattern. This relation was
the opposite in the non-shaded areas. Therefore, subtracting one response from another
evoked by orthogonal orientation stimuli gave black and white patches, corresponding to
electrophysiologically identifiable orientation-selective columns (Fig. 1d). In summary,
intrinsic signals consist of stimulus-specific and -non-specific parts. The spatial layout of
the stimulus-specific part can be visualized with a differential image in primary visual
cortex. Taking into account the fact that deoxyHb has larger absorption at 620 nm than that
of oxyHb (Fig. 1f), intrinsic signals at 620 nm suggest that there are stimulus-specific and -
non-specific increases of deoxyHb concentration evoked by neural activation.

3.2. Intrinsic signals with other wavelengths

Stimulus-specific and -non-specific parts of the signals were observed at other wavelengths as well. Fig. 2a shows intrinsic signals at 540 and 570 nm recorded from the same
cortex shown in Fig. 1a. Similar to the intrinsic signal at 620 nm, we observed a non-
specific part of the intrinsic signals as global darkening of the entire cortex, and a stimulus-
specific part as differential images. The spatial patterns in these differential images were
almost identical to the image at 620 nm, which is frequently used in intrinsic signal
imaging and empirically gives a higher quality. Since oxyHb and deoxyHb have the same
absorption coefficients at 570 nm, we believe the stimulus-specific and -non-specific
increases in the blood volume were induced by neural activation. To quantitatively
examine this possibility, we recorded intrinsic signals at 540, 570 and 620 nm simultaneously, and decomposed the results into individual components.

3.3. Spectroscopic analysis of intrinsic signals

Fig. 2b shows the results obtained from the spectroscopic analysis of the intrinsic
signals in Figs. 1 and 2a. As expected from the intrinsic signals at 620 nm, the stimuli
evoked a global increase in the deoxyHb concentration across the entire primary visual
cortex, and the differential images of the deoxyHb component were stimulus specific. The
analysis also showed stimulus-specific and -non-specific changes in the blood volume
evoked by neural activation. The differential images of deoxyHb and the blood volume
components (right panels in Fig. 2b) were almost identical to the differential image at 620
nm (Fig. 1d). This suggests deoxyHb and the blood volume components had enough
precision to allow visualization of orientation-selective columns. However, spectroscopic
analysis is not accurate enough to conclude that deoxyHb and the blood volume
components have such a high spatial resolution. This is because, the model is for
transmitted light, and we do not know how well the same equation would apply in the
case of reflected light. Furthermore, the path length may not be the same among different
wavelengths. Therefore, it is necessary to confirm the results obtained from spectroscopic
analysis with other measurements [6,7], we carried out another experiment, in which, we
injected a dye intravenously and measured changes in the blood volume as dye-specific
absorption changes.

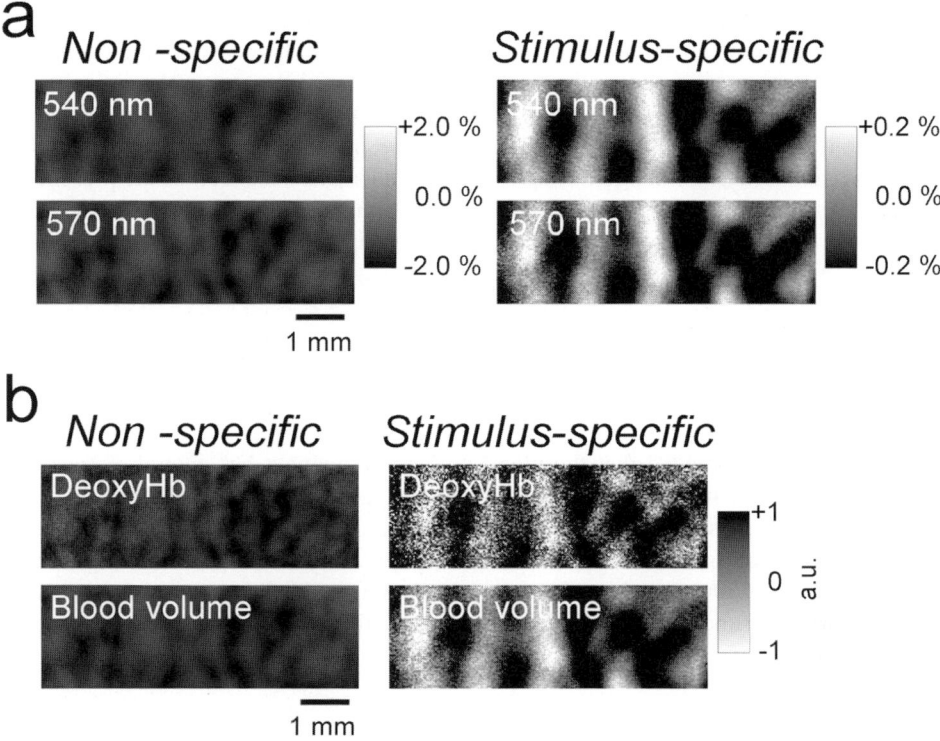

Fig. 2. (a) The intrinsic signals at 2.0 s after the stimulus onset, recorded with 540 and 570 nm. Dark gray indicates a decrease of reflection. (b) Results of spectroscopic analysis of the intrinsic signals in Fig. 1 and (a). Dark gray indicates an increase of concentration.

3.4. Measurement of plasma volume changes in the blood vessels

Injection of the dye into the bloodstream caused an absorption increase in the cortex ($17\pm3\%$, mean$\pm$SD, $n=5$). This suggests that the dye in the blood vessels contributed to

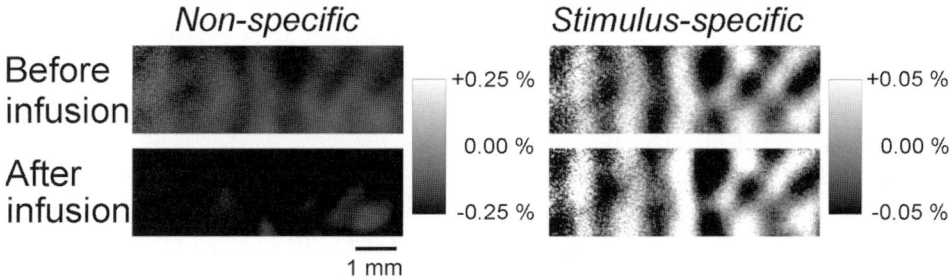

Fig. 3. Contributions of dye-specific absorption change due to the intrinsic signals at 620 nm. The images of stimulus-specific parts were band pass filtered. Other conventions as shown in Fig. 1.

the light reflection from the cortex. The results of the measurements taken of the changes in the plasma volume, as an indication of the changes in the blood volume are shown in Fig. 3. In the non-specific part of the intrinsic signals, initial decreases of light reflection doubled in size as a result of the dye injection (left panels in Fig. 3), suggesting the contribution of changes in the blood volume to the intrinsic signals. Furthermore, the contrast of the differential image of the intrinsic signals was enhanced in the presence of the dye (right panel in Fig. 3). If there were no stimulus-specific changes in the blood volume, the differential image after injection of the dye should be less clear than that before the injection. Similar results were also obtained from four other felines (data not shown).

4. Conclusion

Altogether, we concluded that the blood volume component has enough precision to allow visualization of sub-millimeter-scale functional structures. In general, the blood flow is controlled by arteries, which cause non-specific changes in the blood volume. However, the spatial separation of arteries is not enough to explain stimulus-specific changes in the blood volume at the 500-m scales. This suggests that the capillary bed exerts a fine control of blood flow that supplements the global control by the arteries.

2.3.5.6. On-Site Discussion

2.3.5.6.1. *Question: (Tomita)* The magnitude of light scattering by blood is flow-dependent. When you compare the flow in the activated condition with that of the control, there must be an enhancement. How do you compensate for this factor?

Answer: (Fukuda) As you pointed out the effect of blood flow on light transmittance in your in vitro paper (Tomita et al., Biorheology 1983; 20 (5): 485), light scattering changes by flow changes may be critical factor even in vivo. Although it's probably important to include this factor, there are, so far, no good models where this factor is incorporated. So, we took a different approach, such as direct measurement of change in blood volume to confirm our result. And we obtained a similar result by this measurement to the result obtained from our spectroscopic analysis.

Comment: (Tomita) Flow-dependent light scattering changes by blood are far larger than expected. When measured with blood in a transparent tube, the factor reached ca. 20% in terms of the extinction coefficient when the flow was increased from 50 s^{-1} (average control shear rate of blood in the microvasculature) to 80 s^{-1} (that in the core of an activated area). In the brain tissue in situ, there is no escape from this influence since blood is the largest chromophore in the tissue, and the flow-dependent optical density changes of the tissue expressed on a logarithmic scale will be of the same order of magnitude, if the optical density of the nonvascular components remains unchanged.

2.3.5.6.2. *Question: (Bandettini)* What are the dynamics of the blood volume signals? (Both with dye and without dye)

Answer: (Fukuda) We evaluated the time course of changes in blood volume in three cases: the intrinsic signals at 570 nm, decomposed signals according to Beer–Lambert equations and the dye specific changes. The dye specific changes were obtained by subtracting the intrinsic signal before dye injection from the signal after the injection. Almost identical time courses are obtained in these three cases, where the blood volume increased after the stimulus onset, reached the peak at 3.5 s, and gradually return to the baseline.

2.3.5.6.3. *Question: (Dirnangl)* Thank you for pointing out that the brain cannot be treated as a cuvette because of the wavelength-dependent deflection of photons in the tissue. One word of caution: The signal at 620 nm should not be labelled "deoxyhemoglobin", because at this wavelength the ratio of the absorption of HbR/HbO_2 is still 5/1, meaning that there is a strong interbution? by oxyhemoglobin. More sophisticated models and measurement over a wide wavelength range are needed to resolve the hemoglobin chromophores.

Answer: (Fukuda) Since, as you pointed out, the model based on Beer–Lambert equation is not accurate enough, we further examined the involvement of blood volume by the dye injection. The result showed stimulus specific changes in blood volume.

References

[1] A. Villringer, U. Dirnagl, Coupling of brain activity and cerebral blood flow: basis of functional neuroimaging, Cerebrovasc. Brain Metab. Rev. 7 (3) (1995) 240–276.
[2] D. Malonek, A. Grinvald, Interactions between electrical activity and cortical microcirculation revealed by imaging spectroscopy: implications for functional brain mapping, Science 272 (5261) (1996) 551–554.
[3] D.S. Kim, et al., High-resolution mapping of iso-orientation columns by fMRI, Nat. Neurosci. 3 (2) (2000) 164–169.
[4] N. Logothetis, Can current fMRI techniques reveal the micro-architecture of cortex? Nat. Neurosci. 3 (5) (2000) 413.
[5] A. Villringer, et al., Capillary perfusion of the rat brain cortex. An in vivo confocal microscopy study, Circ. Res. 75 (1) (1994) 55–62.
[6] U. Lindauer, et al., No evidence for early decrease in blood oxygenation in rat whisker cortex in response to functional activation, NeuroImage 13 (6) (2001) 988–1001.
[7] I. Vanzetta, A. Grinvald, Increased cortical oxidative metabolism due to sensory stimulation: implications for functional brain imaging, Science 286 (5444) (1999) 1555–1558.

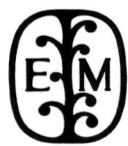

International Congress Series 1235 (2002) 173–179

Sustained microvascular flow response to functional activation in rat cerebral cortex

István Schiszler [a,*], Minoru Tomita [b], Koji Inoue [b],
Norio Tanahashi [b], Yasuo Fukuuchi [b]

[a]*Department of Physiology, Semmelweis University, Budapest, Hungary*
[b]*Department of Neurology, School of Medicine, Keio University, 35-Shinanomachi, Shinjuku, Tokyo-160, Japan*

Abstract

The flow response in the cerebral cortex with high spatial resolution during functional activation was examined employing our new optical method. We found that electrical stimulation (ES) of a hind limb increased localized microvascular flow in the contralateral somatosensory cortex in α-chloralose-anesthetized SD rats. The spatial microflow increase patterns were heterogeneous, but the size of the increased flow area was almost the same in all five cases studied. The microvascular flow increase was approximately 25% (50% at the central peak decreasing to 5% in the margin) over the cortical area of ca. 1.8 ± 0.1 mm in diameter. We also found that the time-sequential spatial extents of the activated area of the two-dimensional (2-D) flow maps were coincident with the activated area determined by changes in reflected light intensity. The local microvascular flow increase triggered by cell activation appeared to induce sustained (mismatched) flow in the associated area, even when the activated state of the neurons subsided immediately after the elimination of the peripheral stimuli. © 2002 Elsevier Science B.V. All rights reserved.

Keywords: Electrical stimulation; Intrinsic optical signal; Somatosensory cortex; Coupling between function and flow; Microflow; Two-dimensional flow map

1. Introduction

Recent studies of Malonek and Grinvald [1], Malonek et al. [2], and Nemoto et al. [3] using optical imaging revealed millisecond order of response of the cerebral cortex to peripheral sensory stimulation. Based on the activity-dependent changes in oxy- and

* Corresponding author. Tel.: +81-3-3353-1211x2316; fax: +81-3-3353-1272.
E-mail address: office@schiszler.hu (I. Schiszler).

deoxyhemoglobin, the blood volume and light scattering, sensory stimulation of the functional cortical columns were concluded by them to initiate tissue hypoxia and vascular responses. Malonek and Grinvald [1] also observed that the vascular responses were highly localized to individual cortical columns only in the early phase, and in the latter phase, they became poorly localized, spreading over distances of 2–4 mm. On the other hand, Yang et al. [4] reported that a positive BOLD signal prevailed throughout the stimulation and its location correlated well with the barrel activation determined by electrophysiological studies. Thus, the late positive BOLD signal has the same spatial pattern and dimension as the electrical activity. The imaging spectroscopy detects oxy- (HBO) and deoxyhemoglobin (HBR) concentration, but the data analysis is biased by light scattering changes observed during functional activation. The alterations in light scattering might be related to the flow-dependent light scattering alterations described by Tomita et al. [5]. The imaging spectroscopy thus detects signals of deoxyhemoglobin (HBR) and light scattering and, therefore, displays changes of metabolism and flow indiscriminately. The source of the BOLD signal is said to be from the HBR, but collocation of HBR to the metabolic site is blurred because of dilution by arterial blood or HBR spread into the venous blood. Again, it detects metabolism and flow parameters together. To solve such a complexity, the measurement of blood flow alone is indispensable. Although concomitant flow studies with optical signal detection have been carried out by Malonek et al. [2] and Nemoto et al. [3], employing laser Doppler flowmetry during activation, the poor collocation and poor spatial resolution of LDF does not satisfy the demand for detailed flow maps during activation. The present study was designed to measure only changes in microvascular flow using a new optical method [6], which permits us to display 2-D flow maps with 500 times higher spatial resolution than that of laser flowmetry. In addition, the present study allows us to compare the result with data provided by optical imaging of intrinsic signals, which can be obtained simultaneously from exactly the same location.

2. Materials and methods

Experiments were carried out on male SD rats weighing 300–350 g ($n = 10$), anesthetized by i.p. administration of 70 mg/kg α-chloralose and 0.7 g/kg urethan. The anesthesia was maintained via continuous intravenous infusion of α-chloralose at a rate of 15 mg/kg/h. Detailed techniques for measuring two-dimensional (2-D) flow maps were reported elsewhere [6–8]. One modification of the technique was that glass fiber was not inserted into the brain and the noninvasive "light reflection method" was adopted instead of the original rather invasive "light transmission method". This modification was necessary for the complete agreement with the conventional technique of optical imaging. The data acquisition and analysis were the same as those in the original method. The animals were placed on a head holder with ear bars and the right parietal region of the skull was thinned to transparency above the right parietal cortex using a dental drill. The thinned bone was covered with immersion oil and a cover glass. The region of interest (ROI) was epiilluminated using a halogen lamp through a band pass filter ($\lambda = 550 \pm 15$ nm at half maximum). An SIT camera with Nikon lens focused on the pial vessels was used to monitor the reflected light. The output of the camera was directly connected to a personal computer through an 8-bit Scion LG-3 frame grabber card so that the intensity of the reflected light (intensity of intrinsic signal at 550 nm) was continuously stored in the RAM disc. The somatosensory cortex was activated by electrical stimulation (Nihonkoden, Electronic Stimulator, SEN-3201) of the hind paw for 5 s with rectangular pulses (2 ms, 5 Hz, 2 V) through a pair of needle electrodes inserted under the skin of the left limb. To determine the regional MTT, 200 consecutive frames of saline transit (RBC transit) in each of the pixels of a 50×50 matrix in a 2×2 mm ROI were grabbed and individual hemodilution curves were analyzed by MATLAB employing a home-written algorithm. The MTTs were calculated in all 2500 pixels based on a conventional formula and arranged into 2-D flow maps. Since reciprocal MTT (or velocity) was a major factor of flow, we regarded 1/MTT in small pixels as microvascular flow and was, therefore, termed as "microflow". The spatial resolution of the flow map thus obtained with our new method is 525 microflow elements per 1 mm^2, which is almost 500 times higher than that of LDF with a 1-mm diameter flow probe. In four rats, 2-D activated microflow maps were expressed in relative flow changes from the control for standardization (2-D flow map$_{activation}$/2-D flow map$_{control}$). The flow values were not influenced by the brightness of the location since the flow values were comparable with those obtained by our light transmission method, in which we confirmed the linearity of the dye–concentration curve or the principle of superposition.

The experimental protocol started with laser Doppler flowmetry (Advance Laser Flowmeter 21R—0.5-mm probe). The position of the LDF probe was fine-tuned for

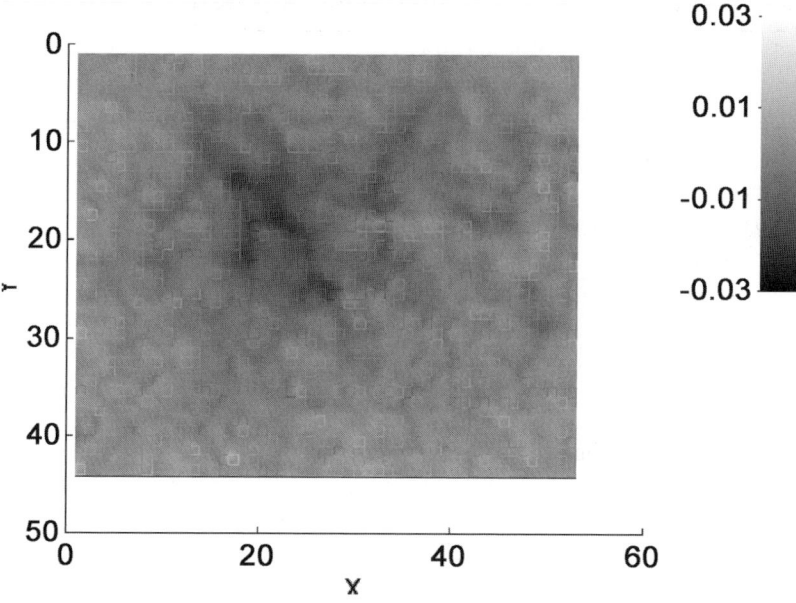

Fig. 1. Δ reflectance after 5 s of electrical stimulation of the hind paw.

maximal signal response during stimulation avoiding large pial vessels. Next, the cortical blood flow response to electrical stimulation was determined by averaging 20 trials using a Biopac MP100 AD board.

If the LDF response was acceptable (15–25% maximal increase), optical imaging was performed. The reflected light intensity was recorded for 20 s and electrical stimulation

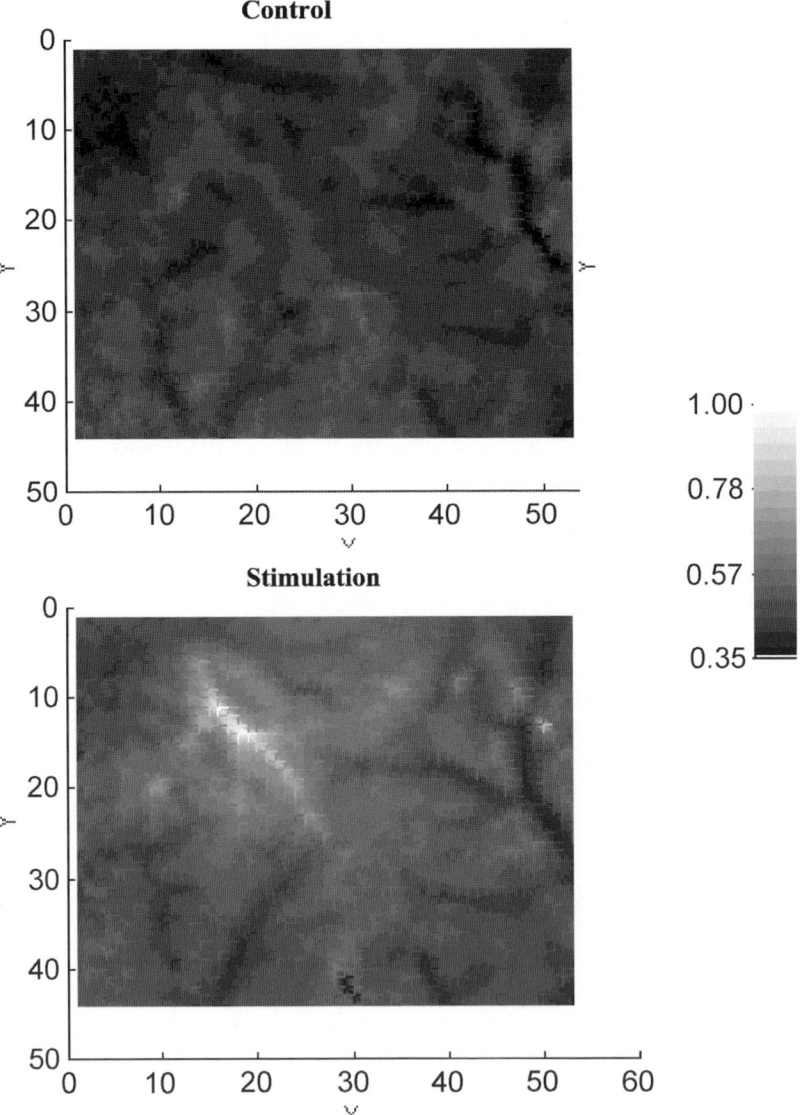

Fig. 2. 2-D velocity maps in control and after 5 s of electrical stimulation of the hind paw.

was performed during the first 5 s. The reflectance change in the ROI was calculated as follows:

$$\Delta \text{ reflectance}(t) = \log\{I_0/I_s(t)\},$$

where I_0 is the reflected light intensity in the prestimulus state and $I_s(t)$ is the reflected light intensity t seconds after the stimulus onset. The Δ reflectance images were averaged across three trials to improve the signal–noise ratio.

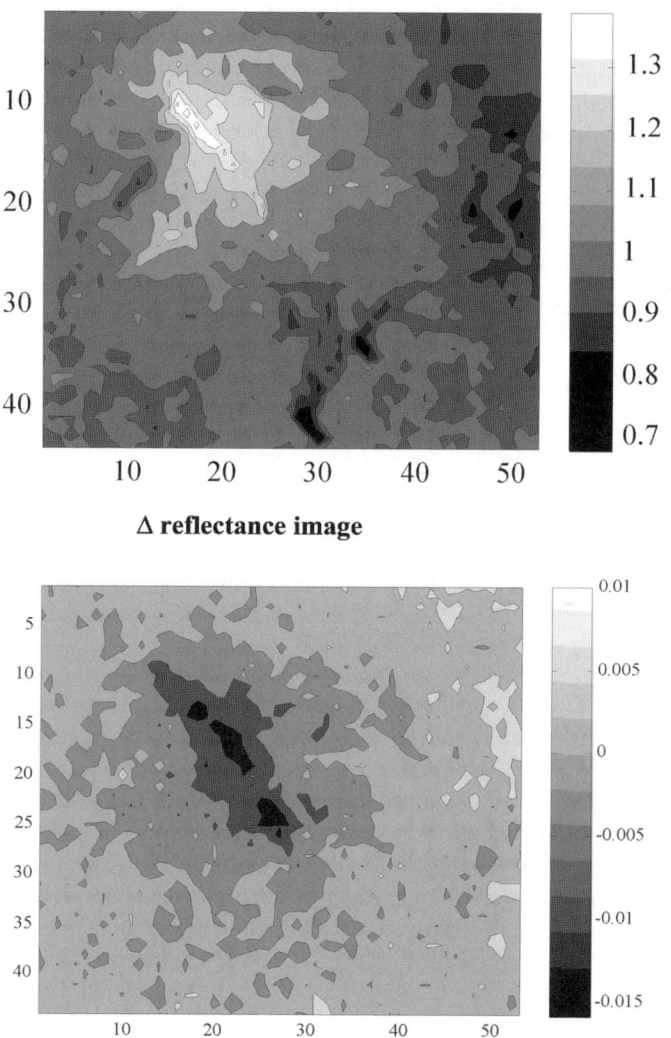

Fig. 3. Relative microflow map calculated as $MTT_{control}/MTT_{stim}$ and Δ reflectance image after 5-s stimulation.

In the last step of the experiment, MTT measurements were carried out as described above. The saline injection was performed 5 s after the stimulus onset. The 2-D MTT maps were again averaged across three trials in each animal.

3. Results

LDF: Electrical stimulation (ES) of the hind limb produced an increase in the cortical LDF in six rats and failed in four rats. After the onset of electrical stimulation, the LDF signal started to rise at 0.87 ± 0.14 s, reached a peak at 4.82 ± 1.39 s, and disappeared 9.35 ± 1.33 s, as the mean and standard deviation of the positive cases. The average LDF increase was 25%. The time courses of the LDF increase were in accord with those reported in the literature [3]. Based on the LDF activation curves, the time of saline injection was decided to be 5 s after the onset of ES.

Intrinsic signals: Activation was detected in four animals out of the six cases studied. In the tissue, the intrinsic signal at 550 nm showed a monophasic characteristic: an early increase in reflectance that started at 1.5 s after the stimulus onset and peaked at 6 s. The reflectance increase was diffuse and its spatial extent was approximately 1.2–1.8 mm. The amplitude was maximal near the center and progressively diminished peripherally (Fig. 1).

2-D flow maps: The 2-D MTT maps (Fig. 2) revealed diffuse heterogeneous flow increases. Its pattern was variable between individual cases. Similar to the intrinsic signal, the amplitude was maximal at the center of the signal ($160 \pm 19\%$, mean $\pm$ S.D.: $p < 0.01$ when compared with the control) and gradually decreased. The spatial extent was again similar with a diameter of 1.3–1.6 mm.

It was noted that the vascular geometry in the ROI was variable in all cases studied. In Fig. 3, contour plots of reflectance and relative flow maps are shown for comparison. A similar coincidence was observed in all four cases. Albeit statistical analysis was not carried out, we think the figure is convincing enough because the spatial extents of the activated area determined by the two different methods were comparable.

4. Discussion

Although the optical imaging of reflectance and the 2-D flow map were both obtained by our new optical method [6], it must be noted that they are constituted from independent elements: the optical imaging comprised optical brightness due to reflectance of the tissue in the ROI, whereas the 2-D flow map consists of reciprocal transit times of RBC (a negative tracer) through element pixels which are independent from the local brightness. The method has the merit that two independent parameters represent simultaneous changes collocated in the same ROI. We showed that the spatial extent of activation in the relative flow maps was comparable with the size of the intrinsic signals. This could partly be explained by the changes in the cerebral blood volume exaggerated by flow-dependent intravascular RBC desegregations, increasing the tissue scattering coefficient with the increase in flow during functional activation. One may argue whether intravascular RBC aggregation is present in normal conditions, but it definitely exists in the venous side of the microcirculation where the linear flow velocity is physiologically lower [9]. On the other hand, Andrew et al. [10] showed a focal increase in light transmittance across the neocortical gray slice during potassium-induced spreading depression. Neuronal activation must be accompanied by neuronal depolarization and, therefore, light transmission changes. However, the nature of the intrinsic optical signal changes in light transmission reported here must have been included in quantitative changes in deoxyhemoglobin reported in the literature.

References

[1] D. Malonek, A. Grinvald, Interactions between electrical activity and cortical microcirculation revealed by imaging spectroscopy: implications for functional brain mapping, Science 272 (5261) (1996) 551–554.

[2] D. Malonek, U. Dirnagl, U. Lindauer, K. Yamada, I. Kanno, A. Grinvald, Vascular imprints of neuronal activity: relationships between the dynamics of cortical blood flow, oxygenation, and volume changes following sensory stimulation, Proc. Natl. Acad. Sci. U. S. A. 94 (1997) 14826–14831.

[3] M. Nemoto, Y. Nomura, C. Sato, M. Tamura, K. Houkin, I. Koyanagi, H. Abe, Analysis of optical signals evoked by peripheral nerve stimulation in rat somatosensory cortex: dynamic changes in hemoglobin concentration and oxygenation, J. Cereb. Blood Flow Metab. 19 (3) (1999) 246–259.

[4] X. Yang, F. Hyder, R.G. Shulman, Functional MRI BOLD signal coincides with electrical activity in the rat whisker barrels, Magn. Reson. Med. 38 (1997) 874–877.

[5] M. Tomita, Y. Fukuuchi, N. Tanahashi, M. Kobari, M. Takao, Y. Tomita, Flow-dependent light scattering by the blood in the brain (abstract), J. Cereb. Blood Flow Metab. 19 (Suppl. 1) (1999) S722.

[6] I. Schiszler, M. Tomita, Y. Fukuuchi, N. Tanahashi, K. Inoue, New optical method for analyzing cortical blood flow heterogeneity in small animals—validation of the method, Am. J. Physiol. 279 (2000) H1291–H1298.

[7] M. Tomita, F. Gotoh, T. Amano, N. Tanahashi, M. Kobari, T. Shinohara, B. Mihara, Transfer function through regional cerebral cortex evaluated by a photoelectric method, Am. J. Physiol. 245 (3) (1983) H385–H398.

[8] M. Tomita, F. Gotoh, T. Sato, T. Amano, N. Tanahashi, K. Tanaka, M. Yamamoto, Photoelectric method for estimating hemodynamic changes in regional cerebral tissue, Am. J. Physiol. 235 (1) (1978) H56–H63.

[9] M. Cabel, H.J. Meiselman, A.S. Popel, P.C. Johnson, Contribution of red blood cell aggregation to venous vascular resistance in skeletal muscle, Am. J. Physiol. 272 (2, Pt. 2) (1997) H1020–H1032.

[10] R.D. Andrew, C.R. Jarvis, A.S. Obeidat, Potential sources of intrinsic optical signals imaged in live brain slices, Methods 18 (2) (1999) 185–196.

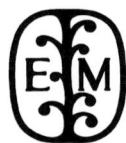

International Congress Series 1235 (2002) 181–188

Quantitative optical imaging of brain activity—human and animal studies

M. Tamura [a,*], Y. Hoshi [b], M. Nemoto [c], C. Sato [a], S. Kohri [a]

[a]Biophysics Division, Research Institute for Electronic Science, Hokkaido University, N12 W6, Kita, Sapporo 060-0812, Japan
[b]Tokyo Institute for Psychiatric Research, Tokyo, Japan
[c]Department of Neurosurgery, School of Medicine, Hokkaido University, Sapporo, Japan

Abstract

In order to overcome the problems associated with near-infrared optical imaging (NIR-imaging) such as the lack of the quantification and poor spatial resolution, we developed a 64-channel time-resolved optical imaging system, by which we could obtain quantitative functional images of human brain activity. Reflectance tomographic images of the changes in oxy-hemoglobin [oxy-Hb], deoxy-hemoglobin [deoxy-Hb], and total-hemoglobin [t-Hb] associated with neural activation were obtained, and given as absolute concentration changes. Then, the obtained optical functional images were superimposed on 3-D images of the subject's brain reconstructed from MRI, on which fMRI images were also superimposed. Very interestingly, but curiously, we found that the activation maps of [oxy-Hb] rather than [deoxy-Hb] were very reasonable and similar to those of the fMRI. The maximum increase in [oxy-Hb] due to finger tapping was about 1 μM, whereas in several cognitive tasks such as the digit span task, the increase was much larger, at 3–8 μM. The optical imaging system employed here can be applied to the subjects of all ages and be used at the bedside as well. By simplifying and miniaturizing the imaging system, we could construct a conventional single channel oxygen monitor for clinical use, by which we could quantify the changes of [oxy-, deoxy- and total Hb] during neuronal activation in each subject and, therefore, statistical analysis became possible. © 2002 Elsevier Science B.V. All rights reserved.

Keywords: Optical imaging; Near-infrared spectrophotometry; Optical computed tomography; Light scattering; Time-resolved spectrophotometry

* Corresponding author. Tel.: +81-11-706-2410; fax: +81-11-706-4964.
E-mail address: mtamura@imd.es.hokudai.ac.jp (M. Tamura).

0531-5131/02 © 2002 Elsevier Science B.V. All rights reserved.
PII: S 0 5 3 1 - 5 1 3 1 (0 2) 0 0 1 8 5 - 1

1. Introduction

The high transparency of near-infrared light into living tissue has made possible the use of near-infrared spectroscopy (NIRS) for functional mapping of the human brain [1–3]. The successful application of multichannel recording of various and specific regions has been done using simple physiological stimuli and cognitive studies [4,5]. Near-infrared spectroscopy (NIRS) measures the changes in the concentration of oxy-hemoglobin [oxy-Hb] and deoxy-hemoglobin [deoxy-Hb], mainly in cerebral mixed venous blood. The total-hemoglobin [t-Hb] is given as the summation of the changes in [oxy-Hb] and [deoxy-Hb], which reflect those in the blood volume. The changes in [oxy-Hb] and [deoxy-Hb] are related to the changes in the cerebral metabolic rates (CMRO$_2$), and the changes in [t-Hb] are related to those in the cerebral blood flow (CBF). Thus, NIRS can give us information related to CMRO$_2$ and CBF simultaneously when the brain tissue is activated.

The many problems with NIRS are, however, also clear. These are the lack of quantification, poor spatial resolution and contamination of non-specific optical signals overlapping true absorption changes. All these must be overcome, and in this paper, we summarize several problems mentioned above and show how to overcome them. Our final goal for functional optical imaging of the human brain is to construct an optical imaging system that will enable us to visualize the dynamic features of quantitative spatio-temporal variations of hemoglobin oxygenation, and blood volume.

2. Results

2.1. Tissue light scattering — animal study

Using a cranial window in a thinned skull, we analyzed the changes in optical signals associated with neuronal activity, employing multi-component analysis to obtain the changes in [oxy-], [deoxy-Hb] and tissue scattering [6]. We found that there is a large change in tissue scattering during the transition from the resting state to the activated state, which must be eliminated from the observed absorption changes due to the hemoglobin changes. A successful procedure for eliminating the artifacts of tissue scattering involved in the reflectance change was the incorporation of the wavelength-dependent optical path length into the analysis. We found that there is a so-called "initial dip" of early, small but distinct deoxygenation of the hemoglobin just after the onset of the stimulus [7]. These animal studies strongly warned us of the necessity for the correction of the wavelength dependence of tissue scattering in the absorption measurements, which must be incorporated into the algorithm of near-infrared spectroscopy and imaging of the human brain.

2.2. Scattering corrected algorithms for NIRS and NIR-imaging

In general, attenuation of the incident light in turbid media like living tissue is due to the sum of the light scattering and absorption. Therefore, the observed absorbance can be written as

$$\log(I_\lambda^0/I_\lambda) = \varepsilon_\lambda C\beta_\lambda L + S_\lambda \tag{1}$$

where I_λ^0, and I_λ are the light intensities of illuminating and transmitted, and the reflected light, respectively. ε_λ, C are the absorption coefficient and concentration of the chromophores. β_λ is the wavelength-dependent path length factor due to scattering, and L is the physical or geometrical optical path influenced by factors such as the thickness of the tissue. $\beta_\lambda L$ is the true optical path length, and S_λ is the attenuation due to light scattering.

In our activation studies, we followed the changes of [oxy- and deoxy-Hb] before and during neuronal activation. Then, we obtained the formula of Eq. (2)

$$\Delta A_\lambda(t) = \{\varepsilon_\lambda^{oxy}\Delta[\text{oxy}-\text{Hb}] + \varepsilon_\lambda^{deoxy}\Delta[\text{deoxy}-\text{Hb}](t)\}\beta_\lambda L + \Delta S_\lambda(t) \qquad (2)$$

where $\Delta A_\lambda(t)$ is the absorbance difference between the resting state (before the stimulus onset) and activated state at time t. $\Delta S_\lambda(t)$ is the difference of scattering between the two states.

In constructing our NIRS algorithm, β_λ was incorporated into the apparent absorption coefficients of [oxy-] and [deoxy-Hb], which were determined experimentally in vivo. The scattering change, $\Delta S_\lambda(t)$, could be removed by the introduction of dual-wavelength photometry [8]. Furthermore, we used three wavelengths for the measurement of [oxy-] and [deoxy-Hbs]. This is due to the fact that there are three unknown parameters in the activation study of [oxy-], [deoxy-Hbs] and scattering.

Finally, we used Eq. (3) for the NIRS and NIR-imaging of continuous wave measurements.

$$\Delta[\text{oxy}-\text{Hb}] = -3.0\Delta A_{805} + 3.0\Delta A_{830}$$

$$\Delta[\text{deoxy}-\text{Hb}] = 1.6\Delta A_{780} - 2.8\Delta A_{805} + 1.2\Delta A_{870} \qquad (3)$$

$$\Delta[\text{t}-\text{Hb}] = \Delta[\text{oxy}-\text{Hb}] + \Delta[\text{deoxy}-\text{Hb}]$$

Using Eq. (3), we systematically measured the hemodynamic responses of the human brain in response to various physiological stimuli and higher order cognitive tasks [4]. Then, we examined the fundamental questions underlying the studies of fMRI. An example is given in Fig. 1. During the neuronal activation induced by a cognitive task, the left frontal (LF) region showed the typical responses of increased [t-Hb], [oxy-Hb], and a decrease in [deoxy-Hb]. The left temporal region showed increases in [oxy-Hb] [deoxy-Hb] and [t-Hb], whereas the left occipital showed increases in [oxy-Hb] and [deoxy-Hb] but no increase in [deoxy-Hb]. These observations raised a question. Do increases in neuronal activity always accompany decreases in [deoxy-Hb]? We concluded that oxy-Hb is the best indicator for detecting neuronal activation, as it is very sensitive to the change in cerebral blood flow. An animal study using rats confirmed this [9].

2.3. Quantitative optical mapping of brain activity

To obtain the absolute values of the hemoglobin changes during neuronal activation, we must know the path length, βL, of Eq. (2) at each optode spacing. Time-resolved spec-

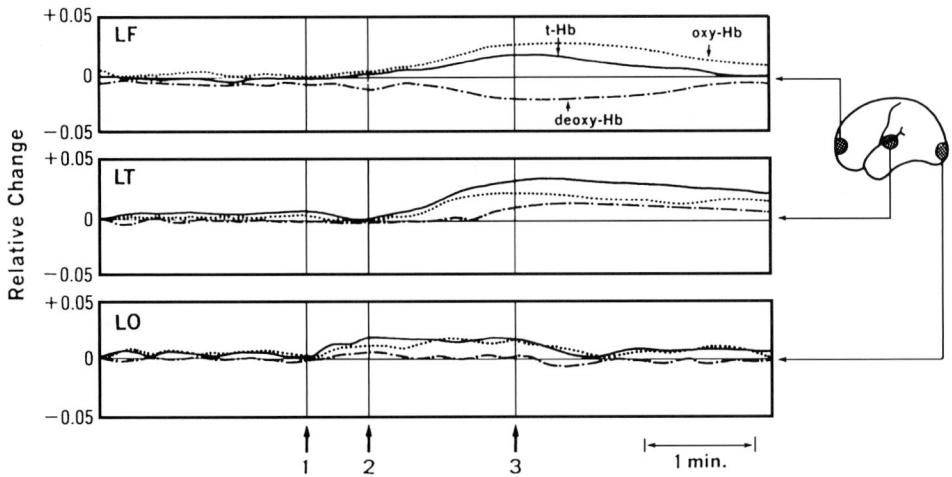

Fig. 1. Changes in regional cerebral oxygenation during the arithmetic task. Changes in the concentrations of [oxy-Hb], [deoxy-Hb] and [t-Hb] in several regions in the dominant hemisphere of a right-handed man. The ordinate is the relative amount, and abscissa is a time. Baselines were selected from the resting state, and the values were taken as zero in each signal. The upward (plus) and the downward (minus) trends show the increase and the decrease in values, respectively. The arithmetic problem was read out between the points shown by arrows 1 and 2. At the point shown by arrow 2, he started to solve it. Arrow 3 denotes the end of solving the problems. LF, LT and LO are left frontal, left temporal and left occipital, respectively [5].

troscopy, TRS, meets this demand, as time can be converted to the path length of each photon traveling through the turbid media by Eq. (4).

$$l = vt \qquad (4)$$

Where l is the optical path and v the speed of photons in the medium, i.e., 0.23 mm/ps, βL can be obtained by the mean transit time, $\langle t \rangle$, as Eq. (5)

$$\beta L = \langle L \rangle = v\langle t \rangle = v \cdot \frac{\int F(t)t\,\mathrm{d}t}{\int F(t)\,\mathrm{d}t} \qquad (5)$$

where $F(t)$ is the observed temporal profile of the time of flight of the transmitted photons.

Combined use of Eqs. (3) and (5) can, therefore, give us the absolute values of the changes in [oxy-], [deoxy-], and [t-Hb] during neuronal activation. Recently, we have developed a new 64-channel time-resolved optical tomographic imaging system, which has 3-ps pulsed laser diodes as light sources, and 64 fiber bundles that are connected to 64 corresponding time-resolved detection systems. Time-resolved measurements of each channel enabled us to determine each mean optical path length by Eq. (5), which gives quantitative values of the concentration changes of [oxy-], [deoxy-] and [t-Hb] in the brain. Then, we reconstructed the image from the multichannel data using several algebraic reconstruction algorithms.

Here, we employed our optical imaging system to show that the backward digit span (DB) task activated the dorsolateral prefrontal cortex (DLPEC) of each hemisphere more than the forward digit span (DF) task in healthy adult volunteers, and the higher performance of the DB task was closely related to the activation of the right DLPEC

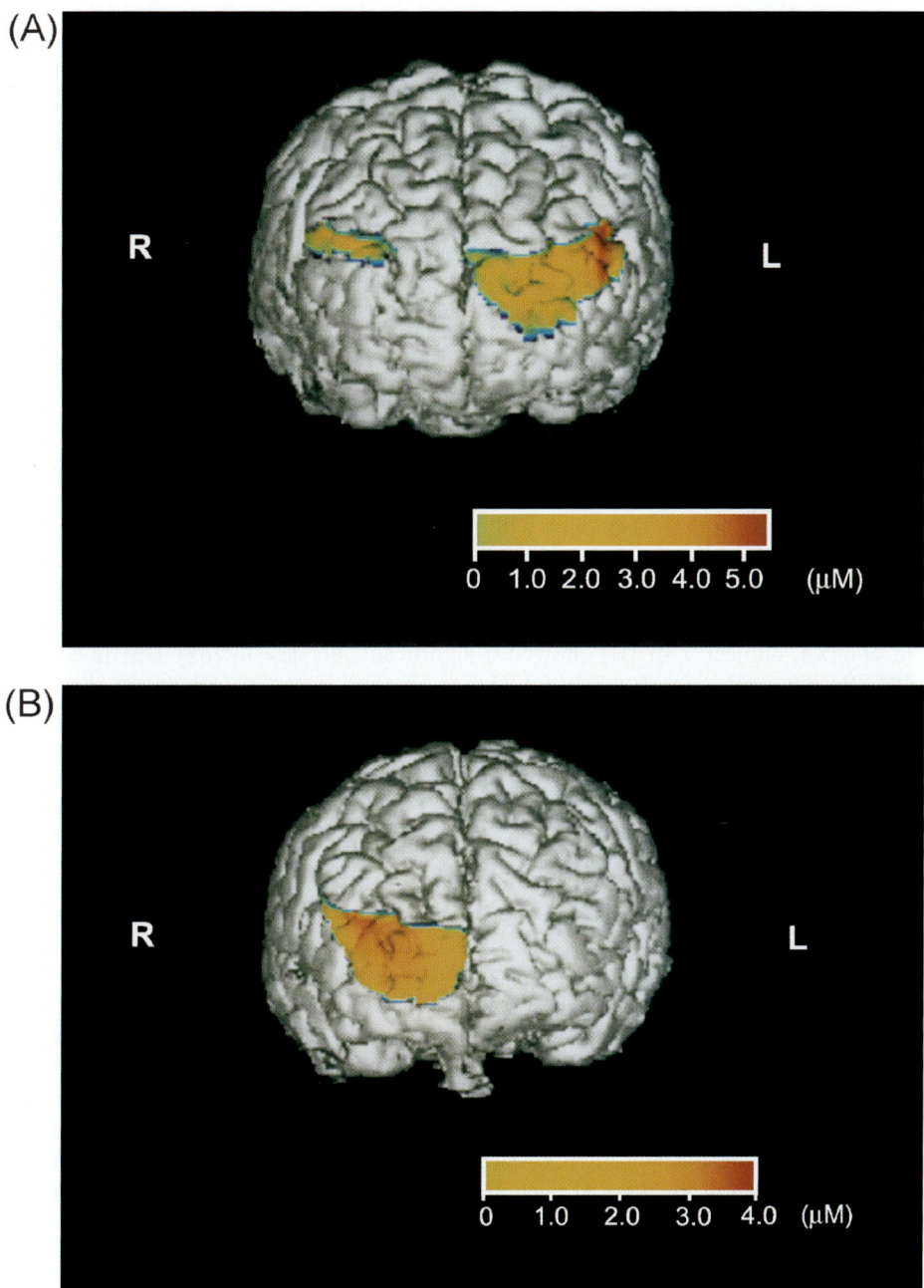

Fig. 2. (A) Subtraction images of [oxy-Hb] between the DB and DF tasks obtained from subject 6. Areas with increases in [oxy-Hb] are shown. (B) Subtraction images of [oxy-Hb] between the DB and DF tasks obtained from subjection [10].

Table 1
Foci maximal activation and task performance [10]

Subject	L/R	Brodmann's area	Δ[oxy-Hb] (μM, mean±S.D.)	Task performance (the longest digits)	
				DF	DB
1	L	9/46	3.16±0.62	7	4
2	R	9/46	1.95±0.29	8	7
3	L	9	1.27±0.22	7	4
4	R	46/45	5.95±0.83	8	7
5	L	46/45	4.81±1.16	7	3
6	L	8/9	1.49±0.24	8	4
7	R	9	2.80±0.7	7	7
8	R	9	2.69±0.66	8	5

[10]. Fig. 2 shows the subtraction images of [oxy-Hb] between the DB and DF tasks obtained from subject 6 (A) and subject 7 (B), respectively. Areas with increases in [oxy-Hb] are shown, since [oxy-Hb] is much more sensitive than [deoxy-] or [t-Hb] to the changes of hemodynamics associated with neuronal activation [10]. In Fig. 2A, it can be seen that [oxy-Hb] increased significantly in the left DLPC (Broadman's areas 9 and 8) in subject 6, compared with other areas in which [oxy-Hb] increased ($p<0.001$, Student's t-test).

In contrast, subject 7 of (B) showed a significant increase in [oxy-Hb] in the right DLPC (Broadmann's area 9). Table 1 shows areas in each subject where there were significant increases in [oxy-Hb] (μM, mean±S.D.). The degree of increase in [oxy-Hb] in these areas, which varied in each subject ($1.49\pm0.24-5.95\pm0.83$ μM), was not correlated with either laterality of the activated brain areas or task performance. Instead, higher performance in the DB task was closely related to the activation of the right DLPEC, suggesting that visuospatial imagery is a useful strategy for the DB task.

3. Conclusion

The lack of quantification and poor spatial resolution of the NIRS are now being overcome by introducing the technique of time-resolved optical tomography. As seen in Table 1, we can compare the degrees of hemodynamic changes and the degree of neuronal activation, i.e., performance. We found that there was no correlation between [oxy-Hb] and performance. In addition, we can introduce statistical analysis into NIRS and NIR-imaging because the changes in [oxy-Hb], [deoxy-Hb] and [t-Hb] can be obtained as absolute concentration changes in each subject. The true three-dimensional imaging of NIR is now in progress using a monkey, and will be reported very soon.

2.3.7.5. On-Site Discussion

2.3.7.5.1. **Question: (Tomita)** Light scattering by blood is flow-dependent and angle-dependent. How did you correct for these factors?

Answer: (Tamura) The light scattering change can be reflected by the values of reduced scattering coefficient, μ's. The solution of the photon diffusion equation can give continuously the μ's and μ'a during the activation. In conclusion, our approach for solving the photon diffusion equation automatically corrects the tissue scattering change.

2.3.7.5.2. *Question: (Dirnagl)* This is pioneering work. NIRS without quantification will be of not use, and TRS is a very good way to go. Are there any future perspectives for improving the sensitivity of TRS, which is inherently low since you have to throwaway most of the photons that have interacted with the tissue?

Answer: (Tamura) Yes, qualification is critical for NIRS. We are now improving the time-resolved imaging system, and sensitivity for collecting the photon increased more than 10-fold, and the many others. We can obtain the photons traveled more than 20 cm in adult head. Thus, TRS sensitivity is much more improved.

2.3.7.5.3. *Question: (Grinvald)* Can you speculate on the ultimate spatial resolution of this approach?

Answer: (Tamura) Spatial resolution seems the function of measuring time and size of the object. For new-born baby, at least 1 cm^3 of the resolution is possible. For adult head, we believe the resolution similar to PET is our final goal.

2.3.7.5.4. *Question: (Kleinfeld)* Is there a possibility to use very short pulses, ~ 10 fs, with concomitantly broad spectra (> 200 nm) so that you can resolve absorption on a function of wavelength as well as time? Namely, one would think that this will help determine the ratio [Hb-O$_2$]/[Hb].

Answer: (Tamura) Yes, using such ultrafast pulse, we can obtain the time-resolved snap shot of absorption spectra which transmitted through the head. We tried to use picosecond white light generated by non-linear materials such as D$_2$O or alcohol. Problem is too complicate system for medical use.

2.3.7.5.5. *Question: (Kleinfeld)* What spatial details do you put in your absorption/diffusion equation? Do you use, e.g., MRI data to incorporate an anatomically correct model of tissue? Do you use different diffusion values for different parts of the tissue, e.g., white matter versus gray matter?

Answer: (Tamura) At moment, we did not put on the actual anatomical data of human head. But, we are now trying to use MRI data for boundary conditions of each pixel during the solving inverse problem. The reduced scattering coefficient of white matter, etc., also should be used for increase in spatial resolution.

2.3.7.5.6. *Question: (Nemoto)* (1) I would like to take issue with the comment that NIRs are useless without quantification. Although there are qualifications, the use of the ratio related to the isosbestic point enables the detection of cerebral desaturation and oxygenation. (2) What is the average value that you observed of both hemoglobin saturation in the basal state and the response to activation in % hemoglobin saturation?

Answer: (Tamura) (1) The absorption ratio between the isosbestic point and another wavelength cannot give the oxygen saturation, since we need the true absorption due to hemoglobin in the light scattering media. (2) The lowest is $\sim 65\%$ and the highest $\sim 70\%$ saturation.

References

[1] Y. Hoshi, M. Tamura, Detection of dynamic charges in cerebral oxygenation coupled to neuronal function during mental work in man, Neurosci. Lett. 150 (1993) 5–8.

[2] T. Kato, A. Kamia, S. Takashima, T. Oyagi, Human visual cortical function during photic stimulation monitoring by means of near infrared spectroscopy, J. Cereb. Blood Flow Metab. 13 (1993) 516–520.

[3] A. Villringer, J. Plank, C. Hock, S. Schelinkfer, U. Dirnagle, Near infrared spectroscopy (NIRS): a new tool to study hemodynamic changes during activation of brain function in human adults, Neurosci. Lett. 154 (1933) 101–104.

[4] M. Tamura, Y. Hoshi, F. Okada, Localized near-infrared spectroscopy and functional optical imaging of brain functional optical imaging of brain activity, Phil. Trans. R. Soc. London, Ser. B 352 (1977) 737–742.

[5] Y. Hoshi, M. Tamura, Dynamic multichannel near-infrared optical imaging of human brain activity, J. Appl. Physiol. 74 (1993) 1842–1846.

[6] M. Nemoto, Y. Nomura, C. Sato, M. Tamura, K. Houkin, I. Koyanagi, H. Abe, Analysis of optical signals evoked by peripheral nerve stimulation in rat somatosensory cortex: dynamic changes in oxyhemoglobin concentration and oxygenation, J. Cereb. Blood Flow Metab. 19 (1999) 246–259.

[7] C. Sato, M. Nemoto, T. Nojo, M. Tamura, Analysis of the scattering component in early phase of intrinsic optical signals induced by neural activation, J. Cereb. Blood Flow Metab. 19 (1999) S-89, (Suppl).

[8] Y. Hoshi, O. Hazeki, Y. Kakihana, M. Tamura, Redox behavior of cytochrome oxidase in the rat brain measured by near-infrared spectroscopy, J. Appl. Physiol. 83 (1997) 1842–1848.

[9] Y. Hoshi, N. Kobayashi, M. Tamura, Interpretation of near-infrared spectroscopy signals: a study with a newly developed perfused rat brain model, J. Appl. Physiol. 90 (2001) 1657–1662.

[10] Y. Hoshi, I. Oda, Y. Wada, Y. Ito, Y. Yamashita, M. Oda, K. Ohta, Y. Yamada, M. Tamura, Visuospatial imagery is a fruitful strategy for the digit span backward task: a study with near infrared optical tomography, Cognit. Brain Res. 9 (2000) 339–342.

Neuronal activity induced effects

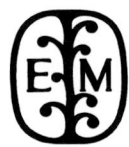

International Congress Series 1235 (2002) 189–196

Role of astrocytes in coupling synaptic activity to glucose utilization

Luc Pellerin [a,*], Gilles Bonvento [b], Brigitte Voutsinos-Porche [b],
Kohichi Tanaka [c], Jean-Yves Chatton [a], Jean-François Brunet [d],
Pierre J. Magistretti [a]

[a]Institut de Physiologie, 7 rue du Bugnon, 1005 Lausanne, Switzerland
[b]Laboratoire de Recherches Cérébrovasculaires, CNRS FRE 2363, 10 avenue de Verdun, 75010 Paris, France
[c]Medical Research Institute, Tokyo Medical and Dental University, Bunkyo-Ku, Tokyo 113-8510, Japan
[d]Service de Neurochirurgie, Centre Hospitalier Universitaire Vaudois, 1011 Lausanne, Switzerland

Abstract

Recently, in vitro evidence has suggested that astrocytes might play an important role in coupling neuronal activity to glucose utilization. The mechanism proposed to explain such coupling involves the uptake of glutamate by astrocytes via specific transporters. Here, we have taken advantage of the existence of knockout (KO) mice for each glial glutamate transporter to further explore the underpinnings of this mechanism, both in vitro and in vivo. Experiments performed on cultured cortical astrocytes from these mice indicate that an increase in intracellular Na^+ concentration caused by glutamate transport via the glutamate transporter GLAST is necessary to induce an increase in glucose utilization and lactate production. In vivo, the role of glial glutamate transporters in coupling neuronal activity to energy metabolism was further explored using the whisker-to-barrel pathway. Specific stimulation of the whiskers caused an accumulation of ^{14}C-2-deoxyglucose in related areas of the somatosensory cortex in wild type mice at the age of postnatal day 10. In both GLAST and GLT-1 transporter knockout mice, the metabolic response was strongly reduced. These data further emphasized the prominent role of astrocytes in the regulation of brain energy metabolism and identify glial glutamate transporters as key elements. © 2002 Elsevier Science B.V. All rights reserved.

Keywords: Astrocyte; Deoxyglucose; Glutamate transporter; Lactate; Barrel

* Corresponding author. Tel.: +41-21-692-5547; fax: +41-21-692-5595.
  E-mail addresses: Luc.Pellerin@iphysiol.unil.ch (L. Pellerin), bonvento@ext.jussieu.fr (G. Bonvento),
voutsinos@ext.jussieu.fr (B. Voutsinos-Porche), tanaka.aud@mri.tmd.ac.jp (K. Tanaka),
Jean-Yves.Chatton@iphysiol.unil.ch (J.-Y. Chatton), Jean-François.Brunet@chuv.hospvd.ch (J.-F. Brunet),
Pierre.Magistretti@iphysiol.unil.ch (P.J. Magistretti).

0531-5131/02 © 2002 Elsevier Science B.V. All rights reserved.
PII: S 0 5 3 1 - 5 1 3 1 (0 2) 0 0 1 8 6 - 3

1. Introduction

Neuro-metabolic coupling, i.e., an increase in glucose use anatomically restricted to the activated neural structure, is a fundamental feature of brain function and has provided the basis for functional brain imaging. The cellular and molecular mechanisms that link glucose metabolism and functional neuronal activity are still largely unknown. In addition to neurons, the possibility that astrocytes may participate in this process has been raised. A signaling pathway has been proposed by which glutamate, following its uptake by the astrocytes, exerts a metabolic action, i.e., increased glucose uptake and lactate production [1]. Using transgenic KO mice, the present study was designed to evaluate the involvement of both glial transporters GLAST and GLT-1 in signaling the metabolic response, using both an in vitro and an in vivo approach.

2. Materials and methods

Primary cultures of cortical astrocytes were prepared from GLAST and GLT-1 wild type (+/+), heterozygote (+/−) and knockout (−/−) mice [2,3] as previously described [1]. For RT-PCR, the total RNA was extracted with Trizol® (Gibco BRL) and 5 µg were used for the first strand synthesis using Sensiscript® RT (Qiagen) with 5 pmol of NV (dT)18 oligonucleotides as described by the suppliers. PCR was done on cDNA with rTaq polymerase (Pharmacia) using sets of mouse cDNA primers specific for each target sequence. Immunocytochemistry was performed with polyclonal GLAST and GLT-1 antibodies [4,5] and detected using fluorescence microscopy. ^{3}H-2-Deoxyglucose (2-DG) and ^{3}H-D-Aspartate uptake as well as lactate release measurements in vitro were done as previously described [1,6]. In vivo physiological neuronal activation was performed by stimulating the left C1, C2 whiskers in the awake P10 KO GLAST (n=7), P10 KO GLT-1 (n=6) and littermate control wild type mice (n=7 and n=5, respectively) as described [7]. Activity-dependent 2-DG uptake in vivo was measured using the autoradiographic technique on serial coronal sections [8].

3. Results

We first sought to determine the level of expression of the glial glutamate transporters GLAST and GLT-1 in cortical astrocyte cultures prepared from wild type (+/+), heterozygote (+/−) and knockout (−/−) newborn mice for either GLAST or GLT-1. Using RT-PCR, it could be demonstrated, using two different sets of primers, that GLAST is expressed in cultures from GLT-1 +/+, +/− and −/− mice (Fig. 1). GLAST was also found to be present in cultures from GLAST +/+ and +/− mice, but, as expected, not from GLAST −/− cultures. Similar results were obtained with GLT-1, with the difference that the expression of GLT-1 was found in all cultures except in astrocytes from GLT-1 −/− mice. These observations were confirmed at the protein level using immunocytochemistry. In addition, as a control, the level of expression of the astrocytic marker GFAP was assessed and no significant differences were found between

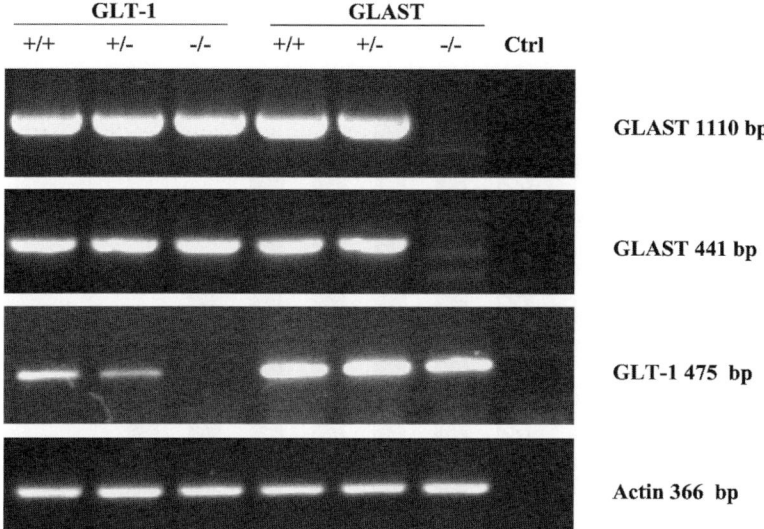

Fig. 1. Expression of glial glutamate transporters in primary cultures of cortical astrocytes from GLT-1 and GLAST transgenic mice determined by RT-PCR. Two sets of primers specific for the mouse GLAST sequence and giving rise to two bands of 1110 and 441 bp, respectively, were used to detect the presence of GLAST mRNA in astrocyte cultures prepared from wild type (+/+), heterozygote (+/−) and knockout (−/−) mice for either GLAST or GLT-1. Identification of GLT-1 mRNA expression in the same preparations was done with the use of two primers designed for the mouse GLT-1 sequence and was revealed as a single band of 475 bp. The expression of actin mRNA was used as a positive control, which was revealed by a band of 366 bp using an appropriate set of primers for the mouse sequence. As a negative control, a reaction was carried out without cDNA (Ctrl).

the different cultures. The importance of each transporter for the overall glutamate uptake was then determined. The uptake rate, as assessed with the analog D-aspartate did not significantly differ between cultured astrocytes prepared from GLT-1 +/+, +/− and −/− mice. In contrast, the uptake rate was significantly reduced in astrocytes from GLAST +/− and −/− mice, reaching 72.8±8.6% and 33.9±4.6%, respectively, of the uptake measured in GLAST +/+ astrocytes. In order to evaluate the contribution of GLT-1 to the residual uptake observed in astrocytes from GLAST −/− mice, the specific GLT-1 inhibitor dihydrokainate (DHK) was tested (Fig. 2). A concentration-dependent reduction in uptake was found with maximal effect observed at 500 μM DHK. These results indicate that although the transporter GLAST is responsible for most of the glutamate uptake in the cultured cortical astrocytes from neonatal mice, GLT-1 is at least in part responsible for the remaining uptake in the astrocytes prepared from GLAST −/− mice.

The next step was to measure the changes in intracellular Na^+ concentration in response to glutamate application in astrocyte cultures from mice with different genotypes. The astrocytes prepared from GLT-1 mice all displayed a robust increase in intracellular Na^+ concentration from a basal level of 10–15 up to 35–40 mM upon application of 100 μM glutamate. No significant differences were observed between GLT-1 +/+, +/− and −/− cultures. When Na^+ responses to glutamate were evaluated in astrocytes from GLAST mice, striking differences were observed. When compared to strong response in the

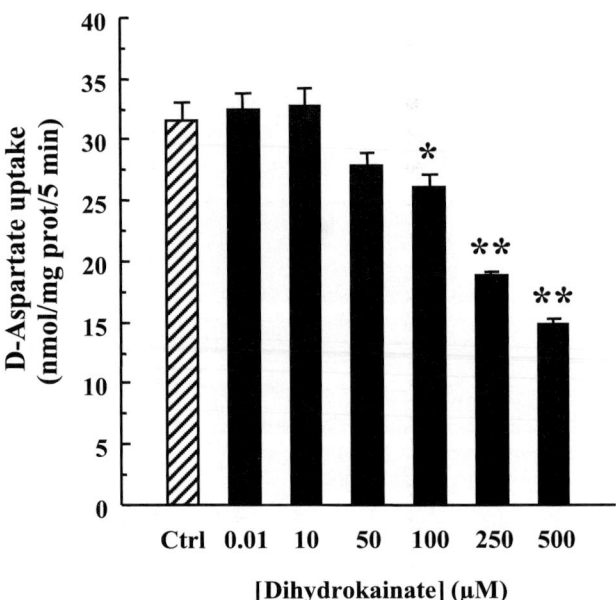

Fig. 2. The effect of dihydrokainate, a specific inhibitor of the glial glutamate transporter GLT-1, on D-aspartate uptake in cultured astrocytes prepared from GLAST knockout mice. Accumulation of ^{3}H-D-aspartate in primary cultures of cortical astrocytes was assessed over a 5-min period in the presence of increasing concentrations of dihydrokainate. Each bar represents the mean±S.E.M. of three determinations. Data were statistically analyzed with ANOVA followed by the Dunnett's test. Asterisks indicate D-aspartate uptake which are significantly different from the basal uptake (Ctrl) at *$p<0.05$ and **$p<0.01$.

astrocytes from GLAST +/+ mice, concentration changes in the intracellular Na$^+$ concentration for the +/− astrocytes represented only 43.2±10.8% of the wild type response, while it was almost abolished in the −/− astrocytes (9.9±0.9% of the wild type response). The effect of glutamate exposure on both glucose utilization and lactate production was then evaluated. The results obtained were very analogous compared to those found on Na$^+$ responses. Thus, an increase in both glucose utilization and lactate production was observed upon exposure to 200 μM glutamate (from 73% to 101% increase over the basal level), while no significant differences were observed between the astrocytes prepared from the GLT-1 +/+, +/− and −/− mice. In contrast, both the enhanced glucose utilization and lactate production responses were reduced by about half in astrocytes from the GLAST +/− as compared to the GLAST +/+ astrocytes (−43% for glucose utilization and −66% for lactate production, respectively), while they were completely abolished in astrocytes from GLAST −/− mice.

Finally, accumulation of ^{14}C-2-deoxyglucose in the somatosensory cortex of GLAST and GLT-1 transgenic mice following whisker stimulation was evaluated by autoradiography. A significant increase in 2-DG uptake was obtained in postnatal day 10 GLT-1 and GLAST +/+ mice (22–32% increase above basal level). In contrast, an important reduction of the metabolic response to whisker stimulation was observed in the corresponding activated cortical area of both postnatal day 10 GLAST and GLT-1 −/− mice.

4. Discussion

It has been previously demonstrated that glutamate, the major excitatory neurotransmitter of the central nervous system, promotes glucose utilization and lactate production in cultured cortical astrocytes [1,9]. A pharmacological analysis had revealed that the effect of glutamate was not receptor-mediated but suggested that glutamate transporters might be involved. Here, we have provided evidence, using cultured astrocytes prepared from transgenic animals, that glutamate uptake via at least one of these transporters is essential to obtain the metabolic response. Moreover, the influence of glutamate uptake on glucose utilization and lactate production by the astrocytes was paralleled by changes in the intracellular Na^+ concentration, consistent with a role for sodium as an intracellular metabolic signal in astrocytes as previously suggested [9]. These changes in intracellular Na^+ concentration upon exposure to glutamate have been shown to be largely associated with the operation of glutamate transporters [10]. One consequence of these important Na^+ fluxes is an activation of the Na^+/K^+ ATPase. Indeed, it was previously shown that glutamate stimulates the activity of the Na^+/K^+ ATPase and this effect was essential to induce the enhancement in glucose utilization and lactate utilization [11]. In addition, it was also suggested that the effect of glutamate involved the mobilization of a specific subunit of the Na^+/K^+ ATPase called the α_2, which is found primarily in astrocytes in the central nervous system [12]. These data provide strong evidence that glutamate transporters constitute key elements in the mechanism that could link detection of synaptic activity by astrocytes to enhanced glucose utilization. As a corollary, these observations strongly emphasize the potential role of the astrocytes in vivo, in mediating the neurometabolic coupling observed under so many different conditions of stimulation, modalities and in various areas of the brain.

The whisker-to-barrel pathway in rodents has been a very popular system to study the coupling between neuronal activation and either blood flow or metabolism [13,14]. By combining the use of ^{14}C-2-deoxyglucose and autoradiography, it is thus possible to visualize and work out the increase in glucose utilization occurring within restricted areas of the somatosensory cortex (known as barrels) following vibrissal stimulation [15–17]. This system appears ideal to investigate the potential role of astrocytes in this metabolic response. Our results using transgenic mice for both glial glutamate transporters GLAST and GLT-1, showing a reduction of whisker-stimulated response in knockout animals, are consistent with the involvement of astrocytes. Moreover, it was recently shown that 24 h after the local injection of antisense oligonucleotides designed to target GLAST mRNA in adult rats, and despite the presence of normal whisker-related neuronal activity, the metabolic response to whisker stimulation decreased by more than 50% [8]. These in vivo observations strongly argue in favour of a role of astrocytes in coupling neuronal activity to glucose utilization. An important issue to be resolved now would be the metabolic fate of glucose consumed by the astrocytes. It was previously shown that glutamate increases lactate formation and release by cultured astrocytes in a concentration-dependent manner, with a pharmacology consistent with a glutamate transporter-mediated mechanism [1]. The possibility that lactate could be exported by astrocytes to be used as an energy substrate by neurons was also raised. This hypothesis implies the presence of specific transporters to allow the release of lactate by the astrocytes and its uptake by neurons. In situ hybridization and immunohistochemical studies have revealed the expression of monocarbox-ylate transporters (MCTs), which are capable of transporting lactate in various regions of the brain [18,19]. Moreover, it was shown both from cultured cells and in vivo, that astrocytes were found to strongly express the monocarboxylate transporter MCT1, while neurons predominantly expressed another subtype, MCT2 [19,20]. In summary, both in vitro and in vivo evidence strongly suggest that astrocytes contribute to the coupling between glucose utilization and neuronal activity, and glial glutamate transporters represent a critical component of the mechanism.

2.4.1.7. On-Site Discussion

2.4.1.7.1. *Question: (Gjedde)* Is the presence of transporters of pyruvate and lactate not equally consistent with a transport of pyruvate from neurons to astrocytes?

Answer: (Pellerin) It could be, but since both lactate and pyruvate will compete for the same transporter and lactate is always in higher concentration than pyruvate, lactate transport might be quantitatively more important, especially during phases of activation where lactate concentration was shown to transiently increase. In addition, a net transfer of lactate (or pyruvate) from one cell type to another will require, in addition to the presence of transporters, that one cell type act as a "source" and produce the exchanged metabolite while the other cell type act as a "sink" and consumes it. Available in vitro data point to astrocytes as being lactate producers while neurons can utilize lactate as an energy substrate. Thus, although it does not exclude other possibilities, available data are consistent with a possible transfer of lactate from astrocytes to neurons.

2.4.1.7.2. *Question: (Harder)* Astrocytes are excitable cells with voltage gated K^+ channels.

Answer: (Pellerin) In our case, it is the increase in intracellular Na^+ concentration and not a change in membrane potential which represents the critical step, leading to an activation of the Na^+,K^+ ATPase and triggering the metabolic response.

2.4.1.7.3. *Question: (Iadecola)* What is resting glucose utilization in the glucose trans-porter null mice? It seems that it is not affected suggesting that this system is not active in the resting state.

Answer: (Pellerin) Only 2-DG uptake was performed. Therefore, no quantitative compar-ison can be done. However, the overall pattern of 2-DG uptake seems not to be affected in both KO mice. Resting glucose uptake does not appear different between wild type and glutamate transporter null mice. Absence of one of the two glial glutamate transporter might not be a limiting factor for glutamate uptake under resting state but it might become under activated state.

2.4.1.7.4. *Question: (Kuschinsky)* I do not understand that both the knockout of GLAST and of GLT-1 both can completely block the effect of whisker stimulation on local glucose utilization. These should be some residual effect in each of the knockout models.

Answer: (Pellerin) We do not have for the moment a definitive answer to this observation. It looks as if the two transporters act in a coordinated manner to trigger the metabolic response.

Or it could be that missing one or the other transporter becomes a limiting factor and under activation glial glutamate uptake fails to keep up with enhanced glutamate release.

Acknowledgements

This work was supported by a grant from the Human Frontier Science Program Organization (RG118/1998-B). The authors wish to acknowledge the excellent technical assistance provided by Mrs. Mauricette Maillard and Mr. Didier Foretay.

References

[1] L. Pellerin, P.J. Magistretti, Glutamate uptake into astrocytes stimulates aerobic glycolysis: a mechanism coupling neuronal activity to glucose utilization, Proc. Natl. Acad. Sci. U. S. A. 91 (1994) 10625–10629.

[2] K. Tanaka, K. Watase, T. Manabe, K. Yamada, M. Watanabe, K. Takahashi, H. Iwama, T. Nishikawa, N. Ichihara, T. Kikuchi, S. Okuyama, N. Kawashima, S. Hori, M. Takimoto, K. Wada, Epilepsy and exacerbation of brain injury in mice lacking the glutamate transporter GLT-1, Science 276 (1997) 1699–1702.

[3] K. Watase, K. Hashimoto, M. Kano, K. Yamada, M. Watanabe, Y. Inoue, S. Okuyama, T. Sakagawa, S.-I. Ogawa, N. Kawashima, S. Hori, M. Takimoto, K. Wada, K. Tanaka, Motor discoordination and increased susceptibility to cerebellar injury in GLAST mutant mice, Eur. J. Neurosci. 10 (1998) 976–988.

[4] T. Shibata, K. Yamada, M. Watanabe, K. Ikenaka, K. Wada, K. Tanaka, Y. Inoue, Glutamate transporter GLAST is expressed in the radial glia–astrocyte lineage of developing mouse spinal cord, J. Neurosci. 17 (1997) 9212–9219.

[5] K. Yamada, M. Watanabe, T. Shibata, M. Nagashima, K. Tanaka, Y. Inoue, Glutamate transporter GLT-1 is transiently localized on growing axons of the spinal cord before establishing astrocytic expression, J. Neurosci. 18 (1998) 5706–5713.

[6] R. Debernardi, P.J. Magistretti, L. Pellerin, Trans-inhibition of glutamate transport prevents excitatory amino acid-induced glycolysis in astrocytes, Brain Res. 850 (1999) 39–46.

[7] E. Welker, S.B. Rao, J. Dorfl, P. Melzer, H. van der Loos, Plasticity in the barrel cortex of the adult mouse: effects of chronic stimulation upon deoxyglucose uptake in behaving animal, J. Neurosci. 12 (1992) 153–170.

[8] N. Cholet, L. Pellerin, E. Welker, P. Lacombe, J. Seylaz, P.J. Magistretti, G. Bonvento, Local injection of antisense oligonucleotides targeted to the glial glutamate transporter GLAST decreases the metabolic response to somatosensory activation, J. Cereb. Blood Flow Metab. 21 (2001) 404–412.

[9] S. Takahashi, B.F. Driscoll, M.J. Law, L. Sokoloff, Role of sodium and potassium ions in regulation of glucose metabolism in cultured astroglia, Proc. Natl. Acad. Sci. USA 92 (1995) 4616–4620.

[10] J-Y. Chatton, P. Marquet, P.J. Magistretti, A quantitative analysis of L-glutamate-regulated Na$^+$ dynamics in mouse cortical astrocytes: implications for cellular bioenergetics, Eur. J. Neurosci. 12 (2000) 3843–3853.

[11] L. Pellerin, P.J. Magistretti, Glutamate uptake stimulates Na$^+$,K$^+$-ATPase activity in astrocytes via activation of a distinct subunit highly sensitive to ouabain, J. Neurochem. 69 (1997) 2132–2137.

[12] R. Cameron, L. Klein, A.W. Shyjan, P. Rakic, R. Levenson, Neurons and astroglia express distinct subsets of Na,K-ATPase a and b subunits, Mol. Brain Res. 21 (1994) 333–343.

[13] T.A. Woolsey, C.M. Rovainen, S.B. Cox, M.H. Henegar, G.E. Liang, D. Liu, Y.E. Moskalenko, J. Sui, L. Wei, Neuronal units linked to microvascular modules in cerebral cortex: response elements for imaging the brain, Cereb. Cortex. 6 (1996) 647–660.

[14] N. Cholet, J. Seylaz, P. Lacombe, G. Bonvento, Local uncoupling of the cerebrovascular and metabolic responses to somatosensory stimulation after neuronal nitric oxide synthase inhibition, J. Cereb. Blood Flow Metab. 17 (1997) 1191–1201.

[15] J. Chmielowska, M. Kossut, M. Chmielowski, Single vibrissal cortical column in the mouse labeled with 2-deoxyglucose, Exp. Brain Res. 63 (1986) 607–619.

[16] J.S. McCaslands, T.A. Woolsey, High-resolution 2-deoxyglucose mapping of functional cortical columns in mouse barrel cortex, J. Comp. Neurol. 278 (1988) 555–569.

[17] M. Kossut, P.J. Hand, J. Greenberg, C.L. Hand, Single vibrissal cortical column in SI cortex of rat and its alterations in neonatal and adult vibrissa-deafferented animals: a quantitative 2-DG study, J. Neurophysiol. 60 (1988) 829–852.

[18] L. Pellerin, G. Pellegri, J-L. Martin, P.J. Magistretti, Expression of monocarboxylate transporter mRNAs in mouse brain: support for a distinct role of lactate as an energy substrate for the neonatal vs. adult brain, Proc. Natl. Acad. Sci. U. S. A. 95 (1998) 3990–3995.

[19] K. Pierre, L. Pellerin, R. Debernardi, B.M. Riederer, P.J. Magistretti, Cell-specific localization of monocarboxylate transporters, MCT1 and MCT2, in the adult mouse brain revealed by double immunohistochemical labeling and confocal microscopy, Neuroscience 100 (2000) 617–627.

[20] S. Bröer, B. Rahman, G. Pellegri, L. Pellerin, J-L. Martin, S. Verleysdonk, B. Hamprecht, P.J. Magistretti, Comparison of lactate transport in astroglial cells and monocarboxylate transporter 1 (MCT1) expressing *Xenopus laevis* oocytes, Expression of two different monocarboxylate transporters in astroglial cells and neurons, J. Biol. Chem. 272 (1997) 30096–30102.

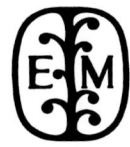

International Congress Series 1235 (2002) 197–204

The role of neuronal nitric oxide in the regional neurovascular coupling. Voxel-based comparison between perfusion and metabolic PET images

Takuya Hayashi [a,*], Yukinori Katsumi [a], Manabu Inoue [b],
Yasuhiro Nagahama [c], Chisako Oyanagi [a], Hiroshi Yamauchi [c],
Hidenao Fukuyama [b], Hiroshi Shibasaki [a,b]

[a]*Department of Neurology, Kyoto University Graduate School of Medicine,
54 Shogoinkawahara-cho, Sakyo-ku, Kyoto 606-8507, Japan*
[b]*Brain Pathophysiology, Kyoto University Graduate School of Medicine,
54 Shogoinkawahara-cho, Sakyo-ku, Kyoto 606-8507, Japan*
[c]*Shiga Medical Center for Adults, Moriyama, Shiga, Japan*

Abstract

In order to clarify the role of neuronal nitric oxide in cerebral neurovascular coupling, we measured the CBF and CMRglc with PET in α-chloralose anesthetized cats during electrical somatosensory stimulation, and under the treatment of a neuronal nitric oxide inhibitor, 7-nitroindazole (7-NI). The voxel-based analysis was performed with the use of globally normalized CBF and CMRglc values to identify the increased areas of CBF and CMRglc produced by somatosensory stimulation, and the uncoupled areas between their changes induced by the 7-NI. Somatosensory stimulation in the left forepaw elicited an increase in both the CBF and CMRglc in the left cerebellum, the right thalamus and the right somatosensory cortex. Injection of 7-NI induced global uncoupling (20% decrease in the global CBF, but not in the global CMRglc), whereas the regional uncoupling during activation was observed in the ipsilateral cerebellum. Thus, neuronal nitric oxide may play a predominant role in the coupling of the regional perfusion and metabolism in the cerebellum, but less so in the neocortex. © 2002 Elsevier Science B.V. All rights reserved.

Keywords: Cat; Cerebral blood flow; Nitric oxide; Cerebral glucose metabolism; Neurovascular coupling

* Corresponding author. Present address: Department of Investigative Radiology, National Cardiovascular Center, Research Institute, 5-7-1 Fujishirodai, Suita, Osaka 565-8565, Japan. Tel.: +81-6-6833-5004-2559; fax: +81-6-6872-7485.

E-mail address: thayashi@ri.ncvc.go.jp (T. Hayashi).

0531-5131/02 © 2002 Elsevier Science B.V. All rights reserved.
PII: S 0 5 3 1 - 5 1 3 1 (0 2) 0 0 1 8 7 - 5

1. Introduction

Nitric oxide (NO) has long been a candidate as a mediator of neurovascular coupling in the central nervous system [1,2]. However, several studies using knockout mice with a lack of NO synthase (NOS) showed normal CBF responses during somatosensory stimulation [3,4]. Studies that tested the pharmacological effect of the inhibitor of endothelial (eNOS) or neuronal NOS (nNOS) also failed to show any perturbations on the CBF increase produced by somatosensory activation in rats [5,6] or in humans [7]. In addition, another possible role of NO, is in the modulation of the synaptic function, which is related directly to neuronal activity [8], therefore, it makes it more difficult to consolidate the role of NO in the regulation of CBF. Thus, we assumed that the estimation of the quantitative changes in the CBF, as well as in the neuronal activity might be inevitable for evaluating the NO-related pharmacological perturbations on flow-metabolism coupling.

PET enabled us to estimate not only the CBF but also cerebral glucose metabolism (CMRglc), which are tightly coupled to synaptic activity [9]. Recent advances in the resolution of the PET scanner allowed us to perform repeated measurements of multiple physiological parameters in the same animal. In order to examine the role of neuronal-derived NO in neurovascular coupling during neuronal activation, we measured the CBF and CMRglc using PET before and after infusion of the NOS inhibitor specific to nNOS, 7-nitroindazole (7-NI); during the somatosensory activation in α-chloralose anesthetized cats. The voxel-based analysis was performed in order to identify any regions where changes of CBF and CMRglc did not couple.

2. Methods and materials

Fourteen adult male cats weighing 3.32 ± 0.3 kg (mean $\pm$ S.D.) were used for this experiment (Liberty Research, NY, USA). The experiments were performed under anesthesia with 50 mg/kg (i.p.) α-chloralose at the beginning and a continuous intravenous infusion of 10 mg/kg of α-chloralose and muscle relaxant with gallamine triethiodide (5 mg/kg/h). The femoral artery was cannulated for sampling the arterial blood, monitoring the physiological variables (blood pressure, pO_2, pCO_2, pH, and the blood glucose level) and the ante-tibial vein for injecting radiopharmaceuticals. The regional CBF was determined using an intravenous bolus injection of 30 mCi ^{15}O-labeled water, followed by dynamic PET image acquisition and arterial blood sampling over a period of 3 min [10,11]. The regional CMRglc was measured using a conventional autoradiographic method for 20 min PET scanning, initiated 30 min after the 5 mCi ^{18}F-FDG injection [9,12]. The regional CMRglc images were generated using an operational equation belonging to Sokoloff et al. [9], using known lumped constants and transfer rate constants for the ^{18}F-FDG in the cat brain [13]. In addition, using the plasma ^{18}F activity time, activity curve and plasma glucose concentration. The PET data were collected with a high-resolution PET scanner developed for animal experiments (SHR7700, Hamamatsu Photonics, Hamamatsu, Japan), with an intrinsic resolution of 2.6 mm in a plane and 3.3 mm axially in full width at half of the maximum.

2.1. Experimental design

The animals were divided into two groups: the somatosensory group (Study I, $n = 8$) and the nNOS inhibition group (Study II, $n = 6$). In Study I, the change in rCBF or rCMRglc produced by somatosensory activation was studied and their relationships were compared. The experiments were performed in a darkened room with the animals eyes closed. Activation was performed by electrical stimulation of the left forepaw given with a pair of subcutaneous electrodes delivering recto-angular pulses (0.5 ms, 180 mV, 3 Hz) with an electric generator (Electric Stimulator, Nihon Kohden, Tokyo, Japan), and it was started 30 s before the PET measurement and was continued throughout the measurement. One hour after the induction of anesthesia, four sequential measurements of the CBF were repeatedly carried out during the alternative states of rest and the activation. The interval of each measurement of the CBF was set for at least 15 min to ensure decay of any residual ^{15}O activity. The two sequential measurements of the CMRglc during rest and activation were performed on the same animal. After the first CMRglc measurement, at least 1 h was allowed to minimize any residual ^{18}F activity, and the correction of residual ^{18}F activity at the start of the second scan was achieved by the assumption of linear decay from the last 10 min of the data from the first scan to the 10 min of scan data before the second injection of ^{18}F-FDG. Study II was arranged to elucidate the effect of 7-NI on the CBF and the CMRglc during activation, including three protocols for each animal: CBF/7-NI, CMRglc/7-NI, and Control. In the CBF/7-NI, the CBF during the rest and activation conditions was measured before and after infusion of the 7-NI (50 mg/kg, i.p., Nakarai Task, Kyoto, Japan) and after that, a donor of NO, L-arginine, was injected intravenously (10 mg/kg) and the fifth measurement of the CBF was performed. In the CMRglc/7-NI, two sequential CMRglc measurements during activation were undertaken before and after the infusion of 7-NI. In the Control experiment, the CBF and CMRglc were measured with infusion of the vehicle alone instead of the 7-NI.

2.2. Data processing and analysis

Global CBF and CMRglc were calculated in the brain regions of interest. The global CBF values were compared among images before and after the infusion of the 7-NI, and after L-arginine. The global CMRglc values were compared before and after the infusion of the 7-NI. To find out significant the changes in rCBF and rCMRglc, the statistical parametric mapping software (SPM99, Wellcome Department of Cognitive Neurology, London, UK) was used for the analysis. First, we created an atlas of the cat brain for both the CMRglc and T1-weighted MRI images using dPETMac [14] and AIR3.0 software [15], oriented in a standard space of the cat brain [16] to enable the data to be transformed and analyzed in the same space, and the statistical results to be displayed on the atlas. Then, the CMRglc image for each animal was edited to remove the non-brain structure, and co-registered and normalized anatomically to fit the cat CMRglc atlas using linear and non-linear three-dimensional transformation on a slice-by-slice basis. All sets of the CBF images were co-registered to the CMRglc image for each animal, masked by the edited CMRglc image and transformed to the standard space using a transformation parameter for the CMRglc image. Smoothing with an isotropic Gaussian filter of 5 mm was performed to

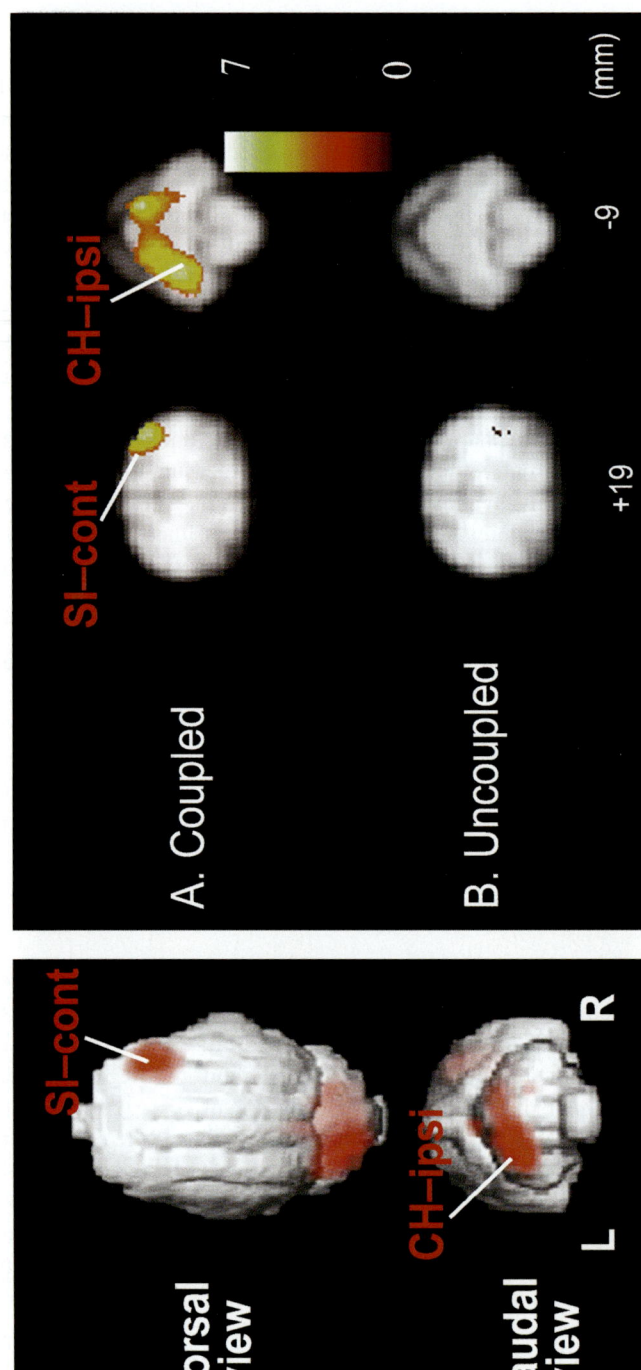

Fig. 1. Left: The somatosensory-activated areas were the primary somatosensory area contralateral to the stimulation (SI-cont) and the ipsilateral cerebellum (CH-ipsi) on the voxel-based analysis of CBF data (*shown in red on the brain surface of the cat*). Right: Coupled areas of CBF-CMRglc changes during the unilateral electrical somatosensory stimulation revealed by conjunction analysis between them (*P* < 0.001, uncorrected) (A). Uncoupled areas with relatively less change in the CBF compared to that of the CMRglc during somatosensory stimulation, revealed with the interaction analysis (*P* < 0.001, uncorrected) (B).

enhance the signal-to-noise ratio. To test the hypothesis about the regional effects of somatosensory activation or 7-NI, a general linear model was employed at each and every voxel. The obtained values were then globally normalized by scaling, and the mean global value of both rCBF and rCMRglc images were proportionally adjusted to 100 to observe the regional change as a proportion (%). In order to find out the areas where coupling or uncoupling exist, conjunction and interaction analysis was performed between the rCMRglc and rCBF changes induced by activation or 7-NI. Analysis of the volumes of interest (VOI) were also performed by placing the VOI with a 3-mm diameter sphere in relation to the primary sensory cortex (SI), and the cerebellar cortical areas.

3. Results

Global CBF decreased by 20% (pre 7-NI: 34.2 ± 4.4; post 7-NI: 28.3 ± 4.2 ml/100 g/min, $P < 0.01$) after the infusion of 7-NI and was recovered by the infusion of L-arginine (32.7 ± 5.4 ml/100 g/min), whereas global CMRglc did not change before or after the infusion of the 7-NI (23.4 ± 5.5, 22.1 ± 4.0 μmol/100 g/min). These findings are

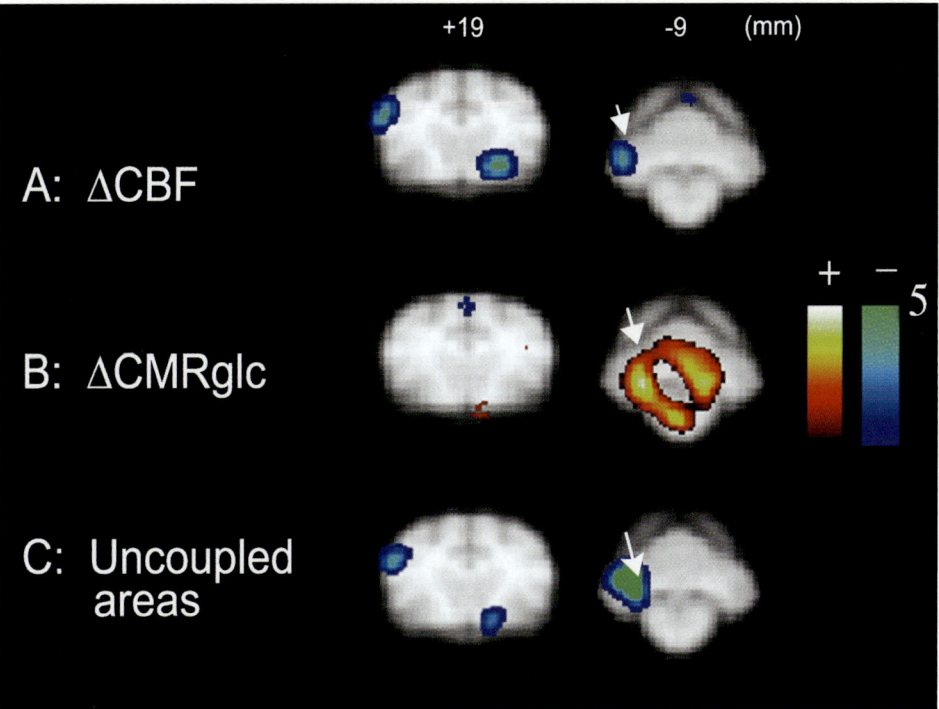

Fig. 2. The effect of the nNOS inhibitor (7-nitroindazole) on CBF and CMRglc during somatosensory activation. Neuronal NOS inhibition decreased the CBF at CH-ipsi and increased the CMRglc at the same region (arrows). Thus, their uncoupling was observed at this site ($P < 0.001$, uncorrected), however, and not at the SI-cont where activation by somatosensory stimulation occurred as shown in Fig. 1.

consistent with prior studies carried out on cats in which 7-NI was used [17]. Somato-sensory activation elicited an increase in CBF and CMRglc at the ipsilateral lobe of the cerebellum (CH-ipsi), and the primary somatosensory cortex (SI-cont) ($P < 0.05$, corrected). Regional CBF increased by 7.2% at SI-cont and by 8.2% at CH-ipsi, and rCMRglc increased by 8.2% and 7.9%, respectively (corrected, $P < 0.05$, Fig. 1). Conjunction analysis also revealed that the coupled increase of rCBF and rCMRglc at these areas and interaction analysis did not reveal any voxels. In addition, whereas the 7-NI induced a decrease in the rCBF at CH-ipsi, there was a tendency for rCMRglc to increase. Interaction analysis revealed that there was relatively lower rCBF than rCMRglc at CH-ipsi ($P < 0.001$, uncorrected), but not at the SI-cont (Fig. 2). In the Control experiment, interaction analysis did not show any areas of uncoupling between the rCBF and rCMRglc among the activated areas. Volumes of interest (VOI) analysis also showed dissociated changes between rCBF and rCMRglc at CH-ipsi after the infusion of 7-NI.

4. Discussion

The present study was the first to investigate the effect of neuronal activation or pharmaceuticals on the coupling of CBF and CMRglc during activation in the same animal. Somatosensory electrical stimulation in the unilateral forepaw in cats elicited coupled increases of the normalized CBF and CMRglc in the SI-cont and CH-ipsi. The activated areas were predicted form the known anatomical connections for the somato-sensory pathway and were also consistent with prior studies carried out in rodents or humans. Both voxel-based and VOI analysis on the perfusion and metabolic images confirmed the coupled increase of normalized CBF and CMRglc values in the neocortex and cerebellum. Similarly, we tested if the inhibition of neuronal NOS using 7-NI resulted in the regional uncoupling of normalized CBF and CMRglc, and we found uncoupling of the CBF and CMRglc (relative low perfusion) in the ipsilateral CH but not in the contralateral SI.

We measured both CBF and CMRglc in the present study to find out the role NO plays in coupling. Different from the classical neurotransmitter, NO has unique properties: extreme diffusibility in both aqueous and lipid environments, allowing the generation of NO at the single point source to influence the function within a sphere with a diameter of approximately 0.3 mm, which includes a large amount of cerebral capillaries and synapses. Therefore, NO generated by the NOS neuron is not targeted to the specific anatomical and functional structure, but it can act on any of the neurons and capillaries surrounding the NOS neuron. Thus, it may serve as a modulator of local overall neuronal activity and hemodynamics. In fact, in the present study, CMRglc at CH-ipsi increased after the infusion of 7-NI, whereas the CBF decreased. Thus, it seems that the inhibition of neuronal NO augments synaptic activity with an insufficient CBF response in the cerebellum, which may suggest that NO plays a substantial role as a mediator in coupling.

The present study showed that NO may play a major role in coupling in the cerebellar cortex, and less so in the cerebral cortex. The regional diversity in the concentration of NOS neurons in the brain has been made known by histological studies with NADPH staining or immunohistochemistry. However, the regional difference of the function of NO or the NOS neuron is not yet fully understood. As regards the role in the regulation of CBF, Cholet et al. [18] first described that there is more substantial role in the somatosensory area and the thalamus, then in the trigeminal primary nucleus in the brainstem in rats under peri-oral somatosensory stimulation. Recently, Yang et al. [1] found that 7-NI totally abolished the functional hyperemia in the cerebellum but attenuated less the increase of neocortical CBF produced by perioral somatosensory stimulation in rats. The present study supports the predominant role of NO in the cerebellum as compared to the cerebral cortex, and clarified the regional difference in the mechanism of coupling at least between the neocortex and the cerebellum.

In conclusion, normalized CBF and CMRglc incremental responses produced by somatosensory stimulation were coupled in α-chloralose anesthetized cats. The neuronal-derived NO participates in the maintenance of global cerebral blood flow. Furthermore, the neuronal-derived NO may act as a predominant mediator in neurovascular coupling in the cerebellum, but less so in the neocortex.

2.4.2.7. On-Site Discussion

2.4.2.7.1. *Comment: (Lauritzen)* Comment with respect to the properties of callossal fibres connecting the hemispheres. They are in all main excitatory, glutamatergic, but GABAergic tissues do exist although they are rare. Excitation of the intrahemispheric fibers will excite both inhibition neurons in the opposite hemisphere that might or might not release NO, and pyramidal cells that were previously located in cortical layer III.

Acknowledgements

This work was supported by the Research for the Future Program (RFTF) JSPS-RFTF97L00201 from the Japan Society for the Promotion of Science, and General Research Grant for Aging and Health 'Analysis of aged brain function with neuroimaging.'

References

[1] G. Yang, et al., Nitric oxide is the predominant mediator of cerebellar hyperemia during somatosensory activation in rats, Am. J. Physiol. 277 (6 Pt 2) (1999) R1760–R1770.

[2] T.J. Lee, Nitric oxide and the cerebral vascular function, J. Biomed. Sci. 7 (1) (2000) 16–26.

[3] C. Ayata, et al., L-NA-sensitive rCBF augmentation during vibrissal stimulation in type III nitric oxide synthase mutant mice, J. Cereb. Blood Flow Metab. 16 (4) (1996) 539–541.

[4] J. Ma, et al., Regional cerebral blood flow response to vibrissal stimulation in mice lacking type I NOS gene expression, Am. J. Physiol. 270 (3 Pt 2) (1996) H1085–H1090.

[5] K. Adachi, et al., Increases in local cerebral blood flow associated with somatosensory activation are not mediated by NO, Am. J. Physiol. 267 (6 Pt 2) (1994) H2155–H2162.

[6] J.H. Greenberg, N.W. Sohn, P.J. Hand, Nitric oxide and the cerebral-blood-flow response to somatosensory activation following deafferentation, Exp. Brain Res. 129 (4) (1999) 541–550.

[7] R.P. White, et al., The effect of the nitric oxide synthase inhibitor L-NMMA on basal CBF and vasoneuronal coupling in man: a PET study, J. Cereb. Blood Flow Metab. 19 (6) (1999) 673–678.

[8] J.P. Kiss, E.S. Vizi, Nitric oxide: a novel link between synaptic and nonsynaptic transmission, Trends Neurosci. 24 (4) (2001) 211–215.

[9] L. Sokoloff, et al., The [^{14}C]deoxyglucose method for the measurement of local cerebral glucose utilization: theory, procedure, and normal values in the conscious and anesthetized albino rat, J. Neurochem. 28 (5) (1977) 897–916.

[10] P. Herscovitch, J. Markham, M.E. Raichle, Brain blood flow measured with intravenous H$_2$(15)O: I. Theory and error analysis, J. Nucl. Med. 24 (9) (1983) 782–789.

[11] M.E. Raichle, et al., Brain blood flow measured with intravenous H$_2$(15)O: II. Implementation and validation, J. Nucl. Med. 24 (9) (1983) 790–798.

[12] M.E. Phelps, et al., Tomographic measurement of local cerebral glucose metabolic rate in humans with (F-18)2-fluoro-2-deoxy-D-glucose: validation of method, Ann. Neurol. 6 (5) (1979) 371–388.

[13] H. Nakai, et al., Time-dependent changes of lumped and rate constants in the deoxyglucose method in experimental cerebral ischemia, J. Cereb. Blood Flow Metab. 7 (5) (1987) 640–648.

[14] H. Fukuyama, et al., Coronal reconstruction images of glucose metabolism in Alzheimer's disease, J. Neurol. Sci. 106 (2) (1991) 128–134.

[15] R.P. Woods, et al., Automated image registration: I. General methods and intrasubject, intramodality validation, J. Comput.-Assist. Tomogr. 22 (1) (1998) 139–152.

[16] F. Reinoso-Suarez, Topographischer Hirnatlas der Katze fur Experimental-Physiologische Untersuchungen, E. Merk, Darmstadt, 1979.

[17] A.G. Kovach, et al., The effect of hemorrhagic hypotension and retransfusion and 7-nitro-indazole on rCBF, NOS catalytic activity, and cortical NO content in the cat, Ann. N. Y. Acad. Sci. 738 (1994) 348–368.

[18] N. Cholet, et al., Local uncoupling of the cerebrovascular and metabolic responses to somatosensory stimulation after neuronal nitric oxide synthase inhibition, J. Cereb. Blood Flow Metab. 17 (11) (1997) 1191–1201.

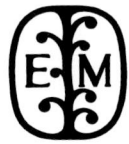

International Congress Series 1235 (2002) 205–212

Hemodynamic and metabolic features of cerebral activation

Olaf B. Paulson*, Ian Law

Neurobiology Research Unit, Copenhagen University Hospital, N 9201 Rigshospitalet, 9 Blegdamsvej, DK-2100 Copenhagen, Denmark

Abstract

It is well established that cerebral activation is accompanied by an increase of cerebral blood flow (CBF) and glucose metabolism which exceeds a smaller increase in oxygen consumption. Thus, cerebral activation is accompanied by an uncoupling of the normal relations between blood flow and oxygen metabolism as well as of the ratio between oxygen and glucose consumption. The present communication discusses the physiological relevance of these changes and whether or not they are necessary in order to maintain an adequate brain function. Experimental studies in rat demonstrated that the uncoupling of the ratio between oxygen and glucose consumption during activation is reset by β-adrenergic blockade with Propranolol. © 2002 Elsevier Science B.V. All rights reserved.

Keywords: Activation; Uncoupling; Glucose/oxygen index; Cerebral metabolism; Cerebral blood flow; Propranolol; Lactate

1. Introduction

Changes in the cerebral hemodynamics and/or metabolism during activation had been suggested and supported by scarce studies in the more ancient literature. But, it was first in the 1970s that it became apparent that mapping of regional cerebral blood flow (CBF) changes could be used to map cerebral activation. Niels A. Lassen and David H. Ingvar had in the 1960s introduced the radioemitting inert gasses for regional CBF measurements. These techniques were now used for mapping of cerebral activation [1,2]. This field of research has since expanded dramatically and uses today the more atraumatic methods, functional magnetic resonance imaging (fMRI) and positron emission tomography (PET) with the flow tracer $H_2^{15}O$.

---

* Corresponding author.
E-mail address: paulson@nru.dk (O.B. Paulson).

0531-5131/02 © 2002 Elsevier Science B.V. All rights reserved.
PII: S 0 5 3 1 - 5 1 3 1 (0 2) 0 0 1 8 8 - 7

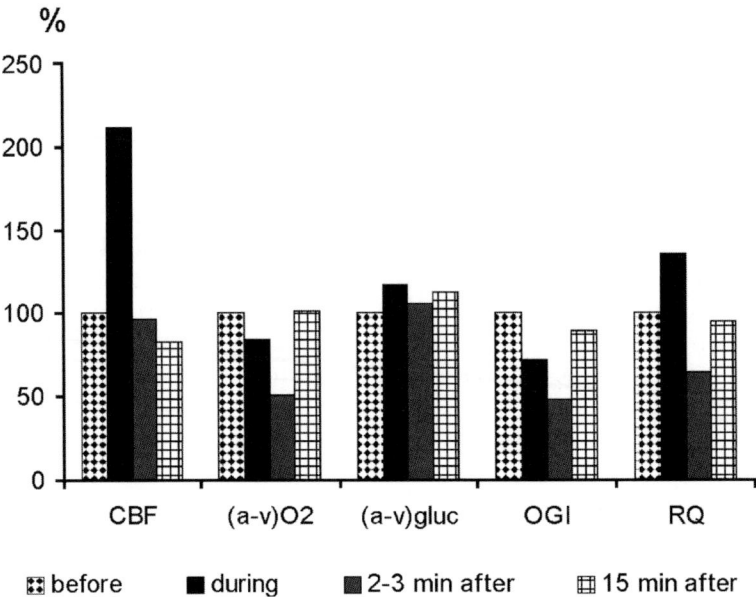

Fig. 1. During generalized seizures, there is a marked increase in cerebral blood flow (CBF) which exceeds the increase in oxygen consumption as (a-v)O₂ drops. The oxygen/glucose index (OGI) drops markedly. The respiratory coefficient increases indicating production of lactic acid in the brain. (Based on results from Brodersen et al. [3].)

Wonderful tools have thus been developed allowing to investigate the function of the brain in the intact living subject. But, why is flow increased in activated area and which metabolic aspects are involved? Let us first look at what might be called extreme activation, the epileptic seizure. Here both flow oxygen and glucose consumption are markedly increased. However, flow and glucose consumption increase more than the oxygen consumption and part of the glucose is converted to lactate resulting in a pH decrease and thereby release of carbondioxide with an increase in the respiratory coefficient of the brain (Fig. 1) [3]. In this study, the arterial oxygen tension was kept constant during the seizure and corresponding to the larger increase in flow than in oxygen consumption, there was a significant increase in the oxygen tension and saturation in the venous outflow from the brain. New major attention was focused on the topic when it was demonstrated that uncoupling of flow and glucose consumption versus oxygen consumption also takes place during normal physiological activation [4,5].

2. Oxygen and lactate

Why does the organism need an increased flow during activation? Is it necessary in order to maintain an adequate oxygen or an adequate glucose supply? The above mentioned anaerobic glucose metabolism with lactate production could favor a shortage of oxygen, but the increased oxygen tension in the venous outflow from the brain would contradict such a hypothesis. Further experimental studies had demonstrated that more physiological activation is accompanied by an increase of the average oxygen tension in the activated cerebral tissue [6,7]. However, these studies do not take into account possibilities of heterogeneity in oxygen tension at the cellular level. With a large oxygen consumption of the brain diffusion gradients will be present in the cerebral tissue and it might be that cells far away from the capillaries might have a critical low oxygen supply compared to other cells in the brain. It might be calculated that sufficient steep gradients of the oxygen tension in a situation with increased oxygen consumption might lead to critical low values distant from the capillaries simultaneous to average tissue and venous outflow oxygen tensions that were increased rather than decreased [8].

For the sake of argument, attention should also be drawn to another hypothesis which might favor an increased lactate production. Magistretti's group [9] has forwarded theories according to which glucose in the brain is consumed by the glia cells which release lactate, which in turn is used as the metabolic substrate for the neurons. In case of a metabolic increase of the neurons, then the brain could need a higher lactate concentration in order to allow sufficient rapid diffusion. With such a theory, the increased lactate production would reflect an increased demand of the neurons and not a lack of oxygen. However, Shulman suggested that the glial cells have a function clearing neurotransmitters during activation. This requires increased anaerobic glucose metabolism with increased lactate production and lactate efflux [10].

Under normal baseline conditions, a small efflux of lactate from the brain is observed, i.e., a slightly higher concentration in the venous outflow as compared to the arterial inflow. This efflux may increase slightly during physiological activation. But, if the activation involves motor activity with increased arterial lactate concentration, then the efflux is reversed to a slight uptake [11,12]. These changes of the flux of lactate across the blood–brain barrier can be considered as a simple reflection of diffusion gradients, lactate being transported across the blood–brain barrier by a mechanism of facilitated diffusion similar to the glucose transport.

3. Glucose

The glucose supply to the brain might seem to have a reasonable safety margin. Normally, about 15% of the glucose in the arterial blood will diffuse across the capillary wall into the cerebral tissue. About 1/3 of the glucose that has entered the brain will later diffuse back to the capillary blood resulting in an arteriovenous difference of about 10% and in an extracellular glucose concentration in the brain and the cerebrospinal fluid of about 40% of the concentration in the blood [13]. But if glucose consumption is suddenly increased, then back diffusion to the blood would decrease and so would the extracellular glucose concentration in the brain.

This might, at least theoretically, imply risks of insufficient glucose concentration gradients to secure an adequate glucose supply to all parts of the cells. How could an increased flow increase the glucose supply to the brain in the form of an increased glucose diffusion across the blood–brain barrier? A simple linear flow increase in the capillaries would not be very efficient. With an (a-v) difference of only 10%, the average capillary glucose concentration could hardly increase by more than a few percent with an even marked flow increase. This would be quite insufficient to account for a larger glucose diffusion from blood to brain. On the contrary, if the flow increase involved a recruitment of additional capillaries with an increase of the efficient capillary surface area, then the diffusion capacity from blood to brain of glucose could increase substantially. These aspects have been reviewed in details by Kuschinsky and Paulson [14] and later confirmed in other studies [15,16]. Recruitment of capillaries is its classical sense as opening of previous closed capillaries seems not to take place in the brain. However, under normal circumstances, the capillary perfusion in the brain is rather heterogenous with shorter and longer transit times and this heterogeneity seems to vanish with flow increase resulting in a larger efficient capillary surface area.

4. Oxygen/glucose index (OGI)

Which changes are seen in the metabolic pattern during activation? In the normal brain under baseline conditions, the molar ratio between oxygen and glucose consumption, the OGI is very close to 6 as essentially all glucose is metabolized to water and carbon dioxide with the exception of the minimal release of lactate mentioned above. This changes during activation where glucose consumption increase in excess of oxygen consumption as mentioned above. Recent studies performed in rats in our laboratory showed that activation reduced (a-v)O_2 by 25% while (a-v)gluc remained unchanged [11,12]. The molar uptake ratio between the cerebral uptake of oxygen and glucose was reduced from about 6 during baseline to about 4 during activation (Fig. 2). From these values observed during activation, it can be calculated that oxidative metabolism only accounted for 60% of the glucose that was taken up by the brain. The metabolic fate of the activation-induced cerebral glucose

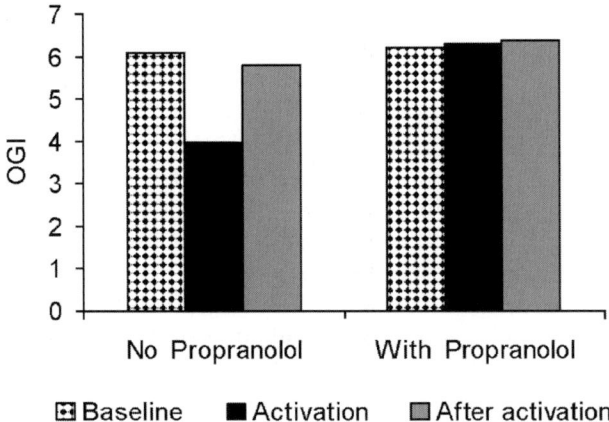

Fig. 2. During physiological activation in rats, the molar oxygen/glucose consumption ratio (index, OGI) drops markedly. (Based on results from Schmalbruch et al. [12].)

accumulation is unknown and some of the excess glucose uptake may have been converted to lactate that was accumulated in the brain. However, previous data that have addressed this problem directly indicates that only approximately 50% of the activation-induced excess glucose uptake can be accounted for by anaerobic conversion to lactate [17].

5. β-Adrenergic blockade

In the context of the evaluation of these metabolic changes during activation, the influence of β-adrenergic blockade becomes of major interest. It has previously been shown that severe immobilization stress in rats will increase global $CMRO_2$ and CBF up to 90% and this cerebral activation response could be totally abolished by β-adrenergic blockade with Propranolol [18]. A recent study from our group evaluated the effect on the activation response of β-adrenergic blockade in rats (Propranolol hydrochloride, 2 to 3 mg kg^{-1}, i.v.). Activation was induced by opening the shelter box, exposing the rat to the environment for 10 min. The behavioral degree of activation as assessed by monitoring sniffing and body movements was not reduced by the administration of Propranolol. Further blood pressure during activation was the same in control and in Propanolol-treated animals and in both groups activation induced an increase in the arterial glucose concentration. Thus, the rats that received Propranolol were activated to a comparable degree as compared to the rats that not did receive any Propranolol. The β-adrenergic blockade totally abolished the activation-induced uncoupling of oxygen consumption from glucose consumption and CBF [12]. Thus, with β-adrenergic blockade, the OGI remained close to 6 (Fig. 2) and the $(a-v)O_2$ was unchanged indicating an unchanged CBF. All glucose taken up by the brain during activation following β-adrenergic blockade could thus be fully accounted for by oxidation and a small efflux of lactate.

It raises the important question of how β-adrenergic blockade with Propranolol can be tolerated without serious cognitive side effects. If Propranolol abolishes the activation-induced increase in cerebral metabolism and this does not cause serious cerebral side effects, what is then the purpose of the activation-induced increased cerebral metabolism. This observation is important because it may bear significant information on the subject of mechanism responsible for the coupling between cerebral blood flow and cerebral metabolism.

6. Conclusion

It remains still a puzzle whether the brain is at the borderline of starvation during activation for which reason changes in flow are necessary in order to meet metabolic demand. Or if the flow and metabolism changes are more like to be an epiphenomenon accompanying activation but not of essential importance for the brain function. This latter question has been further investigated by studies in sea level and after being acclimatized at high altitude in the Andes (5260 m over sea level). Here the arterial oxygen tension under baseline condition is close to the venous oxygen tension at sea level. Despite this normal activation occurs at exercise at high altitude and normal quantitative flow increase is observed during activation in the settings of PET scanning. These results are reported further in a separate communication to this symposium [19].

In conclusion, we may state that it might be that the brain needs additional flow and changes in metabolism in order to optimize its function during activation. However, the brain is doing pretty well without such changes and we have still got a puzzle.

Further, if Propranolol abolishes the uncoupling between CBF and $CMRO_2$, it would also be expected to abolish the activation response as detected by f-MRI.

2.4.3.9. On-Site Discussion

2.4.3.9.1. *Question: (Traystman)* The confluence of the sinuses has extracranial contamination so the venous 02 measured may be erroneous. Did the β-blocker decrease blood pressure, and result in an autoregulatory response?

Answer: (Paulson) We, and especially Bolwig and Hertz from our Hospital, have carefully investigated how to collect blood flow the confluence sinus. We have set up a reliable sampling method with very slow blood sampling. In the control state, blood pressure dropped only 4–5 mm Hg, and during activation, blood pressure increased on the average 1 mm Hg. Thus, blood pressure changes were without significance for the findings.

2.4.3.9.2. *Question: (Dreier)* You reported that blockade with Propranolol abolishes the uncoupling of cerebral glucose and oxygen metabolism during activation. Shulman suggested that the uncoupling of cerebral glucose and oxygen metabolism during activation is related to an astrocytic glycogen shunt. Propranolol has been reported to inhibit cerebral glycogenolysis. I would like to suggest the hypothesis that Propranolol abolishes the uncoupling of cerebral glucose and oxygen metabolism during activation by blocking the astrocytic glycogen shunt.

Answer: (Paulson) Your suggested mechanism is really interesting. It cannot be answered from our present study. Further investigation clarifying this question would be highly interesting.

2.4.3.9.3. *Question: (Busch)* Propanolol is one of the drugs which works for prophylaxis of migraene. On the other side, migraine is related to flow changes in the brain. Do you see any relation of your findings to the condition of migraine?

Answer: (Paulson) In migraine with aura, flow is markedly decreased in the initial phase. The flow changes are probably an epiphenomenona and not the cause of the migraine attack. The prophylactic effect of propanolol is therefore likely independent of the flow changes. Further propanolol may very well be without influence on the flow changes in migraine, but this has not been studied.

2.4.3.9.4. *Question: (Gjedde)* Do you intend to test the elimination of the "BOLD" response in rats with the administration of a β-blocked in human fMRI?

Answer: (Paulson) BOLD fMRI studies and results will soon be ready!

2.4.3.9.5. *Question: (Jones)* In view of our future activities tonight, could you comment on the β-blocker effects of alcohol ingestion?

Answer: (Paulson) It seems not to disturb cerebral activation. It might, in fact, enhance it, at least at moderate doses—let us see at the party.

Acknowledgements

This work was supported by a research grant from The 1991 Pharmacy Foundation, Health Insurance Fund and The Lundbeck Foundation.

References

[1] J. Olesen, Contralateral focal increase of cerebral blood flow in man during arm work, Brain 94 (1971) 635–646.

[2] N.A. Lassen, D.H. Ingvar, E. Skinhøj, Brain function and blood flow, Changes in the amount of blood flowing in areas of the human cerebral cortex, reflecting changes in the activity of those areas, are graphically revealed with the aid of radioactive isotopes, Sci. Am. 239 (1978) 62–71.

[3] P. Brodersen, O.B. Paulson, T.G. Bolwig, Z.E. Rogon, O.J. Rafaelsen, N.A. Lassen, Cerebral hyperemia in electrically induced epileptic seizures, Arch. Neurol. 28 (1973) 334–338.

[4] P.T. Fox, M.E. Raichle, Focal physiological uncoupling of cerebral blood flow and oxidative metabolism during somatosensory stimulation in human subjects, Proc. Natl. Acad. Sci. U. S. A. 83 (1986) 1140–1144.

[5] P.T. Fox, M.E. Raichle, M.A. Mintun, C. Dence, Nonoxidative glucose consumption during focal physiologic neural activation, Science 241 (1988) 462–464.

[6] R. Cooper, H.J. Crow, W.G. Walter, A.L. Winter, Regional control of cerebral vascular reactivity and oxygen supply in man, Brain Res. 3 (1966) 174–191.

[7] R. Cooper, H.J. Crow, Changes of cerebral oxygenation during motor and mental tasks, in: D.I. Ingvar, N.A. Lassen (Eds.), Brain Work: The Coupling of Function, Metabolism and Blood Flow in the Brain, Alfred Benzon Symposium VIII, Munksgaard, Copenhagen, 1975, pp. 389–392.

[8] R. Buxton, Coupling Between CBF and CMRO2 During Neuronal Activity, Contribution to the present symposium, 2001.

[9] L. Pellerin, G. Pellegri, P.G. Bittar, Y. Charnay, C. Bouras, J.L. Martin, N. Stella, P.J. Magistretti, Evidence supporting the existence of an activity-dependent astrocyte-neuron lactate shuttle, Dev. Neurosci. 20 (1998) 291–299.

[10] R.G. Shulman, Cerebral Energetics and the Glycogen Shunt, Contribution to the present symposium, 2001.

[11] P.L. Madsen, R. Linde, S.G. Hasselbalch, O.B. Paulson, N.A. Lassen, Activation-induced resetting of cerebral oxygen and glucose uptake in the rat, J. Cereb. Blood Flow Metab. 18 (1998) 742–748.

[12] I.K. Schmalbruch, R. Linde, O.B. Paulson, P.L. Madsen, The activation-induced resetting of cerebral blood flow and metabolism is abolished by β-blockade with Propranolol. In preparation.

[13] G.M. Knudsen, K.D. Pettigrew, O.B. Paulson, M.M. Hertz, C.S. Patlak, Kinetic analysis of blood–brain barrier transport of D-glucose in man: quantitative evaluation in the presence of tracer backflux and capillary heterogeneity, Microvasc. Res., 39 (1990) 28–49.

[14] W. Kuschinsky, O.B. Paulson, Capillary circulation in the brain, Cerebrovasc. Brain Metab. Rev. 4 (1992) 261–286.

[15] G.M. Knudsen, K.D. Pettigrew, C.S. Patlak, O.B. Paulson, Blood–brain barrier permeability measurements by double-indicator method using intravenous injection, Am. J. Physiol. 266 (1994) H987–H999 (Heart Circ. Physiol. 1994, 35).

[16] W. Kuschinsky, Heterogeneity of Cerebral Microvascular Flow: Relationship to CBF, Contribution to the present symposium, 2001.

[17] P.L. Madsen, N.F. Cruz, L. Sokoloff, G. Dienel, Cerebral oxygen/glucose ratio is low during sensory stimulation and rises above normal during recovery: excess glucose consumption during stimulation is not accounted for by lactate efflux from or accumulation in brain tissue, J. Cereb. Blood Flow Metab. 19 (1999) 393–400.

[18] C. Carlsson, M. Hägerdal, A.E. Kaasik, B.K. Siesjö, A catecholamine-mediated increase in cerebral oxygen uptake during immobilization stress in rats, Brain Res. 119 (1977) 223–231.

[19] I. Law, R.C. Roach, N.V. Olsen, S. Holm, M. Nowak, T.F. Hornbein, O.B. Paulson, Oxygen Delivery to the Brain During Behavioral Activation at Acute Normobaric Hypoxemia, Contribution to the present symposium, 2001.

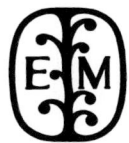

International Congress Series 1235 (2002) 213–222

Inhibition and functional magnetic resonance imaging

Petra Ritter*, Arno Villringer

*Division of Neuroimaging, Department of Neurology, Neurologische Klinik, Charité,
Schumannstraße 20-21, 10117 Berlin, Germany*

Abstract

This review summarizes our current knowledge on how inhibitory phenomena are reflected in the functional magnetic resonance imaging (fMRI) signal. It is well-established that activity-related changes of brain metabolism and blood flow are dominated by changes in synaptic activity. Both excitatory and inhibitory synaptic activities are associated with increased metabolic demands. The amount of energy consumption associated with inhibition vs. excitation is reflected in metabolism- and blood flow-related neuroimaging signals such as the blood oxygen level-dependent (BOLD) contrast; the relationship between the different "signals", however, may not be linear. The influence on these signals depends on the number of active inhibiting synapses, the duration of inhibition and the degree of propagation within subsequent neuronal circuits. The relative influence of inhibition as compared to excitation on the metabolism/blood flow may also vary in different neuronal circuits. Inhibition leads to locally decreased discharge activity, which does not have a significant effect on the cerebral blood flow (CBF)/BOLD images. However, inhibition may also result in suppression of complex neuronal circuits, leading to a decrease in excitatory as well as inhibitory synaptic activity, and therewith, to a decreased metabolism and blood flow within those complex neuronal networks. The available fMRI data indicate that, depending on the abovementioned factors, inhibition may be reflected in positive, negative or no BOLD-signal at all. Thus, the BOLD-signal is ambiguous with respect to the underlying electrophysiological event. In the future, combining fMRI with electrophysiological methods will strengthen neuroimaging studies. © 2002 Elsevier Science B.V. All rights reserved.

Keywords: Functional magnetic resonance imaging; Blood oxygen level-dependent (BOLD); Metabolism; BOLD-signal

* Corresponding author.
E-mail addresses: Petra.Ritter@charite.de (P. Ritter), Arno.Villringer@charite.de (A. Villringer).

0531-5131/02 © 2002 Elsevier Science B.V. All rights reserved.
PII: S 0 5 3 1 - 5 1 3 1 (0 2) 0 0 1 8 9 - 9

1. Introduction

Several neuroimaging techniques assess neuronal activation indirectly after translation by neurovascular and neuro-metabolic coupling into a physiologic (vascular or metabolic) signal, which can be measured by the respective technique.

The blood oxygen level-dependent (BOLD) and functional magnetic resonance imaging (fMRI) techniques are currently the most widely used methods for indirect mapping of neuronal activity. The BOLD-signal has an inverse relationship to changes in the local deoxyhemoglobin concentration, which result from changes in the local cerebral metabolic rate of oxygen ($CMRO_2$), cerebral blood flow (CBF) and cerebral blood volume (CBV) associated with neuronal activity.

In "activated" brain areas, the BOLD-signal intensity increases within a few seconds after the onset of stimulation as a consequence of an increase in the regional CBF, exceeding the increase in oxygen utilization. After the termination of the stimuli, the signal decays in several seconds. It should be emphasized, however, that the term "activation" is only defined by the behavior of the BOLD-signal and is not a priori equivalent with any event (e.g., action potential, excitatory or inhibitory synaptic activity, etc.) occurring on a neuronal level.

If the underlying situation is characterized by an increase in synaptic activity and an increased neuronal firing rate, then there is general consensus that this is reflected in a BOLD-signal increase, i.e., "activation". However, there are other situations in which these neuronal events are not in "synchrony". An increase in synaptic activity may also be due to an increase in excitatory (as in the case above) or inhibitory activity. In the latter case, synaptic activity and local firing rate of the neurons may actually diverge [1]. It is discussed controversially, whether the decreased neuronal activity of certain brain areas resulting from the inhibition leads to a drop in the BOLD-signal intensity below the baseline, or to an increase of the BOLD-signal intensity (similar to activation) due to an increase in energy metabolism, or whether it cannot be detected at all by functional neuroimaging methods due to negligible effects on local brain metabolism.

2. Spikes vs. synaptic potentials—what causes gross metabolic changes?

In order to allow the predictions of the respective effects of neuronal spikes and of neuronal synaptic activity on regional brain metabolism, knowledge of the ratio between the energy requirements of both types of neuronal activity is critical. The complex reactions surrounding synaptic activity including transmitter cycling, transmitter–receptor reactions, second messenger activities (in contrast to the only reestablishment of ion equilibrium during discharge activity), as well as the mitochondrial distribution within a neuron, suggest synaptic activity to be the greater energy consumer.

These hypotheses are supported by several studies, e.g., [^{14}C]-2-deoxyglucose (2-DG) distribution [2] matched the distribution of the activated synapses and not the distribution of the discharging postsynaptic membrane, and during the stimulation of the excitatory afferents of the nucleus laminaris of a chick [3]. It follows that local changes in glucose consumption are not evidence of changes in local neuronal discharge activity, but instead evidence of alterations in synaptic activity.

3. Glucose metabolism during excitatory and inhibitory activity

Inhibitory postsynaptic potentials are caused by energy-requiring mechanisms. Using 2-DG labeling increased glucose metabolism during the inhibition of the hippocampal pyramidal cells induced by low frequency stimulation of the fornix in rats and has been shown in Ref. [4]. Increased glucose uptake occurred particularly in the stratum pyramidale, which contains a dense plexus of inhibitory interneuronal terminals upon pyramidal cells.

Another group also employing [^{14}C]-2-DG labeling investigated glucose metabolism of: (1) synaptic activity in the absence of postsynaptic cell discharge (active inhibitory synapses); (2) cell discharge in the absence of synaptic activity. Also, they addressed the question whether increased glucose metabolism is caused predominantly by cell discharge or by synaptic activity [3].

It is well known from neuroanatomical experiments that lateral superior olives (LSOs) in the brainstem auditory system receive each of the afferents from both ears. According to electrophysiological, pharmacological and anatomical reports, afferents from the ipsilateral ear are excitatory, and those from the contralateral ear are inhibitory.

After the destruction of the left cochlea in cats, auditory stimulation did result in heavy 2-DG labeling in the left as well as in the inhibited right LSO.

In order to estimate the degree of 2-DG labeling contributed by the discharging membrane, the medial superior olive (MSO) in cats was stimulated antidromically, avoiding synaptic activity. No significant 2-DG labeling was produced. However, microphotodensitometry indicated that antidromic stimulation of the MSO did result in a slightly elevated glucose metabolism, too small to be assessed by the untrained eye.

Finally, the group found that synaptic activity dominated the changes in glucose metabolism, and that discharges of neuronal membranes are not sufficient by themselves to produce obvious 2-DG labeling. To show this, researchers took advantage of the bipolar structure of the nucleus laminaris in the chicks. The nucleus laminaris is composed of two dendritic cells with a dorsoventral orientation. One set of afferents (from the ipsilateral ear) predominantly ends on the dorsal dendrites of the somata, the other set of afferents (from the contralateral ear) predominantly ends on the ventral dendrites. Exciting the nucleus laminaris yielded a dorsoventral asymmetry of 2-DG labeling, depending on whether it was stimulated via one set of afferents or the other.

4. Changes in cerebral metabolism vs. changes in cerebral blood flow

Can data on changes that occur in cerebral metabolism (e.g., glucose consumption and oxygen consumption) be linked to the changes in the cerebral blood flow and in the BOLD-signal. Ever since the landmark reports by Fox and Raichle [5,6] on a "focal" uncoupling during transient changes in brain activity, this issue has been discussed controversially. In those studies, a large mismatch between the changes in oxygen consumption and the cerebral blood flow during increased brain activity had been reported. Whereas many other groups have confirmed the finding of a mismatch between $CMRO_2$ and CBF, a consensus is now emerging that this mismatch is quantitative, not qualitative, i.e., there seems to be a tight coupling between the blood flow and metabolism; however, this coupling is not linear.

A mathematical model for the delivery of oxygen to the brain [7] predicts that disproportionately large changes in the blood flow are required to support small changes in the cerebral metabolic rate of oxygen ($CMRO_2$). In fact, the very nature of the positive BOLD-signal during "activation" studies is a consequence of this mismatch between CBF (more precisely, it is the blood flow velocity that matters) and oxygen use. This model also predicts a higher oxygen extraction fraction for decreases in flow. Accordingly, a negative BOLD response during "deactivation" induced by saccades in the striate visual cortex [8] has been reported, indicating a similar type of mismatch between flow and oxygen delivery with decreased neuronal activity.

In conclusion, in healthy brain tissue, it can be expected that increases in brain metabolism (glucose consumption and oxygen consumption) are associated with increases in the local blood flow and local BOLD-signal. The quantitative relationship between these physiological parameters, however, awaits further investigation.

Thus, in situations of inhibition, which are associated with an increase in metabolism, increases in blood flow and the BOLD-signal are to be expected. In an experimental study on the cerebellum, Mathiesen et al. [1] have shown nicely how the inhibitory synaptic activity is associated with a local increase in the cerebral blood flow.

5. Efficiency of excitatory and inhibitory synapses

Excitatory and inhibitory synapses have distinct ultrastructures [9]. Two common morphological types, referred to as Gray type I (excitatory) and type II (inhibitory), differ in the width of the synaptic cleft, the presynaptic active zone and the shape of the synaptic vesicles. The synapses containing round vesicles, which are typical for excitatory synapses, are about five times as frequent as those with flat vesicles, typical for inhibitory synapses in area 17 of the cat [10].

A single hippocampal CA1 pyramidal cell receives around 30,000 excitatory and 1700 inhibitory inputs [11]. The highly convergent excitation arriving onto the distal dendrites of the pyramidal cells is controlled primarily by proximally located inhibition.

The smaller number and higher efficiency [12] of inhibitory as compared to excitatory synapses may result in a lower metabolic demand during inhibition. Since few inhibitory synapses can inhibit large neuronal populations [13,14], such inhibited regions should have a low net regional CBF and regional cerebral metabolism. Due to less excitatory input from the inhibited regions, there might also be a decrease in metabolism in the projection areas.

6. Functional neuroimaging of inhibition

6.1. "Activation" of cerebral structures is accompanied by "deactivations" of other structures

The results of a positron emission tomography (PET) study employing vibratory stimulation of the right hand indicated that the stimulation-induced increases of the regional CBF and $CMRO_2$ in the left SI, left SII, left retroinsular field (RI), left anterior parietal cortex, left MI and left SMA are associated with regional decreases of CBF and $CMRO_2$ in the superior parietal cortex bilaterally (main decrease was adjacent to left SI), paralimbic association areas and the left globus pallidus [15]. The regional changes were balanced, so that the mean global CBF and $CMRO_2$ did not change when compared with the rest.

During the specific tasks, deactivations of areas belonging to the nonrelevant sensory modality have been shown, e.g., decreases in CBF in the visual cortex during somatosensory tasks [16], and decreased CBF in the auditory and prefrontal regions during a visual task [17]. Thus, inhibition may be an essential component of the selective attentional processes playing a complementary role to task-specific activations.

6.2. Transcallosal and cortico–cortical motor system inhibition

Three effects of transcranial magnetic stimulation (TMS) are well-known: (1) cortico–spinally excitatory contralateral tonic motor response mediated by large pyramidal cells and postexcitatory inhibition of these pyramidal cells [18,19]; (2) transcallosal inhibition of the contralateral motor cortex [20–22]; (3) paired-pulse cortico–cortical facilitation at interstimulus intervals (ISI) of 6–20 ms (subthreshold conditioning stimulus) and 10–40 ms (suprathreshold conditioning stimulus) and inhibition at ISI of 1–4 ms/40–200 ms (sub/suprathreshold conditioning stimulus) [23,24]. These phenomena provide experimentally and neurophysiologically well-defined mechanisms inducing cortico–cortically mediated inhibitory and excitatory effects, which can be evaluated by neuroimaging methods like PET or BOLD-sensitive fMRI.

Based on the findings described above, a recent study employing positron emission tomography (PET) and transcranial magnetic stimulation (TMS) of the left primary motor cortex (M1) evaluated the correlation between the local CBF and contralateral motor-evoked potentials (MEPs) induced by paired-pulse stimuli (subthreshold conditioning stimulus, suprathreshold test stimulus), with ISIs of 3 and 12 ms [25]. A significant positive correlation was observed between the CBF changes (activation) in the left M1 and in the amount of suppression, as well as facilitation of the electromyographic (EMG) response for both ISIs. As the CBF changes in the left M1 for 3 and 12 ms, ISIs did not overlap, supporting the hypotheses that early inhibition and late facilitation arise from separate pools of cortical interneurons [23].

By using a combination of transcranial stimulation (TES) and fMRI as recently established by our group [26,27], we have recently shown that TES-stimulation of the motor cortex on one hemisphere (associated with transcallosal inhibition) leads to a BOLD–fMRI signal intensity increase in the somatomotor cortex of the other (presumably inhibited) hemisphere ([28] (Abstract) and unpublished results). Another physiological setting, in which transcallosal inhibition has been reported, is in finger/thumb tapping. Using this paradigm, a decrease of the BOLD-signal in the ipsilateral (presumably inhibited) sensorimotor cortex has been reported [29]. One intriguing interpretation of these diverging findings is that they are due to the different forms of transcallosal inhibition in the two settings. Studies in which electrophysiological recordings are performed simultaneously to the fMRI are needed to further clarify these points.

6.3. Motor system inhibition by go/no-go task

Employing a go/no-go auditory reaction time paradigm, simultaneously TMS-induced MEPs in the bilateral extensor pollicis brevis muscles were evaluated [30]. After the no-go tones, bilateral inhibition occurred at a time corresponding to the mean reaction time to the go tones. Using the go/no-go paradigm in combination with the event-related fMRI, it has recently been shown that there is no significant change in the BOLD-signal intensity from the baseline for the no-go task in M1 [31]. Based on these results, Waldvogel et al. [31] drew the conclusion that "when blood flow is increased, it is very likely that this represents predominant excitatory synaptic activity".

6.4. 'Saccadic suppression'—inhibition of the primary visual cortex during saccades

'Saccadic suppression'—the phenomenon of an elevated visual threshold associated with voluntary saccadic eye movement—has been quantitatively demonstrated by both psychophysical and electrophysiological techniques. The absence of any alteration in LGN cell activity during directionally specific inhibition of the striate visual cortex neurons, was recorded by microelectrodes in encéphale isolé monkeys, with a short latency of inhibition of only 20–30 ms (the latency of the first component (P3a), the human visual-evoked response (VER) is approximately 40 ms). This supports the concept of a central mechanism (corollary discharge) playing a significant role in saccadic suppression [32]. Several facts suggest the superior colliculus (SC) to be a generator of corollary discharge [33–35]. Other possible sources for corollary discharge are the frontal cortical eye fields, which fire in association with eye movements [36].

With the use of PET, changes in regional CBF during the execution of saccades with varying frequencies (40–140 saccades per minute) were measured in complete darkness [37]. With increasing numbers of saccades, the regional CBF increased in the frontal eye field, the superior colliculus and the cerebellar vermis. In parallel, the regional CBF decreased (in comparison to the baseline) in the striate cortex, the adjacent extrastriate cortex and the parietal cortex, indicating a decrease in the net amount of synaptic neurotransmission. In accordance with these results, the regional BOLD decreases measured by fMRI and the regional increases of [deoxyhemoglobin] measured by near infrared spectroscopy (NIRS)—both indicating deactivation—in the primary and adjacent secondary visual areas have been shown [8].

6.5. A model for deactivation: reversal of the common stimulus design

The majority of the MR mapping studies employed paradigms that led to "brain activation", implying a change from low degree neuronal activity to a high degree of neuronal activity. In the BOLD–fMRI, "activation" simply refers to a positive BOLD effect.

A general practice is the analysis of the switches in neuronal activity between arbitrary steady-state conditions and functional states.

In a BOLD–fMRI study, "activation" (BOLD–fMRI signal increase) and "deactivation" (BOLD fMRI signal decrease) in the human visual cortex were accomplished by reversing the order of the baseline/stimulation condition [38]. All activation protocols employed a gray light stimulus as the baseline condition and a checkerboard stimulus as the activation condition. All the deactivation protocols employed the checkerboard as a baseline condition (corresponding to sustained visual stimulation). The steady-state conditions were established by presenting the "baseline stimulus" for 60–120 s. Decreased neuronal activity resulted in an initial 5% drop in the BOLD-signal corresponding to the poststimulus undershoot, followed by a small 1.5–2% increase up to a new steady-state in sustained "deactivation". Furthermore, the activation paradigm induced a 4.5–5% BOLD-signal increase and a poststimulus 1.5–2% undershoot.

These results from the PET and fMRI studies indicate that deactivation following inhibition might be regarded as less activation due to a decrease in neuronal synaptic activity.

7. Conclusions—inhibition can result in "activation" or "deactivation"

The activity-related changes of brain metabolism and the blood flow are dominated by changes in synaptic activity. Both excitatory and inhibitory synaptic activities are associated with increased metabolic demands, increased blood flow and the BOLD-signal, and the quantitative relationship between these parameters is probably nonlinear. The difference in energy consumption associated with inhibition vs. excitation is probably reflected in metabolism- and blood flow-related neuroimaging signals such as the BOLD contrast. The influence on these signals depends on the number of active inhibiting synapses, the duration of inhibition and the degree of propagation within subsequent neuronal circuits. The relative influence of inhibition as compared to excitation on metabolism/blood flow may also vary in the different neuronal circuits. Inhibition leads to locally decreased discharge activity, which does not have a significant effect on the CBF/BOLD images. However, inhibition may also result in the suppression of the complex neuronal circuits, leading to a decrease in excitatory as well as inhibitory synaptic activity, and therewith, to decreased metabolism and blood flow within those complex neuronal networks.

These considerations may explain why in the abovementioned TMS study, cortico–cortical inhibition is associated with increased CBF [25], whereas the fMRI–BOLD-signal decreases during transcallosal inhibition [29], which indicates a decrease in the CBF. Thus, inhibitory events may be associated with "activation" as well as "deactivation".

The BOLD-signal is thus ambiguous with respect to the underlying neuronal events. The addition of electrophysiological techniques such as TMS to neuroimaging protocols may be useful in order to elucidate the functional status of the cerebral tissue under investigation.

8. On-Site Discussion

Question: (Heiss) I found your reports of results of transcallosal inhibition very interesting. Collateral and transcallosal inhibition is very important for the development of lateralized function, e.g., for dominance of speech in the left hemisphere. Do you have any data showing disinhibition of collateral or transcallosal inhibition playing a role in compensation for lesions in primary centers? This might be important for recovery from motor deficit or aphasia after stroke. I will discuss some of these effects in my presentation.

Answer: (Villinger) I agree that this may be very interesting to study; however, so far, we do not have our own data on this issue.

Comment: (Hyder) (1) The kind of work being done for an excitatory event and inhibition event is similar at the pre-synaptic terminal (e.g., docking of vesicles, excytosis, vesicular release of transmitter). Since it is work being done, energy is being consumed for both events. Therefore, an energy-based imaging modality (e.g., BOLD) may not be able to dissociate between these two types of events. (2) So the correlation between spiking activity and BOLD found by Hees et al. and Heeger et al. (please see Nat. Neurosci. papers from 2000) will be only true for specific cases. The more likely correlation is to be found between synaptic activity and BOLD (e.g., Hyder et al. (Society for Neuroscience 2001) or Logothetis et al. (Society for Neuroscience 2001).

Question: (Dirnagl) Should we call "saccadic suppression" deactivation (which implies an active process) or just "decrease of activity"?

Answer: (Villinger) In the case of saccadic depression, the decrease of fMRI signal ("deactivation") probably corresponds to a decrease of neuronal activity. This relationship, however, may not necessarily hold in all situations.

Question: (Gjedde) What makes you so sure that an increased BOLD-signal reflects increased (neuronal) work?

Answer: (Villinger) We know this indirectly. In several instances where increased blood flow has been measured, it is known that glucose consumption increases.

Question: (Iadecola) In response to Dr. Gjedde's question, stimulation of the cerebellar parallel fiber increases glucose utilization locally. Concerning the inhibition effects on CBF, we must keep in mind that the withdrawal of vasodilator cannot be the sole mechanism of coupling of CBF to neural activity. Arteriolar diameter is determined by both constrictor and vasodilator influences—constrictor effects may predominate during inhibition.

Answer: (Villinger) Your are right, Costantino.

References

[1] C. Mathiesen, K. Caesar, N. Akgoren, M. Lauritzen, Modification of activity-dependent increases of cerebral blood flow by excitatory synaptic activity and spikes in rat cerebellar cortex, J. Physiol. 512 (1998) 555–566.

[2] L. Sokoloff, M. Reivich, C. Kennedy, M.H. Des Rosiers, C.S. Patlak, K.D. Pettigrew, O. Sakurada, M. Shinohara, The [C-14]deoxyglucose method for measurements of the local cerebral glucose utilization: theory, procedure, and normal values in the conscious and anesthetized albino rat, J. Neurochem. 28 (1977) 897–916.

[3] R.J. Nudo, R.B. Masterton, Stimulation-induced [^{14}C]2-deoxyglucose labeling of synaptic activity in the central auditory system, J. Comp. Neurol. 245 (1986) 553–565.

[4] R.F. Ackerman, D.M. Finch, T.L. Babb, J. Engel, Increased glucose metabolism during long-duration recurrent inhibition of hippocampal pyramidal cells, J. Neurosci. 4 (1984) 251–264.

[5] P.T. Fox, M.E. Raichle, M.A. Mintun, C. Dence, Nonoxidative glucose consumption during focal physiologic neural activity, Science 241 (1988) 462–464.

[6] P.T. Fox, M.E. Raichle, Focal physiological uncoupling of cerebral blood flow and oxidative metabolism during somatosensory stimulation in human subjects, Proc. Natl. Acad. Sci. U. S. A. 83 (1986) 1140–1144.

[7] R.B. Buxton, L.R. Frank, A model for the coupling between cerebral blood flow and oxygen metabolism during neural stimulation, J. Cereb. Blood Flow Metab. 17 (1997) 64–72.

[8] R. Wenzel, P. Wobst, H.H. Heekeren, K.K. Kwong, S.A. Brandt, M. Kohl, H. Obrig, U. Dirnagl, A. Villringer, Saccadic suppression induces focal hypooxygenation in the occipital cortex, J. Cereb. Blood Flow Metab. 7 (2000) 1103–1110.

[9] E.R. Kandel, J.H. Schwartz, Directly gated transmission at central synapses, in: E.R. Kandel, J.H. Schwartz, T.M. Jessell (Eds.), Principles of Neural Science, Appleton & Lange, USA, 1991, pp. 153–172.

[10] C. Beaulieu, M. Colonnier, A laminar analysis of the number of round-asymmetrical and flat-symmetrical synapses on spines, dendritic trunks, and cell bodies in area 17 of the cat, J. Comp. Neurol. 231 (1985) 180–189.

[11] M. Megias, Z. Emri, T.F. Freund, A.I. Gulyas, Total number and distribution of inhibitory and excitatory synapses on hippocampal CA1 pyramidal cells, Neuroscience 102 (2001) 527–540.

[12] T. Koos, J.M. Tepper, Inhibitory control of neostriatal projection neurons by GABAergic interneurons, Nat. Neurosci. 2 (1999) 467–472.

[13] T.F. Freund, M. Antal, GABA-containing neurons in the septum control inhibitory interneurons in the hippocampus, Nature 336 (1988) 170–173.

[14] G.F. Tseng, L.B. Haberly, Characterization of synaptically mediated fast and slow inhibitory processes in piriform cortex in an in vitro slice preparation, J. Neurophysiol. 59 (1988) 1352–1376.

[15] R.J. Seitz, P.E. Roland, Vibratory stimulation increases and decreases the regional cerebral blood flow and oxidative metabolism: a positron emission tomography (PET) study, Acta Neurol. Scand. 86 (1992) 60–67.

[16] R. Kawashima, B.T. O'Sullivan, P.E. Roland, Positron-emission tomography studies of cross-modality inhibition in selective attentional tasks: closing the "mind's eye", Proc. Natl. Acad. Sci. U. S. A. 92 (1995) 5969–5972.

[17] J.V. Haxby, B. Horwitz, L.G. Ungerleider, J.M. Maisog, P. Pietrini, C.L. Grady, The functional organization of human extrastriate cortex: a PET–rCBF study of selective attention to faces and locations, J. Neurosci. 14 (1994) 6336–6353.

[18] J. Classen, R. Benecke, Inhibitory phenomena in individual motor units induced by transcranial magnetic stimulation, Electroencephalogr. Clin. Neurophysiol. 97 (1995) 264–274.

[19] B.U. Meyer, A. Kuehn, S. Roricht, A. Kupsch, Direct activation of corticospinal fibres at the level of the internal capsule in man, Clin. Neurophysiol., Suppl. 12 (2001) 7.

[20] A. Ferbert, A. Priori, J.C. Rothwell, B.L. Day, J.G. Colebatch, C.D. Marsden, Interhemispheric inhibition of the human motor cortex, J. Physiol. 453 (1992) 525–546.

[21] B.U. Meyer, S. Roricht, V.E. Grafin, F. Kruggel, A. Weindl, Inhibitory and excitatory interhemispheric transfers between motor cortical areas in normal humans and patients with abnormalities of the corpus callosum, Brain 118 (1995) 429–440.

[22] B.U. Meyer, S. Roricht, C. Woiciechowsky, Topography of fibers in the human corpus callosum mediating interhemispheric inhibition between the motor cortices, Ann. Neurol. 43 (1998) 360–369.

[23] U. Ziemann, J.C. Rothwell, M.C. Ridding, Interaction between intracortical inhibition and facilitation in human motor cortex, J. Physiol. 496 (1996) 873–881.

[24] U. Ziemann, M. Hallett, Basic neurophysiological studies with TMS, in: M.S. George, R.H. Belmaker (Eds.), Transcranial Magnetic Stimulation in Neuropsychiatry, American Psychiatry Press, Washington, 2000, pp. 45–98.

[25] A.P. Strafella, T. Paus, Cerebral blood-flow changes induced by paired-pulse transcranial magnetic stimulation of the primary motor cortex, J. Neurophysiol. 85 (2001) 2624–2629.

[26] S.A. Brandt, T. Davis, H. Obrig, B.U. Meyer, J.W. Belliveau, B.R. Rosen, A. Villringer, Functional magnetic resonance imaging shows localized brain activation during serial transcranial stimulation in man, NeuroReport 7 (1996) 734–736.

[27] S.A. Brandt, J. Brocke, S. Roricht, C.J. Ploner, A. Villringer, B.U. Meyer, In vivo assessment of human visual system connectivity with transcranial electrical stimulation during functional magnetic resonance imaging, NeuroImage 14 (2001) 366–375.

[28] S.A. Brandt, L. Niehaus, S. Röricht, J. Brocke, A. Villringer, B.U. Meyer, Distant effects from transcranial electrical stimulation (TES) over motor cortex during functional magnetic resonance imaging (f MRI), NeuroImage 9 (6) (1999) 463 (Abstract).

[29] J.D. Allison, K.J. Meador, D.W. Loring, R.E. Figueroa, J.C. Wright, Functional MRI cerebral activation and deactivation during finger movement, Neurology 54 (2000) 135–142.

[30] L. Leocani, L.G. Cohen, E.M. Wassermann, K. Ikoma, M. Hallett, Human corticospinal excitability evaluated with transcranial magnetic stimulation during different reaction time paradigms, Brain 123 (2000) 1161–1173.

[31] D. Waldvogel, P. van Gelderen, W. Muellbacher, U. Ziemann, I. Immisch, M. Hallett, The relative metabolic demand of inhibition and excitation, Nature 406 (2000) 995–998.

[32] F.H. Duffy, J.L. Burchfiel, Eye movement-related inhibition of primate visual neurons, Brain Res. 89 (1975) 121–132.

[33] D.L. Robinson, C.D. Jarvis, Superior colliculus neurons studied during head and eye movements of the behaving monkey, J. Neurophysiol. 37 (1974) 533–540.

[34] P.H. Schiller, F. Koerner, Discharge characteristics of single units in superior colliculus of the alert rhesus monkey, J. Neurophysiol. 34 (1971) 920–936.

[35] R.H. Wurtz, M.E. Goldberg, Activity of superior colliculus in behaving monkey: 3. Cells discharging before eye movements, J. Neurophysiol. 35 (1972) 575–586.

[36] E. Bizzi, P.H. Schiller, Single unit activity in the frontal eye fields of unanesthetized monkeys during eye and head movement, Exp. Brain Res. 10 (1970) 150–158.

[37] T. Paus, S. Marrett, K.J. Worsley, A.C. Evans, Extraretinal modulation of cerebral blood flow in the human visual cortex: implications for saccadic suppression, J. Neurophysiol. 74 (1995) 2179–2183.

[38] P. Fransson, G. Kruger, K.D. Merboldt, J. Frahm, MRI of functional deactivation: temporal and spatial characteristics of oxygenation-sensitive responses in human visual cortex, NeuroImage 9 (1999) 611–618.

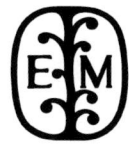

International Congress Series 1235 (2002) 223–229

Dynamic changes of CBF, CMRO$_2$, OEF, CMR$_{glc}$, CBV and ADC during neuronal suppression due to hypothermia

Masaharu Sakoh [a],[*], Leif Østergaard [b], Donald F. Smith [c], Takanori Ohnishi [a], Albert Gjedde [c]

[a]*Department of Neurological Surgery, Ehime University School of Medicine, Shizukawa, Shigenobu-cho, Onsen-gun, Ehime 791-0205, Japan*
[b]*Department of Neuroradiology, Aarhus University Hospital, Aarhus, Denmark*
[c]*PET-Center, Aarhus University Hospital, Aarhus, Denmark*

Abstract

The objective of this study was to test that hypothermia improves the outcome of an acute ischemic stroke. In order to test the hypothesis that hypothermia (32 °C) improves the outcome by effecting the global cerebral reduction of oxygen consumption when the blood flow is already low, we investigated the sequential changes of physiological variables during hypothermia using positron emission tomography (PET) and diffusion-weighted magnetic resonance imaging (DW-MRI) in pigs. The cerebral blood flow (CBF) and cerebral metabolic rate of oxygen (CMRO$_2$) decreased significantly to within 50% of the baseline in 3 and 5 h as functions of time, thereby lowering the viability threshold of the brain tissue. The oxygen extraction fraction (OEF) was significantly elevated to 140% of the baseline in 4 h, indicating a reduction in the driving pressure of oxygen delivery in response to the reduced metabolic need, and then it gradually returned so that it was once again level with the baseline. The cerebral metabolic rate of glucose (CMR$_{glc}$), the cerebral blood volume (CBV), and apparent diffusion coefficient (ADC) decreased to 75%, 72% and 80% of the baseline after 6 h of hypothermia in response to the lowered metabolism for maintenance of cellular integrity, and the diminution of intracranial pressure. The results of ischemia show that rapid cooling of the brain to 32 °C significantly increases the survival of tissue at risk. © 2002 Elsevier Science B.V. All rights reserved.

Keywords: Hypothermia; CBF; CMRO$_2$; OEF; ADC

[*] Corresponding author. Tel.: +81-89-960-5338; fax: +81-89-960-5340.
E-mail address: sakoh@m.ehime-u.ac.jp (M. Sakoh).

0531-5131/02 © 2002 Elsevier Science B.V. All rights reserved.
PII: S 0 5 3 1 - 5 1 3 1 (0 2) 0 0 1 9 0 - 5

1. Introduction

Hypothermia has improved the outcome of acute cerebral ischemia in laboratory animals [1,2]. In humans, hypothermia is an established tool for the protection of brain tissue during surgery [3], and it seems to improve the outcome of patients, which have suffered an acute ischemic stroke [4]. At normal temperature, the brain tissue at risk does not survive when metabolic variables decline below a specific threshold [5–7]. The duration of this decline is often referred to as the critical time window of therapeutics. A critical time-window of less than 3 h is too narrow for the reperfusion of severely ischemic tissue in clinical situations, unless hypothermia is introduced preoperatively [7–9]. Thus, the time required for initiating the cooling and the subsequent duration of hypothermia, both play roles in determining the efficacy of this treatment. The present studies with positron emission tomography (PET) and diffusion weighted-magnetic resonance imaging (DW-MRI) tested the hypothesis that, the effect of hypothermia is a function of the degree to which it causes a global lowering of cerebral metabolism and perfusion.

2. Materials and methods

The Danish National Committee on Ethics in Animal Research (DaNCARE) approved the research project. Of the 20 female country-bred Yorkshire pigs weighing 38–45 kg, 10 pigs underwent the sequential measurement of physiological variables after hypothermia, five pigs underwent the baseline measurement of cerebral metabolic rate of glucose (CMR_{glc}) and apparent diffusion coefficient (ADC) and five pigs underwent the combination therapy of hypothermia and reperfusion after middle cerebral artery occlusion (MCAO).

Hypothermia was induced for 8 h by a forced air-cooling system (Bair Hugger Model 600 PolarAir Hyper/Hypothermia System, Augustine Medical, USA). The air in the cooling system was additionally cooled to -20 °C by dry ice. The brain temperature was reduced to 32 °C and maintained at that level during the experiments. For the combination therapy, the hypothermia was initiated 30 min after MCAO and continued for 8 h, whereas reperfusion began 2 h after the MCAO.

The cerebral blood flow (CBF) (by intravenous bolus injection of 800 MBq $H_2^{15}O$), the cerebral metabolic rate of oxygen ($CMRO_2$) (by single-breath inhalation (1 l) of 1200 MBq $^{15}O_2$), and oxygen extraction fraction (OEF) were measured before and every hour up until 6 h after the initiation of hypothermia using PET (Siemens/CTI ECAT EXACT HR). The CMR_{glc} (by intravenous bolus injection of 300 MBq ^{18}F-fluorodeoxyglucose), the cerebral blood volume (CBV) (by single-breath inhalation (1 l) of 1200 MBq $C^{15}O$), were carried out while the ADC was measured before and for 6 h after the initiation of hypothermia using PET and a Horizon 1.0 Tesla MR Imager (GE Medical Systems, Milwaukee, WI, USA). The ADC was measured by multislice DW spin-echo echo-planar imaging (EPI), with diffusion-sensitising gradients in three orthogonal directions (b=1000 s/mm^2).

Statistical analysis was carried out by one-way repeated-measures, and analysis of variance (ANOVA) in order to determine whether absolute values for CBF, $CMRO_2$,

OEF, CMR_{glc}, CBV and ADC changed significantly over time, and whether the volume of infarction was affected significantly by the combination therapy.

3. Results

Within 3 h, the brain temperature declined significantly to 32 °C ($p<0.01$), where it remained stable for the duration of the experiment (Fig. 1). Under baseline conditions, all physiologic variables remained stable in the normal range. However, pCO_2 declined significantly 3 h after the initiation of hypothermia. The sequential changes of CBF, $CMRO_2$ and OEF before and after hypothermia are illustrated in Fig. 1. In 3 h, the CBF declined significantly to within 50% of the baseline ($p<0.01$), where it remained stable. The cerebral metabolic rate of oxygen ($CMRO_2$) declined significantly to 50% of the baseline in 5 h ($p<0.01$), the OEF rose significantly to 140% of the baseline in 3 h ($p<0.01$), and gradually returned to the baseline level thereafter. The cerebral metabolic rate of glucose (CMR_{glc}), ADC and CBV decreased significantly to 75%, 80% and 72% of the baseline, 6 h after initiation of hypothermia, respectively (Table 1).

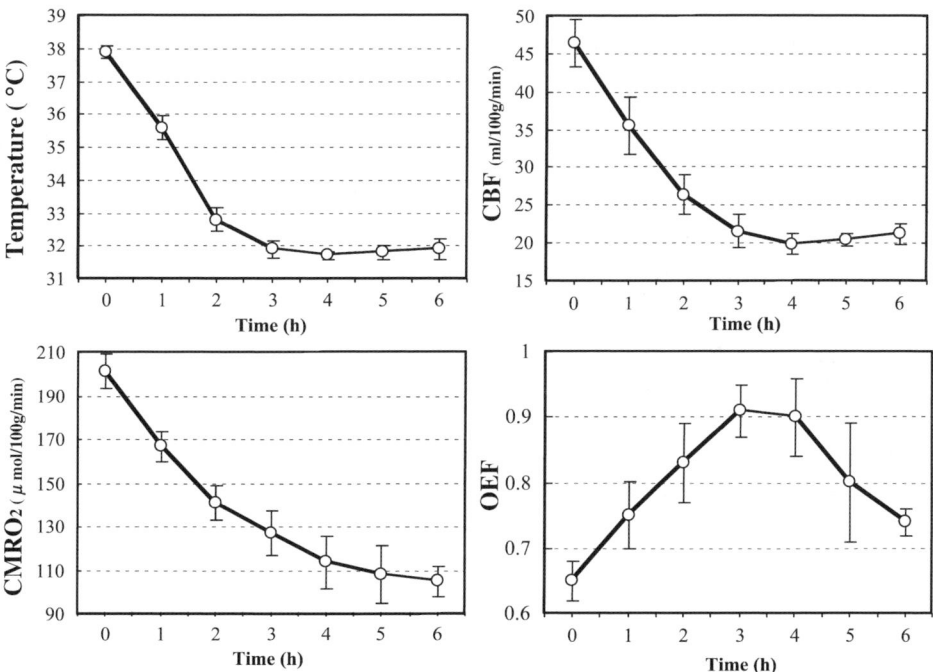

Fig. 1. Sequential changes in brain temperature, CBF, $CMRO_2$ and OEF before and after hypothermia in intact brains. Hypothermia decreased the CBF and $CMRO_2$ to 50% of the baseline as a function of time. OEF was significantly elevated to 140% of the control in 3 h.

Table 1
Changes of CMR_{glc}, ADC and CBV before and 6 h after hypothermia in intact brains

	Control	Hypothermia
CMR_{glc} (μmol/100 g/min)	26.2±1.0	19.5±1.6* (75%)
ADC ($\times 10^{-6}$ mm²/s)	940±41	750±31* (80%)
CBV (ml/m)	322±27	232±12* (72%)

Values are means±S.D. Hypothermia decreased CMR_{glc}, ADC and CBV to 75%, 80% and 72% of the baseline 6 h after hypothermia in intact brains, respectively.
   * Significantly different from baseline values ($p<0.01$, ANOVA).

The combination therapy of severe ischemia significantly decreased the volume of infarction from MCAO compared with the reperfusion therapy (Table 2). The therapy also suppressed the postischemic hyperperfusion and maintained the $CMRO_2$ in the ischemic cortex; outside the ischemic core, which was not affected (Fig. 2).

4. Discussion

The results of the present study confirmed the predicted 50% reduction in $CMRO_2$ and CBF over time after the initiation of hypothermia. The OEF was significantly elevated during the first 4 h of hypothermia as the decrease of CBF occurred more rapidly than the decline of $CMRO_2$ as predicted by the oxygen delivery model of Vafaee and Gjedde [10]. Thereafter, the OEF showed a tendency to return to the baseline, suggesting only temporary uncoupling between the CBF and $CMRO_2$. The increase of OEF reduces the partial pressure of oxygen in the capillaries, and hence the driving pressure for oxygen delivery in the hypothermic brain tissue, in keeping with the lowered oxygen consumption. The suppression of CMR_{glc} and $CMRO_2$ in hypothermia explains the neuroprotective effect in brain tissue at risk as a reduction of the energy consuming processes, for both the activation mechanism of neuronal function and the residual metabolism of maintenance of cellular integrity [11,12]. The reductions of CBF and CBV could also diminish the intracranial pressure (ICP) and eliminate intracranial hypertension, which clinically are life-threatening complications of damaged brain tissue [13–15]. In the ischemic cortex, however, not in the ischemic core, the combination therapy of hypothermia and reperfusion significantly reduced the volume of infarction in MCAO when compared with reperfusion alone, by suppressing the postischemic hyperperfusion and maintaining

Table 2
Volume of infarction of the cerebral hemisphere after MCAO with severe ischemia according to therapy

	Permanent MCAO	Reperfusion only	Combination therapy
Infarction volume (ml)	18.8±1.7	13.2±4.0	6.1±4.7*
Ipsilateral hemisphere	52.6±2.5 (n=4)	52.7±3.4 (n=3)	53.0±3.0 (n=5)

Values are means±S.D. MCAO=middle cerebral artery occlusion. Severe ischemia was selected according to the CBF values of less than 12 ml/100 g/min in the ischemic core. The combination therapy significantly reduced the volume of infarction to 32% of them after permanent MCAO.
   * Significantly different from baseline values ($p<0.05$, ANOVA).

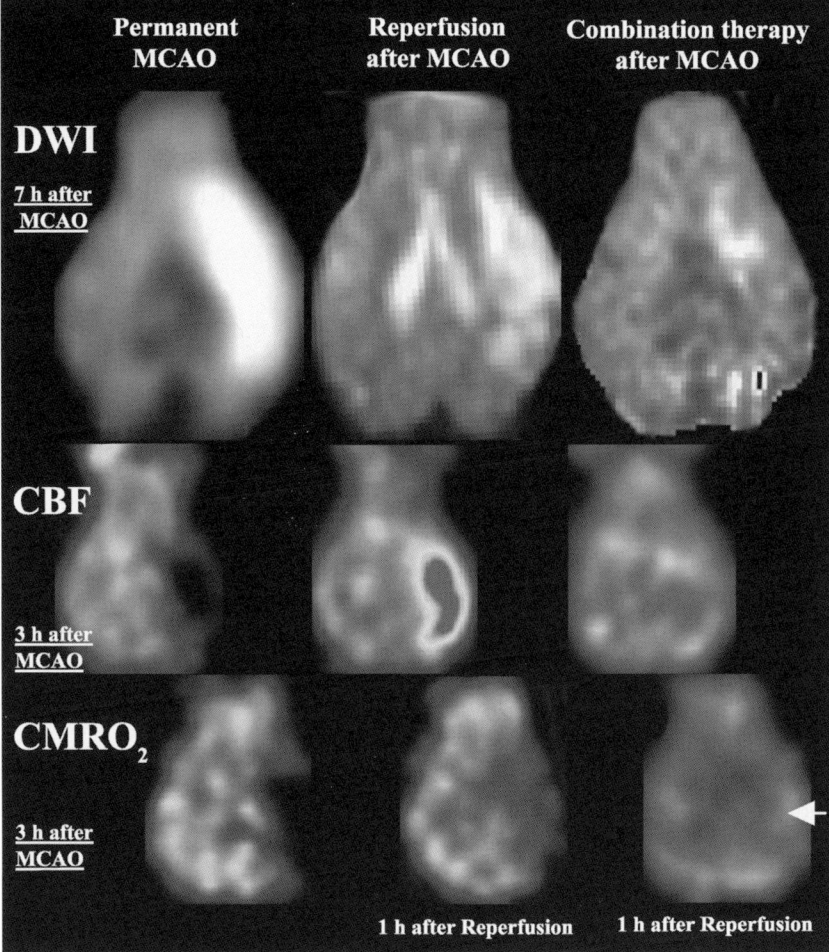

Fig. 2. Combination therapy of hypothermia and reperfusion for severe Ischemia after MCAO. The combination therapy significantly reduced the volume of infarction, because it suppressed the postischemic hyperperfusion and preserved CMRO$_2$ in the ischemic cortex, but not in the ischemic core.

CMRO$_2$. In addition, hypothermia prolonged the time window open to reperfusion therapy. We conclude that rapid cooling of the brain to 32 °C is reliably neuroprotective in that it reduces cerebral metabolism and perfusion.

On-Site Discussion

Question: (Strong) To my knowledge this is the first study examining the effect of hypothermia on ADC. How do values of ADC compare in lesioned and nonlesioned animals under hypothermia?

Answer: (Sakob) In the study, we measured ADC at 6 h of hypothermia in the intact brain. 32 °C hypothermia decreased ADC to 80% of the baseline. We did not compare the ADC values in lesioned and nonlesioned brains under hypothermia.

However, in the reperfusion study, we could rescue the ischemic regions of ADC more than 75% of the baseline by the reperfusion at 2 h of MCAO at normal temperature. So our results show that ADC threshold of the ischemic tissue viability is 75% of the baseline at normal temperature.

Acknowledgements

This study was funded by the Scandinavia-Japan Sasakawa Foundation, the Danish Medical Research Council grants 9305246, 9305247, 9601888, and 9802833, and the Institute of Experimental Clinical Research, and the University of Aarhus, Denmark.

References

[1] R. Busto, M.Y. Globus, W.D. Dietrich, E. Martinez, I. Valdes, M.D. Ginsberg, Effect of mild hypothermia on ischemia-induced release of neurotransmitters and free fatty acids in rat brain, Stroke 20 (7) (1989) 904–910.

[2] P.W. Huh, L. Belayev, W. Zhao, S. Koch, R. Busto, M.D. Ginsberg, Comparative neuroprotective efficacy of prolonged moderate intraischemic and postischemic hypothermia in focal cerebral ischemia, J. Neurosurg. 92 (1) (2000) 91–99.

[3] D.I. Sessler, Deliberate mild hypothermia, J. Neurosurg. Anesthesiol. 7 (1) (1995) 38–46.

[4] J. Reith, H.S. Jorgensen, P.M. Pedersen, H. Nakayama, H.O. Raaschou, L.L. Jeppesen, T.S. Olsen, Body temperature in acute stroke: relation to stroke severity, infarct size, mortality, and outcome, Lancet 347 (8999) (1996) 422–425.

[5] W.J. Powers, R.L. Grubb Jr., D. Darriet, M.E. Raichle, Cerebral blood flow and cerebral metabolic rate of oxygen requirements for cerebral function and viability in humans, J. Cereb. Blood Flow Metab. 5 (4) (1985) 600–608.

[6] O. Touzani, A.R. Young, J.M. Derlon, V. Beaudouin, G. Marchal, P. Rioux, F. Mezenge, J.C. Baron, E.T. MacKenzie, Sequential studies of severely hypometabolic tissue volumes after permanent middle cerebral artery occlusion. A positron emission tomographic investigation in anesthetized baboons, Stroke 26 (11) (1995) 2112–2119.

[7] M. Sakoh, L. Ostergaard, L. Rohl, D.F. Smith, C.Z. Simonsen, J.C. Sorensen, P.V. Poulsen, C. Gyldensted, S. Sakaki, A. Gjedde, Relationship between residual cerebral blood flow and oxygen metabolism as predictive of ischemic tissue viability: sequential multitracer positron emission tomography scanning of middle cerebral artery occlusion during the critical first 6 hours after stroke in pigs, J. Neurosurg. 93 (4) (2000) 647–657.

[8] T. Ueda, S. Sakaki, W.T. Yuh, I. Nochide, S. Ohta, Outcome in acute stroke with successful intra-arterial thrombolysis and predictive value of initial single-photon emission-computed tomography, J. Cereb. Blood Flow Metab. 19 (1) (1999) 99–108.

[9] The National Institute of Neurological Disorders and Stroke rt-PA Stroke Study Group, Tissue plasminogen activator for acute ischemic stroke, N. Engl. J. Med. 333 (24) (1995) 1581–1587.

[10] M.S. Vafaee, A. Gjedde, Model of blood–brain transfer of oxygen explains nonlinear flow–metabolism coupling during stimulation of visual cortex, J. Cereb. Blood Flow Metab. 20 (4) (2000) 747–754.

[11] J. Astrup, B.K. Siesjo, L. Symon, Thresholds in cerebral ischemia—the ischemic penumbra, Stroke 12 (6) (1981) 723–725.

[12] E.M. Nemoto, R. Klementavicius, J.A. Melick, H. Yonas, Suppression of cerebral metabolic rate for oxygen ($CMRO_2$) by mild hypothermia compared with thiopental, J. Neurosurg. Anesthesiol. 8 (1) (1996) 52–59.

[13] D.W. Marion, W.D. Obrist, P.M. Carlier, L.E. Penrod, J.M. Darby, The use of moderate therapeutic hypothermia for patients with severe head injuries: a preliminary report, J. Neurosurg. 79 (3) (1993) 354–362.

[14] C. Metz, M. Holzschuh, T. Bein, C. Woertgen, A. Frey, I. Frey, K. Taeger, A. Brawanski, Moderate hypothermia in patients with severe head injury: cerebral and extracerebral effects, J. Neurosurg. 85 (4) (1996) 533–541.

[15] K. Angstwurm, S. Reuss, D. Freyer, G. Arnold, U. Dirnagl, R.R. Schumann, J.R. Weber, Induced hypothermia in experimental pneumococcal meningitis, J. Cereb. Blood Flow Metab. 20 (5) (2000) 834–838.

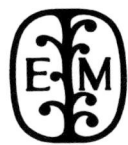

International Congress Series 1235 (2002) 231–242

Cerebral metabolic compartmentation: the effects of hypothermia and metabolic activation

Edwin M. Nemoto [a,*], Howard Yonas [a],
Frank Pigula [b], Simon Watkins [c]

[a]*Department of Neurological Surgery, Suite B-400, Presbyterian University Hospital,
200 Lothrop St., Pittsburgh, PA 15213, USA*
[b]*Cardiothoracic Surgery, Children's Hospital, 2 Main, Children's Hospital of Pittsburgh,
Pittsburgh, PA 15213, USA*
[c]*Department of Cell Biology and Physiology, BSTWR S225, University of Pittsburgh,
Pittsburgh, PA 15261, USA*

Abstract

The cerebral metabolic rate for oxygen ($CMRO_2$) is separable into two compartments: (1) $CMRO_2$ associated with the electroencephalogram (EEG) or functional ($fCMRO_2$); and (2) $CMRO_2$ for all other metabolic processes or basal $CMRO_2$ ($bCMRO_2$). These compartments were separated by $CMRO_2$ measurements with and without total thiopental suppression of EEG activity. $CMRO_2$ without EEG is $bCMRO_2$ and that which was suppressed is $fCMRO_2$, each representing about 50% of total $CMRO_2$ ($tCMRO_2$). Hypothermia differentially affects the $CMRO_2$ compartments. The 15–20% reduction in $tCMRO_2$ at 34 °C is due to a 50% reduction in $bCMRO_2$, suggesting a greater sensitivity to temperature than $fCMRO_2$. The Q_{10} for $tCMRO_2$ was about 2.5, whereas the Q_{10} for $bCMRO_2$ was 5.2, which could be further separated into a high temperature sensitivity component with a Q_{10} of 12.1 and a low temperature sensitivity component with a Q_{10} of 2.1. Norepinephrine metabolic activation of $CMRO_2$ occurs entirely by an increase in $bCMRO_2$. During hypothermia, GLUT-3 immunostaining showed greater staining in axons and dendrites versus neuronal perikarya. The relevance of these cerebral metabolic compartments for oxygen and glucose in altered physiological states remains to be elucidated. © 2002 Elsevier Science B.V. All rights reserved.

Keywords: Brain activation; Cerebral metabolic rate for oxygen ($CMRO_2$); Glucose transporter protein; Hypothermia; Norepinephrine

* Corresponding author. Tel.: +1-412-648-9654; fax: +1-412-648-3326.
E-mail addresses: nemoto@neuronet.pitt.edu (E.M. Nemoto), hyonas@neuronet.pitt.edu (H. Yonas), pigulaf@heart.chp.edu (F. Pigula), swatkins@pitt.edu (S. Watkins).

0531-5131/02 © 2002 Elsevier Science B.V. All rights reserved.
PII: S 0 5 3 1 - 5 1 3 1 (0 2) 0 0 1 9 2 - 9

1. Introduction

"Since anesthetics act by the reversible inhibition of synaptic transmission suppression of $CMRO_2$ by anesthetics should be only that associated with synaptic transmission", said Kety [1]. This suggestion led to the definition for the separation of the cerebral metabolic rate for oxygen ($CMRO_2$) into a functional, EEG associated component ($fCMRO_2$) and a basal ($bCMRO_2$) component by complete suppression of the EEG with sodium thiopental [2,3]. Astrup et al. [4] showed that about 50% of $bCMRO_2$ or 25% of total $CMRO_2$ could be associated with active Na^+-K^+ transport. This is where this topic was left in the early 1980s.

Although it had already been recognized that there was a discrepancy between the $CMRO_2$ depressant effects of barbiturates compared to hypothermia and their relative protective effect in ischemic brain damage, it was not until the early 1990s that this was really brought to fore. In 1990, Minamisawa et al. [5] said, "Thus, a 10 °C reduction in body temperature dramatically reduced the susceptibility of the brain ischemia/hypoxia while deep barbiturate anesthesia which reduces it equally has no such effect or only a minor one". Others have made the same observation [6]. Thus, the question remained as to how this apparent discrepancy can be explained.

This paper presents a synopsis of what we have done over the past several years to further develop the concept of functional and basal $CMRO_2$ and its application in understanding alterations in these two compartments in various states. In particular, we were interested in the insight that it may shed on the greater protective effect of hypothermia against ischemic brain injury compared to barbiturate suppression of $CMRO_2$.

In the early 1990s, we began the application of the concept of functional and basal $CMRO_2$ by verifying that these metabolic compartments could be demonstrated in monkeys where we found a 50:50 ratio of these compartments [7]. We also showed that as expected, the functional $CMRO_2$ compartment was suppressed early postischemia whereas basal $CMRO_2$ was elevated [8]. Thus, despite a reduced total $CMRO_2$, $bCMRO_2$ was hypermetabolic and metabolic activity was high despite the reduced total $CMRO_2$.

Following these studies, we noted in a report by Steen at al. [9] that the EEG did not become isoelectric until temperature reached 14 °C, at which point $tCMRO_2$ was less than 10% of normal. This led us to the realization that the EEG must be very insensitive to hypothermia. Therefore, we hypothesized that hypothermia preferentially attenuates basal as opposed to functional $CMRO_2$, which may also explain the greater protective effect of hypothermia compared to barbiturate despite the equal or greater reduction in $CMRO_2$ by barbiturates. The studies described below were designed to test this hypothesis.

2. Differential effects of hypothermia on functional and basal $CMRO_2$ [10]

2.1. Methods

To test the hypothesis that hypothermia selectively suppresses $bCMRO_2$ as opposed to $fCMRO_2$, rats were anesthetized and mechanically ventilated with 1% halothane/70% nitrous oxide/30% oxygen. The rats were instrumented for measurement of whole brain

CBF by H_2 clearance (platinum microelectrode in the superior sagittal sinus) and $CMRO_2$ with cerebral venous sampling from the transverse sinus. Baseline CBF and $CMRO_2$ measurements were made at 38 °C during 1% halothane/70% nitrous oxide/30% oxygen anesthesia. Thereafter, in one group of rats, cortical temperature (<1-mm diameter thermocouple, Physitemp, Clifton, NJ) was reduced to 34 °C and maintained at 38 °C in the other group. After stabilization of temperature at 34 °C, an isoelectric EEG (at a sensitivity of 50 μV/cm) was induced by titrated thiopental (TP) infusion (50 mg/ml). During TP infusion, the inspired gas was changed to 70% nitrogen/30% oxygen and a second set of two CBF and $CMRO_2$ measurements were made during TP-induced isoelectric EEG. Heparin anticoagulated, filtered blood from a donor rat was infused i.v. during TP infusion to maintain mean arterial blood pressure between 80 and 100 mm Hg. All blood volumes withdrawn for arterial and cerebral venous blood gases and oxygen content were replaced with an equal volume of donor blood.

2.2. Results

The results showed that in the normothermic rats, TP suppression of EEG accounted for a 50% reduction in both $tCMRO_2$ and tCBF, indicating maintained coupling of flow and metabolism during deep TP anesthesia (Table 1). During mild hypothermia at 34 °C, TP isoelectric EEG revealed a 64% decrease in $tCMRO_2$ to 36% of control before TP at 34 °C (Table 2). Therefore, the suppression of $tCMRO_2$ by TP revealed that whereas $fCMRO_2$ accounted for 64% of $tCMRO_2$ at 34 °C, $bCMRO_2$ represented 36% of $tCMRO_2$, indicating that the reduction in $tCMRO_2$ by mild hypothermia was entirely due to a reduction in $bCMRO_2$.

2.3. Discussion

Our data support the hypothesis that $bCMRO_2$ is more sensitive to hypothermia than $fCMRO_2$. At mild hypothermia of 34 °C, the 20% reduction in $tCMRO_2$ is entirely due to suppression of $bCMRO_2$ which actually represents a 50% reduction in $bCMRO_2$. From these data, we hypothesized that the Q_{10} for $bCMRO_2$ must be higher than that for

Table 1
Cerebral variables in normothermic rats ($n = 7$)

Variable	N_2O/O_2	TP	$N_2O/O_2 - TP^a$
Tb (°C)	37.9 ± 1.05	37.8 ± 0.4	
$CMRO_2$ (ml 100 g^{-1} min^{-1})	7.92 ± 1.05	3.95 ± 0.70	3.79 ± 0.51
Percentage of N_2O/O_2		50 ± 4	50 ± 4
CBF (ml 100 g^{-1} min^{-1})	125 ± 26	63 ± 10	62 ± 17
Percentage of N_2O/O_2		51 ± 4	49 ± 4

N_2O/O_2, 70% nitrous oxide in 30% oxygen; TP, thiopental; Tb, brain temperature; $CMRO_2$, cerebral metabolic rate for oxygen; CBF, cerebral blood flow.
Reproduced with permission from the Editor of J. Neurosurg. Anesthesiol.
[a] TP-suppressible component was calculated as the difference between the value obtained during N_2O/O_2 analgesia minus the value obtained during TP-induced isoelectric EEG.

Table 2
Cerebral variables in hypothermic rats ($n=7$)

Variable	N_2O/O_2	N_2O/O_2	TP	N_2O/O_2-TP^a
Tb (°C)	38.0 ± 0.2	34.0 ± 0.07	33.9 ± 0.09	
$CMRO_2$ (ml 100 g^{-1} min^{-1})	7.62 ± 1.92	6.28 ± 1.22	2.15 ± 0.46^b	4.13 ± 1.11
Percentage of N_2O/O_2			36 ± 8^b	64 ± 7^c
CBF (ml 100 g^{-1} min^{-1})	96 ± 30	98 ± 25	38 ± 12^b	60 ± 27
Percentage of N_2O/O_2			44 ± 14	56 ± 14

N_2O/O_2, 70% nitrous oxide in 30% oxygen; TP, thiopental; Tb, brain temperature; $CMRO_2$, cerebral metabolic rate for oxygen; CBF, cerebral blood flow.
Reproduced with permission from the Editor of J. Neurosurg. Anesthesiol.
[a] TP-suppressible component was calculated as the difference at 34 °C between the value obtained during N_2O/O_2 analgesia minus the value obtained during TP-induced isoelectric EEG.
[b] $p<0.01$ compared with corresponding value in TP at 38 °C in Table 1.
[c] $p<0.01$ compared with corresponding value in N_2O/O_2-TP in Table 1.

$fCMRO_2$. A hypothetical diagram of the partition between $fCMRO_2$ and $bCMRO_2$ is shown in Fig. 1.

3. Differential Q_{10} values for basal and functional $CMRO_2$

3.1. Introduction

The studies described above showed that $bCMRO_2$ was selectively inhibited by hypothermia compared to $fCMRO_2$, suggesting a relatively greater sensitivity of $bCMRO_2$

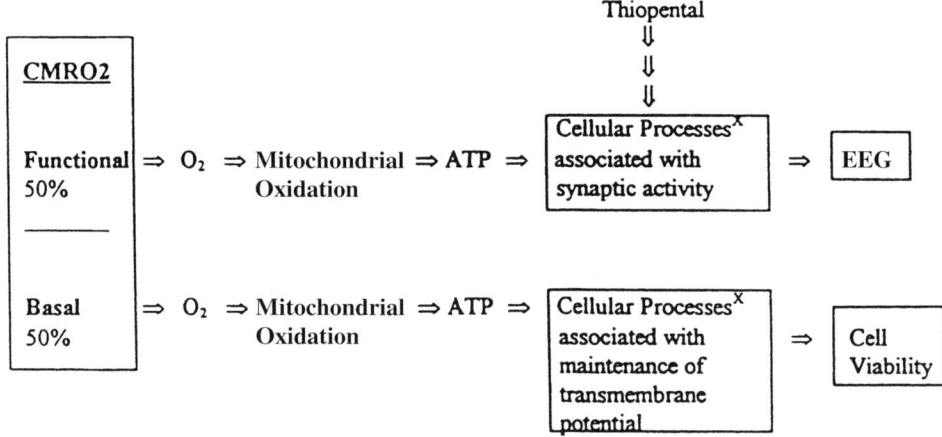

Fig. 1. Illustration of the concept of the components of functional and basal brain oxygen uptake ($CMRO_2$) relative to cellular processes and energy (ATP) utilization. The X marks the cellular processes of neurotransmitter synthesis, protein synthesis, astrocytic K$^+$ and glutamate uptake, synaptic membrane replenishment, lipid and carbohydrate synthesis, Na$^+$–K$^+$ ATPase ion pumping, Ca^{2+} ATPase ion pumping and microtubular transport, i.e. all cellular energy-requiring processes. Reproduced with permission from the Editor of J. Neurosurg. Anesthesiol.

to hypothermia. The objective of this study was to quantify this difference by measuring the Q_{10} for bCMRO$_2$ compared to that for tCMRO$_2$.

3.2. Methods

Rats were mechanically ventilated on 0.5% isoflurane/70% nitrous oxide/30% oxygen and prepared as described above for measurements of CBF, CMRO$_2$ and epidural temperature. The studies were done on three groups of rats, all groups first, beginning with two baseline measurements at a brain temperature of 38 °C. Thereafter, the rats were divided into three different experimental protocols: (1) a normothermic control group with brain temperature maintained at 38 °C for 3 h over which six sets of CBF and CMRO$_2$ measurements were made; (2) a normothermic thiopental group in whom after the two baseline measurements, TP was infused to render the EEG isoelectric followed by six sets of CBF and CMRO$_2$ measurements over 3 h; and (3) a hypothermic TP group in whom brain temperature was reduced to 34, 30 and 28 °C with CBF and CMRO$_2$ measurements at each temperature. Temperature was reduced by ice packs on the back of the rats. During TP infusion to produce an isoelectric EEG, the inspired gas was changed to 70% nitrogen/30% oxygen.

3.3. Results

The decrease in bCMRO$_2$ with temperature appeared to be biphasic with an overall Q_{10} of 5.2 (Fig. 2). The separation of the high temperature sensitivity component of bCMRO$_2$ revealed a Q_{10} of 12.1 and the low sensitivity component with a Q_{10} of 2.8 (Fig. 3). Thus, bCMRO$_2$ has two components of metabolic processes markedly different in their Q_{10} values that differ by a factor of 4.

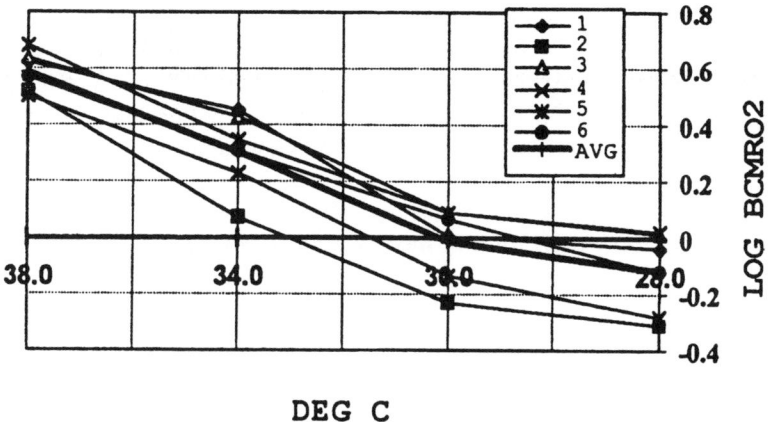

Fig. 2. Graph showing the $\log_{10}$ bCMRO$_2$ (y-axis) versus brain temperature (x-axis in °C) in six rats during progressive cooling. Reproduced with permission from the Editor of J. Neurosurg. Anesthesiol.

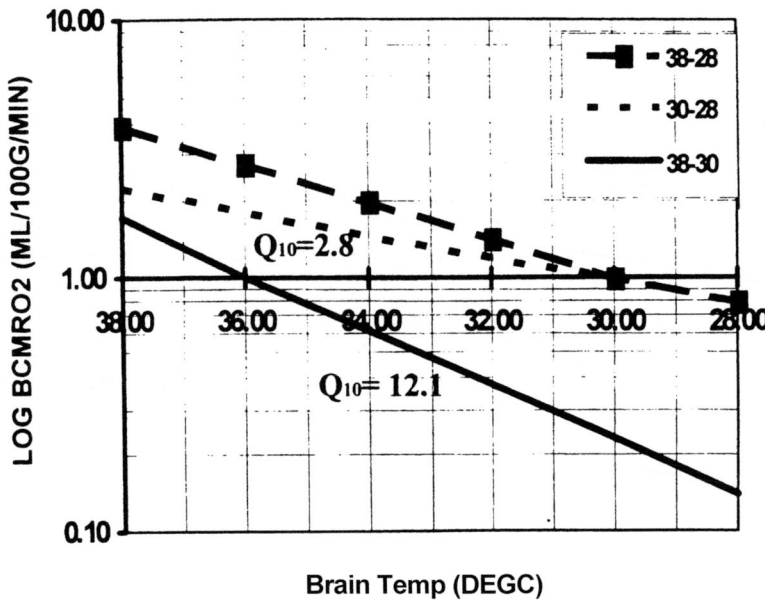

Fig. 3. Graph showing the separation of high and low temperature sensitivity components in the basal cerebral metabolic rate for oxygen ($bCMRO_2$) in a semilog plot. The Q_{10} values (ratio of $bCMRO_2$ over temperature) for the high and low temperature sensitivity components were 12.1 and 2.8, respectively, with an overall Q_{10} for basal $CMRO_2$ of 5.2. DEGC = degrees centigrade.

3.4. Discussion

The results show that $bCMRO_2$ is composed of two temperature-sensitive components that differ in temperature sensitivity by a factor of 4. The metabolic processes associated with these high sensitivity temperature components are unknown. However, the greater sensitivity of $bCMRO_2$ to temperature and the fact that TP suppresses $fCMRO_2$ alone suggests that the greater protective effect of hypothermia may be due to its suppression of $bCMRO_2$ as opposed to $fCMRO_2$. The reduction in $bCMRO_2$ on a speculative vein, which is proven to be protective, could be due to a decrease in the "resting" permeability of the neuronal membrane to Na^+-K^+, thereby requiring less energy to maintain the ionic gradient.

4. Norepinephrine (NE) activation of basal $CMRO_2$ during hypothermia

4.1. Introduction

In the studies described under Section 1, we began at first by using NE to maintain mean arterial blood pressure between 80 and 100 mm Hg during TP infusion. However, we found that after TP infusion, $CMRO_2$ was increased and not reduced, which was not what we had expected. We subsequently used blood infusion to maintain arterial blood pressure and observed the expected decrease in $CMRO_2$. The aim of this series of studies was to determine whether NE infusion increases $CMRO_2$ and whether its effects are on basal as opposed to functional $CMRO_2$.

4.2. Methods

Rats were anesthetized and mechanically ventilated on 1% halothane/70% nitrous oxide/30% oxygen and instrumented for measurements of brain temperature and CBF and $CMRO_2$ as described above. Two successive sets of baseline CBF and $CMRO_2$ measurements were made at 38 °C. Thereafter, the rats were divided into two groups, one group with brain temperature kept at 38 °C and the other group brought to a brain temperature of 34 °C. After achieving these temperatures, two additional baseline CBF and $CMRO_2$ measurements were made at these two different temperatures. Subsequently, TP was infused to render the EEG isoelectric. During TP infusion, mean arterial blood pressure was kept between 80 and 100 mm Hg, be it either the infusion of blood from a donor rat or by the infusion of NE. During TP infusion as before, the inspired gas was changed to 70% nitrogen/30% oxygen. During the period of TP infusion and isoelectric EEG, two additional sets of CBF and $CMRO_2$ were made.

4.3. Results

During normothermia of 38 °C, NE had no effect on either functional or basal $CMRO_2$ (Table 3). However, there was a significant effect of NE on CBF with a reduction in bCBF and an increase in fCBF.

During hypothermia of 34 °C, however, NE infusion during TP-induced isoelectric EEG significantly increased basal as opposed to functional $CMRO_2$ (Table 4). CBF, on the other hand, was not significantly affected by NE infusion.

Table 3
Cerebral metabolic rate for oxygen ($CMRO_2$) and cerebral blood flow (CBF) compartments (mean ± S.D.) at 38 °C in rats using norepinephrine infusion ($n = 5$) or DB transfusion ($n = 7$) to maintain mean arterial blood pressure during TP-induced isoelectric EEG for measurement of the basal compartment

	(Total) N_2O/O_2 (ml 100 g^{-1} min^{-1})	Basal TP	Functional N_2O/O_2–TP
CMRO_2			
DB	7.92 ± 1.05	3.95 ± 0.70[a]	3.97 ± 0.50[a]
Percentage of N_2O/O_2		50 ± 4	50 ± 4
NE	6.4 ± 0.80	3.32 ± 0.41[a]	3.11 ± 0.54[a]
Percentage of N_2O/O_2		51 ± 3	48 ± 3
CBF			
DB	125 ± 26	63 ± 10[a]	62 ± 17[a]
Percentage of N_2O/O_2		51 ± 4	49 ± 4
NE	141 ± 22	50 ± 5	90 ± 25[a]
Percentage of N_2O/O_2		37 ± 8	63 ± 8 *

DB = donor blood; TP = thiopental.

[a] These values are in ml 100 g^{-1} min^{-1}.

* $p < 0.05$ compared with DB distribution.

Table 4
Functional/basal $CMRO_2$ and CBF compartments (mean ± S.D.) in rats at 34 °C with norepinephrine infusion ($n = 9$) or DB transfusion ($n = 10$) to maintain mean arterial blood pressure during TP-induced isoelectric EEG to measure basal $CMRO_2$

	(Total) N_2O/O_2 (ml 100 g^{-1} min^{-1})	(Total) N_2O/O_2 (ml 100 g^{-1} min^{-1})	Basal TP	Functional N_2O/O_2–TP
$CMRO_2$				
DB	7.41 ± 1.78	6.31 ± 1.41 *	$2.37 \pm 0.63^{a,+}$	$3.94 \pm 1.38^{a,+,\psi}$
Percentage of N_2O/O_2 at 34 °C			$38 \pm 10^{+,\varphi}$	$61 \pm 10^{+,\psi,\varphi}$
NE	7.48 ± 2.49	5.41 ± 2.02 *	3.85 ± 1.27^a	$1.56 \pm 1.26^{a,\psi}$
Percentage of N_2O/O_2 at 34 °C			$73 \pm 16^+$	$27 \pm 16^{+,\psi}$
CBF				
DB	98 ± 28	101 ± 32	$39 \pm 10^{a,+}$	62 ± 31^a
Percentage of N_2O/O_2 at 34 °C			42 ± 15	58 ± 15
NE	132 ± 27	121 ± 24	68 ± 25	52 ± 21^a
Percentage of N_2O/O_2 at 34 °C			56 ± 16	44 ± 16

$CMRO_2$ = cerebral metabolic rate for oxygen; CBF = cerebral blood flow; TP = thiopental; DB = donor blood. Reproduced with permission from the Editor of Anesth. Analg.
  [a] These values are in ml 100 g^{-1} min^{-1}.
  * $p < 0.001$ compared with the value at 38 °C.
  [+] $p < 0.05$ compared with values for the compartments at 38 °C.
  [ψ] $p < 0.05$ compared with corresponding basal value.
  [φ] $p < 0.05$ compared with corresponding values during norepinephrine infusion at 34 °C.

4.4. Discussion

The results show that NE infusion during hypothermia in the anesthetized rat increased $bCMRO_2$ relative to $fCMRO_2$, suggesting that NE infusion during hypothermia may attenuate a protective effect of hypothermia in ischemic brain damage. NE selectively stimulates $bCMRO_2$ as opposed to $fCMRO_2$. This may explain the observation that increased $CMRO_2$ by catecholamine does not cause electrocortical activation, i.e. seizure states, but rather high amplitude, slow-wave activity [11]. The relevance of an increase in $bCMRO_2$ as opposed to $fCMRO_2$ with respect to cerebral cortical EEG activity remains to be defined.

5. Subcellular verification of basal versus functional $CMRO_2$

5.1. Introduction

The observation that brain glucose uptake in neonates undergoing deep hypothermic cardiopulmonary bypass (DHCPB) exceeded that of oxygen uptake suggested either anerobiosis, metabolic shunting or sequestering of glucose rather than aerobic oxidation [12]. We hypothesized that hypothermia may activate glucose transport or uptake relative to oxygen uptake. To test this hypothesis, we subjected rats to deep hypothermia of 18 °C and compared the glucose transporter protein (GLUT-3) immunostaining compared to that at 38 °C.

5.2. Methods

Six rats were anesthetized and mechanically ventilated on 1% halothane/70% nitrous oxide/30% oxygen. Three rats were maintained at 38 °C and their brains perfused and fixed in situ with 2% buffered glutaraldehyde. Three rats were cooled to 18 °C with ice packs on their backs and their brains perfused and fixed. The brains were then processed for immunostaining for GLUT-3.

5.3. Results

With the rats at 38 °C, GLUT-3 staining was clearly evident on neuronal cell bodies as well as on dendrites and axons (Fig. 4). On the other hand, at 18 °C, the GLUT-3 staining of neuronal cell bodies was difficult to find whereas the staining on dendrites was easily visualized (Fig. 5).

5.4. Discussion

If it can be assumed that metabolic coupling between oxygen and glucose uptake is maintained during deep hypothermia, then the translocation of GLUT-3 would correlate with an increased oxygen uptake. The observation that during deep hypothermia the visualization of GLUT-3 is more intense on dendrites and axons than on cell bodies

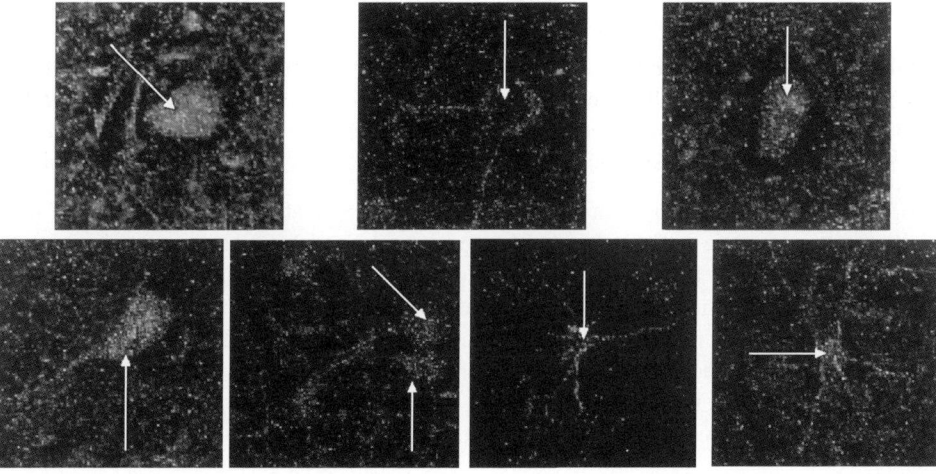

Fig. 4. Glucose transporter 3 (GLUT-3) staining of the rat brain at 38 °C.

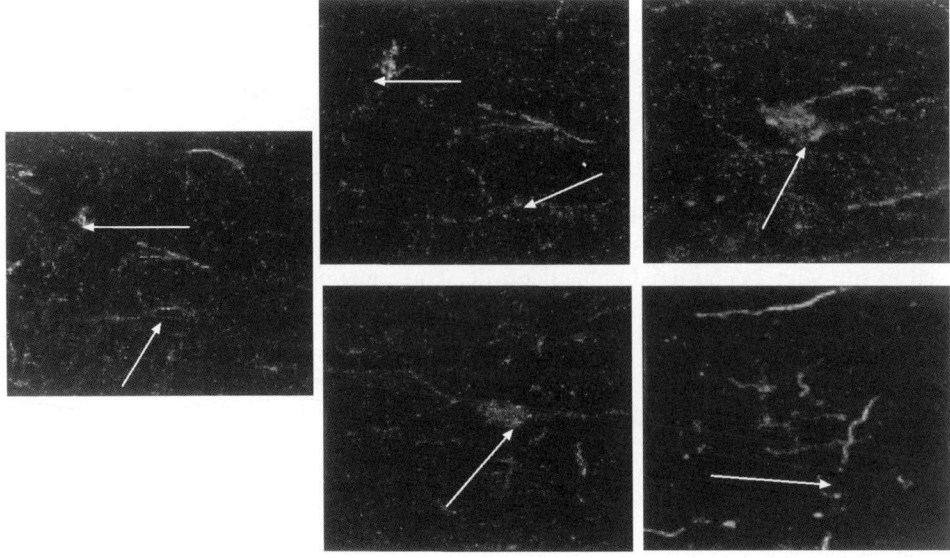

Fig. 5. Glucose transporter 3 (GLUT-3) staining of the rat brain at 18 °C.

whereas at 38 °C the staining of neuronal cell bodies is more prevalent suggests that hypothermia selectively suppresses $bCMRO_2$, as shown by our oxygen uptake data.

2.4.6.7. On-Site Discussion

2.4.6.7.1. **Question: (Gjedde)** How did you distinguish between "basal" and "functional" $CMRO_2$, particular in relation to anesthesia?

Answer: (Nemoto) The baseline $CMRO_2$ measurements were made on 1% halothane/70% N_2O/30% O_2 which was corrected for the depression of $CMRO_2$ by this baseline anesthesia of 20%. When thiopental was infused to render the EEG isoelectricity, the holocrine/N_2O/O_2 anesthesia was replaced by 70% N_2/30% O_2.

2.4.6.7.2. **Question: (Hyder)** I think the prediction of S. Kety about the action of most anesthetics on synaptic activity has held true as evidenced by recent molecular biology studies (e.g. Richards (1998) Toxicology Letters). We are familiar with Michenfelder studies with thiopental in dog brain, where $CMRO_2$ was depressed by 50% at flat EEG. An important point about degree of suppression in $CMRO_2$ is that the older studies were whole brain measurements whereas same of the recent 13C studies from Yale (where cortical measurements were made, Rothman (2001) NMR Biomedicine) show $CMRO_2$ superior by about 80% for $CMRO_2$ in cortex.

Answer: (Nemoto) Thank you for your comment and for the information. It is true that we should do and plan to do studies using PET to look at regional suppression of $CMRO_2$ by thiopental along with the effect of hypothermia on functional and basal $CMRO_2$ at the regional level.

2.4.6.7.3. **Question: (Traystman)** Since hypothermia may inhibit glutamate release following injury (ischemia) and be neuroprotective from this aspect, which compartment would be effected here, i.e. basal or active? If you used ketamine, would the hypothermia's effect to protect be less?

Answer: (Nemoto) The inhibition of glutamate release by hypothermia in ischemia, I believe, would reduce the basal $CMRO_2$ compartment. Yes, I would guess that ketamine would reduce the protective effects of hypothermia.

2.4.6.7.4. **Question: (Andrew)** In terms of being therapeutically useful, what factors determine how early and how late hypothermia may be protective following stroke onset?

Answer: (Nemoto) Hypothermia could be protective as early as possible. That is to say, the earlier the better. As far as how late hypothermia may be protective would depend on the severity of the stroke and whether the stroke is evolving. If it is a completed? stroke that has stabilized, I believe that hypothermia would not be useful. I believe that CT and, if possible, stable XE/CT CBF or MR1 evaluation would be important to help decide whether hypothermia would be useful.

2.4.6.7.5. **Question: (Golanov)** Have you tried to correlate EEG components (α, θ rhythms, etc.) with $CMRO_2$ level?

Answer: (Nemoto) No, we have not.

References

[1] S.S. Kety, Discussion, Pharmacol. Rev. 17 (1965) 230–233.
[2] J.D. Michenfelder, The in vivo effects of massive concentrations of anesthetics on canine cerebral metabolism, in: B.R. Fink (Ed.), Molecular Mechanisms of Anesthesia, Progress in Anesthesiology, vol. 1, Raven Press, New York, 1975, pp. 537–543.
[3] J.D. Michenfelder, The interdependency of cerebral functional and metabolic effects following massive doses of thiopental in the dog, Anesthesiology 41 (1974) 231–236.
[4] J. Astrup, P.M. Sorensen, H.R. Sorensen, Oxygen and glucose consumption related to $Na^+ - K^+$ transport in canine brain, Stroke 12 (1981) 726–730.
[5] H. Minamisawa, C.H. Nordstrom, M.L. Smith, B.K. Siesjo, The influence of mild body and brain hypothermia on ischemic brain damage, J. Cereb. Blood Flow Metab. 10 (1990) 365–374.
[6] G.L. Clifton, J.Y. Jiang, B.G. Lyeth, L.W. Jenkins, R.J. Hamm, R.L. Hayes, Marked protection by moderate hypothermia after experimental traumatic brain injury, J. Cereb. Blood Flow Metab. 11 (1991) 114–121.
[7] E.M. Nemoto, L. Yao, H. Yonas, J. Darby, Compartmentation of whole brain blood flow and oxygen and glucose metabolism in monkeys, J. Neurosurg. Anesthesiol. 6 (1994) 170–174.
[8] E.M. Nemoto, R. Klementavicius, H. Yonas, Functional and basal cerebral metabolic rate for oxygen ($CMRO_2$) and its relevance to the pathogenesis and therapy of brain injury, in: A. Hudetz, D. Bruley (Eds.), Oxygen Transport to Tissue XX, Advances in Exptl. Med., vol. 454, Plenum Press, New York, 1998, pp. 235–242.
[9] P.A. Steen, L. Newberg, J.H. Milde, J.D. Michenfelder, Hypothermia and barbiturates: individual and combined effects on canine cerebral oxygen consumption, Anesthesiology 58 (1983) 527–532.

[10] E.M. Nemoto, R. Klementavicius, J.A. Melick, H. Yonas, Suppression of cerebral metabolic rate for oxygen (CMRO$_2$) by mild hypothermia compared to thiopental, J. Neurosurg. Anesthesiol. 8 (1996) 52–59.

[11] N. Dahlgren, I. Rosen, T. Sakabe, B.K. Siesjo, Cerebral functional, metabolic, and circulatory effects of intravenous infusion of adrenaline in the rat, Brain Res. 184 (1980) 143–152.

[12] F. Pigula, R.D. Siewers, E.M. Nemoto, Hypothermic cardiopulmonary bypass alters oxygen/glucose uptake in pediatric brain, J. Thorac. Cardiovasc. Surg. 121 (2001) 366–373.

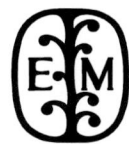

International Congress Series 1235 (2002) 243–248

Intrinsic optical recording of somatosensory responses in the human cerebral cortex during brain tumor surgery

Tadashi Nariai [a,*], Yoshihisa Ohta [a], Kimiyoshi Hirakawa [a],
Katsushige Sato [b], Itaru Yazawa [b], Shin-ichi Sasaki [b],
Kohtaro Kamino [b], Kikuo Ohno [a]

[a] Department of Neurosurgery, Graduate School, Tokyo Medical and Dental University, 1-5-45 Yushima,
Bunkyo-ku, Tokyo 113-8519 Japan
[b] Department of Physiology, Graduate School, Tokyo Medical and Dental University, Tokyo, Japan

Abstract

Intrinsic optical signals to electrical stimulation of the face and hand were recorded from the human primary sensory cortex. Somatotopic representation of optical recording was compared with that of MEG. The recordings were carried out on 10 patients bearing tumors, adjacent to the sensorimotor cortex. The cortical surface was illuminated with voltage-stabilized Xe white light. The reflected light passed through a band-pass filter (605 nm), and eight functional images were acquired during 5 s using the intrinsic optical imaging system (Imager 2001). The median nerve, the first and the fifth digits or the first and the third branches of the trigeminal nerve were electrically stimulated. In all patients, the somatosensory optical signals were recorded on the primary sensory cortex. The location of the optical signals corresponded with that of the dipole estimation of the cortical sensory responses in MEG. The optical signals to the stimulation of the first and the fifth digits, and the first and the third branches of the trigeminal nerve were recorded on different locations among the sensory strip. These results indicated that the intrinsic optical signal recorded from the human primary sensory cortex represented somatotopic representation well, and could be a useful technique in monitoring human cortical neuronal activity. © 2002 Elsevier Science B.V. All rights reserved.

Keywords: Intrinsic optical signal; Somatosensory response; Human cerebral cortex; MEG; 3D image

---

* Corresponding author. Fax: +81-3-5803-0140.
E-mail address: nariai.nsrg@tmd.ac.jp (T. Nariai).

0531-5131/02 © 2002 Elsevier Science B.V. All rights reserved.
PII: S 0 5 3 1 - 5 1 3 1 (0 2) 0 0 1 9 4 - 2

1. Background

The optical method has proven to be a useful technique for monitoring neural responses in the central nervous system in vivo condition [1–3], and has been applied for investigating the functional organization of the visual [4–6] and somatosensory systems [7–10] in animal brains.

Some research groups have applied this technique to the human brain during neuro-surgical operations [11–15]. However, they have not yet obtained detailed functional maps of the human brain in comparison with various noninvasive preoperative brain mapping techniques.

In the present study, we applied the optical imaging technique to brain tumor patients during neurosurgical operations and examined whether it corresponds with the intra-operative cortical electrophysiological data, and the preoperative noninvasive brain mapping data with MEG.

2. Methods

We measured intrinsic optical signals from the somatosensory cortex in 10 patients who underwent resection of a brain tumor located adjacent to the primary sensory cortex (postcentral gyrus) (Table 1). Informed consent was obtained from all patients prior to the operation. All the patients needed localization of the sensorimotor cortex by means of the classical electrophysiological method. The anesthesia and surgical strategy were not modified in order to perform the optical imaging, and the recording was performed under general anesthesia with isoflurane.

For the optical imaging, the median nerve, Digits I and V or the supraorbital branch of the ophthalmic nerve (N. V_1) and the mental branch of the mandibular nerve (N. V_3) were stimulated transcutaneously with surface electrodes driven by an electrical stimulator. The

Table 1
Patients list

Case no.	Patient	Age/sex	Diagnosis	Location	Stimulation	Methods for validation
1	S.K.	52/M	meningioma	left parietal	right median nerve	MEG, CorSEP
2	H.K.	75/M	metastatic brain tumor	right parietal	left median nerve	CorSEP
3	S.K.	61/M	anaplastic oligodendroglioma	right parietal	left median nerve	MEG, CorSEP
4	T.A.	68/M	meningioma	left parietal	right median nerve	CorSEP
5	H.N.	57/M	anaplastic oligodendroglioma	right parietal	left 1st/5th digit	fMRI, CorSEP
6	T.K.	71/M	metastatic brain tumor	right frontal	left 1st/5th digit	MEG, CorSEP
7	K.M.	47/M	oligodendroglioma	left temporal	right V1/V2 nerve	subdural electrode
8	M.N.	63/F	metastatic brain tumor	left parietal	right 1st/5th digit	MEG, CorSEP
9	Y.Y.	44/M	metastatic brain tumor	left frontal	right 1st/5th digit	MEG, CorSEP
10	E.A.	51/F	glioblastoma	right parietotemporal	left V1/V2 nerve, left median nerve	MEG, CorSEP

stimulus, consisting of 10 pulses, was delivered at 5 Hz for 2 s with an interstimulus interval of 20 s.

After identifying the central sulcus, the recording site of the cerebral cortex was stabilized with a glass plate. The somatosensory cortex was illuminated using a Xenon lamp driven by a stable DC power supply via an operating microscope (Carl Zeiss, Thornwood, NY). The reflected light from the cortex was passed through interference filters of different wavelengths. The filter used for visualizing the surface of the cortex and its vascular pattern had a transmission maximum of 540 ± 30 nm, and the filter used for intrinsic imaging had a passband at 605 ± 5 nm (Asahi Spectra, Tokyo, Japan). In our previous studies on the rat somatosensory cortex [9,10], we detected the largest intrinsic signal at a wavelength of 605 nm. In the intraoperative recording, we used this single wavelength (605 ± 5 nm) to detect the optical signals. The depth of focus of the operating microscope was set to about 500 μm under the cortical surface. Intrinsic imaging was performed using a differential video acquisition system, Imager 2001 (Optical Imaging, Germantown, NY) via a charge coupled device camera fitted to an operating microscope. During each trial, eight optical images were collected over 5.0 s and stored on a computer with data acquisition software, VDAQ (Optical Imaging). The optical reflectance images were represented by the fractional change ($\Delta R/R$) to correct for uneven illumination using a data-analyzing software program, TVMix (Optical Imaging). It usually took about 15 min to obtain the functional map.

We recorded somatosensory-evoked fields (SEFs) in six patients before the operations using a whole head-type MEG system with 148 channel magnetometers (Magnes,

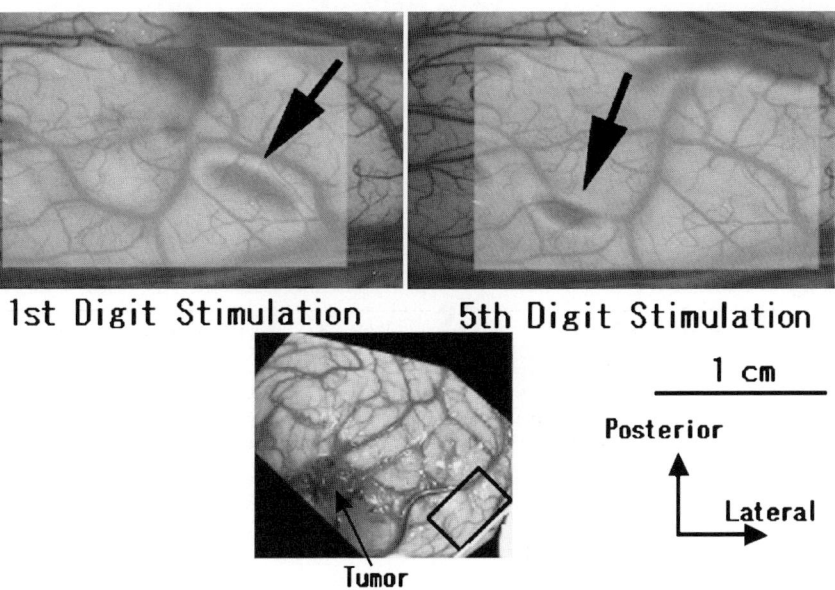

Fig. 1. Intrinsic optical signal by stimulation of Digits I and V recorded in a patient with a left parietal metastatic tumor (Case 8). Black arrows indicate the optical signals. Stimulation of the different digits evoked optical signals in different locations, and the result of the Digit I stimulation is lower than that of the Digit V stimulation along the axis of the central sulcus (CS).

Biomagnetic Technologies, San Diego, CA). Following the recording, the source current locations in the three dimensions of SEFs and the equivalent current dipole (ECD) moments were calculated using a single dipole model, assuming the brain to be a sphere. The ECD that best explained the most dominant sources were determined using data recorded from a subset of channels, and the ECD were superimposed on a three-dimensionally reconstructed MR image of the brain.

3. Results

In our initial four patients, the recording was carried out to examine whether the optical signal could be obtained by median nerve simulation. In all these, the signal was obtained on the surface of the postcentral gyrus but not on the surface of pre-central gyrus. The location of the signal was at the anterior edge of the gyrus, close to the central sulcus. The location of the signal corresponded with the most prominent N20 response in the cortical SEP, and the cortical surface projection of the N20 ECD in MEG.

In the latter six patients, the focus was put mainly on whether the somatotopic representation of the primary sensory cortex could be visualized by optical recording. As is shown in Figs. 1 and 2, the signals by the stimulations of V1 and V3, and of Digits I

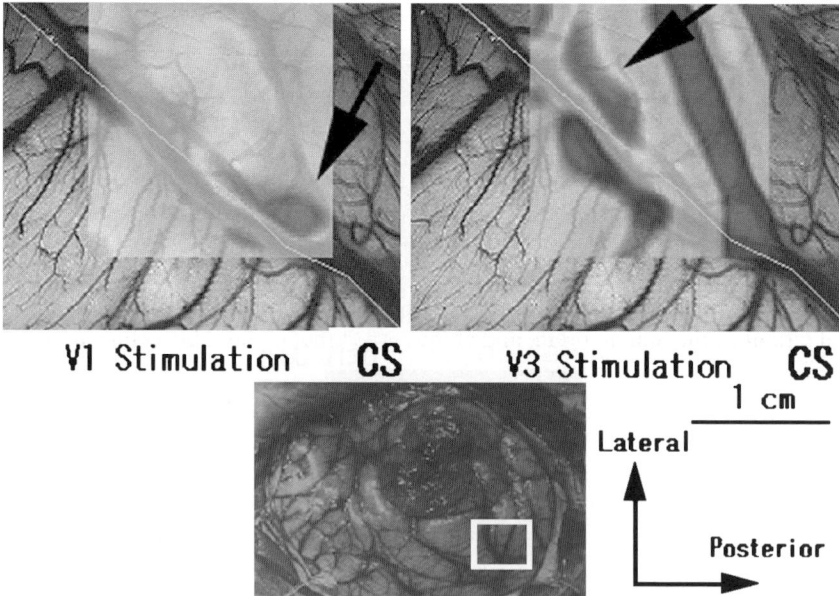

Fig. 2. Intrinsic optical signal by stimulations of the first branch of the trigeminal nerve (V1) and the third branch of the trigeminal nerve (V3) recorded in a patient with right parietotemporal glioblastoma (Case 10). Black arrows indicated the optical signals. Stimulation of the different branches of the trigeminal nerve evoked optical signals in different locations and the result of the V3 stimulation is lower than that of the V1 stimulation along the axis of the central sulcus (CS).

and V, were traced in the different locations among the postcentral gyrus. There were no overlaps of signals in each patient. In all patients, signals created by the stimulations of V3 and V1, and of Digits I and V, were located along the central sulcus in this order from lower to upper portion. The somatotopic representation observed by the optical method corresponded well with "homunculus" figure presented by Penfield and Boldray [16]. It was also confirmed that the brain surface projection of the N20 ECD by the stimulation of Digits I and V recorded with MEG, corresponded with the location of the optical signal along the axis of the central sulcus in three patients.

4. Discussion

The intrinsic optical imaging of neural activities is an excellent technique to obtain functional maps of the central nervous system. Application of this method in order to map the function of the human brain was first reported by Haglund et al. [11], who recorded stimulation-evoked epileptiform after-discharges and cognitively evoked functional activity. Since then, there have been several reports of applying this method to map the human brain function [12–15]. However, detailed comparison of the optical method to the other noninvasive functional mapping techniques, and to the symptoms of patients, has not yet been conducted.

In this report, we showed the correspondence between the ECD estimation with MEG and the optical signal along the axis of the somatosensory cortex. From a neurosurgeon's point of view, the optical recording was more useful than MEG because the former can delineate the group of neurons significantly activated by certain stimuli, but the latter can estimate the activated area only as a single point. Spatial resolution in the optical method is far superior to electrophysiological recording with a cortical electrode because the latter cannot visualize the activated area; however, it can only draw the topographical map using electrodes placed at 1-cm intervals.

In conclusion, the intrinsic optical signal recorded from the human primary sensory cortex represented somatotopic representation well, and could delineate the area of human cortical neuronal activity. Moreover, it could be a useful technique to investigate the neuronal circuit of the human brain, and at the same time, it could be a clinical monitoring tool during neurosurgical operations.

2.4.7.6. On-Site Discussion

2.4.7.6.1. *Question: (Fukuda)* What about the picture signal polarity?

Answer: (Nariai) Our color scale is expressed as $-\Delta R/R$. Thus, a decrease in signal is expressed with red colour. Concerning the technical details, please refer to the published reference (Tanaka et al., Neurovasc. Res. 2000; 36: 193).

References

[1] A. Grinvald, E. Lieke, R.D. Frostig, C.D. Gilbert, T.N. Wiesel, Functional architecture of cortex revealed by optical imaging of intrinsic signals, Nature 324 (6095) (1986) 361–364.

[2] I. Godecke, T. Bonhoeffer, Development of identical orientation maps for two eyes without common visual experience, Nature 379 (6562) (1996) 251–254.

[3] B. Chapman, M.P. Stryker, T. Bonhoeffer, Development of orientation preference maps in ferret primary visual cortex, J. Neurosci. 16 (20) (1996) 6443–6453.

[4] D.Y. Ts'o, R.D. Frostig, E.E. Lieke, A. Grinvald, Functional organization of primate visual cortex revealed by high resolution optical imaging, Science 249 (4967) (1990) 417–420.

[5] T. Bonhoeffer, A. Grinvald, Iso-orientation domains in cat visual cortex are arranged in pinwheel-like patterns, Nature 353 (6343) (1991) 429–431.

[6] A. Shmuel, A. Grinvald, Functional organization for direction of motion and its relationship to orientation maps in cat area 18, J. Neurosci. 16 (21) (1996) 6945–6964.

[7] S.A. Masino, M.C. Kwon, Y. Dory, R.D. Frostig, Characterization of functional organization within rat barrel cortex using intrinsic signal optical imaging through a thinned skull, Proc. Natl. Acad. Sci. U. S. A. 90 (21) (1993) 9998–10002.

[8] J.L. Dowling, M.M. Henegar, D. Liu, C.M. Rovainen, T.A. Woolsey, Rapid optical imaging of whisker responses in the rat barrel cortex, J. Neurosci. Methods 66 (2) (1996) 113–122.

[9] T. Tanaka, I. Yazawa, K. Sato, Y. Momose-Sato, K. Kamino, Consistency behind trial-to-trial variation in intrinsic optical responses to single-whisker movement in the rat D1-barrel cortex, Neurosci. Res. 36 (3) (2000) 193–207.

[10] I. Yazawa, S. Sasaki, H. Mochida, K. Kamino, Y. Momose-Sato, K. Sato, Developmental changes in trial-to-trial variations in whisker barrel responses studied using intrinsic optical imaging: comparison between normal and de-whiskered rats, J. Neurophysiol. 86 (1) (2001) 392–401.

[11] M.M. Haglund, G.A. Ojemann, D.W. Hochman, Optical imaging of epileptiform and functional activity in human cerebral cortex, Nature 358 (6388) (1992) 668–671.

[12] A.F. Cannestra, K.L. Black, N.A. Martin, T. Cloughesy, J.S. Burton, E. Rubinstein, et al., Topographical and temporal specificity of human intraoperative optical intrinsic signals, NeuroReport 9 (11) (1998) 2557–2563.

[13] A.F. Cannestra, S.Y. Bookheimer, N. Pouratian, A. O'Farrell, N. Sicotte, N.A. Martin, et al., Temporal and topographical characterization of language cortices using intraoperative optical intrinsic signals, Neuroimage 12 (1) (2000) 41–54.

[14] N. Pouratian, S.Y. Bookheimer, A.M. O'Farrell, N.L. Sicotte, A.F. Cannestra, D. Becker, et al., Optical imaging of bilingual cortical representations. Case report, J. Neurosurg. 93 (4) (2000) 676–681.

[15] A.W. Toga, A.F. Cannestra, K.L. Black, The temporal/spatial evolution of optical signals in human cortex, Cereb. Cortex 5 (6) (1995) 561–565.

[16] W. Penfield, E. Boldray, Somatic motor and sensory representation in the cerebral cortex of man as studied by electrical stimulation, Brain 60 (1937) 389–443.

Mediators

Neuronal, astroglial and other mediators

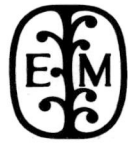

International Congress Series 1235 (2002) 251–257

Activity-induced changes in cerebellar blood flow

M. Lauritzen [a,*], K. Caesar [b]

[a]*Department of Clinical Neurophysiology, Glostrup Hospital, Denmark*
[b]*Department of Medical Physiology, Panum Institute, University of Copenhagen, Copenhagen, Denmark*

Abstract

Changes in brain cellular activity are accompanied almost invariably by changes in the local cerebral blood flow (CBF). In most functional imaging studies, the increase in local blood flow is assumed to correlate with an increase in the net spike activity of the neurons in the activated region. The question raised in this work is whether the increase in perfusion correlates to spike activity or synaptic transmission, or both. By utilizing measurements of neuronal activity, i.e., single-cell spike activity and synaptic activity of ensembles of neurons (i.e., field potentials), we were able to show that activity-dependent increases in CBF are independent of spiking activity; however, it can be explained by active and passive pre- and postsynaptic mechanisms distinct from spiking. Our work has primarily been focused on the cerebellar cortex where CBF was monitored by laser-Doppler flowmetry and neuronal activity was measured using a glass electrode positioned close to the Purkinje cell. © 2002 Elsevier Science B.V. All rights reserved.

Keywords: Cerebral blood flow; Electrophysiology; Cerebellum; Glutamate; GABA

1. Introduction

Neurovascular coupling is a fundamental feature of the brain and is traditionally seen as an increase in spike activity in the principal target cells or interneurons of the active brain region, accompanied by an increase in metabolism and CBF [1]. The issue addressed in this study is whether the increase in perfusion correlates to spike activity, or rather to synaptic transmission, or both. Our working hypothesis is that events related to passive and active postsynaptic events trigger and determine the amplitude of the blood-flow increase. These events are the interaction of the neurotransmitter with the receptor, external and internal gating of ion conductance and the production of second messengers (including calcium),

* Corresponding author.
E-mail address: mlauritz@mfi.ku.dk (M. Lauritzen).

0531-5131/02 © 2002 Elsevier Science B.V. All rights reserved.
PII: S0531-5131(02)00197-8

the generation of the action potential, neurotransmitter re-uptake, and recovery of intra-cellular and transmembrane ionic gradients [2]. Clearly, the relative requirements of these events in terms of energy metabolism and blood flow differ among neuronal circuits and regions, depending on the properties of the neuronal circuits being stimulated. Any measure of electrical activity of a neuron represents a complex of cellular properties, both anatomical and physiological; our study required a model in which the afferent input(s) to a target cell could be easily separated. Therefore, we used the cerebellar cortex. The neuronal circuits of the cerebellar cortex are well defined and the basic electrophysiology is well established. Purkinje neurons, the principal target neurons of this system, have a monosynaptic excitatory input and a disynaptic excitatory/inhibitory input that can be separated exper-imentally [3]. Due to the absence of excitatory collaterals from Purkinje cell axons, the cerebellar cortex is incapable of generating epileptic neuronal activity. Furthermore, the elicitation of cortical spreading depression requires conditioning of the tissue so as to decrease the chloride concentration in the interstitial fluid, and in consequence, the influence of synaptic inhibitory activity. These intrinsic properties of the cerebellar cortex have been essential for our experiments, since it has been possible to control the stimulus-response paradigms even at high levels of electrical stimulation. We stimulated both climbing and parallel fibres, which allowed us to examine the neurovascular coupling, secondary to activation of a monosynaptic excitatory pathway and a disynaptic excitatory/inhibitory pathway.

2. Methods

Male Wistar rats (300–350 g, Panum Institute, Copenhagen) were anaesthetised with halothane (Vapor, Dräger; 4% at induction and 1.5% during surgery) in O_2 30%–N_2O 70%. Lidocaine (5 mg ml^{-1} s.c.) was used at the operation sites and at the contact spots for the ear pins. Catheters were inserted into the femoral artery for recording of arterial blood pressure, and in the femoral vein. The rats were tracheotomized and artificially ventilated to maintain arterial pH at 7.35–7.40, $PaCO_2$ at approximately 39 mm Hg, and PaO_2 at approximately 100 mm Hg (measured by ABL 715, Radiometer, Denmark). The head was placed in a stereotactic head holder. The cranial bone and the dura were carefully removed over the cerebellar cortex. A pool of 5% agar in Ringer solution was made around the craniotomy for continuous superfusion with aerated (95% air, 5% CO_2) artificial cerebrospinal fluid (aCSF) at 37 °C (composition in mM: 120 NaCl, 2.8 KCl, 22 $NaHCO_3$, 1.45 $CaCl_2$, 1.0 Na_2HPO_4, and 0.876 $MgCl_2$). The temperature of the animal was monitored with a rectal thermometer and kept at 37 °C by a heating pad (custom made). The level of anaesthesia was checked continuously by observing the arterial blood pressure during stimulation, and by a tail pinch. At the end of the experiment, the rats were killed by an intravenous injection of air. The National Animal Ethics Committee approved all surgical and anaesthetic procedures.

The CBF was assessed by laser-Doppler flowmetry [4]. Single-unit activity in Purkinje cells and synaptic field potentials was recorded with glass microelectrodes positioned near the cell body. Increases in CBF or neuronal activity were evoked by stimulation of the parallel or climbing fibre systems.

3. Results and discussion

3.1. Cerebellar blood flow and spike activity

In the absence of stimulation, Purkinje neurons spontaneously produce regular Na^+-action potentials, termed simple spikes. Stimulating the parallel fibres by direct electrical stimulation of the cerebellar cortical surface causes glutamate release from the parallel fibres that interacts with AMPA receptors on Purkinje cells, and with interneurons that in turn release GABA which inhibits the Purkinje cells [5]. This is an example of a complex disynaptic circuit that gives rise to both monosynaptic excitatory and inhibitory post-synaptic potentials (EPSPs and IPSPs) in the Purkinje neurons, the combination of which results in a net inhibition of the simple spikes. However, a significant increase in cerebellar blood flow is still apparent. Therefore, in this system, the increase in blood flow does not correlate with an increase in spike rate in the principal target neuron [6]. In contrast, stimulation of the climbing fibres in the brain stem activates Purkinje cells in the cerebellar cortex, directly, via a monosynaptic excitatory input produced by the interaction of glutamate with an AMPA receptor on the postsynaptic membrane. This is an example of a relatively simple monosynaptic system. Furthermore, stimulation of the climbing fibres produces high-frequency bursts of both Na^+- and Ca^{2+}-action potentials in Purkinje neurons, termed complex spikes. These spikes reflect both passive and active membrane properties of the Purkinje cells. By passive membrane mechanisms, we mean the extrinsically gated conductance that binds neurotransmitters and receives and reports activity of presynaptic neurons. The active membrane mechanisms refer to the plethora of conductance gated by changes of the membrane potential, and for some, also by changes in the intracellular calcium concentration [2]. Triggering these passive and active membrane mechanisms of the Purkinje cells by climbing fibre stimulation gives rise to a large increase in blood flow.

Thus, the changes of spike activity of individual Purkinje neurons underlying the changes in blood flow differ, depending on whether climbing fibres or parallel fibres are stimulated [6,7].

3.2. Synaptic activity and cerebellar blood flow

A different measure of electrical activity is obtained by recording the field potentials that are evoked by stimulation of either of the two pathways.

Neuronal activity gives rise to transmembrane ion-fluxes that produce a current flow in the extracellular space, and since the extracellular space has a defined electrical resistance, this gives rise to a field potential. Thus, a field potential is produced by the activity of ensembles of cells close to the recording electrode and gives information about the synchronised neuronal activity in the stimulated region.

Climbing fibre stimulation generates a slow field potential with a large postsynaptic component. The contribution from the presynaptic structures to the extracellular ion fluxes, i.e., field potentials, is negligible in this pathway.

Parallel fibre stimulation generates a field potential that can be divided into a large presynaptic component and a small postsynaptic component. The inhibitory postsynaptic potential cannot be visualized in the FP due to the functional anatomy of the stellate cells. In examining the coupling between neuronal activity and cerebellar blood flow, we compared the field-potential records with the real time flow measurements by correlating the overall electrical and CBF responses for the different stimulation frequencies. Summing up the amplitudes of each FP generated within a stimulation period and multiplying this value with the stimulation frequency assessed the electrical activity. A stimulation period of 30 s and a stimulation frequency of 5 Hz generated 150 FPs. Correlating the value of summated FPs to the maximal CBF response evoked at 5, 10, and 20 Hz revealed a linear relation with respect to climbing fibre stimulation, and a sigmoidal relation with respect to parallel fibre stimulation (Fig. 1) [6].

The linear relationship in the climbing fibre system suggests that there is a direct link between blood flow and the postsynaptic activity in Purkinje neurons. The sigmoidal relationship in the parallel fibre system indicates that the link between the extracellular current flow and cerebellar blood flow is more complex in this system. First, it consists of a level of neuronal activity which is not accompanied by an increase in flow, followed by a range of neuronal activity for which the flow increase is linear and ending with a level of activity for which there is no further increase in blood flow. Both climbing fibre and parallel fibre stimulations result in glutamate release that activates Purkinje neurons by interacting with AMPA receptors on the postsynaptic membrane [8,9]. Using an AMPA receptor antagonist to block transmission during climbing fibre stimulation causes a reduction in both the size of the evoked field potentials and the blood-flow response. This emphasises

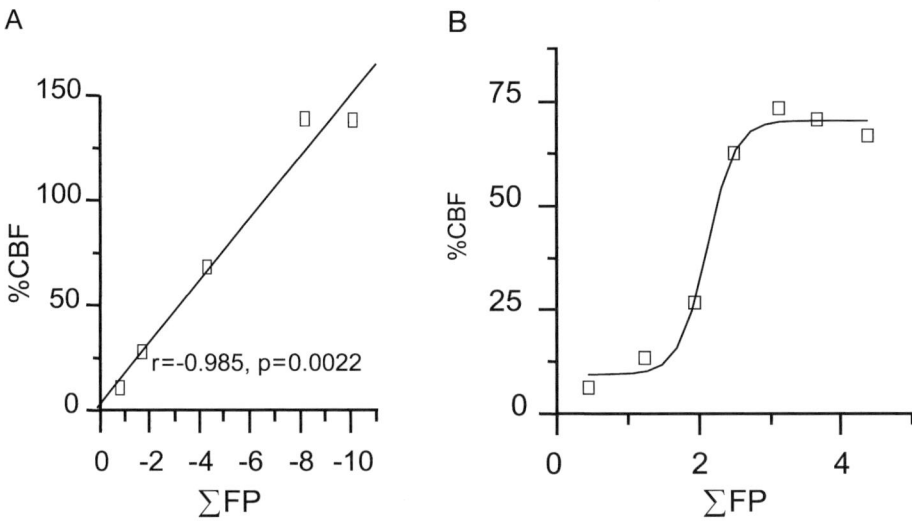

Fig. 1. Correlation between changes in cerebellar blood flow (CBF) and electrical field potential in response to stimulation of either climbing fibres or parallel fibres. (A) Following climbing fibre stimulation, there is a linear correlation between the increase in cerebellar blood flow and summed field potential. The summed field potential is the product of the field potential amplitude (in mV) and stimulus rate (in Hz) and represents total synaptic activity during stimulation. (B) There is a sigmoid relationship between synaptic activity and cerebellar blood flow following stimulation of the parallel fibre system. See text and Mathiesen et al. [6] for details.

the robust relationship between the increase in synaptic activity and blood flow, and confirms that the increase in blood flow is linked to the postsynaptic activity in this monosynaptic system. In response to parallel fibre stimulation, the blockade of AMPA receptors only inhibited 50% of the CBF increase, emphasising the fact that blood-flow regulation in this system is partly governed by mechanisms other than postsynaptic events. Thus, in this system, both presynaptic and synaptic events are important for the blood-flow increase.

4. Conclusion

Activity-dependent increases in CBF are independent of spike activity in the principal target cells of the activated region. This observation breaks with the common notion that increased CBF indicates increased impulse traffic in and out of a region, and the study demonstrates for the first time the importance of interneurons for the control of CBF. Investigating neuronal activity in terms of field potentials showed that the changes in blood flow correlated with the postsynaptic activity within a monosynaptic system, however, with changes of the overall pre- and postsynaptic neuronal activity in a disynaptic system. Thus, the coupling between activity of the principal neurons and vascular responses is more complex than is usually assumed. Complementary studies of the somatosensory cortex by others and by us indicated that functional activation works differently in different brain regions, suggesting that several neuronal circuits need to be studied if we want to explain the electrophysiological basis of functional activation.

3.1.1.7. On-Site Discussion

3.1.1.7.1. **Comment: (Heiss)** I was intrigued by your sophisticated techniques and by the results you presented. However, one of the causes of the discrepancies among changes in neuronal activity and changes in flow could be the different volumes you are recording from. If you use a small microelectrode to record from neurons and use the same microelectrode for determination of flow, the results might be completely different. Probably in most of the examples, you discussed the volume from which perfusion was determined was much larger—and additionally different—from that the neuronal activity was originating. For climbing fibre stimulations, almost the whole cerebellum was stimulated. For parallel fibre stimulation, the width of the activated beam of fibres was adjusted so as to be appropriate for the LDF probe. The microelectrode was positioned immediately below the LDF probe. For field potentials, the sampling volume is approximately the same as the LDF. For spike measurements, the volume is clearly smaller.

Answer: (Lauritzen) I agree with your statement that microelectrodes record from much smaller volumes than laser-Doppler probes. The important issue is however whether the electrical recording is representative for neuronal activity in a much larger volume of brain cells, or in other words whether the electrophysiological events at the level of the single nerve cell is reproduced in a stereotyped fashion throughout the volume from which the laser-Doppler probe is sampling. We suggest that this ideal situation has been accomplished in our experiments using the cerebellar cortex.

3.1.1.7.2. **Question: (Benyó)** Is it possible that the neuronal synaptic transmitter influences blood flow by a direct action on blood vessels?

Answer: (Lauritzen) Yes, this is possible, but it is more likely that the transmitters work via a second messenger mechanism such as nitric oxide or adenosine.

3.1.1.7.3. **Question: (Dreier)** The extracellular field potential is not only connected to synaptic activity but also to glial functions such as glial buffering. Does the correlation between changes of the extracellular field potential and CBF in the cerebellar system support an important role of glial cells?

Answer: (Lauritzen) The field potential mainly created by the neurons not the glial cells. The scannering role of glial cells with respect to maintenance of extracellular K^+ of concentration and glutamate uptake is, however, well known. Therefore, it is certainly likely that glial cells contribute to the CBF response.

3.1.1.7.4. **Question: (Gjedde)** Would you care to speculate about the expectation to be made about metabolism in the case of increased blood flow and complete absence of postsynaptic spiking?

Answer: (Lauritzen) The drive for metabolism under these conditions will be the ionic fluxes that are produced by the active and passive postsynaptic ion fluxes that are distinct from spiking. The cellular elements that will contribute to this will be the principal target cell itself, inhibitory interneurons and glial cells. The fact that the principal target cell—the Purkinje cell in the cerebellum—stops spiking does not mean that ionic fluxes are absent. Indeed, the postsynaptic activity is intense, but does not lead to spiking.

Acknowledgements

This study was supported in part by Neuro Science Pharma Biotech, The Danish Medical Research Council, The Carlsberg Foundation, The Brødrene Hartmanns foundation, and the NOVO-Nordisk Foundation. The expert technical assistance of Ms. Lillian Grøndahl is gratefully acknowledged.

References

[1] M.E. Raichle, Behind the scenes of functional brain imaging: a historical and physiological perspective, Proc. Natl. Acad. Sci. U. S. A. 95 (3) (1998) 765–772.
[2] J. Midtgaard, Processing of information from different sources: spatial synaptic integration in the dendrites of vertebrate CNS neurons, Trends Neurosci. 17 (4) (1994) 166–173.
[3] R.R. Llinas, M. Sugimori, The electrophysiology of the cerebellar Purkinje cell revisited, in: R.R. Llinas, C. Sotelo (Eds.), The Cerebellum Revisited, Springer, New York, 1992, pp. 167–181.
[4] M. Fabricius, M. Lauritzen, Laser-Doppler evaluation of rat brain microcirculation: comparison with the [C-14]-iodoantipyrine method suggests discordance during cerebral blood flow increases, J. Cereb. Blood Flow Metab. 16 (1) (1996) 156–161.
[5] R. Llinas, M. Sugimori, Electrophysiological properties of in vitro Purkinje cell dendrites in mammalian cerebellar slices, J. Physiol. (London) 305 (1980) 197–213.

[6] C. Mathiesen, K. Caesar, N. Akgoren, M. Lauritzen, Modification of activity-dependent increases of cerebral blood flow by excitatory synaptic activity and spikes in rat cerebellar cortex, J. Physiol. 512 (2) (1998) 555–566.

[7] C. Mathiesen, K. Caesar, M. Lauritzen, Temporal coupling between neuronal activity and blood flow in rat cerebellar cortex as indicated by field potential analysis, J. Physiol. 523 (Pt. 1) (2000) 235–246.

[8] T. Hirano, S. Hagiwara, Synaptic transmission between rat cerebellar granule and Purkinje cells in dissociated cell culture: effects of excitatory-amino acid transmitter antagonists, Proc. Natl. Acad. Sci. U. S. A. 85 (1988) 934–938.

[9] K. Okamoto, M. Sekiguchi, Synaptic receptors and intracellular signal transduction in the cerebellum, Neurosci. Res. 9 (1991) 213–237.

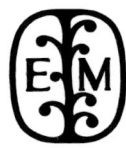

International Congress Series 1235 (2002) 259–266

Neurovascular coupling in health and disease: lessons from transgenic mice

Costantino Iadecola*, Kiyoshi Niwa, Yi Zhang, Ken Kazama

Department of Neurology, Center for Clinical and Molecular Neurobiology, University of Minnesota, MMC 295, 516 Delaware Street S.E., Minneapolis, MN, USA

Abstract

Neuronal activity is one of the major factors regulating the cerebral circulation. Synaptic activity produces increases in blood flow that are spatially restricted to the activated region and temporally related to the period of activation, a phenomenon termed functional hyperemia. The cellular and molecular factors linking synaptic activity to cerebral blood flow (CBF) and the mechanisms of their alteration in disease states are not well understood. The introduction of genetically engineered mice with overexpression or deletion of selected gene products provides a powerful tool to investigate the mechanisms of functional hyperemia. In this work, we will review the contributions to this field provided by transgenic mouse models, focusing on the role of nitric oxide (NO) and cyclooxygenase (COX) in cerebral cortex and/or cerebellum. Furthermore, the alterations in functional hyperemia produced by β-amyloid, a peptide that accumulates in the brain of patients with Alzheimer's disease, will also be examined. © 2002 Elsevier Science B.V. All rights reserved.

Keywords: Nitric oxide; Cyclooxygenase-1; Cyclooxygenase-2; Cerebellum; Alzheimer's disease

1. Introduction

Evidence accumulated over the past 100 years indicates that cerebral blood vessels are endowed with complex regulatory systems that allow the brain to finely regulate its own blood supply. One of the major factors that regulates cerebral blood flow (CBF) is neuronal activity. In this work, we will focus on the mechanisms governing the relationship between neural activity and blood flow highlighting the contributions derived from genetically engineered mouse models. In particular, we will examine the role of nitric oxide (NO) and cyclooxygenase (COX)-1 and -2 in functional hyperemia, and the

---

* Corresponding author. Tel.: +1-612-624-1902; fax: +1-612-625-7950.
 E-mail address: iadec001@tc.umn.edu (C. Iadecola).

0531-5131/02 © 2002 Elsevier Science B.V. All rights reserved.
PII: S 0 5 3 1 - 5 1 3 1 (0 2) 0 0 1 9 1 - 7

alterations in the coupling between neocortical CBF and energy demands that occur in mouse models of Alzheimer's dementia (AD).

2. Neural activity is one of the major factors controlling cerebral blood flow

It has long been known that increases in brain activity are associated with increases in CBF restricted to the activated areas (see Ref. [1] for a review). However, the mechanisms of this fundamental characteristic of the cerebral circulation remain to be clearly elucidated. One widely accepted hypothesis, stemming from the work of Roy and Sherrington, is that active neurons release vasoactive factors that reach local blood vessels and mediate smooth muscle relaxation (see Ref. [2] for a review). A number of vasoactive agents have been identified that are either released by depolarizing neurons, e.g., neurotransmitters or K^+ and H^+ ions, or depleted from the extracellular and perivascular environment during brain activity, e.g., O_2, Ca^+ [2]. In models of activity-dependent CBF increases in cerebral cortex and cerebellum, adenosine, a nucleoside that has long been implicated in vascular regulation, mediates a component of the vascular response [3]. Neurotransmitters and neuropeptides, such as catecholamines and the vasoactive intestinal peptide, have also been

Table 1
Selected transgenic mouse models used in studies of functional hyperemia

Transgenic mouse model	Genetic defect/ phenotype	Brain region activated	Activation paradigm	Effect on functional hyperemia	Reference
nNOS-null mice	lack of nNOS	Whisker barrel cortex	Vibrissal stimulation	no change	[28]
		Cerebellar cortex (crus II)	electrical stimulation of upper lip	attenuation	[29]
eNOS-null mice	lack of eNOS	Whisker barrel cortex	Vibrissal stimulation	no change	[30]
iNOS-null mice	lack of iNOS	Whisker barrel cortex	Vibrissal stimulation	no change	[31]
Cyclin D2-null mice	lack of cyclin D2; no stellate interneurons in cerebellum	Cerebellar cortex (crus II)	electrical stimulation of upper lip	attenuation	[21]
		Whisker barrel cortex	electrical stimulation of upper lip	no change	[21]
COX-2-null mice	lack of COX-2	Whisker barrel cortex	Vibrissal stimulation	attenuation	[12]
COX-1-null mice	lack of COX-1	Whisker barrel cortex	Vibrissal stimulation	no change	[13]
APP transgenics	Aß-peptide accumulation	Whisker barrel cortex	Vibrissal stimulation	attenuation	[26]
PO3 transgenics	disrupted development of Purkinje neurons	cerebellar molecular layer	electrical stimulation of parallel fibers	attenuation	[17]

proposed to participate in activity-induced CBF changes [2]. In addition, it has been proposed that epoxygenated products of arachidonic acid formed by P450 enzymes participate in coupling neural activity to blood flow (see Ref. [4] for a review).

3. Genetically engineered mice and neurovascular coupling

Mice lacking or overexpressing a certain gene product have provided a new and powerful tool to investigate the factors regulating the cerebral circulation during neural activity. As illustrated in Table 1, several genetically engineered mice have been used for studies of functional hyperemia. These are described in detail below.

4. Nitric oxide and nitric oxide synthase null mice

NO is a short-lived and diffusible vasodilator that is released by active neurons, and has been implicated in the mechanisms of functional hyperemia [2]. A number of studies using models of activation in cerebral cortex and cerebellum have provided evidence that inhibition of NO synthase (NOS), the enzyme that synthesizes NO, attenuates activation-induced increases in CBF, usually by 50% (see Ref. [5] for a review). Some studies, however, have failed to find a relationship between NO and the vasodilation evoked by neural activity [6]. The role of NO has also been examined with mice lacking the neuronal (nNOS), endothelial (eNOS) or immunological (iNOS) isoform of NOS. These mice did not have an attenuation in the increase of neocortical CBF produced by somatosensory activation (Table 1), suggesting that the role of neurally derived NO was compensated for by other vasodilators released by neural activity (see Section 2). These findings support the hypothesis, suggested also by studies using pharmacological inhibitors [7], that NO is not absolutely required for the vasodilation to occur. However, in cerebellum, the increase in blood flow produced by somatosensory stimuli was attenuated in nNOS null mice (Table 1). Therefore, in the cerebellum of nNOS mice, the lack of neurally derived NO cannot be adequately compensated for. These observations suggest that, in cerebellum, NO produced by synaptic activity is absolutely required for the vasodilation to occur. The difference in the role of NO in the response to activation in cerebral cortex and cerebellum suggests that the role of NO in the mechanisms of functional hyperemia is regionally specific.

5. Cylooxygenase-1 and -2

COX, an enzyme involved in the synthesis of prostaglandins and thromboxanes from arachidonic acid, is present in two isoforms COX-1 and COX-2 (see Ref. [8] for a review). COX-1 is present in most organs and produces prostanoids involved in normal cellular function. In brain, COX-1 is present in some neurons and in blood vessels [9]. COX-2 is expressed in the normal state only in selected organs, including the brain, but its expression is ubiquitously upregulated by inflammatory stimuli or mitogens [8]. In brain, COX-2 is localized to dendritic arborizations and spines of excitatory neurons [10,11]. Its synaptic localization raises the possibility that COX-2 is involved in activity-dependent processes and synaptic signaling [10].

The development of selective pharmacological inhibitors and the introduction of COX-1 and COX-2 null mice have provided the opportunity to investigate the role of these enzymes in cerebrovascular regulation. Using activation of the rodent's whisker–barrel cortex as a model of functional hyperemia, we found that the selective COX-2 inhibitor NS-398 attenuates the increase in neocortical blood flow produced by vibrissal stimulation [12]. Furthermore, the hyperemic response is impaired in mutant mice lacking COX-2, whereas the associated increase in cerebral glucose utilization (CGU), a variable that reflects neural activity, is not affected [12]. Interestingly, COX-2 inhibition with NS398 or COX-2 deletion in null mice does not affect cerebrovascular responses elicited by systemic hypercapnia or by topical application of endothelium-dependent vasodilators such as acetylcholine, bradykinin or the calcium ionophore A23187 [12]. Therefore, the evidence suggests that COX-2 contributes to the hyperemia produced by neural activity, but not by endothelium-dependent vasodilators.

On the other hand, inhibition of COX-1 with SC-560 or genetic deletion in COX-2 null mice reduces resting CBF and attenuates the increase in CBF produced by hypercapnia, bradykinin or arachidonic acid [13]. However, COX-1 inhibition or genetic deletion does not affect the increase in CBF produced by vibrissal stimulation [13]. These findings suggest that COX-1 and COX-2 are both involved in the regulation of the cerebral circulation. However, they subserve markedly distinct roles: while COX-1 participates in responses initiated at the vascular level (hypercapnia, endothelium-dependent vasodilation), COX-2 contributes to responses initiated by neural activity.

6. Genetically engineered mice with cerebellar alterations

The cerebellum has emerged as an important brain region to investigate the relationship between synaptic activity and blood flow [14,15]. Due to its relative simplicity, compared to the cerebral cortex, the cerebellum offers the opportunity to approach the cellular and molecular correlates of functional hyperemia. Furthermore, there are several transgenic and knockout mice with cerebellar alterations that are useful in studies of activity-induced changes in blood flow.

7. PO3 mice with Purkinje cell dysfunction

Transgenic mice in which the expression of a mutant form of the large T-antigen is targeted to cerebellar Purkinje cells exhibit arrested Purkinje cell development [16]. This mouse line, termed PO3, has abnormal Purkinje cell morphology with shrunken cell bodies and stunted dendrites. The number of synaptic contacts between Purkinje cell dendrites and cerebellar parallel fibers (PF), the axons of granule cells, is dramatically reduced, while molecular layer interneurons are not affected [17]. Activation of PF depolarizes Purkinje cells and molecular layer interneurons and increases local BFcrb, an effect mediated, in part, by neuronal NO [18]. We employed PO3 mice to determine the component of the response to PF stimulation that is attributable to Purkinje cells. PF stimulation in PO3 mice produces field potentials lacking the component dependent on Purkinje cell depolarization [17]. The BFcrb increase evoked by PF stimulation is reduced in PO3 mice compared to nontransgenic littermates [17]. The residual BFcrb increase in PO3 mice is blocked by the NO synthase (NOS) inhibitor L-NA [17]. These data suggest that Purkinje cells are responsible for a component of the BFcrb response evoked from PF stimulation.

8. Cyclin D2-null mice lack stellate interneurons

To study more closely the role in cerebellar interneurons in the mechanisms of functional hyperemia, we used cyclin D2 null mice. These mice lack stellate interneurons in the cerebellar molecular layer [19]. To produce a more "natural" pattern of cerebellar activation we stimulated the upper lip, which produces localized increases in BFcrb in a region of the cerebellar hemisphere termed crus II [20]. We found that crus II activation produces substantially smaller increases in BFcrb in D2 −/− mice than in D2 +/+ littermates [21]. However, the increase in BFcrb produced by vasodilators that do not depend in neural activity, e.g., hypercapnia or adenosine, was not altered in D2 −/− mice. Administration of the nNOS inhibitor 7-nitroindazole did not attenuate the residual response in D2 null mice. These findings suggest that most of the NO responsible for the vasodilation in this model originates from stellate neurons.

9. APP mice

Mice overexpressing the amyloid precursor protein (APP) have been a valuable model of Alzheimer disease (AD), a disease characterized by the accumulation of β-amyloid (Aβ) in brain and cerebral blood vessels [22]. APP mice have increased Aβ in their brain and have cognitive deficits resembling those of AD [23,24]. Cerebrovascular factors have long been thought to contribute to the mechanisms of AD [25]. However, in human studies, it has been difficult to determine whether the cerebrovascular alterations observed in patients with AD are the cause or the effect of the neuropathological changes, such as amyloid plaques, that characterize the disease. APP mice offer the opportunity to investigate the cerebrovascular dysfunction produced by Aβ before the onset of neuropathological alterations. We used the activation of the whisker barrel cortex as a model to study functional hyperemia in APP mice. We found that the increase in somatosensory cortex CBF produced by whisker stimulation is attenuated in APP mice and that the magnitude of the attenuation is proportional to the amount of Aβ present in brain [26]. The increase in CGU produced by whisker stimulation was not attenuated in APP mice. We also found that APP mice have a profound deficit in the increase in CBF produced by endothelium-dependent vasodilators, such as acetylcholine and bradykinin, but not by hypercapnia [27]. The data suggest that Aβ produces a marked vascular dysregulation that affects many aspects of the regulation of the cerebral circulation. In particular, the mismatch between CBF and energy demands during activation could produce neuronal dysfunction and contribute to the mechanisms of the disease.

10. Summary and conclusions

Transgenic mice have provided a new and powerful tool to study the mechanisms of functional hyperemia in brain. Studies in COX-1 and COX-2 null mice have begun to define the relative contribution of these enzymes in cerebrovascular regulation. Thus, COX-1 has emerged as an important factor in the vasodilation produced by hypercapnia and selected endothelium-dependent vasodilators, whereas COX-2 is critical for functional hyperemia produced by whisker stimulation. Mouse mutants with cerebellar alterations have helped define the cellular basis of the increase in flow produced by cerebellar activation. In particular, D2 cyclin null mice, which lack cerebellar stellate interneurons, have indicated that these neurons are a critical link for the flow increase produced by somatosensory activation of the cerebellar cortex. The increase in flow produced by functional activation is attenuated in mice overexpressing APP, suggesting that direct vascular effects of Aβ, rather than amyloid plaques or neurodegeneration, are responsible for the alterations in cerebrovascular regulation reported in patients with AD. Cerebrovascular dysregulation could play a role in the mechanisms of brain dysfunction associated with AD.

3.1.2.8. On-Site Discussion

3.1.2.8.1. *Question: (Bryan)* 1) Could you speculate on how the Cox-2 metabolite signals the vascular smooth muscle? Is it direct or is there an intermediate step? 2) What price do these COX-2 null mice play for having an attenuated flow-metabolism couple?
Answer: (Iadecola) 1) Possible reaction—products include superoxide and PGE2-COX2 reaction products could mediate vasodilation by inducing the release of another vasodilator from other cells, for example glia. 2) This is an interesting possibility—COX2 null mice may develop neuronal dysfunction over time because of chronic failure of blood supply.
3.1.2.8.2. *Question: (Harder)* Is β-amyloid a cause or consequence of Alzheimer's dementia?
Answer: (Iadecola) This is an important question of critical significance to the field. There is relative consensus that β-amyloid is linked to Alzheimer. However, deposition of β-amyloid in amyloid plaques is seen by some scientists as a "tombstone", rather than an active mechanism of brain dysfunction. On going studies on β-amyloid immunization to clear plaques in Alzheimer's mice and patients, will help clarify this important issue.
3.1.2.8.3. *Question: (Lauritzen)* The use of the field potential to indicate the state of activation of the cerebellum following stimulations of the upper lip may be dubious. The celluler elements that contribute to the field potential is unknown under these conditions but most likely stellate cells do not contribute due to their spherical shape. The expectation is therefore that in KO mice lacking stellate cells the field potential is unchanged. One way to assess the impact of stimulation is to measure glucose consumption. Do you have data using e.g., 2-DG?
Answer: (Iadecola) I agree that field potential may not reflect the activity of stellate neurons. The 2-DG experiments are under way.

3.1.2.8.4. ***Question: (Hamel)*** Is COX-2 expressed in a specific population of neurons? ***Answer: (Iadecola)*** Yes, COX-2 is expressed in the synaptic terminals of glutamatergic neurons.

Acknowledgements

Supported by NIH grants NS31318, NS38252, and NS37853. C.I. is the recipient of a Javits Award from NIH/NINDS. The editorial assistance of Andrea Hyde is gratefully acknowledged.

References

[1] M.E. Raichle, Behind the scenes of functional brain imaging: a historical and physiological perspective, Proc. Natl. Acad. Sci. U. S. A. 95 (3) (1998) 765–772.

[2] C. Iadecola, Regulation of the cerebral microcirculation during neural activity: is nitric oxide the missing link?, Trends Neurosci. 16 (1993) 206–214.

[3] J. Li, C. Iadecola, Nitric oxide and adenosine mediate vasodilation during functional activation in cerebellar cortex, Neuropharmacology 33 (1994) 1453–1461.

[4] D.R. Harder, R.J. Roman, D. Gebremedhin, Molecular mechanisms controlling nutritive blood flow: role of cytochrome P450 enzymes, Acta Physiol. Scand. 168 (4) (2000) 543–549.

[5] C. Iadecola, in: R.T. Mathie, T.M. Griffith (Eds.), The Role of NO in Cerebrovascular Regulation and Stroke, Imperial College Press, London, 1999, pp. 202–225.

[6] K. Adachi, S. Takahashi, P. Melzer, K.L. Campos, T. Nelson, C. Kennedy, et al., Increases in local cerebral blood flow associated with somatosensory activation are not mediated by NO, Am. J. Physiol. 267 (1994) H2155–H2162.

[7] U. Lindauer, D. Megow, H. Matsuda, U. Dirnagl, Nitric oxide: a modulator, but not a mediator, of neuro-vascular coupling in rat somatosensory cortex, Am. J. Physiol. 277 (2 Pt 2) (1999) H799–H811.

[8] J.R. Vane, Y.S. Bakhle, R.M. Botting, Cyclooxygenases 1 and 2, Annu. Rev. Pharmacol. Toxicol. 38 (1998) 97–120.

[9] C.D. Breder, W.L. Smith, A. Raz, J. Masferrer, K. Seibert, P. Needleman, et al., Distribution and character-ization of cyclooxygenase immunoreactivity in the ovine brain, J. Comp. Neurol. 322 (3) (1992) 409–438.

[10] W.E. Kaufmann, P.F. Worley, J. Pegg, M. Bremer, P. Isakson, COX-2, a synaptically induced enzyme, is expressed by excitatory neurons at postsynaptic sites in rat cerebral cortex, Proc. Natl. Acad. Sci. U. S. A. 93 (6) (1996) 2317–2321.

[11] K. Yamagata, K.I. Andreasson, W.E. Kaufmann, C.A. Barnes, P.F. Worley, Expression of a mitogen-indu-cible cyclooxygenase in brain neurons: regulation by synaptic activity and glucocorticoids, Neuron 11 (2) (1993) 371–386.

[12] K. Niwa, E. Araki, S.G. Morham, M.E. Ross, C. Iadecola, Cyclooxygenase-2 contributes to functional hyperemia in whisker–barrel cortex, J Neurosci. 20 (2) (2000) 763–770.

[13] K. Niwa, C. Haensel, M.E. Ross, C. Iadecola, Cyclooxygenase-1 participates in selected vasodilator re-sponses of the cerebral circulation, Circ. Res. 88 (6) (2001) 600–608.

[14] N. Akgören, M. Fabricius, M. Lauritzen, Importance of nitric oxide for local increases of blood flow in rat cerebellar cortex during electrical stimulation, Proc. Natl. Acad. Sci. U. S. A. 91 (1994) 5903–5907.

[15] C. Iadecola, J. Li, T.J. Ebner, S. Xu, Nitric oxide contributes to functional hyperemia in cerebellar cortex, Am. J. Physiol.: Regul., Integr. Comp. Physiol. 268 (37) (1995) R1153–R1162.

[16] R.M. Feddersen, W.S. Yunis, M.A. O'Donnell, T.J. Ebner, L. Shen, C. Iadecola, et al., Susceptibility to cell death induced by mutant SV40 T-antigen correlates with Purkinje neuron functional development, Mol. Cell. Neurosci. 9 (1) (1997) 42–62.

[17] G. Yang, R.M. Feddersen, F. Zhang, H.B. Clark, A.J. Beitz, C. Iadecola, Cerebellar vascular and synaptic

responses in transgenic mice with Purkinje cell dysfunction, Am. J. Physiol.: Regul., Integr. Comp. Physiol. 274 (43) (1998) R529–R540.

[18] C. Iadecola, G. Yang, S. Xu, 7-Nitroindazole attenuates vasodilation from cerebellar parallel fiber stimulation but not acetylcholine, Am. J. Physiol.: Regul., Integr. Comp. Physiol. 270 (39) (1996) R914–R919.

[19] J.M. Huard, C.C. Forster, M.L. Carter, P. Sicinski, M.E. Ross, Cerebellar histogenesis is disturbed in mice lacking cyclin D2, Development 126 (9) (1999) 1927–1935.

[20] G. Yang, G. Chen, T.J. Ebner, C. Iadecola, Nitric oxide is the predominant mediator of cerebellar hyperemia during somatosensory activation in rats, Am. J. Physiol.: Regul., Integr. Comp. Physiol. 277 (46) (1999) R1760–R1770.

[21] G. Yang, J.M. Huard, A.J. Beitz, M.E. Ross, C. Iadecola, Stellate neurons mediate functional hyperemia in the cerebellar molecular layer, J. Neurosci. 20 (18) (2000) 6968–6973.

[22] D.J. Selkoe, Translating cell biology into therapeutic advances in Alzheimer's disease, Nature 399 (Suppl. 6738) (1999) A23–A31.

[23] K.K. Hsiao, D.R. Borchelt, K. Olson, R. Johannsdottir, C. Kitt, W. Yunis, et al., Age-related CNS disorder and early death in transgenic FVB/N mice overexpressing Alzheimer amyloid precursor proteins, Neuron 15 (1995) 1203–1218.

[24] K. Hsiao, P. Chapman, S. Nilsen, C. Eckman, Y. Harigaya, S. Younkin, et al., Correlative memory deficits, Aβ elevation, and amyloid plaques in transgenic mice, Science 274 (5284) (1996) 99–102.

[25] R.N. Kalaria, Cerebral vessels in ageing and Alzheimer's disease, Pharmacol. Ther. 72 (3) (1996) 193–214.

[26] K. Niwa, L. Younkin, C. Ebeling, S.K. Turner, D. Westaway, S. Younkin, et al., Abeta 1–40-related reduction in functional hyperemia in mouse neocortex during somatosensory activation, Proc. Natl. Acad. Sci. U. S. A. 97 (17) (2000) 9735–9740.

[27] C. Iadecola, F. Zhang, K. Niwa, C. Eckman, S.K. Turner, E. Fischer, et al., SOD1 rescues cerebral endothelial dysfunction in mice overexpressing amyloid precursor protein, Nat. Neurosci. 2 (2) (1999) 157–161.

[28] J. Ma, C. Ayata, P.L. Huang, M.C. Fishman, M.A. Moskowitz, Regional cerebral blood flow response to vibrissal stimulation in mice lacking type I NOS gene expression, Am. J. Physiol.: Heart Circ. Physiol. 270 (39) (1996) H1085–H1090.

[29] G. Yang, C. Haensel, M.E. Ross, C. Iadecola, Attenuation of activity-induced increases in cerebellar blood flow in neuronal nitric oxide synthase-null mice, Soc. Neurosci. Abstr. (2000) 26.

[30] C. Ayata, J. Ma, W. Meng, P. Huang, M.A. Moskowitz, L-NA-sensitive rCBF augmentation during vibrissal stimulation in type III nitric oxide synthase mutant mice, J. Cereb. Blood Flow Metab. 16 (4) (1996) 539–541.

[31] C. Iadecola, K. Niwa, Nitric oxide, in: L. Edvinsson, D.N. Krause (Eds.), Cerebral Blood Flow and Metabolism, Lippincott, Williams & Wilkins, Philadelphia, 2002, in press.

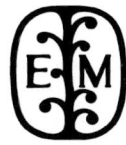

International Congress Series 1235 (2002) 267–276

Neuronal messengers as mediators of microvascular tone in the cerebral cortex

E. Hamel*, E. Vaucher, X.-K. Tong, M. St-Georges

Laboratory of Cerebrovascular Research, Montreal Neurological Institute, McGill University, 3801 University Street, Montreal, Quebec, Canada H3A 2B4

Abstract

Changes in regional neuronal activity are accompanied by concurrent temporal and spatial changes in the cerebral blood flow and these form the basis of modern brain imaging techniques used to map the functional neuronal activity. This neurovascular coupling is achieved by several mechanisms that are still poorly understood but ionic, glial, metabolic, and neuronal factors have been involved. In the present investigation, we provide evidence that specific populations of cortical interneurons, which play a central role in integrating multiple incoming local and afferent synaptic and paracrine signals, could act as local integrators of the neuronal activity and cerebral blood flow. We suggest that different subpopulations of cortical γ-amino-butyric acid (GABA) interneurons, which colocalize specific vasoactive substances such as nitric oxide (NO), vasoactive intestinal polypeptide (VIP), and neuropeptide Y (NPY), could serve as a functional relay in the neurovascular coupling that accompanies the activation of basal forebrain acetylcholine (ACh) and brainstem raphe nucleus serotonin (5-HT)-neurons. Thus, in addition to direct changes in the microvascular tone induced by ACh and 5-HT fibers projecting to cortical microvessels, these neurons also send projections to NO, VIP and/or NPY interneurons which, via their direct neurovascular projections, could affect the microvascular tone and therein adapt changes in perfusion to the local changes in neuronal activity. The results suggest that specific populations of GABA interneurons constitute a functional unit with their respective neuronal and vascular effects. © 2002 Elsevier Science B.V. All rights reserved.

Keywords: Neurovascular coupling; Intracortical arterioles; Microvascular receptors; Vasomotricity; Cerebral blood flow

Abbreviations: ACh, acetylcholine; GABA, γ-Amino-butyric acid; NO, nitric oxide; NPY, neuropeptide Y; VIP, vasoactive intestinal polypeptide; 5-HT, serotonin.
* Corresponding author. Tel.: +1-514-398-8928; fax: +1-514-398-8106.
E-mail address: edith.hamel@mcgill.ca (E. Hamel).

1. Introduction

Changes in the cortical cerebral blood flow have been documented following the electrical or chemical stimulation of basal forebrain cholinergic (acetylcholine (ACh)) [1] and brainstem serotonergic (serotonin (5-HT)) [2] neurons, or the fastigial nucleus of the cerebellum through a relay via the nucleus basalis [3]. Depending on the neuronal pathway stimulated, the perfusion responses were selectively blocked by antagonizing the neurotransmitter system activated (i.e. antagonists of ACh or 5-HT receptors) (for review, see Refs. [1,2]) and, in some cases, by inhibitors of nitric oxide (NO) synthase, suggesting a role for NO in the blood flow changes, at least in those mediated through basal forebrain neurons [4]. Morphological evidence has confirmed that basal ACh [5] and brainstem 5-HT [2] neurons project to intracortical microvessels including penetrating arteries and small arterioles, thus providing means to directly modify the blood flow in cortical areas. Additionally, NO neurons were identified as cholinoceptive cells in the cerebral cortex [6,7], and were shown to be innervated by basal ACh fibers [8,9]. Interestingly, cortical NO neurons, as well as those containing the vasoactive peptides vasoactive intestinal polypeptide (VIP) and neuropeptide Y (NPY) are intimately associated with cortical microvessels [10–13] and they all belong to distinct subpopulations of γ-amino-butyric acid (GABA) interneurons [14]. As GABA interneurons are the local integrator of cortical activity [15,16], we suggest that they be strategically positioned to translate incoming neuronal signal from subcortical afferents into adapted local neuronal and vascular responses. More specifically, we suggest that GABA neurons which activity is modulated by both ACh [17] and 5-HT through different 5-HT receptor populations [18,19], act as a functional relay in the coupling of cerebral blood flow to neuronal activity. In the present study, we present evidence that changes in the neuronal activity of basal forebrain ACh and brainstem 5-HT neurons may be translated into cortical vascular responses, not only by their direct effects on the cortical microcirculation but also via specific populations of cortical GABA interneurons.

2. Materials and methods

2.1. Immunocytochemical staining and NADPH-D histochemistry

All anatomical studies were performed as described in detail in our previous publications. In short, rats (male, Sprague–Dawley, 250–300 g) were perfused under deep anesthesia (Somnotol, 65 mg/kg, i.p.) through the ascending aorta with a 4% paraformaldehyde ($\pm 0.05\%$ glutaraldehyde) buffered solution. Brains were removed, post-fixed (2 h, 4 °C) in the same solution, cryoprotected and sliced (20 μm thick) on a freezing microtome. Free-floating sections were then processed for single or double immunocytochemistry for GABA (single labeling) or ACh nerve terminals and intracortical VIP or NO neuronal (identified histochemically for NADPH-D) cell bodies, or for 5-HT nerve terminals and NO/NADPH-D neurons. For this purpose, sections were first incubated (overnight, room temperature) with either a mouse antibody directed against the terminal isoform of the GABA synthesizing enzyme glutamic acid decarboxylase

(GAD65, 1/3000, Boehringer) [20], a monoclonal antibody against the ACh synthesizing enzyme choline acetyltransferase (ChAT, anti-ChAT17, 2 μg/ml) [5] or a rabbit polyclonal anti-5-HT antibody (1/10,000). Tissue sections were then incubated with appropriate secondary antibodies, the ABC kit and the reaction product revealed a 3,3′-diaminoben-zidine tetrachloride (DAB) (brown reaction). For double-immunocytochemistry, following the revelation of the first antibody, the sections were then subsequently incubated (overnight, room temperature) with the anti-VIP antibody (rabbit polyclonal antibody, 1:5000, Peninsula) [11], appropriate secondary antibodies, the ABC kit and the reaction visualized with the SG reagent kit (Vector Labs) (blue-grey reaction). Other sections were incubated (~ 30 min) for NADPH-D histochemistry with 0.01% nitroblue tetrazolium chloride and 0.1% β-NADPH-D, as we described previously [9]. Sections were embedded into Araldite and semithin sections (1–2 μm) obtained on an ultramicrotome for the quantitative analysis of the interactions between ACh, 5-HT and/or GABA nerve terminals with VIP and/or NO/NADPH-D neurons, as described in detail before [8,20]. In some rats, a unilateral neurotoxic lesion of the substantia innominata was performed with quisqualic acid [20] in order to identify the basal origin of the cortical fibers.

2.2. Expression of receptors in intracortical microvascular smooth muscle and endothelial cells

Expression of receptors for vasoactive peptides such as VIP was determined by RT-PCR in cultures of human cerebromicrovascular smooth muscle cells generated from tissues obtained at surgery for the treatment of epilepsy, as previously described [21]. After the RNA extraction, some samples were reverse transcribed while others were not to monitor for possible DNA contamination. Primers were either designed with the Oligo5 program or taken from previous publications [22]. PCR products were identified by gel electrophoresis and/or sequencing.

2.3. Microvascular reactivity in isolated intracortical arterioles

The vasomotor responses to neurotransmitters were evaluated on isolated bovine and/or human intracortical arterioles (luminal diameter ~ 48–50 μm), as we described recently [23,24]. In short, penetrating arteries were isolated from the cortical parenchyma, cannulated and pressurized as described originally [25] and the reactivity of the micro-vessels to ACh or 5-HT and specific agonists and/or antagonists tested. The receptors involved were characterized pharmacologically with appropriate antagonists and their potency compared to previously published data at the cloned receptors.

3. Results

In sections that were single-labeled for the GABA synthesizing enzyme, a very dense network of cortical punctate fibers was present and several of these neuronal varicosities were in direct contact with the local intracortical microvessels, including penetrating arteries, intraparenchymal arterioles and capillaries. More importantly, effective lesion (i.e.

inducing ~ 80% decrease in ChAT nerve terminals) of the substantia innominata had no significant effect on the number of cortical GABAergic nerve fibers, including those associated with the microvessels. These findings clearly indicated that the vast majority of GABAergic nerve terminals in the cerebral cortex originated from the local intracortical interneurons [20]. Such findings are consistent with the central role of GABA interneurons in the regulation of cortical activity. In this respect, in sections double-labeled for cholinergic (ChAT) or serotonergic (5-HT) nerve terminals and NO neurons, it was apparent that NO neurons were richly innervated by both basalocortical ACh fibers [8] and brainstem 5-HT nerve fibers [this presentation]. In fact, about half of the NO neurons in the cerebral cortex were reached by either ACh or 5-HT (53% or 56% of all NO neurons, respectively) nerve terminals on their cell soma and proximal dendrites. In the case of cortical VIP neurons, we found that about 28% of all cortical VIP neurons are contacted by cholinergic nerve terminals immunoreactive for ChAT (Fig. 1).

We previously reported the expression of specific subtypes of receptors for ACh and 5-HT in the endothelial and/or smooth muscle cells of cortical microarterioles and capillaries [26,27] and suggested that ACh and 5-HT can exert direct microvascular effects. We recently provided evidence that intracortical arterioles either at spontaneously developed tone or after a pharmacologically induced tone can dilate in response to ACh, an effect blocked by inhibitors of NO synthase and by muscarinic receptor antagonists with affinity

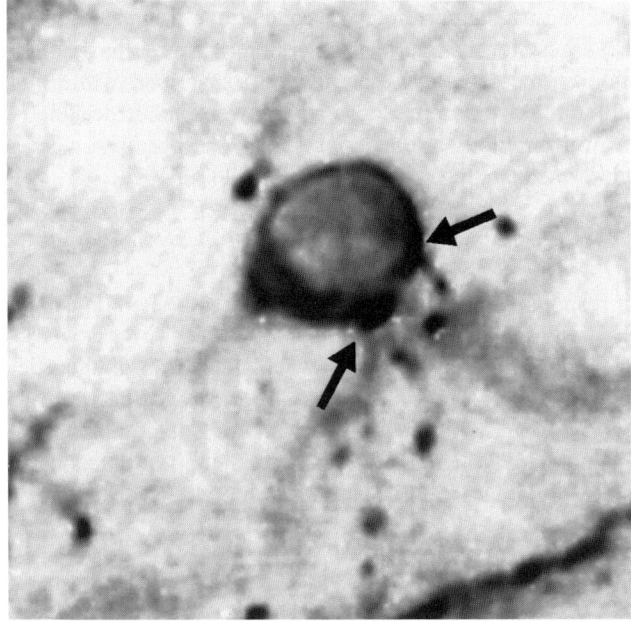

Fig. 1. Double immunocytochemistry showing the innervation of VIP neurons (dark blue in original staining) by ACh nerve terminals (immunolabeled for ACh-synthesizing enzyme ChAT, brown reaction in original staining). The ACh nerve terminals (arrows) can be seen on the cell soma of the VIP neurons. Quantitative analysis revealed that about 28% of all cortical VIP neurons are innervated by ACh nerve terminals.

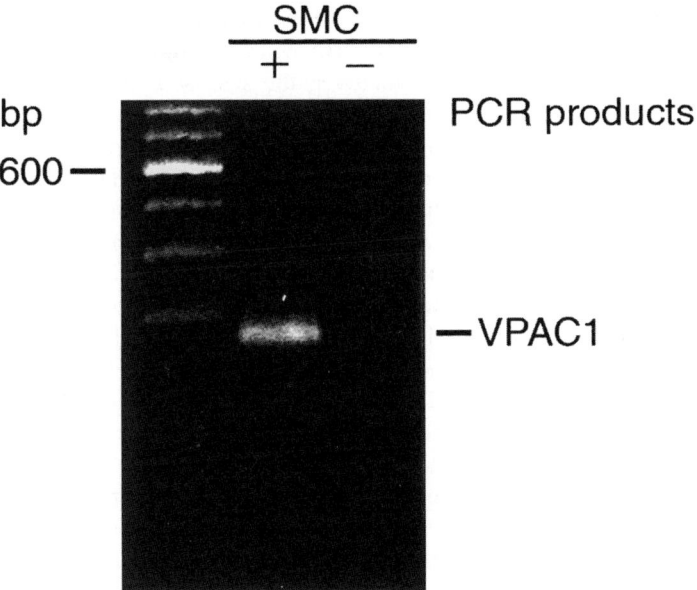

Fig. 2. Gel electrophoresis of PCR products for the VIP1 (VPAC1) receptors expression in primary cultures of the human cerebromicrovascular smooth muscle cells (SMC). Samples with (+) and without (−) reverse transcriptase were run in parallel to monitor for possible DNA contamination.

at the M5 receptors but not at the M1 or M2 muscarinic receptor subtypes [23]. In contrast, intracortical arterioles constricted in response to 5-HT, an effect which was antagonized by the 5-HT1 receptor antagonist GR127935. Interestingly, when 5-HT1 receptors agonists were tested, only those with affinity at the 5-HT1B receptor subtype, which is highly expressed in the cerebromicrovascular smooth muscle cells [27], were able to induce a vasocontractile response [24], therefore indicating that this receptor is the mediator of the local decrease in tone of microarterioles following the perivascular release of 5-HT. With regards to the neuropeptide receptors, the vasocontractile NPY-Y1 receptors have been shown to be expressed in cortical microarterioles [21], and more specifically, in those that are surrounded by the NPY-immunoreactive fibers [28]. We now show that VIP receptors of the type 1 (or VPAC1 receptors) are highly expressed in smooth muscle cells of intracortical arterioles (Fig. 2), similar to their localization in cerebral and pial arteries where they are believed to mediate dilation [29].

4. Discussion

Altogether, the anatomical results suggest that several of the intracortical neurotransmitter systems that have been shown to be intimately associated with local microvessels correspond to specific populations of GABA interneurons that are innervated by subcortical basal forebrain ACh and/or brainstem 5-HT nerve fibers. Indeed, VIP and NO neurons belong to distinct populations of GABA neurons while NO and NPY colocalized within the same subpopulation [14]. Moreover, the size of VIP, NOS, and NPY nerve terminals in the cerebral cortex (0.56 ± 0.4, 0.53 ± 0.4, and 0.58 ± 0.2 μm^2, respectively) [10,11,13], corresponded very well to that of GABAergic nerve terminals (0.50 ± 0.3 μm^2) [20], strongly indicating that they belong to common neuronal populations. In this regard, the much smaller size of the subcortical ACh and 5-HT nerve terminals (0.32 ± 0.02 and 0.37 ± 0.02 μm^2, respectively) [2,5] was strongly supportive of their distinct origin. Our results also showed that cortical GABA nerve terminals were the most numerous around blood vessels of all perivascular terminals studied so far (see Ref. [20]), possibly suggesting that they are particularly important in the regulation of cerebrovascular functions. GABA has previously been shown to play a role in local neurovascular signaling in the brain parenchyma, albeit in hippocampal microvessels [30]. Our results would suggest that this role might be fulfilled and/or modulated by the different neuro-peptides that are colocalized within GABA neurons, and also able to modulate the microvascular tone. In fact, the presence of muscarinic M2 receptors on the intracortical NO neurons [6,7], and of nicotinic receptors on a specific population of cortical VIP neurons [31] could explain the modulation of the cortical blood flow response elicited by the basal forebrain stimulation by muscarinic and nicotinic receptor antagonists, and by nitric oxide synthase inhibitors (for review, see Refs. [1,4]). However, a direct neurogenic modulation of the cortical blood flow by basal forebrain NO neurons, which have recently been shown to directly project to cortical microvessels [13], can also participate in the overall perfusion response. Further, the present results show that intracortical NO neurons are a frequent target for brainstem 5-HT nerve terminals. Their activation/inhibition via different 5-HT receptors could possibly explain the dual flow response observed following the stimulation of specific subregions of the dorsal raphe nucleus [32] (for review, see Ref. [2]), a hypothesis that will need to be substantiated. Whether or not VIP neurons are a target for 5-HT terminals still remains to be elucidated.

In addition, our functional data on isolated cortical microarterioles indicate that direct vascular effects exerted by ACh and 5-HT on the cortical microcirculation have to be considered in the global perfusion response to either basal forebrain or dorsal raphe stimulation. ACh, via muscarinic receptors corresponding to the M5 subtype, elicits dilation of intracortical arterioles [23], and 5-HT predominantly constricted the arterioles by acting on 5-HT1B receptors. Interestingly, small size arterioles (<100 μm) dilated at low doses of the 5-HT1B receptor agonist sumatriptan [24]. The presence of VIP1 (VPAC1) (Fig. 2) and NPY-Y1 [21,28] receptors in the intracortical arterioles strongly suggest that these neuropeptides are able to modulate the microvascular tone and/or restrict the extent of an NO-mediated dilation, as suggested for NPY which is colocalized with NO in a subpopulation of GABA neurons [10,33]. The role of these peptides on cortical microarterioles will be an important determinant to conclude that they are local regulators of the intracortical perfusion in response to the neuronal activation.

In conclusion, we suggest that GABA neurons can act as local integrators of the incoming and intrinsic information in the cerebral cortex to adjust and/or maintain local perfusion to the neuronal activity (Fig. 3). Such an organization could be complementary to other mechanisms involving ionic, metabolic, and astroglial factors. These factors could

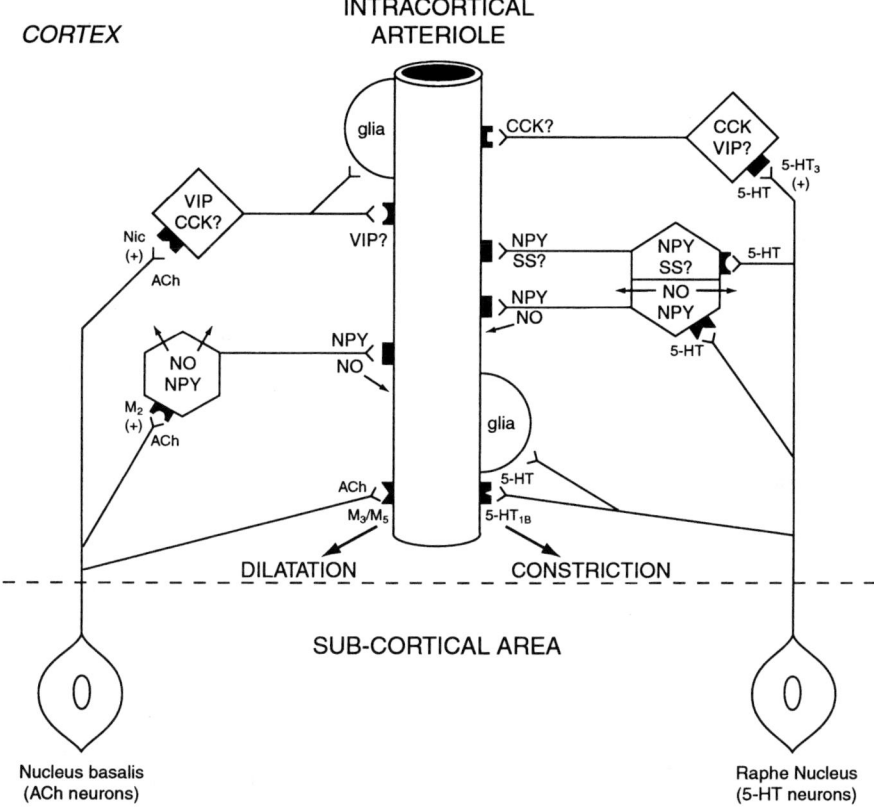

Fig. 3. Schematic representation of the suggested role for different populations of cortical GABA neurons (illustrated here only by their neuropeptide or NO content) in the local control of microvascular tone and how they could act as neurovascular relay for the subcortical ACh and 5-HT neurons. Note also that ACh and 5-HT can directly modulate the microvascular tone via their respective receptors. ACh: acetylcholine; CCK: cholecystokinin; NO: nitric oxide; NPY: neuropeptide Y; SS: somatostatin; VIP: vasoactive intestinal polypeptide.

participate in a fully integrated neurovascular coupling response as a function of increased brain activity.

3.1.3.7. On-Site Discussion

3.1.3.7.1. **Question: (Bryan)** How do these nerves traverse the Virchow–Robin space?

Answer: (Hamel) We believe that the nerves are reaching the lower segment of penetrating arteries when parenchyma and vessel wall are quite closely apposed.

3.1.3.7.2. **Question: (Pelligrino)** What muscarinic receptor mediates acetylcholine effects on arterioles? Your figure suggests M3/M5 but our own immunohistochemical results would indicate that M2 is the major arteriolar receptor, and it seems to be localized to the endothelial/smooth muscle junction. We have never found M3, M4, or M5 on arterioles or venules. Perhaps we need better antibodies but our results seem similar to those of Alan Levy.

Answer: (Hamel) We have found M2 and M5 muscarinic receptor expression in the endothelial cells. However, in dilation, we have a pharmacology, which does not correspond to M2 but to M3/M5 as the dilation is blocked by M3/M5 receptor antagonists but not by antagonist with high affinity for M2 receptors. We never found M4 but M1 and M5 are expressed in the smooth muscle cells and coupled to their signalling pathways.

3.1.3.7.3. *Question: (Kalaria)* Several years ago, we had described that the noradrenergic afferents from the locus coeruleus may innervate cortical microvessels. Therefore, where do the noradrenergic afferents fit into the innervation/modulation of the cerebral arterioles in your scenario?

Answer: (Hamel) When we looked at noradrenergic nerve terminals in the cerebral cortex, we observed that their main targets were astrocytes, whether located in the parenchyma or perivascularly. This is in agreement with the work of others. So, these morphological data suggested that they are not particularly concerned with the microcirculation. This is in agreement with physiological studies, which showed rather small changes in CBF following the locus coeruleus stimulation.

3.1.3.7.4. *Question: (Krause)* It is interesting that GABA interneurons appear to be a major input in the cortical vasculature. Years ago, we showed that GABA produced vasodilation in pial vessels. Thus, GABA may also be a vasodilator in the cortex. Have you looked at the effects of GABA in your cortical microartery preparation?

Answer: (Hamel) No, but the work of K. Lee and A. Fergus has shown that GABA may dilate microvessels in hippocampus (J. Cereb. Blood Flow Metab. 17 (1997) (9) 992; Brain Res. 754 (1997) (1–2) 35).

Acknowledgements

The experiments reported in this short review have been sponsored by grants from the Medical Research Council (MRC) of Canada, the Heart and Stroke Foundation of Quebec and an MRC-Industry grant with Boehringer Ingelheim Pharma, Biberach, Germany.

References

[1] A. Sato, Y. Sato, Cholinergic neural regulation of regional cerebral blood flow, Alzheimer Dis. Assoc. Disord. 9 (1995) 28–38.
[2] Z. Cohen, G. Bonvento, P. Lacombe, E. Hamel, Serotonin in the regulation of brain microcirculation, Prog. Neurobiol. 50 (1996) 335–362.
[3] C. Iadecola, S. Mraovitch, M.P. Meeley, D.J. Reis, Lesions of the basal forebrain in rat selectively impair the cortical vasodilation elicited from cerebellar fastigial nucleus, Brain Res. 279 (1983) 41–52.

[4] J.L. Raszkiewicz, D.G. Linville, J.F. Kerwin Jr., F. Wagenaar, S.P. Arneric, Nitric oxide synthase is critical in mediating basal forebrain regulation of cortical cerebral circulation, J. Neurosci. Res. 33 (1992) 129–135.

[5] E. Vaucher, E. Hamel, Cholinergic basal forebrain neurons project to cortical microvessels in the rat: electron microscopic study with anterogradely transported *Phaseolus vulgaris* leucoagglutinin and choline acetyltransferase immunocytochemistry, J. Neurosci. 15 (1995) 7427–7441.

[6] V. Moro, et al., Regional study of the co-localization of neuronal nitric oxide synthase with muscarinic receptors in the rat cerebral cortex, Neuroscience 69 (1995) 797–805.

[7] J.F. Smiley, A.I. Levey, M.-M. Mesulam, Infracortical interstitial cells concurrently expressing M2-muscarinic receptors, acetylcholinesterase and nicotinamide adenine dinucleotide phosphate-diaphorase in the human and monkey cerebral cortex, Neuroscience 84 (1998) 755–769.

[8] E. Vaucher, D. Linville, E. Hamel, Cholinergic basal forebrain projections to nitric oxide synthase-containing neurons in the rat cerebral cortex, Neuroscience 79 (1997) 827–836.

[9] X.-K. Tong, E. Hamel, Regional cholinergic denervation of cortical microvessels and nitric oxide synthase-containing neurons in Alzheimer's disease, Neuroscience 92 (1999) 163–175.

[10] R. Abounader, E. Hamel, Associations between Neuropeptide Y nerve terminals and intraparenchymal microvessels in rat and human cerebral cortex, J. Comp. Neurol. 388 (1997) 444–453.

[11] A. Chedotal, D. Umbriaco, L. Descarries, B.K. Hartman, E. Hamel, Neurovascular relationship of cholinergic and VIPergic nerve terminals in rat cerebral cortex, J. Comp. Neurol. 343 (1994) 57–71.

[12] C. Iadecola, Regulation of the cerebral microcirculation during neural activity: is nitric oxide the missing link? TINS 16 (1993) 206–214.

[13] X.-K. Tong, E. Hamel, Basal forebrain nitric oxide synthase (NOS)-containing neurons project to microvessels and NOS neurons in the rat neocortex: cellular basis for cortical blood flow regulation, Eur. J. Neurosci. 12 (2000) 2769–2780.

[14] Y. Kubota, R. Hattori, Y. Yui, Three distinct subpopulations of GABAergic neurons in rat frontal agranular cortex, Brain Res. 649 (1994) 159–173.

[15] Y. Kawaguchi, Y. Kubota, Neurochemical features and synaptic connections of large physiologically identified GABAergic cells in the rat frontal cortex, Neuroscience 85 (1998) 677–701.

[16] Y. Kawaguchi, Y. Kubota, GABAergic cell subtypes and their synaptic connections in rat frontal cortex, Cereb. Cortex 7 (1997) 476–486.

[17] Y. Kawaguchi, Selective cholinergic modulation of cortical GABAergic cell subtypes, J. Neurophysiol. 78 (1997) 1743–1747.

[18] M. Morales, E. Battenberg, L. de Lecea, F.E. Bloom, The type 3 serotonin receptor is expressed in a subpopulation of GABAergic neurons in the rat neocortex and hippocampus, Brain Res. 731 (1996) 199–202.

[19] W.M. Abi-Saab, M. Bubser, R.H. Roth, A.Y. Deutch, 5-HT2 receptor regulation of extracellular GABA levels in the prefrontal cortex, Neuropsychopharmacology 20 (1999) 92–96.

[20] E. Vaucher, X.-K. Tong, N. Cholet, S. Lantin, E. Hamel, GABA neurons provide a rich input to microvessels but not nitric oxide neurons in the rat cerebral cortex: a means for direct regulation of local cerebral blood flow, J. Comp. Neurol. 421 (2000) 161–171.

[21] R. Abounader, et al., Expression of Neuropeptide Y receptors mRNA and protein in human brain vessels and cerebromicrovascular cells in culture, J. Cereb. Blood Flow Metab. 19 (1999) 155–163.

[22] R. Uddman, J. Tajti, S. Moller, F. Sundler, L. Edvinsson, Neuronal messengers and peptide receptors in the human spenopalatine and otic ganglia, Brain Res. 826 (1999) 193–199.

[23] A. Elhusseiny, E. Hamel, Muscarinic — but not nicotinic — acetylcholine receptors mediate a nitric oxide (NO)-dependent dilation in brain cortical arterioles: a possible role for the M5 receptor subtype, J. Cereb. Blood Flow Metab. 20 (2000) 298–305.

[24] A. Elhusseiny, E. Hamel, Sumatriptan elicits both constriction and dilation in human and bovine brain intracortical arterioles, Br. J. Pharmacol. 132 (2001) 55–62.

[25] R.G. Dacey Jr., J.E. Bassett, Histaminergic vasodilation of intracerebral arterioles in the rat, J. Cereb. Blood Flow Metab. 7 (1987) 327–331.

[26] A. Elhusseiny, Z. Cohen, A. Olivier, D.B. Stanimirovic, E. Hamel, Functional acetylcholine muscarinic receptor subtypes in human brain microcirculation: identification and cellular localization, J. Cereb. Blood Flow Metab. 19 (1999) 794–802.

[27] Z. Cohen, et al., Multiple microvascular and astroglial 5-hydroxytryptamine receptor subtypes in human brain: molecular and pharmacologic characterization, J. Cereb. Blood Flow Metab. 19 (1999) 908–917.

[28] L. Bao, et al., Localization of neuropeptide Y Y1 receptors in cerebral blood vessels, Proc. Natl. Acad. Sci. U. S. A. 94 (1997) 12661–12666.

[29] J. Fahrenkrug, J. Hannibal, J. Tams, B. Georg, Immunohistochemical localization of the VIP_1 receptor ($VPAC_1R$) in rat cerebral blood vessels: relation to PACAP and VIP containing nerves, J. Cereb. Blood Flow Metab. 20 (2000) 1205–1214.

[30] A. Fergus, K.S. Lee, GABAergic regulation of cerebral microvascular tone in the rat, J. Cereb. Blood Flow Metab. 17 (1997) 992–1003.

[31] J.T. Porter, et al., Properties of bipolar VIPergic interneurons and their excitation by pyramidal neurons in the rat neocortex, Eur. J. Neurosci. 10 (1998) 3617–3628.

[32] M.D. Underwood, M.J. Bakalian, V. Arango, J.J. Mann, Effect of chemical stimulation of the dorsal raphe nucleus on cerebral blood flow in rat, Neurosci. Lett. 199 (1995) 228–230.

[33] C. Estrada, J. DeFelipe, Nitric oxide-producing neurons in the neocortex: morphological and functional relationship with intraparenchymal microvasculature, Cereb. Cortex 8 (1998) 193–203.

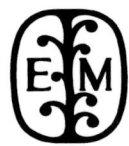

International Congress Series 1235 (2002) 277–287

The red blood cell, ATP and integrated vascular responses to neuronal stimulation

Hans H. Dietrich [a],*, Mary L. Ellsworth [b], Ralph G. Dacey Jr. [a]

[a]*Department of Neurological Surgery, Washington University School of Medicine, 660 South Euclid Avenue, St. Louis, MO 63110, USA*
[b]*Department of Pharmacological and Physiological Science, Saint Louis University School of Medicine, 1402 South Grand Boulevard, St. Louis, MO 63104, USA*

Abstract

Purpose: To provide new insights for linking neuronal activation, local sensing of metabolic need and adenosine triphosphate (ATP) release from red blood cells to conducted vasomotor responses as a mechanism to regulate cerebral microvascular blood flow according to the local tissue needs as seen after, e.g., whisker barrel stimulation [J. Cereb. Blood Flow Metab. 13 (1993) 899]. *Methods*: We measured low PO_2 and/or acidosis-induced ATP release from red blood cells. In isolated and pressurized rat-penetrating arterioles, we simulated neuronal ATP release with local microapplication to study local and conducted vasomotor responses [Am. J. Physiol.: Heart Circ. Physiol. 271 (1996) H1109]. In arterioles of hamster retractor muscle, we microinfused ATP to simulate ATP release from red blood cells. Finally, we measured low PO_2-induced ATP release in red blood cell-perfused cerebral arterioles. *Results*: Red blood cells release ATP in response to low PO_2 and/or acidosis. Extraluminally applied ATP causes constriction (via smooth muscle cell P_{2X1} receptor) with subsequent dilation (via endothelial P_{2Y2} stimulation), with the dilation conducted along the vessel. Microinfused ATP causes retrogradely conducted vasodilation, which is blunted with high ATP doses. Only in red blood cell-perfused arterioles does low PO_2 causes vasodilation coincident with an increase in ATP in the perfusate. *Conclusion*: Local release of ATP either from neurons or from red blood cells (as a sensor for oxygen need) or both may cause local microvascular vessel dilation which is conducted retrogradely to precisely adjust local microvascular flow to metabolic tissue need. © 2002 Elsevier Science B.V. All rights reserved.

Keywords: Conducted vasomotor responses; Cerebral-penetrating arteriole; Skeletal muscle arteriole purinergic receptors; Microvascular regulation; Oxygen sensing; Metabolic coupling

---

* Corresponding author. Tel.: +1-314-362-3648; fax: +1-314-362-2107.
E-mail address: DietrichH@Nsurg.wustl.edu (H.H. Dietrich).

0531-5131/02 © 2002 Elsevier Science B.V. All rights reserved.
PII: S0531-5131(02)00195-4

1. Introduction

The brain microcirculation demonstrates the ability to redistribute local blood flow within the brain tissue according to local metabolic demands without the need to increase total cerebral blood flow. A tight and rapid coupling of neuronal activity with local cortical blood flow is evident. This is elegantly shown in the regulation of blood flow in the whisker barrel of rodents. Woolsey and Van der Loos [3] found that the arrangement of the whisker in the rodent's face is precisely mirrored in the opposite sensory cortex as represented by the whisker barrels. These barrels represent a neuronal column to which the sensory whisker nerves project [4]. Later, Cox et al. [1] and Dowling et al. [5] showed that stimulation of a single row of whiskers caused an increase in blood flow only in the cortical area encompassing the stimulated whisker barrels. Further studies by this group showed that the greatest metabolic activity occurs in layer IV of the cortex, which coincides with the greatest density of capillaries supplying the tissue [6,7]. Thus, there appears to be a correlation between neuronal activity, capillary blood supply and metabolism. Furthermore, stimulation of the whisker leads to a quick increase in blood flow within seconds of the onset of stimulation, leading to the question what mechanism(s) could explain such a local and fast regulatory response and more importantly, how such a local signal is transmitted to the supplying microvessels.

2. Mechanisms that could explain regulation of blood flow to meet local metabolic need

Several mechanisms are commonly cited to contribute to local cerebral blood flow regulation.

2.1. Neuronal influences including sympathetic perivascular nerves or nerves projecting from central nuclei or forebrain

The principal sympathetic perivascular nerves originate from the superior cervical and stellate ganglia and innervate the major cerebral arteries. Clearly, such nerves envelop the arterial vessels but sensitivity to principal neurotransmitters decreases towards arteriolar vessels [8]. The main transmitters found in these nerves are norepinephrine and neuropeptide Y [9,10]. Neuropeptide Y is a potent vasoconstrictor and is found in sympathetic ganglia innervating cerebral arteries and veins. The vasoconstrictor effect is stronger and lasts longer than that of norepinephrine. In addition, co-transmission of adenosine triphosphate (ATP) has been found [11] and sympathetic stimulation causes only small changes in CBF under normal physiological conditions [12]. For perivascular nerves to regulate microvascular flow, there has to be a local sensing system allowing the central regulatory systems to respond to metabolic changes and stimulate perivascular nerve fibers projecting only to the area of metabolic demand. Such a system has not been shown yet and the usually sporadic detection of perivascular nerves surrounding pial and cortical microvessels [13] makes such a mechanism less likely.

2.2. Locally released/sensed metabolites including adenosine, CO_2, pH, low PO_2 or potassium

Locally released metabolites/mediators such as adenosine, potassium and many others have undoubtedly a strong effect on arterial cerebral macro- and microvessel diameter [14]. The question arises on how a vasodilatory signal originating in the vicinity of activated neurons in the depth of the cortex can reach vessels at the surface of the brain. Since increase in local blood flow occurs within seconds after neuronal activation, diffusion of such mediators to the supplying vessels appears unlikely since diffusion of even small molecules would take several minutes to spread 500 um or less [15]. One possibility could be that mediators are picked up by the venous blood stream and influence the supplying vessel by a counter-current exchange as suggested by Hester [16]. However, this system requires that draining venules and supplying arterioles run in parallel which is not present in the cortical microcirculation.

2.3. Shear stress which causes the release of EDRFs

Since locally released metabolites/mediators can reach the terminal end of a supplying arteriole, it is possible that a local dilation occurs. This would cause a decrease in vessel resistance and a possible small increase in blood velocity and thus shear stress. Shear does induce release of endothelium-derived relaxation factors and dilation of a number of vessels including cerebral macrovessels [17] and arterioles [18]. Furthermore, adenosine triphosphate, a potent intraluminal vasodilator [19], is released from the endothelium by shear stress [20]. As such, a local dilation could cause the release of endothelial relaxation factors at the site of initial dilation which could feed back to the adjacent, still constricted vessel causing a dilation there and so on. However, such a saltatory retrograde ascension of vasodilation due to shear has not been shown. Indeed, studies by Kurjiaka and Segal [21] showed that just dilating terminal arterioles locally does not significantly increase blood flow to the tissue. Thus, another mechanism has to be postulated that translates metabolic need into a highly specific vascular response and increased blood flow.

3. The conducted vasomotor response

A candidate that could provide such a connection between the tissue and the supplying arterial vessels is the conducted vasomotor response. Krogh [22] found that stimulation of frog tissue caused a spread of local vasoactivity far greater than the area of stimulation. Muscle stimulation caused an ascending vasodilation as observed by Schretzenmayr [23] and Fleisch [24] which was not dependent on perivascular nerves [25]. Such spread of local vasoactivity was also observed in microvessels in many preparations [49]. This phenomenon was named conducted vasomotor responses to indicate a spread of local vasomotor responses along a blood vessel over distances greater than the area of the local stimulus with spreads measuring in millimeters (Fig. 1). Only with conducted vasomotor response does a local dilation cause an increase in local

Conduction of Vasomotor Responses

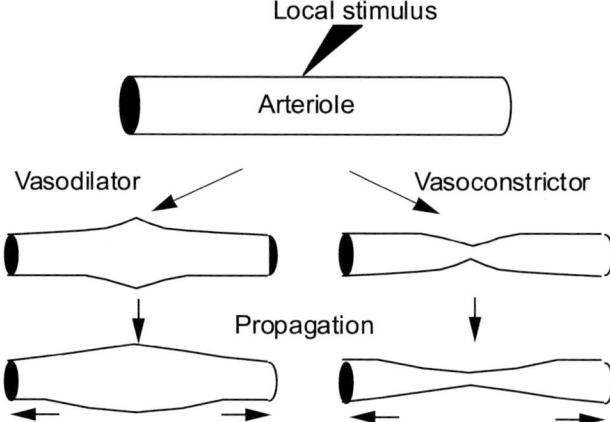

Fig. 1. Schematic of conducted vasomotor responses. A local vasomotor response to, e.g., microapplication of vasoactive substances or tissue activation, travels along the vessel to adjust vascular resistance according to the vascular needs of the tissue.

blood flow [21]. Not only stimulation of arterioles but also stimulation of capillaries [15,26] and venules [27] resulted in conducted responses indicating that the vascular tree has the ability to respond to stimuli and transmit these responses along the blood vessels to cause vasomotor responses to adjust local blood flow precisely to the needs of the supplied tissue. In addition to adjusting local cortical blood flow to the precise needs of the supplied tissue, conducted vasomotor responses would also prevent cerebral microvascular steal [28] which would drain blood to the vessel with low resistance if no adjustment of the vessel diameter in the higher order vessels via conducted responses would occur. Conducted vasomotor responses thus could provide the means to communicate local metabolic need to the supplying vessels in a direct manner.

3.1. Observation of conducted vasomotor responses in brain

Although not recognized at the time, a study by Herz et al. [29] may be the first to show conducted vasoconstriction due to pial vessel puncture and bleeding. Later, Rosenblum et al. [30] demonstrated conducted pial arteriolar constriction in mouse in vivo. Our laboratory demonstrated conducted responses in isolated and cannulated rat cortical arterioles to a variety of vasoactive substances [2].

The question arises which agonist/metabolite is the physiological correlate responsible for conducted vasomotor responses due to metabolic need. From the stimuli tested, all phosphorylated purines (ATP, ADP and AMP) caused consistently conducted vasodilation [2,31,32] while adenosine either did not [2,31]. Acidic pH also did not cause conducted responses [2,31]. The consistent responses to phosphorylated purines caught our attention.

4. Physiological ATP activity and sources for ATP in the brain

Muramatsu et al. [33] reported that perivascular stimulation of sympathetic nerves causes a biphasic vessel response with a transient constriction followed by a subsequent dilation similar to our experiments in penetrating arterioles [2,31]. Muramatsu et al. [11] and Muramatsu and Kigoshi [34] concluded that sympathetic stimulation co-released ATP, which caused an endothelium-dependent dilation after the transient constriction indicating a role for ATP as a vasoactive agent.

ATP is also basally released from platelets [35,36] which may prevent platelet aggregation [37] due to nitric oxide release [38]. Platelet activation causes massive ATP release [39]. ATP is also released in cerebral tissue after neuronal stimulation [40], which either could directly diffuse to nearby microvessels or act indirectly on them via astrocyte stimulation [41,42]. Earlier, Forrester et al. [19] reported that intraluminal ATP is a potent vasodilator in the cerebral circulation. Subsequently, Bergfeld and Forrester [43] and Ellsworth et al. [44] found that red blood cells, which contain millimolar concentrations of ATP, can release this ATP in response to acidic and/or low PO_2 conditions. They hypothesized that the red blood cell not only could be the vehicle to transport oxygen to the tissue, but also a sensor of metabolic tissue need and by releasing ATP, it causes an increase in local blood flow. In concert with conducted vasomotor responses, this would provide a simple but direct mechanism to regulate local blood flow precisely to the tissue needs.

5. Physiological activity of ATP in isolated and cannulated penetrating arterioles

Locally applied ATP causes a biphasic vasomotor response with a transient constriction followed by a vasodilation. Only the vasodilation is conducted over distances greater than

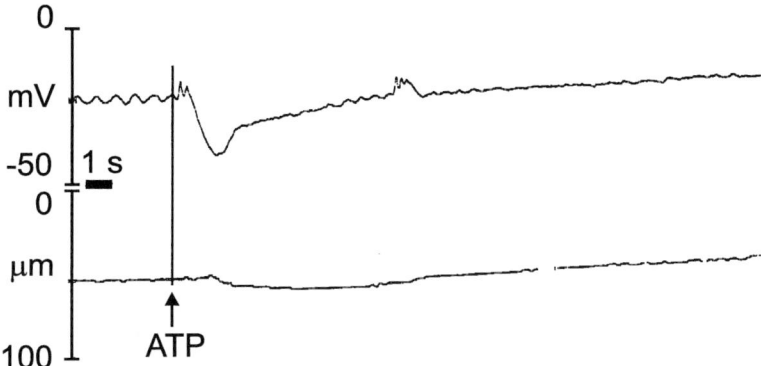

Fig. 2. Trace of conducted membrane potential and diameter response to a 450-ms ATP pulse (arrow). The electrical response (upper trace, intracellular single smooth muscle cell recording) precedes the mechanical trace (lower trace, vessel diameter measured online with Diamtrak, Montech, Australia).

500 um [2,32]. Intraluminal application causes dilation [45]. We measured the membrane potential in smooth muscle cells distant (> 500 um) from the site of stimulation [46] and found that local ATP stimulation caused a hyperpolarization which precedes the vessels dilation (Fig. 2) in a dose-dependent manner (Fig. 3). By measuring the time it takes from the moment of ejecting ATP to the time when a change of either membrane potential or vessel diameter occurred and the distance between stimulation and observation site, we estimated the conduction velocities. This conduction is very fast, with the electrical conduction speed estimated at 1500 um/s and a mechanical conduction speed of 500 um/s (Fig. 4), proving that conducted vasomotor responses are able to transmit a vasomotor signal quickly, thus allowing it to be a fast regulatory mechanism.

We studied the purinergic receptor composition of rat-penetrating arterioles and found that ATP causes a transient constriction via P_{2X1} receptors and vasodilation via endothelial P_{2Y2} receptors [47]. Damage of the endothelium attenuates vessel dilation to ATP [47].

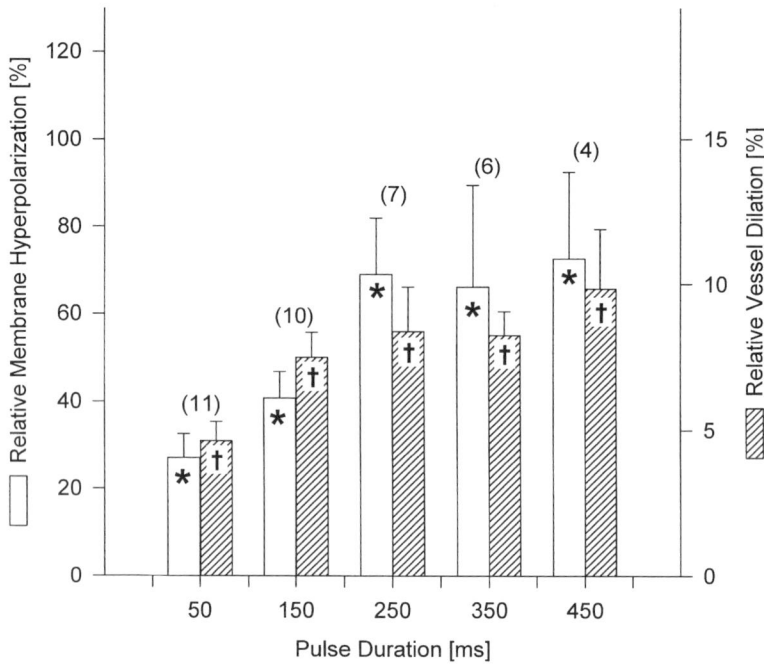

Fig. 3. Dose–response of smooth muscle membrane hyperpolarization and vessel dilation at the conducted site. Increase in ATP pulse duration leads to increased electrical and diameter responses. Numbers in parentheses indicate the number of vessels.

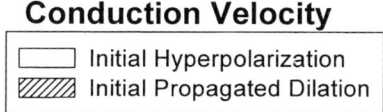

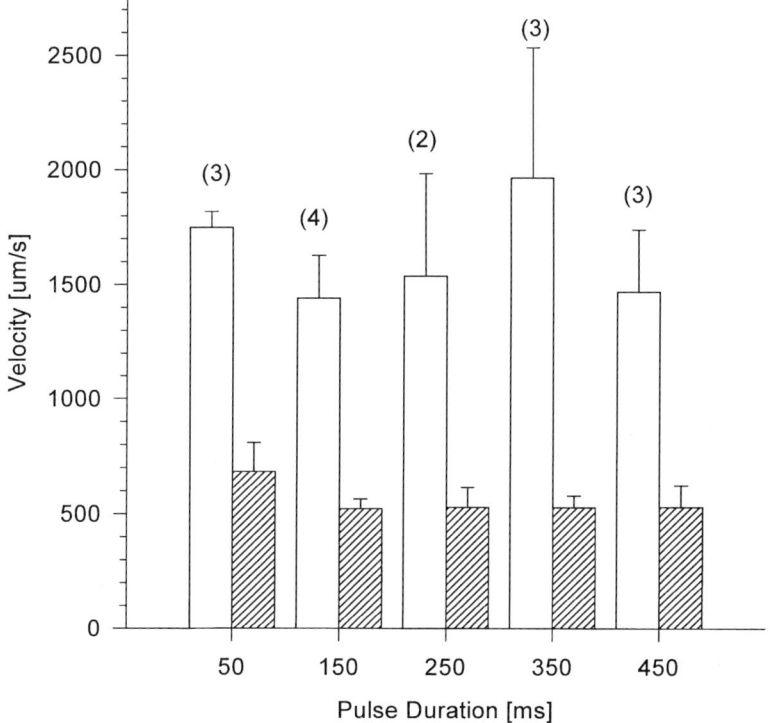

Fig. 4. Electrical and mechanical conduction velocity estimated as time from stimulus application to first measurable deviation of membrane potential or diameter from control per vessel length. The electrical conduction is three times faster than the mechanical one.

Further simulating subarachnoid hemorrhage with oxyhemoglobin greatly reduced conducted vasomotor responses [32].

6. Vessel response to low oxygen environment and red blood cell perfusion

To test if ATP released from red blood cells can alter the diameter of isolated and perfused penetrating arterioles, we measured arteriolar diameter at normal PO_2 (21%) and low PO_2 (~10%) [48]. In addition, we measured ATP content in the effluent using a sensitive luciferin–luciferase assay. We found that only blood vessels perfused with red blood cells dilate to low oxygen [48]. Buffer or dextran-perfused vessels did not dilate nor did the effluent contain any appreciable amount of ATP [48].

7. Conclusion

Conducted vasomotor responses may represent a mechanism that allows the cerebral microcirculation to adjust local blood flow in single arterioles precisely to the metabolic needs of the supplied tissue. Such responses are fast and concur with the need to utilize a mechanism that can respond within seconds to a neuronal tissue activation. ATP released from red blood cells, in addition to other parenchymal tissue sources, may serve as a sensor for local metabolic need and, in concert with conducted vasomotor responses, provide a mechanism to adjust local blood flow quickly and efficiently. Since conducted vasomotor responses are attenuated by oxyhemoglobin failure of the conduction, mechanism may contribute to the vascular insufficiency observed after subarachnoid hemorrhage.

3.1.4.10. On-Site Discussion

3.1.4.10.1. *Question: (Pelligrino)* Is your propagated response to ATP a function of gap junctional communication? Have you, for example, tried octanol, the gap junctional inhibitor?

Answer: (Dietrich) We have tried octanol in skeletal muscle and it suppresses conduction. One of the many functions of oxyhemoglobin is to act as a gap junction uncoupler. There were oxy-Hb data that may indicate on effect of oxy-Hb as a gap junction uncouples.

3.1.4.10.2. *Question: (Busija)* (1) Are the penetrating arterioles that you study normally surrounded by glia end feet in vivo? (2) Does it matter which direction the propagated response goes along the arteriole?

Answer: (Dietrich) (1) Penetrating arterioles are in close proximity to the surrounding tissue through reported by the Virchow-Robin space. However, mediators or metabolites released from parenchymal cells would largely influence arteriolar tone and conduct a vasomotor response to the surface of the brain. (2) The stimulation will travel equally well up or downstream.

3.1.4.10.3. *Question: (Busija)* With propagated impulses, signals originating in paren-chymal or capillary segments could be transferred to surface arteries?

Answer: (Dietrich) The capillary bed and/or venules are the vessels most likely to experience vasoactive stimuli or metabolites representing metabolic need. These signals have to be conducted from these vessels to the penetrating arteriole and higher vessels to adjust vessel resistance to allow an increase in vessel blood flow.

3.1.4.10.4. *Question: (Dirnagl)* If release of ATP from erythrocytes is the mechanism coupling metabolism to blood flow in the brain, what is the signal causing the release of ATP? Is intravascular hypoxia required, and would that imply that an "initial dip" is needed for regulation?

Answer: (Dietrich) Red blood cells release ATP not only to low PO_2 but also under acidotic conditions as well due to deformation. Thus, even if there is only a small or no decrease in PO_2, also neuronal activation, release of lactate would still raise release of ATP.

3.1.4.10.5. **Question: (Iadecola)** Stamler has pointed evidence that Hb releases NO at low PO_2 [Nature 391(6663) (1998) 169]. Could NO play a role in the vasodilation of low PO_2 when RBCs are run through the arterioles?

Answer: (Dietrich) Possibly, but less likely under physiological condition, more likely under pathophysiological condition such as sepsis. However, due to the strong binding of NO to Hb, Vaugln et al. [Am. J. Physiol. 274(5 Pt. 2) (1998) H1705] computed that NO released from Hb may have only a small effect at the smallest terminal arterioles. Relationship of NO to Hb seems to be important for NO cleared, though.

3.1.4.10.6. **Question: (Ances)** Please discuss the role of shear stress and could shear stress lead to deformation of RBC and therefore lead to the release of ATP?

Answer: (Dietrich) Yes, shear stress-induced deformation in capillaries could release ATP as shown in vitro. This is how red blood cells seem to potentiate in lung to reduce pulmonary resistance.

Acknowledgements

This study was supported by National Institutes of Health Grants HL-57540 (to H.H. Dietrich), HL-39226 and HL-54629 (to M.L. Ellsworth) and NS-30555 (to R.G. Dacey, Jr. and H.H. Dietrich).

References

[1] S.B. Cox, T.A. Woolsey, C.M. Rovainen, Localized dynamic changes in cortical blood flow with whisker stimulation corresponds to matched vascular and neuronal architecture of rat barrels, J. Cereb. Blood Flow Metab. 13 (1993) 899–913.

[2] H.H. Dietrich, Y. Kajita, R.G. Dacey Jr., Local and conducted vasomotor responses in isolated rat cerebral arterioles, Am. J. Physiol.: Heart Circ. Physiol. 271 (1996) H1109–H1116.

[3] T.A. Woolsey, H. Van der Loos, The structural organization of layer IV in the somatosensory region (SI) of mouse cerebral cortex. The description of a cortical field composed of discrete cytoarchitectonic units, Brain Res. 17 (2) (1970) 205–242.

[4] J. Greenberg, P.J. Hand, A. Sylvestro, M. Reivich, Localized metabolic-flow couple during functional activity, Acta Neurol. Scand., Suppl. 72 (1979) 12–13.

[5] J.L. Dowling, M.M. Henegar, D.Q. Liu, C.M. Rovainen, T.A. Woolsey, Rapid optical imaging of whisker responses in the rat barrel cortex, J. Neurosci. Methods 66 (1996) 113–122.

[6] J.S. McCasland, T.A. Woolsey, New high-resolution 2-deoxyglucose method featuring double labeling and automated data collection, J. Comp. Neurol. 278 (1988) 543–554.

[7] J.S. McCasland, T.A. Woolsey, High-resolution 2-deoxyglucose mapping of functional cortical columns in mouse barrel cortex, J. Comp. Neurol. 278 (1988) 555–569.

[8] J.A. Bevan, Sites of transition between functional systemic and cerebral arteries of rabbits occur at embryo-logical junctional sites, Science 204 (1979) 635–637.

[9] W. Kuschinsky, M. Wahl, Alpha-receptor stimulation by endogenous and exogenous norepinephrine and blockade by phentolamine in pial arteries of cats, Circ. Res. 37 (1975) 168–174.

[10] J.A. Mejia, J. Pernow, H. von Holst, A. Rudehill, J.M. Lundberg, Effects of neuropeptide Y, calcitonin gene-

related peptide, substance P, and capsaicin on cerebral arteries in man and animals, J. Neurosurg. 69 (1988) 913–918.

[11] I. Muramatsu, T. Ohmura, M. Oshita, Comparison between sympathetic adrenergic and purinergic transmission in the dog mesenteric artery, J. Physiol. 411 (1989) 227–243.

[12] G.L. Baumbach, D.D. Heistad, Effects of sympathetic stimulation and changes in arterial pressure on segmental resistance of cerebral vessels in rabbits and cats, Circ. Res. 52 (1983) 527–533.

[13] F.R. Edwards, D. Hards, G.D. Hirst, G.D. Silverberg, Noradrenaline (gamma) and ATP responses of innervated and non-innervated rat cerebral arteries, Br. J. Pharmacol. 96 (1989) 785–788.

[14] D.D. Heistad, H.A. Kontos, Cerebral circulation, in: J.T. Shepherd, F.M. Abboud (Eds.), Handbook of Physiology: Section 2: The Cardiovascular System vol. III, American Physiological Society, Bethesda, 1983, pp. 137–182.

[15] H.H. Dietrich, Effect of locally applied epinephrine and norepinephrine on blood flow and diameter in capillaries of rat mesentery, Microvasc. Res. 38 (1989) 125–135.

[16] R.L. Hester, Venular–arteriolar diffusion of adenosine in hamster cremaster microcirculation, Am. J. Physiol. 258 (1990) H1918–H1924.

[17] J.L. Garcia-Roldan, J.A. Bevan, Flow-induced constriction and dilation of cerebral resistance arteries, Circ. Res. 66 (1990) 1445–1448.

[18] A.C. Ngai, H.R. Winn, Modulation of cerebral arteriolar diameter by intraluminal flow and pressure, Circ. Res. 77 (1995) 832–840.

[19] T. Forrester, A.M. Harper, E.T. MacKenzie, Effects of intracarotid adenosine triphosphate infusions on cerebral blood flow and metabolism in the anaesthetized baboon, J. Physiol. 250 (1975) 38P–39P.

[20] P. Bodin, G. Burnstock, Synergistic effect of acute hypoxia on flow-induced release of ATP from cultured endothelial cells, Experientia 51 (1995) 256–259.

[21] D.T. Kurjiaka, S.S. Segal, Conducted vasodilation elevates flow in arteriole networks of hamster striated muscle, Am. J. Physiol. 269 (1995) H1723–H1728.

[22] A. Krogh, Studies on the capillariomotor mechanism, J. Physiol. (London) 53 (1920) 399–419.

[23] A. Schretzenmayr, Über kreislaufregulatorische Vorgänge an den groben Arterien bei der Muskelarbeit, Pfluegers Arch. Gesamte Physiol. 232 (1933) 743–748.

[24] A. Fleisch, Les réflexes nutritifs ascendant producteurs de dilation artérielle, Arch. Int. Physiol. 41 (1935) 141–167.

[25] M. Lie, O.M. Sejersted, F. Kiil, Local regulation of vascular cross section during changes in femoral arterial blood flow in dogs, Circ. Res. 27 (1970) 727–737.

[26] H.H. Dietrich, K. Tyml, Microvascular flow response to localized application of norepinephrine on capillaries in rat and frog skeletal muscle, Microvasc. Res. 43 (1992) 73–86.

[27] D.M. Collins, W.T. McCullough, M.L. Ellsworth, Conducted vascular responses: communication across the capillary bed, Microvasc. Res. 56 (1998) 43–53.

[28] L. Symon, The concept of intracerebral steal, Int. Anesthesiol. Clin. Cereb. Circ. 7 (1969) 597–615.

[29] D.A. Herz, S. Baez, K. Shulman, Pial microcirculation in subarachnoid hemorrhage, Stroke 6 (1975) 417–424.

[30] W.I. Rosenblum, Ph. Weinbrecht, G.H. Nelson, Propagated constriction in mouse pial arterioles: possible role of endothelium in transmitting the propagated response, Microcirc. Endothel. Lymphat. 6 (1990) 369–387.

[31] H.H. Dietrich, R.G. Dacey Jr., Demonstration of propagation of vasomotor responses in isolated rat cerebral arterioles in vitro, FASEB J. 6 (1992) A2072, Ref. Type: Abstract.

[32] Y. Kajita, H.H. Dietrich, R.G. Dacey Jr., Effects of oxyhemoglobin on local and propagated vasodilatory responses induced by adenosine, adenosine diphosphate, and adenosine triphosphate in rat cerebral arterioles, J. Neurosurg. 85 (1996) 908–916.

[33] I. Muramatsu, M. Fujiwara, A. Miura, Y. Sakakibara, Possible involvement of adenine nucleotides in sympathetic neuroeffector mechanisms of dog basilar artery, J. Pharmacol. Exp. Ther. 216 (1981) 401–409.

[34] I. Muramatsu, S. Kigoshi, Purinergic and non-purinergic innervation in the cerebral arteries of the dog, Br. J. Pharmacol. 92 (1987) 901–908.

[35] Md. Prada, A. Pletscher, Identification of guanosine 5′-triphosphate and uridine 5′-triphosphate in subcellular monoamine-storage organelles, Biochem. J. 119 (1970) 117–119.

[36] M.J. Harrison, R. Brossmer, Inhibition of platelet aggregation and the platelet release reaction by alpha, omega diadenosine polyphosphates, FEBS Lett. 54 (1975) 57–60.

[37] G. Soslau, R.J. McKenzie, I. Brodsky, T.M. Devlin, Extracellular ATP inhibits agonist-induced mobilization of internal calcium in human platelets, Biochim. Biophys. Acta 1268 (1995) 73–80.

[38] B.T. Mellion, L.J. Ignarro, E.H. Ohlstein, E.G. Pontecorvo, A.L. Hyman, P.J. Kadowitz, Evidence for the inhibitory role of guanosine $3',5'$-monophosphate in ADP-induced human platelet aggregation in the presence of nitric oxide and related vasodilators, Blood 57 (1981) 946–955.

[39] H. Flodgaard, H. Klenow, Abundant amounts of diadenosine $5',5''$-P1,P4-tetraphosphate are present and releasable, but metabolically inactive, in human platelets, Biochem. J. 208 (1982) 737–742.

[40] Y. Kuroda, H. McIlwain, Uptake and release of (14C) adenine derivatives at beds of mammalian cortical synaptosomes in a superfusion system, J. Neurochem. 22 (1974) 691–699.

[41] C. Centemeri, C. Bolego, M.P. Abbracchio, F. Cattabeni, L. Puglisi, G. Burnstock, S. Nicosia, Character-ization of the Ca^{2+} responses evoked by ATP and other nucleotides in mammalian brain astrocytes, Br. J. Pharmacol. 121 (1997) 1700–1706.

[42] D.R. Harder, N.J. Alkayed, A.R. Lange, D. Gebremedhin, R.J. Roman, Functional hyperemia in the brain— hypothesis for astrocyte-derived vasodilator metabolites, Stroke 29 (1998) 229–234.

[43] G.R. Bergfeld, T. Forrester, Release of ATP from human erythrocytes in response to a brief period of hypoxia and hypercapnia, Cardiovasc. Res. 26 (1992) 40–47.

[44] M.L. Ellsworth, T. Forrester, C.G. Ellis, H.H. Dietrich, The erythrocyte as a regulator of vascular tone, Am. J. Physiol.: Heart Circ. Physiol. 269 (1995) H2155–H2161.

[45] D. Janigro, T.S. Nguyen, J. Meno, G.A. West, H.R. Winn, Endothelium-dependent regulation of cerebro-vascular tone by extracellular and intracellular ATP, Am. J. Physiol.: Heart Circ. Physiol. 273 (1997) H878– H885.

[46] H.H. Dietrich, R.G. Dacey Jr., Propagated vasomotor responses: simultaneous measurement of diameter and membrane potential changes in isolated rat cerebral arterioles, Biorheology 32 (2–3) (1995) 352–353, Ref. Type: Abstract.

[47] T. Horiuchi, H.H. Dietrich, S. Tsugane, R.G. Dacey Jr., Analysis of purine- and pyrimidine-induced vascular responses in the isolated rat cerebral arteriole, Am. J. Physiol.: Heart Circ. Physiol. 280 (2001) H767–H776.

[48] H.H. Dietrich, M.L. Ellsworth, R.S. Sprague, R.G. Dacey Jr., Red blood cell regulation of microvascular tone through adenosine triphosphate, Am. J. Physiol. 278 (2000) H1294–H1298.

[49] F. Gustafsson, N. Holstein-Rathlou, Conducted vasomotor responses in arterioles: characteristics, mecha-nisms and physiological significance, Acta Physiol. Scand. 167 (1999) 11–21.

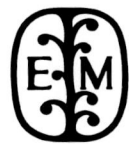

International Congress Series 1235 (2002) 289–295

Regulation of the cerebral circulation by cytochrome P450 epoxygenase activity

Xinqi Peng[a], Juan R. Carhuapoma[b], Anish Bhardwaj[a,b],
Nabil J. Alkayed[a], David R. Harder[c], Richard J. Traystman[a,*],
Raymond C. Koehler[a]

[a]Department of Anesthesiology and Critical Care Medicine, The Johns Hopkins Medical Institutions,
600 North Wolfe Street/Blalock 1408, Baltimore, MD 21287-4961, USA
[b]Department of Neurology, The Johns Hopkins University School of Medicine, Baltimore, MD 21287, USA
[c]The Cardiovascular Research Center, Medical College of Wisconsin, Milwaukee, WI 53226, USA

Abstract

Cytochrome P450 epoxygenases metabolize arachidonic acid into epoxyeicosatrienoic acids (EETs), which can dilate cerebral vessels. In glial cell cultures, glutamate stimulates the release of EETs. Thus, an astrocyte-based epoxygenase pathway could form a link in the coupling of blood flow to neuronal activity. To test this hypothesis, neuronal activation was produced by mechanical displacement of the whiskers of anesthetized rats while monitoring red cell flux by laser-Doppler flowmetry over whisker barrel sensory cortex. N-methylsulfonyl-6-(2-propargyloxyphenol) hexanamide (MS-PPOH) or miconazole, two different types of P450 epoxygenase inhibitors, were superfused over the cortical surface in different groups of rats. Both inhibitors markedly reduced the increase in cortical perfusion during whisker stimulation. To test the effect of these inhibitors on the increase in blood flow evoked by N-methyl-D-aspartate (NMDA), drugs were delivered via microdialysis probes in the striatum, while local blood flow was measured by the hydrogen clearance technique. Both MS-PPOH and miconazole blocked the increase in striatal blood flow during microdialysis perfusion of NMDA. These results support a role for P450 epoxygenase activity in the coupling of cortical blood flow to whisker stimulation and to pharmacological activation of NMDA receptors in striatum. © 2002 Elsevier Science B.V. All rights reserved.

Keywords: Cerebral blood flow; Cytochrome P450; Epoxyeicosatrienoic acid; Epoxygenase; Whisker barrel cortex

* Corresponding author. Tel.: +1-410-955-8157; fax: +1-410-955-7165.
E-mail address: rtraystm@jhmi.edu (R.J. Traystman).

0531-5131/02 © 2002 Elsevier Science B.V. All rights reserved.
PII: S 0 5 3 1 - 5 1 3 1 (0 2) 0 0 1 9 6 - 6

1. Introduction

Sensory stimulation evokes regional increases in cerebral blood flow and glucose consumption. The mechanisms of vasodilation have been studied in rodents using whisker stimulation as a model of physiological sensory activation. Movement of individual whiskers leads to neuronal activation in cortical columns of primary somatosensory cortex (whisker barrel cortex) and to localized increases in cortical blood flow [1].

Several studies have implicated a cyclooxygenase product, adenosine and nitric oxide (NO) in mediating to the cortical vasodilation evoked by whisker stimulation. In mice, cyclooxygenase-2 inhibition or gene deletion reduces the increase in cortical perfusion [2]. In rats, theophylline or adenosine deaminase attenuates the increase in flow, thereby implicating a role for adenosine [3]. In both mice and rats, NO synthase (NOS) inhibitors reduce the increase in cortical perfusion [3,4]. Stimulation of N-methyl-D-aspartate (NMDA) receptors also leads to vasodilation that can be reduced by NO synthase inhibitors [5,6]. These results have led to the concept that glutamate release during neuronal activation generates NO via stimulation of NMDA and possibly other glutamatergic receptors and that neuronally derived NO diffuses to vascular smooth muscle to produce vasodilation. In addition, increased metabolism may lead to adenosine release [7] and calcium influx associated with neuronal activity may lead to mobilization of arachidonic acid and formation of vasodilatory cyclooxygenase products.

However, inhibition of either the NOS, adenosine or cyclooxygenase-2 pathway reduces the flow response to whisker stimulation by 50% or less. Even with the combination of a NOS inhibitor and the adenosine antagonist theophylline, the flow response is reduced by about 60% [3]. Thus, other pathways mediating functional hyperemia probably exist. Existence of redundant pathways is supported by the observations that the flow response to whisker stimulation is normal in neuronal NOS knockout mice and that a NOS inhibitor did not reduce the flow response in these knockout mice [8]. Moreover, Lindauer et al. [9] found that applying a NO donor to restore baseline perfusion after NOS inhibition resulted in full restoration of the blood flow response to whisker stimulation. Similar results were observed when a cyclic GMP (cGMP) analog was used to restore baseline flow after guanylyl cyclase inhibition. Thus, NO may act by enabling other mediators to produce vasodilation in a permissive fashion.

One alternative pathway is the cytochrome P450 epoxygenase pathway [10]. Epoxygenases metabolize arachidonic acid into epoxyeicosatrienoic acids (EETs). Application of EETs to the cortical surface causes pial arteriolar dilation [11,12]. The mechanism involes opening of calcium-sensitive potassium (K_{Ca}) channels [10,13]. In the coronary vascular bed, EETs are synthesized in endothelial cells [14]. In brain, glial cells are capable of synthesizing EETs [15] and cytochrome P450 2C11, which possesses epoxygenase activity, has been found in glial cell cultures [16]. Addition of glutamate to the cell culture medium causes an increase in arachidonic acid and EETs formation in glia and EETs release into the medium [16]. This formation of EETs is inhibited by miconazole, a P450 epoxygenase inhibitor. In vivo, subdural superfusion of miconazole reduces the increase in cortical perfusion evoked by glutamate [17]. Thus, it seems reasonable to postulate that astrocytes sense neuronal activity, possibly through astrocytic glutamatergic [18] or other types of receptors (e.g., purinergic) [19], leading to increases in calcium, mobilization of arachidonic acid [20], formation of EETs, and release of EETs from de nova sysnthesis or from stored phospholipid pools [21]. Because astrocyte processes come into close contact with microvessels in brain parenchyma, release of EETs could contribute to vasodilation of intraparenchymal arterioles that regulate local nutritive blood flow.

The possible role of epoxygenases in the coupling of cortical blood flow to neuronal activation produced by whisker stimulation was tested by using two different types of epoxygenase inhibitors. One inhibitor used was miconazole, which acts at the heme site of the P450. The other inhibitor used was N-methylsulfonyl-6-(2-propargyloxyphenol) hexanamide (MS-PPOH), which acts as a selective substrate inhibitor [22]. The effect of these epoxygenase inhibitors on the increase in striatal blood flow evoked by NMDA stimulation was also evaluated.

2. Methods

Procedures on male Wistar rats were approved by the institutional animal care and use committee. Rats were anesthetized with halothane. Lungs were mechanically ventilated via a tracheostomy to maintain arterial blood gases in the normal physiological range. Arterial blood pressure was monitored via a femoral arterial catheter.

For the whisker stimulation experiments, cortical perfusion was measured by laser-Doppler flowmetry. The skull overlying whisker barrel cortex was thinned by drilling until epidural and pial vessels could be visualized under a dissecting microscope. The laser-Doppler flow probe was placed on the thin layer of bone and a drop of mineral oil was used to provide optical coupling. Drugs were administered topically on the cortical surface underneath the flow probe site by subdural superfusion. Small drill holes were made to expose the dura mater at sites superior and inferior to the probe site. The dura was pierced at these sites and a finely tapered polyethylene catheter was advanced about 1mm subdurally at the superior site. The catheter was perfused at a rate of 5 μl/min with artificial cerebrospinal fluid (CSF). CSF was allowed to drain passively from the inferior site. At the completion of surgery, rats received an intraperitoneal injection of α-chloralose (50 mg/kg) followed by a continuous intravenous infusion (40 mg/kg/min) for the remainder of the experiment. Inhalation of halothane was discontinued.

The whiskers were inserted through a plastic mesh, which was triggered to undergo 7-mm linear displacement at a rate of 3 Hz for 60-s periods. The increase in the laser-Doppler flux signal was averaged over the 60-s stimulation period and expressed as a percent of the previous 60-s baseline mean value. An average of three trails was obtained for every experimental period. A baseline response from three trials was obtained after 1 h of subdural superfusion with CSF containing vehicle (0.5% ethanol) in four groups of rats (n=8 each). During the second hour, the continuous subdural superfusate contained either vehicle, 5 μmol/l MS-PPOH, 20 μmol/l MS-PPOH or 20 μmol/l miconazole. The flow response to whisker stimulation was then repeated.

For testing the effect of epoxygenase inhibitors on the blood flow response to NMDA, MS-PPOH, miconazole and NMDA were delivered intraparenchymally by microdialysis. Microdialysis probes were inserted bilaterally into striatum. Blood flow was measured at

Table 1
Percent increase in laser-Doppler flux signal during 60 s of whisker stimulation

		Baseline	Drug
Vehicle	(0.5% ethanol)	26±12	24±9
MS-PPOH	(5 μmol/l)	25±9	18±8*
MS-PPOH	(20 μmol/l)	28±9	9±4*
Miconazole	(20 μmol/l)	31±6	10±1*

Values are expressed as a percent (means±S.D.; $n=8$ per group).
 * $P<0.05$ from baseline.

the site of drug administration with the hydrogen clearance technique by inserting a fine platinum wire into the tip of the microdialysis probe [6]. The probes were perfused at a rate of 1 μl/min for 1 h with artificial CSF. Then, one probe was perfused with artificial CSF containing vehicle (0.5% ethanol) and the contralateral probe was perfused with either 20 μmol/l MS-PPOH ($n=7$) or 20 μmol/l miconazole ($n=7$). At 1 h of perfusion with vehicle or the epoxygenase inhibitor, NMDA (3 mmol/l) was added to the perfusates at both sides. This design allowed paired comparisons between the vehicle and inhibitor sides under similar conditions of anesthesia, arterial blood gases and blood pressure.

3. Results

Mechanical stimulation of the whiskers resulted in approximately a 25–30% increase in the laser-Doppler flux signal in all groups during subdural superfusion of artificial CSF containing the 0.5% ethanol vehicle (Table 1). In the time-control group receiving vehicle for an additional hour, the increase in perfusion during whisker stimulation remained unchanged. When MS-PPOH was superfused at a dose of 5 μmol/l for 1 h, the response to whisker stimulation was reduced by 28%. When MS-PPOH was superfused at a dose of 20 μmol/l, the response was reduced by 69%. When miconazole was superfused at a dose of 20 μmol/l, the response was reduced by 67%.

Table 2
Striatal blood flow after 1-h microdialysis perfusion with vehicle or epoxygenase inhibitor and during subsequent NMDA perfusion

		Baseline	NMDA
Group 1			
Vehicle	(0.5% ethanol)	68±12	149±24
MS-PPOH	(20 μmol/l)	69±12	69±12*
Group 2			
Vehicle	(0.5% ethanol)	89±19	164±82
Miconazole	(20 μmol/l)	69±12	73±19*

Flows are expressed as ml/min/100 g (means±S.D.; $n=7$).
 * $P<0.05$ from the vehicle group.

When microdialysis probes placed bilaterally in striatum were perfused with artificial CSF, there were no side-to-side differences in the local blood flow measured by hydrogen clearance. With subsequent perfusion of vehicle on one side and of 20 μmol/l of MS-PPOH on the other side, there was no side-to-side difference in blood flow (Table 2). Perfusion of 3 mmol/l of NMDA doubled the blood flow on the side receiving vehicle. However, no increase in blood flow was seen on the side receiving MS-PPOH. In another group of rats in which one microdialysis probe was perfused with 20 μmol/l of miconazole, blood flow also failed to increase during NMDA perfusion, whereas the contralateral side receiving vehicle showed a doubling of blood flow during NMDA perfusion.

4. Discussion

Both MS-PPOH and miconazole, which inhibit cytochrome P450 epoxygenase activity by different mechanisms, substantially reduced the functional hyperemia evoked by whisker stimulation and blocked the increase in blood flow evoked by NMDA in striatum. These results support a role for epoxygenases in the coupling of blood flow to physiological and pharmacological activation in the brain.

Because NOS inhibitors also reduce the vasodilation to NMDA, the NOS and epoxygenase mechanisms probably do not represent simple parallel pathways mediating vasodilation. Rather, there may be complex interactions in the neuronal, glial, endothelial and smooth muscle compartments. Miconazole and MS-PPOH do not inhibit NOS catalytic activity at the concentrations used in these experiments, nor do they prevent increases in blood flow produced by the NO donor nitroprusside [23,24]. Thus, epoxygenase inhibitors do not act by inhibiting NOS or preventing vasodilation to NO. In preliminary work with foreleg stimulation, we did not find any attenuation of somatosensory-evoked potentials by MS-PPOH or miconazole. Hence, the drugs do not appear to act by decreasing neuronal activation. Because Lindauer et al. [9] found that administering a low concentration of an NO donor after NOS inhibition restored the attenuated blood flow response to whisker stimulation seen with NOS inhibition alone, NO may enable dilation to occur via other pathways. NO donors increase blood flow not only by increasing cGMP, but also by inhibiting P450 ω-hydroxylase activity [25]. P450 ω-hydroxylase activity in cerebral arteriolar smooth muscle produces 20-HETE which constricts arterioles by closing K_{ca} channels [26]. By inhibiting 20-HETE production, NO may permit opening of K_{ca} channels by EETs.

In contrast to NOS inhibitors which decrease baseline cerebral blood flow, neither epoxygenase inhibitor reduced baseline perfusion. This finding suggests that EETs may be more important in the signaling process for dynamic changes in blood flow than for regulating basal levels of blood flow. This signaling process may involve not only extracellular release of EETs, but also intracellular signaling by EETs. For example, 5,6-EET appears to serve as a calcium influx factor that helps maintain intracellular calcium stores [27]. If coupling of flow to neuronal activity involves calcium signaling through the astrocyte syncytium for releasing EETs at distant astrocyte processes adjacent to arterioles, EETs might also contribute to flow coupling by enhancing this intracellular calcium signaling. In addition, our results do not exclude a role for EETs from neuronal or endothelial sources. Nevertheless, our results are consistent with an epoxygenase pathway, known to be present in astrocytes, contributing to the coupling of blood flow to neuronal activation.

3.1.5.7. On-Site Discussion

3.1.5.7.1 *Question: (Bryan)* Are the EETs stored and if so can you comment on how they are stored?
Answer: (Traystman) EET's are stored in astrocytes, and released but how they are stored is unclear.
3.1.5.7.2. *Question: (Nemoto)* 1) What evidence is there that the EETs are produced only by the astrocytes? 2) Isn't the SSEP a rather crude method to assess the effect of the epoxygenase inhibitor on brain function? Wouldn't power spectral analysis of the EEGs be preferable?
Answer: (Traystman) 1) In brain they are only in astrocytes (Alkayed et al. Stroke 1996; 27(5): 971. 2) Yes, spectral analysis would be good too.
3.1.5.7.3. *Question: (Gaehtgens)* With respect to the questions of Iadecola and Kuschinsky: In view of the existence of conducted dilation, several systems inducing vasorelaxation do not necessarily have to act in an additive fashion, since some response may be conducted while others are not. Therefore, although causing local relaxation following release from astrocytes, these systems together might not lead to a 300% effect on flow. Do you know whether EET response are conducted?
Answer: (Traystman) EET responses could be conducted and in fact may influence other mediators.

Acknowledgements

This work was supported by a grant from the National Institutes of Health (HL 59996).

References

[1] T.A. Woolsey, C.M. Rovainen, S.B. Cox, M.H. Henegar, G.E. Liang, D. Liu, Y.E. Moskalenko, J. Sui, L. Wei, Neuronal units linked to microvascular modules in cerebral cortex: response elements for imaging the brain, Cereb. Cortex 6 (5) (1996) 647–660.
[2] K. Niwa, E. Araki, S.G. Morham, M.E. Ross, C. Iadecola, Cyclooxygenase-2 contributes to functional hyperemia in whisker-barrel cortex, J. Neurosci. 20 (2) (2000) 763–770.
[3] U. Dirnagl, K. Niwa, U. Lindauer, A. Villringer, Coupling of cerebral blood flow to neuronal activation: role of adenosine and nitric oxide, Am. J. Physiol.: Heart Circ. Physiol. 267 (1994) H296–H301.
[4] K. Irikura, K.I. Maynard, M.A. Moskowitz, Importance of nitric oxide synthase inhibition to the attenuated vascular responses induced by topical L-nitroarginine during vibrissal stimulation, J. Cereb. Blood Flow Metab. 14 (1) (1994) 45–48.
[5] F.M. Faraci, K.R. Breese, Nitric oxide mediates vasodilatation in response to activation of *N*-methyl-D-aspartate receptors in brain, Circ. Res. 72 (1993) 476–480.
[6] F.J. Northington, J.R. Tobin, R.C. Koehler, R.J. Traystman, In vivo production of nitric oxide correlates with NMDA-induced cerebral hyperemia in newborn sheep, Am. J. Physiol.: Heart Circ. Physiol. 269 (1995) H215–H221.

[7] K.R. Ko, A.C. Ngai, H.R. Winn, Role of adenosine in regulation of regional cerebral blood flow in sensory cortex, Am. J. Physiol.: Heart Circ. Physiol. 259 (28) (1990) H1703–H1708.

[8] J. Ma, C. Ayata, P.L. Huang, M.C. Fishman, M.A. Moskowitz, Regional cerebral blood flow response to vibrissal stimulation in mice lacking type I NOS gene expression, Am. J. Physiol.: Heart Circ. Physiol. 270 (1996) H1085–H1090.

[9] U. Lindauer, D. Megow, H. Matsuda, U. Dirnagl, Nitric oxide: a modulator, but not a mediator, of neuro-vascular coupling in rat somatosensory cortex, Am. J. Physiol.: Heart Circ. Physiol. 277 (2 Pt 2) (1999) H799–H811.

[10] D.R. Harder, N.J. Alkayed, A.R. Lange, D. Gebremedhin, R.J. Roman, Functional hyperemia in the brain. Hypothesis for astrocyte-derived vasodilator metabolites, Stroke 28 (1998) 229–234.

[11] E.F. Ellis, R.J. Police, L. Yancey, J.S. McKinney, S.C. Amruthesh, Dilation of cerebral arterioles by cytochrome P-450 metabolites of arachidonic acid, Am. J. Physiol.: Heart Circ. Physiol. 259 (1990) H1171–H1177.

[12] C. Leffler, A.L. Fedinec, Newborn piglet cerebral microvascular responses to epoxyeicosatrienoic acids, Am. J. Physiol.: Heart Circ. Physiol. 273 (42) (1997) H333–H338.

[13] D. Gebremedhin, Y.-H. Ma, J.R. Falck, R.J. Roman, M. VanRollins, D.R. Harder, Mechanism of action of cerebral epoxyeicosatrienoic acids on cerebral arterial smooth muscle, Am. J. Physiol.: Heart Circ. Physiol. 263 (1992) H519–H525.

[14] B. Fisslthaler, R. Popp, L. Kiss, M. Potente, D.R. Harder, I. Fleming, R. Busse, Cytochrome P450 2C is an EDHF synthase in coronary arteries, Nature 401 (6752) (1999) 493–497.

[15] S.C. Amruthesh, M.F. Boerschel, J.S. McKinney, K.A. Willoughby, E.F. Ellis, Metabolism of arachidonic acid to epoxyeicosatrienoic acids, hydroxyeicosatetraenoic acids, and prostaglandins in cultured rat hippocampal astrocytes, J. Neurochem. 61 (1993) 150–159.

[16] N.J. Alkayed, J. Narayanan, D. Gebremedhin, M. Medhora, R.J. Roman, D.R. Harder, Molecular characterization of an arachidonic acid epoxygenase in rat brain astrocytes, Stroke 27 (1996) 971–979.

[17] N.J. Alkayed, E.K. Birks, J. Narayanan, K.A. Petrie, A.E. Kohler-Cabot, D.R. Harder, Role of P-450 arachidonic acid expoygenase in the response of cerebral blood flow to glutamate in rats, Stroke 28 (1997) 1066–1072.

[18] J.A. Holzwarth, S.J. Gibbons, J.R. Brorson, L.H. Philipson, R.J. Miller, Glutamate receptor agonists stimulate diverse calcium responses in different types of cultured rat cortical glial cells, J. Neurosci. 14 (4) (1994) 1879–1891.

[19] M.L. Cotrina, J.H.C. Lin, M. Nedergaard, Cytoskeletal assembly and ATP release regulate astrocytic calcium signaling, J. Neurosci. 18 (1998) 8794–8804.

[20] N. Stella, M. Tence, J. Glowinski, J. Premont, Glutamate-evoked release of arachidonic acid from mouse brain astrocytes, J. Neurosci. 14 (2) (1994) 568–575.

[21] A.C. Shivachar, K.A. Willoughby, E.F. Ellis, Effect of protein kinase C modulators on 14,15-epoxyeicosatrienoic acid incorporation into astroglial phospholipids, J. Neurochem. 65 (1) (1995) 338–346.

[22] M.-H. Wang, E. Brand-Schieber, B.A. Zand, X. Nguyen, J.R. Falck, N. Balu, M.L. Schwartzman, Cytochrome P450-derived arachidonic acid metabolism in the rat kidney: characterization of selective inhibitors, J. Pharmacol. Exp. Ther. 284 (3) (1998) 966–973.

[23] N.J. Alkayed, E.K. Birks, A.G. Hudetz, R.J. Roman, L. Henderson, D.R. Harder, Inhibition of brain P-450 arachidonic acid epoxygenase decreases baseline cerebral blood flow, Am. J. Physiol.: Heart Circ. Physiol. 271 (1996) H1541–H1546.

[24] A. Bhardwaj, F.J. Northington, J.R. Carhuapoma, J.R. Falck, D.R. Harder, R.J. Traystman, R.C. Koehler, P-450 epoxygenase and NO synthase inhibitors reduce cerebral blood flow response to N-methyl-D-aspartate, Am. J. Physiol.: Heart Circ. Physiol. 279 (4) (2000) H1616–H1624.

[25] M. Alonso-Galicia, A.G. Hudetz, H. Shen, D.R. Harder, R.J. Roman, Contribution of 20-HETE to vasodilator actions of nitric oxide in the cerebral microcirculation, Stroke 30 (12) (1999) 2727–2734.

[26] A. Lange, D. Gebremedhin, J. Narayanan, D. Harder, 20-Hydroxyeicosatetraenoic acid-induced vasoconstriction and inhibition of potassium current in cerebral vascular smooth muscle is dependent on activation of protein kinase C, J. Biol. Chem. 272 (43) (1997) 27345–27352.

[27] B.A. Rzigalinski, K.A. Willoughby, S.W. Hoffman, J.R. Falck, E.F. Ellis, Calcium influx factor, further evidence it is 5,6-epoxyeicosatrienoic acid, J. Biol. Chem. 274 (1999) 175–182.

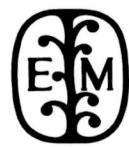

International Congress Series 1235 (2002) 297–304

Epoxyeicosatetrinoic acids released by astrocytes: function in cerebral angiogenesis

Chenyang Zhang *, David R. Harder

Cardiovascular Research Center (CVRC), Medical College of Wisconsin, 8701 Watertown Plank Road, Milwaukee, WI 53226, USA

Abstract

Epoxyeicosatetrinoic acids (EETs) are bioactive metabolites of arachidonic acid (AA). Our laboratory has cloned and sequenced a P450 cDNA from astrocytes which epoxygenate arachidonic acid leading to formation of EETs. The actions of these products include activation of K^+ channels and hyperpolarization of cerebral vascular smooth muscle and induction of mitogenic mechanisms in capillary endothelium resulting in tube formation. This communication focuses on the discussing of angiogenic properties of EETs on cerebral capillary endothelium. © 2002 Elsevier Science B.V. All rights reserved.

Keywords: Cytochrome P450 enzymes; Blood flow; Glutamate; Capillary; Membrane potential

It is obvious that there are gaps in our knowledge regarding many aspects of neurobiology. Among these are understanding the roles played by astrocytes and understanding the mechanisms, which control vascular and capillary density in the brain. This communication summarizes data, which provides a link between neural activity and cerebral capillary density, and defines a role for astrocytes in this process.

1. Arachidonic acid metabolism by astrocytes

Astrocytes express functional metabotropic and ionotropic glutamate receptors which mediate a number of cellular signaling events including: uptake of glutamate and subsequent activation of phospholipase C (PLC) [1], elevation of intracellular Ca [2,3], me-

---

* Corresponding author. Tel.: +1-414-456-5611; fax: +1-414-456-6515.
E-mail address: cyzhang@mcw.edu (C. Zhang).

0531-5131/02 © 2002 Elsevier Science B.V. All rights reserved.
PII: S 0 5 3 1 - 5 1 3 1 (0 2) 0 0 1 9 8 - X

diation of cell–cell signaling [3], and release of arachidonic acid (AA) from bound membrane stores into "free form" and into the cytosol [4]. AA is abundantly stored in estrified form in the cell membrane phospholipid pool from which it is released into soluble and particulate fractions of astrocytes by the action of phospholipases. These phospholipases are regulated by physiological stimuli and ligand–receptor interaction. PLC is activated upon stimulation of metabotropic receptors by glutamate [1]. PLC hydrolysis of PIP2 yields IP3 and DAG. Arachidonyl DAG is the dominant isoform of DAG and free AA is released by the action of monoglycerol lipase [5,6]. Both iontropic and metabotropic receptors can directly increase intracellular Ca^{2+} which activates PLA2, releasing AA from the SN-2 position of membrane phospholipid pools.

Arachidonic acid is metabolized by at least three distinct pathways into autocrine and paracrine signaling molecules. The most well-studied of these pathways are cyclooxyenase and lipoxygenase which metabolize AA into prostaglandins and leucotrienes and related products [7]. Studies from a number of laboratories have defined a third pathway, which metabolizes AA into potent signaling molecules. The peripheral (non-hepatic) P450 family of enzymes consists of numerous isoforms (over 300 in total), many of which use AA as a substrate [8]. Our laboratory has cloned and sequenced several P450 cDNAs from rat astrocytes, at least one of which metabolizes AA into epoxyeicosatrienoic acids (EETs) [9]. P450 2C11 is expressed in cortical astrocytes, and metabolizes AA into four regioisomers of EETs, namely, 5,6-; 8,9-; 11,12-; and 14,15-EET. The structures of these EETs are depicted in Fig. 1.

Glutamate induces release of EETs from astrocytes in culture, and EETs can be measured in cerebral tissue (Fig. 2). The action of EETs when released from astrocytes is to dilate cerebral microvessels by increasing the activity of K^+ channels and hyperpolarizing vascular smooth muscle [10,11]. To date, the primary target for EETs is the large conductance Ca activated K^+ channel (K_{ca}) [12]. It appears that all four isoforms of EETs act similarly, however, 8,9- and 11.12-EETs are the most potent and most stable. With respect to the action of EETs on cerebral arteriolar muscle, it has been hypothesized

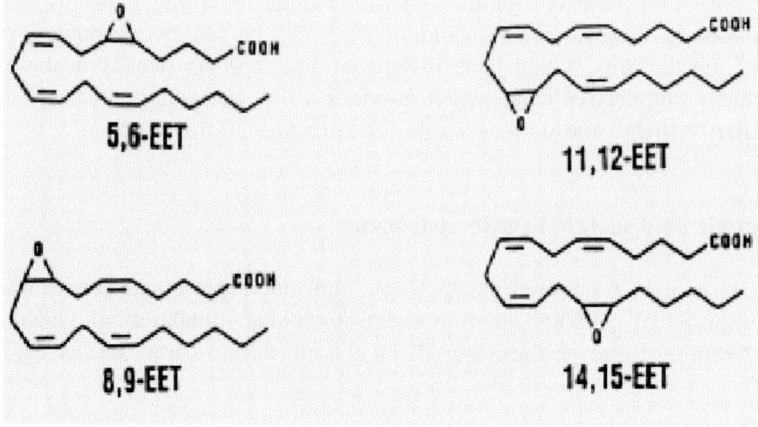

Fig. 1. Structures of the four regioisomers of epoxyeicosatrienoic acids.

A

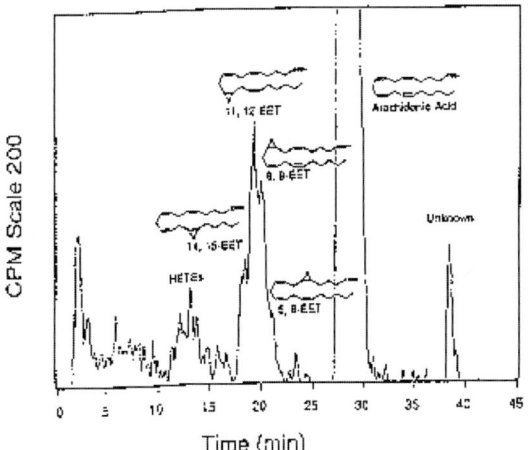

B

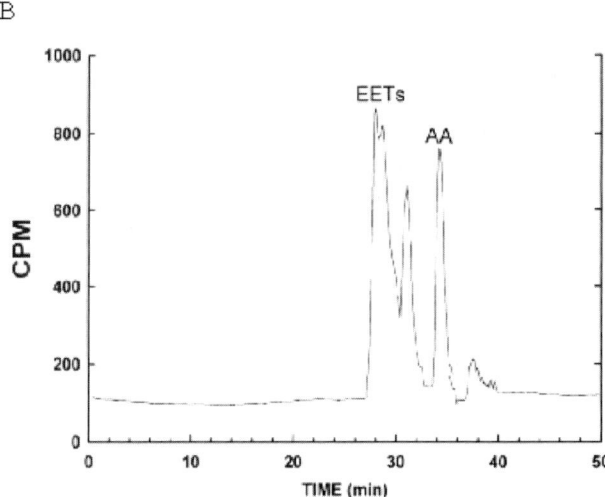

Fig. 2. Representative rpHPLC chromatograms demonstrate the production of EETs from cerebral cortex (A) and cultured astrocytes (B).

that EETs released from astrocytes in response to "spill over" of glutamate during neural activation function mediate/participate in the functional hyperemia observed in response to neural activation. New data have demonstrated that EETs are pre-formed and stored in the plasma membrane to be released upon chemical and/or environmental stimuli. These new findings explain how the vasoactive response to nerve stimulation can occur within fractions of seconds. The topic of this symposium article is not to discuss the role of P450

EETs in functional hyperemia in the brain, but rather to discuss the mitogenic properties of EETs on cerebral capillary endothelium.

2. Mechanisms of cerebral angiogenesis

Cerebral angiogenesis has been shown to be induced by hypoxia, ischemia, physical activity and learning [12,13]. There is indication that increased angiogenesis may have therapeutic effect on the morbidity associated with ischemic insult [14]. While the mechanisms or angiogenesis remain unclear, it is recognized that astrocytes may play a critical role [15]. Brain capillary endothelial cells in culture form tubes when co-cultured with astrocytes. This formation of capillary tubes in co-culture is blocked when P450 enzymes are inhibited [15]. Even though there is a wealth of literature describing growth factors in the brain, identification of factors released by astrocytes under normal conditions remains largely undefined. VEGF does, indeed, induce endothelial tube formation when cells are plated on a matrix such as matrigel. However, release of VEGF from astrocytes occurs only in the presence of hypoxia or other insult [16].

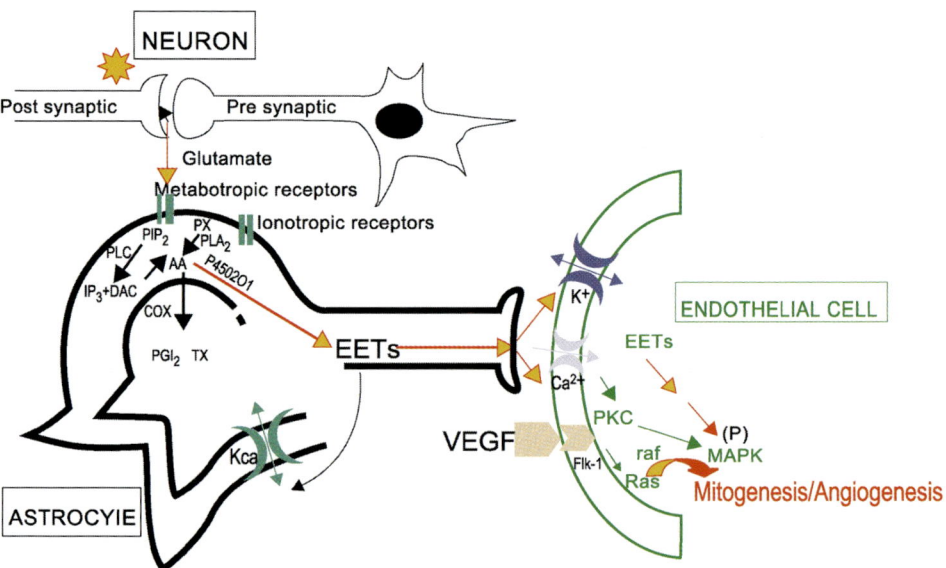

Fig. 3. Schematic representation of overall hypothesis. Glutamate is released from synaptic junctions upon activation of neurons. This "spillover" of glutamate stimulates astrocytes to release AA from the phospholipid pools by action of the lipases. Released free AA in the astrocyte is converted to EETs by microsomal epoxygenases (P450 2C11) or to PGI₂/Tx by cyclooxygenases. The EETs are released from the foot processes of astrocytes onto neighboring endothelial cells, which hyperpolarize endothelial membrane, stimulate proliferation and angiogenesis via tyrosine kinase cascades (Ras-MEK-MAP, etc.). VEGF released by astrocytes following insults activates MAP kinase pathway via binding to its receptor Flk-1 on endothelial cells.

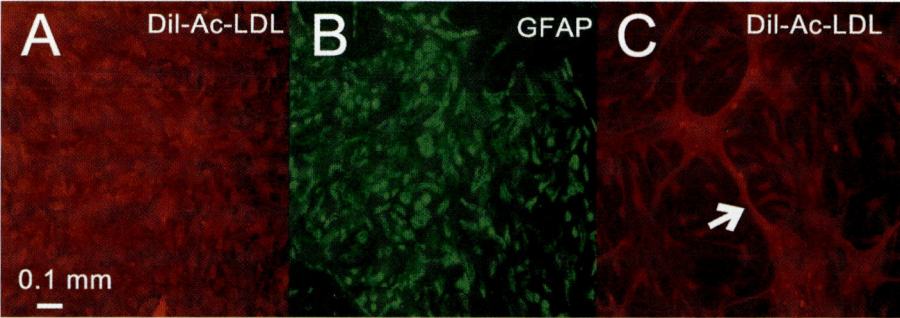

Fig. 4. Changes in morphology of microvascular endothelial cells and astrocytes when co-cultured. (A, B) Show the morphology of microvascular endothelial cells (A) and astrocytes (B) when they were cultured alone. Endothelial cells were stained with Dil-Ac-LDL (red). Astrocytes were immunoreacted with specific antibodies against glial fibrillary acidic protein (GFAP, green). (C) Formation of tubes in co-culture of cerebral capillary endothelial cells and astrocytes. Scale bar, 0.1 mm.

Not all growth factors are peptides. There are a number of reports describing the mitogenic and angiogenic properties of fatty acid metabolites. Among the most potent are AA metabolites of P450 enzymes including EETs [17–19]. Infusion of 11,12-EET into the eye stimulates such intense angiogenic activity that it leads to blindness. The mechanism of action of EETs, with respect to directing endothelial cells to undergo mitogenesis, and ultimately, tube formation appears to involve increased intracellular Ca^{2+}, and activation of Ca^{2+}-dependent 2nd messengers, phosphatases and kinases. Highlighting this point is the observation that depletion of intracellular Ca^{2+} pools in vascular smooth muscle with tahapsigargin block a mitogenic activity [20]. Addition of 11,12-EET completely restored mitogenic activity which was accompanied by increased intracellular Ca^{2+} [21]. Similarly, vasoactive agents such as norepinepherine, angiotensin and others have mitogenic actions which are dependent on AA and elevation of intracellular Ca^{2+}, and which are blocked by pharmacological inhibition of P450 enzyme activity [22]. 14,15-EET induces mitogenic activity in renal epithelial cells [18]. Finally, there is a growing literature regarding the role of P450 metabolites of AA in coronary angiogenesis and collateral vessel development. The scenario depicting the hypothesized actions of EETs on cerebral angiogenesis is shown in Fig. 3. The physical evidence that such a mechanism occurs is seen in Fig. 4. When astrocytes and capillary endothelium are plated separately they exhibit a normal morphology and phenotype. However, when plated together under co-culture conditions there is a dramatic change in morphology of both cell types. Endothelial cells form tubes and astrocytes send projections that make contact with these tubes at discrete locations analogous to the situation which occurs in vivo (Fig. 4A–C).

3. Interaction between VEGF and P450 metabolites

The literature on the vascular biology of growth factors is large. We have provided evidence that P450 metabolites play a role in capillary tube formation—a process which appears to be orchestrated by astrocytes. Embryologically, astrocytes and blood vessels exhibit a similar regional distribution. Vessel encroachment by astrocytic processes increases during fetal life [23]. We know that AA P450 metabolites are potent regulators of ion conductance systems in the cerebral vasculature. We do not know, however, if the action of these fatty acid para- and autocrine metabolites on ion channels and membrane potential function in any way to mediate their potent mitogenic actions. There are suggestions in the literature that the actions of VEGF require, and induce vasodilation [24]. In the cerebral circulation, one of the primary mechanisms of arteriolar dilation is activation of K^+ channels which brings membrane potential toward the equilibrium potential for K^+, thereby, hyperpolarizing cells in the vessel wall [25,26]. Shear stress is the calculated force of fluid and particulate exerted in the vascular wall. Increasing blood flow increases shear stress. Increases in shear function as a precursor to vascular remodeling and capillary formation [27]. One of the mechanisms through which increased arterial/arteriolar wall shear stress transduces signaling events is through hyperpolarization of vascular endothelium which increases intracellular Ca^{2+} and release of nitric oxide (NO) and endothelium-derived hyperpolarizing factor (EDHF). The only EDHF to be chemically identified by analytical biochemical methods are P450-derived EETs [28].

We have chemically identified the structure of hyperpolarizing factors released from astrocytes as P450-derived EETs [9,29]. Inhibition of nitric oxide synthase (NOS) blocks the angiogenic actions of VEGF [30]. EETs and NO have similar actions on vascular cells including activation of K^+ channels and membrane hyperpolarization [31]. At this point, we can only speculate that EETs will have similar actions as NO in facilitating the actions of VEGF. There are, however, a number of reports which speculate that membrane hyperpolarization and/or inhibition of vasoconstriction is requisite for angiogenesis in the brain [24,30]. Even though we have demonstrated that EETs induce cerebral capillary angiogenesis independent of VEGF under normoxic conditions, it is possible to speculate that EETs may function in a manner similar to NO with respect to the mitogenic actions of VEGF in brain capillary endothelium.

Acknowledgements

This work was supported in part by VA Merit Grant 3440 and NHLBI grant 5-RO1-HL33833-17.

References

[1] I. Aramori, S. Nakanishi, Signal transduction and pharmacological characteristics of metabotropic glutamate receptor, mGluR1, in transfected CHO cells, Neuron 8 (1992) 757–765.

[2] S. Miller, R.J. Bridges, A.R. Chamberlin, C.W. Cotman, Pharmacological dissociation of glutamatergic metabotropic signal transduction pathways in cortical astrocytes, Eur. J. Pharmacol. 269 (2) (1994) 235–241.

[3] Z. Cai, H.K. Kimelberg, Glutamate receptor-mediated calcium responses in acutely isolated hippocampal astrocytes, Glia 21 (1997) 380–389.

[4] J. Chen, K.H. Backus, J.W. Deitmer, Intracellular calcium transients and potassium current oscillations evoked by glutamate in cultured rat astrocytes, J. Neurosci. 17 (1997) 7278–7287.

[5] E.A. Dennis, S.G. Rhee, M. Billah, Y.A. Hannun, Role of phospholipases in generating lipid second messengers in signal transduction, FASEB J. 5 (1991) 2068–2077.

[6] M.J. Berridge, Inositol triphosphate and diacylglycerol: two interacting second messengers, Annu. Rev. Biochem. 56 (1987) 159–193.

[7] P. Needleham, J. Turk, B.A. Jakschik, A.R. Morrison, J.B. Lefkowith, Arachidonic acid metabolism, Annu. Rev. Biochem. 55 (1986) 69–102.

[8] D.R. Harder, A.R. Lange, D. Gebremedhin, E.K. Briks, R.J. Roman, Cytochrome P450 metabolites of arachidonic acid as intracellular signaling molecules in vascular tissue, J. Vasc. Res. 34 (1997) 237–243.

[9] N.J. Alkayed, J. Narayanan, D. Gebremedhin, M. Medhora, R.J. Roman, D.R. Harder, Molecular characterization of an arachidonic acid epoxygenase in rat brain astrocytes, Stroke 5 (1996) 971–979.

[10] J.E. Brayden, M.T. Nelson, Regulation of arterial tone by activation of calcium-dependent potassium channels, Science 256 (1992) 532–535.

[11] D. Gebremedhin, Y.-H. Ma, J.R. Falck, R.J. Roman, M. VanRollins, D.R. Harder, Mechanism of action of cerebral epoxyeicosatrienoic acids on cerebral arterial smooth muscle, Am. J. Physiol. 263 (1992) H519–H525.

[12] D. Shweiki, A. Itin, D. Soffer, E. Keshet, Vascular endothelial growth factor induced by hypoxia may mediate hypoxia-initiated angiogenesis, Nature 359 (6398) (1992) 843–845.

[13] K.R. Issacs, B.J. Anderson, A.A. Alcantara, J.E. Black, W.T. Greenough, Exercise and the brain: angiogenesis in the adult rat cerebellum after vigorous physical activity and motor skill learning, J. Cereb. Blood Flow Metab. 12 (1992) 110–119.

[14] R.N. Kalaria, D.L. Cohen, D.R. Premkumar, S. Nag, J.C. LaManna, W.D. Lust, Vascular endothelial growth factor in Alzheimer's disease and experimental cerebral ischemia, Brain Res. Mol. Brain Res. 62 (1) (1998) 101–105.

[15] D.H. Munzenmaier, D.R. Harder, Cerebral microvascular endothelial cell tube formation: role of astrocytic epoxyeicosatrienoic acid release, Am. J. Physiol. 278 (4) (2000) H1163–H1167.

[16] H.H. Mart, W. Risau, Systemic hypoxia changes the organ-specific distribution of vascular endothelial growth factor and its receptors, Proc. Natl. Acad. Sci. U. S. A. 95 (1998) 15809–15814.

[17] R.C. Harris, T. Homma, H.R. Jacobson, J. Capdevila, Epoxyeicosatrienoic acids activate Na^+/H^+ exchange and are mitogenic in cultured rat glomerular messangial cells, J. Cell. Physiol. 144 (3) (1990) 429–437.

[18] J.K. Chen, J.R. Falck, K.M. Reddy, J. Capdevilla, R.C. Harris, Epoxyeicosatrienoic acids and their sulfonamide derivatives stimulate tyrosine phosphorylation and induce mitogenesis in renal epithelial cells, J. Biol. Chem. 273 (44) (1998) 29254–29260.

[19] J.K. Chen, D.W. Wang, J.R. Falck, J. Capdevila, R.C. Harris, Transfection of an active cytochrome P450 arachidonic acid epoxygenase indicates that 14, 15-epoxyeicosatrienoic acid functions as an intracellular second messenger in response to epidermal growth factor, J. Biol. Chem. 274 (1999) 4764–4769.

[20] N. Shukla, N. Freeman, P. Gadsdon, G.D. Angelini, J.Y. Jeremy, Thapsigargin inhibits angiogenesis in the rat isolated aorta: studies on the role of intracellular pools, Cardiovasc. Res. 49 (2001) 681–689.

[21] M.N. Graber, A. Olfanso, D.L. Gill, Recovery of calcium pools and growth-depleted is mediated by specific epoxyeicosatrienoic acids derived from arachidonic acid, J. Biol. Chem. 272 (1997) 29546–29553.

[22] N.O. Dulin, L.D. Alexander, S. Harwalkar, J.R. Falck, J.G. Douglas, Phospholipase A_2 mediated activation of mitogen-activated kinase by angiotensin, Proc. Natl. Acad. Sci. 95 (1998) 80098–80102.

[23] K.H. Plate, Mechanism of angiogenesis in the brain, J. Neuropathol. Exp. Neurol. 58 (1999) 313–320.

[24] M. Ziche, L. Morbidelli, Nitric oxide and angiogenesis, J. Neurooncol. 50 (2000) 139–148.

[25] J.E. Brayden, M.T. Nelson, Regulation of arterial tone by activation of calcium-dependent potassium channels, Science 256 (1992) 532–535.

[26] M.T. Nelson, J.B. Patlak, J.F. Worley, N.B. Standen, Calcium channels, potassium channels, and voltage dependence of arterial smooth muscle tone, Am. J. Physiol. 259 (1990) C3–C18.

[27] D.A. Tulis, J.L. Unthank, R.L. Prewitt, Flow-induced arterial remodeling in rat mesenteric vasculature, Am. J. Physiol. 274 (1998) H874–H882.

[28] W.B. Campbell, D. Gebremedhin, P.F. Pratt, D.R. Harder, Identification of epoxyeicosatrienoic acids as endothelium-derived hyperpolarizing factors, Circ. Res. 78 (1996) 415–423.

[29] S.C. Amruthesh, M.F. Boerschel, J.S. McKinney, K.A. Willoughby, E.F. Ellis, Metabolism of arachidonic

acid to epoxyeicosatrienoic acids, hydroxyeicsatetraenoic acids and prostaglandins in cultured rat hippo-campal astrocytes, J. Neurochem. 61 (1) (1993) 150–159.

[30] A. Papapetropoulos, G. Garcia-Gradena, J.A. Madri, W.C. Sessa, Nitric oxide production contributes to the angiogenic properties of vascular endothelial growth factor in human endothelial cells, J. Clin. Invest. 100 (12) (1997) 3131–3139.

[31] M. Wahl, L. Schilling, Regulation of cerebral blood flow—a brief review, Acta Neurohir., Suppl. 59 (1993) 3–10.

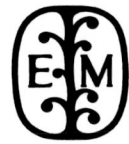

International Congress Series 1235 (2002) 305–312

Effects of activation of glutamate receptors on neurons and blood vessels

David W. Busija [a,*], Ferenc Domoki [b],
Ferenc Bari [b], Thomas M. Louis [c]

[a]*Department of Physiology and Pharmacology School of Medicine, Wake Forest University,
Medical Center Boulevard, Winston-Salem, NC 27157, USA*
[b]*Department of Physiology, University of Szeged, Szeged, Hungary*
[c]*Department of Anatomy and Cell Biology, Brody School of Medicine of East Carolina University,
Greenville, NC, USA*

Abstract

Glutamate dilates pial arterioles in piglets via activation of N-methyl-D-aspartate (NMDA) receptors and increases cortical glucose utilization. Administration of NMDA, the chemical compound which was used to characterize this glutamate receptor subtype, dilates cerebral arteries via activation of nitric oxide synthase (NOS) in neurons and subsequent actions of nitric oxide (NO) on vascular smooth muscle. Thus, administration of inhibitors of NOS attenuates NMDA-induced arteriolar dilation, while inhibitors of cyclooxygenase and cytochrome P-450 epoxygenase do not alter the vascular response. Additionally, inhibition of adenosine receptors and endothelial "stunning" do not alter arteriolar dilation to NMDA. Finally, NO metabolites accumulate on the cortical surface following NMDA application. We conclude that NMDA-induced arteriolar dilation is via direct actions on smooth muscle of NO synthesized and released by cortical neurons. NMDA-induced dilator responses are severely restricted after ischemia-reperfusion. Previous studies have shown that potassium channel activators given prior to ischemia preserve responses after ischemia. However, intracellular localization of this effect is unclear. We provide evidence to indicate that activation of K_{ATP} on mitochondria by diazoxide is able to provide neuroprotection against ischemic stress, probably by restricting calcium entry into mitochondria. Use of selective activators of K_{ATP} on mitochondria could be a new therapeutic approach to protect the brain against ischemic stress.
© 2002 Elsevier Science B.V. All rights reserved.

Keywords: Ischemia; Potassium channels; Mitochondria; N-methyl-D-aspartate; Nitric oxide; Diazoxide; Endothelium

* Corresponding author. Tel.: +1-336-716-4355, fax: +1-336-716-0237.
E-mail address: dbusija@wfubmc.edu (D.W. Busija).

0531-5131/02 © 2002 Elsevier Science B.V. All rights reserved.
PII: S 0 5 3 1 - 5 1 3 1 (0 2) 0 0 1 9 9 - 1

1. Introduction

Glutamate is one of the most prevalent neurotransmitters in the brain and activates at least three different types of receptors on neurons; alpha-amino-3-hydroxy-5-methyl-4-isoxazolepropionate or AMPA, kainate, and N-methyl-D-aspartate (NMDA) receptors. In the newborn pig, glutamate dilates pial arterioles via a mechanism involving activation of NMDA receptors and is associated with increased glucose utilization [1,2] (Fig. 1). Further, the link between glutamate actions on NMDA receptors and increased metabolic rate appears to involve synthesis of nitric oxide (NO) by neurons and subsequent actions of NO on cerebral resistance vessels [1,3] (Fig. 2). However, many elements of this series of events are either unknown or controversial. For example, the disassociation between nitric oxide synthase (NOS) containing neurons and NMDA-positive neurons in the cerebral cortex [4] implies that additional cells and substances might be involved in coupling of NMDA receptor activation and dilation of pial arterioles. Recently, Bhardwaj et al. [5] have found that cytochrome P-450 metabolites of arachidonic acid are essential mediators of blood flow responses in the striatum after infusion of NMDA, the chemical compound that was used to define the receptor subtype. However, this relationship has not been explored adequately in the cerebral cortex or in another species.

Another unique characteristic of NMDA-induced arteriolar dilator responses in the cerebral cortex is its susceptibility to reduced oxygen levels. Thus, even brief periods of arterial hypoxia [4], asphyxia [6], or ischemia [7], followed by reperfusion/reoxygenation, severely reduces arteriolar dilator responses to NMDA (Fig. 2). This attenuation of dilation apparently is at the level of the NMDA receptor [8] and is prevented by administration of oxygen radical scavengers [6,9], cyclooxygenase inhibitors [6], and more recently by activators of potassium channels [10,11] (Fig. 3). While metabolism of arachidonic acid by

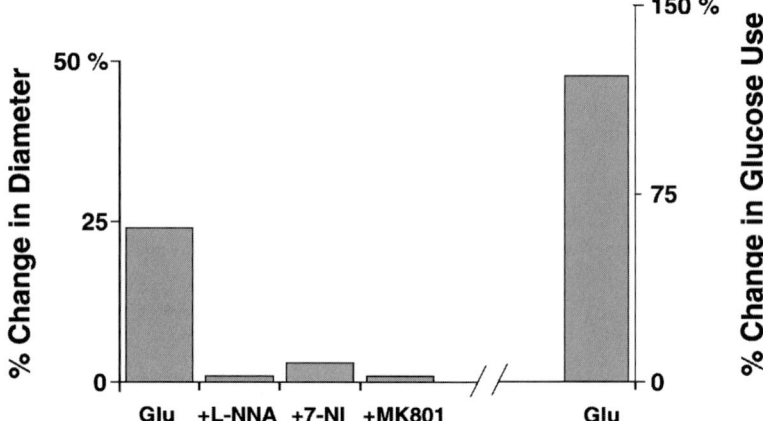

Fig. 1. Glutamate effects on pial arteriolar diameter and glucose utilization in cerebral cortex. Glutamate at 10^{-3} M dilated arterioles, and effects were blocked by N^G-nitro-L-arginine (L-NNA), 7-nitroindazole (7-NI), and MK-801. Further, glutamate increases brain metabolic rate as measured by the ^{14}C-deoxyglucose method. Thus, NO production following activation of NMDA receptors may couple blood flow and metabolism in the cortex. Original data from Refs. [1,2,14].

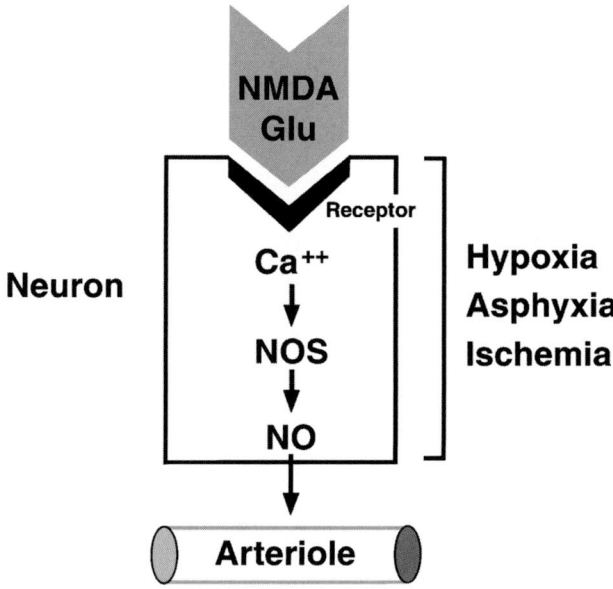

Fig. 2. Schematic illustration depicting generalized sequence of steps involved in NMDA- or glutamate-induced arteriolar dilation and susceptibility of this response to hypoxic or ischemic stress in piglet cortex. Effects of hypoxic or ischemic stress with reoxgenation appear to be localized to the NMDA receptor since NOS activity of cortical cells and sodium nitroprusside-induced dilation are not affected. Supporting data from Refs. [1,3,4,6–9].

cyclooxygenase at the onset of reperfusion has been shown to generate substantial amounts of superoxide anion, which could interfere with receptor function, the mechanism of protection of neuronal function by potassium channel activators is unclear. However, one possible mechanism of protection could involve ATP-sensitive potassium channels (K_{ATP}) located on neuronal mitochondria. Activation of K_{ATP} in cardiac myocytes has been shown to limit infarct volume following ischemia in the heart [12]. However, effects of activation of K_{ATP} on neuronal function in vivo have not been examined thoroughly.

2. Mechanism of dilator responses to NMDA

We made the initial discovery that glutamate or NMDA was able to dilate resistance vessels in the cerebral circulation [13] (Fig. 1). Further, we showed that glutamate was able to increase glucose utilization by the cerebral cortex [2] (Fig. 1). The dilator response to glutamate or NMDA was not reduced by indomethacin [13] or theophylline [4] pretreatment, but has been shown by several investigators starting with Faraci and Breese [3] and Bari et al. [14] to involve synthesis of NO probably from cortical neurons (Figs. 1 and 2). Thus, a simplistic approach suggests that neuronal release and actions of NO directly on resistance vessels could provide the link between coupling of metabolism and blood flow during neuronal activation. If this model was correct, it would indicate that in brain tissue NO could diffuse over considerable distances and affect other cells including vascular

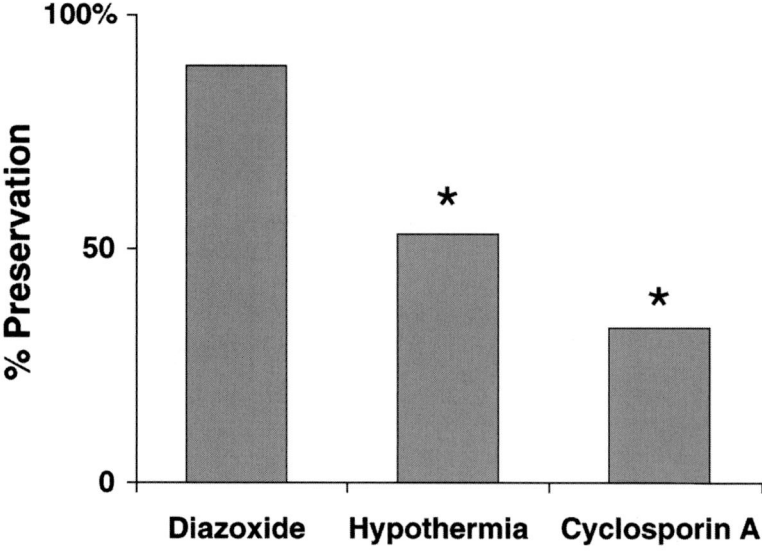

Fig. 3. Specificity of diazoxide effects on preservation of NMDA-induced dilation following ischemia and reperfusion. Pretreatment of diazoxide (10^{-5} M) ($n=5$), but not cyclosporin A (10^{-4} M) ($n=6$) and also not hypothermia (34 °C) ($n=8$), preserved arteriolar dilation to NMDA (ratio of averaged data for first and second dilator responses to NMDA). Unpublished data. *$p<0.05$, compared to vasodilator response to NMDA before ischemia.

smooth muscle. However, there are at least two studies that indicate that this relationship may be more complex. First, we have failed to observe extensive co-localization between bNOS-positive and NMDA-positive neurons in the cerebral cortex of piglets [4], thereby suggesting additional cells and substances may be involved. Second, Bhardwaj et al. [5] have recently shown the presence of a mandatory step involving synthesis and actions of a cytochrome P-450 epoxygenase metabolite in addition to NO production in rat striatum in order for NMDA to increase CBF. Thus, blockade of production of either substance is sufficient to prevent NMDA-induced blood flow changes. Consequently, we extended our earlier studies to investigate this possibility in the piglet cortex.

In contrast to the earlier study in rats, however, we could find no evidence for involvement of cytochrome P-450 epoxygenase metabolites in piglets [15]. Thus, either co-application of miconazole, a potent but nonspecific inhibitor of P-450 epoxygenase, with NMDA or repeated application of miconazole over 60 min prior to co-application with NMDA failed to alter NMDA-induced dilation. Further, NMDA-induced dilation was accompanied with increased accumulation of NO breakdown products on the cortical surface [15]. Lastly, dilation of arteriolar segments over surface veins was reduced compared to segments directly over the cortex, thereby implying that a diffusable substance from the brain parenchyma was involved in mediating dilation to NMDA (data not shown). Transient stunning of the endothelium to remove the influence of flow-mediated dilation of surface arteries fails to change dilator responses to NMDA [15]. Thus, we conclude that NO is the only identified substance mediating NMDA-induced dilation of pial arterioles in pigs, and that synthesis of NO from cortical neurons and diffusion of

NO from deep within the cortex to arterioles mediates dilation. While it is possible that other cell types or substances involve in this response will be identified in the future, we speculate that NO may be relatively stable in brain tissue in vivo and, thus, exert actions at sites quite distant from synthesis.

3. Role of K_{ATP} in neuroprotection against ischemia

We have shown that ischemic stress, as well as arterial hypoxia and asphyxia, followed by reperfusion/reoxygenation are able to severely attenuate arteriolar dilator responses to NMDA [4,6,7] (Fig. 2). Further, we and others have shown that pretreatment with potassium channel activators is able to either reverse this attenuation of vascular dilation or to protect neurons [10]. However, a major drawback of previous studies was the lack of information concerning subcellular localization of actions of potassium channel openers since potassium channels are located on the sarcolemmal as well as mitochondrial membranes.

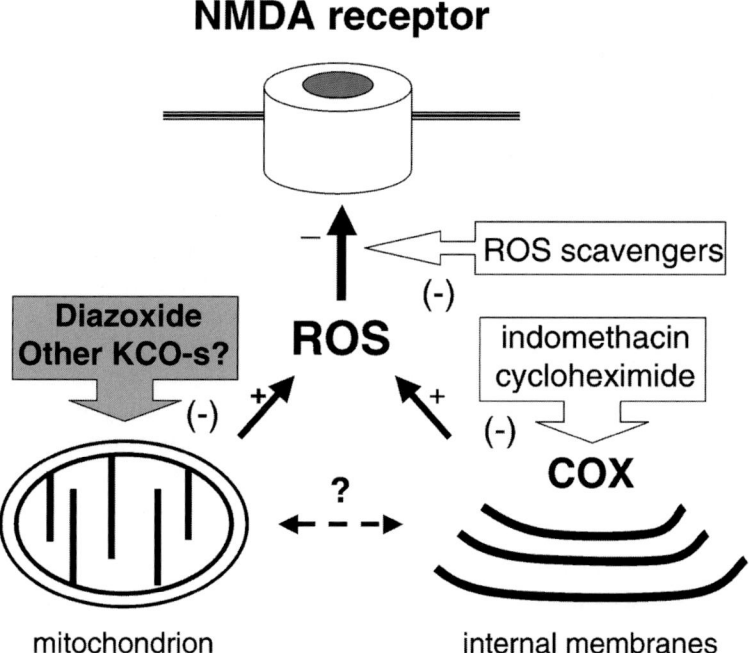

Fig. 4. Schematic illustration concerning mechanism of protection by diazoxide. On the right side is represented the cyclooxygenase pathway for production of reactive oxygen species (ROS) that can depress function of the NMDA receptor. A parallel pathway may involve ROS released by the mitochondria during ischemia/reperfusion (left side). Pretreatment with diazoxide and activation of K_{ATP} would depolarize mitochondria prior to ischemia and perhaps attenuate calcium influx and ROS release during ischemia/reperfusion. We speculate that synergy between the cyclooxygenase and mitochondrial systems is necessary for ROS inhibition of NMDA receptor function either due to total amounts of ROS available or due to facilitatory or permissive effects of one system to the other system.

Following pretreatment with diazoxide, a selective inhibitor of mitochondrial K_{ATP}, we found that we were able to preserve dilator response to NMDA following ischemic stress in a dose-dependent fashion [11]. Additionally, protective actions of diazoxide were reversed by 5-hydroxydecanoic acid, an antagonist of mitochondrial K_{ATP}. Thus, selective activation of potassium channels located on mitochondria offers protection of neurons against ischemic stress as it does in cardiomyocytes [12]. Our previous studies with NS1619 may also indicate that calcium-activated potassium channels may also be located on mitochondria and also serve to protect neurons [10]. Effects of K_{ATP} also appear to be specific since cyclosporin A and hypothermia fail to preserve NMDA-induced dilation after ischemia (Fig. 3). Cyclosporin A blocks the permeability transition pore in mitochondria in damaged neurons and hypothermia nonspecifically decreases brain metabolism and, thus, mitochondrial function in neurons. While the mechanism of protection by activation of K_{ATP} is not known precisely, one possibility is that mitochondrial depolarization prior to ischemia lessens the influx of calcium into this organelle and consequently allows rapid recovery of mitochondrial function during reperfusion (Fig. 4).

4. Summary and conclusions

Application of NMDA to the cortical surface is a useful approach by which to investigate the linkage between neuronal activation, increased metabolism, and resistance vessel responses in the brain. NMDA-induced arteriolar dilation in the cortex is due to synthesis of NO by cortical neurons and subsequent diffusion and actions of NO on vascular smooth muscle. While other substances or additional cells may be involved in mediating overall responses, we have eliminated a significant role of prostanoids, adenosine, and *P*-450 epoxygenase products. Additionally, we have found that NMDA-induced arteriolar dilation is very susceptible to ischemic stress, and that activation of mitochondrial K_{ATP} is able to preserve this response. While the exact mechanism of neuroprotection by activation of mitochondrial K_{ATP} is not know with precision, it appears to be specific and may be related to the prevention of calcium entry into mitochondria during ischemia. Nonetheless, use of pharmacological agents that modulate function of K_{ATP} may provide protection of the brain against ischemic insults or other neuropathological diseases.

3.1.7.7. On-Site Discussion

3.1.7.7.1. *Question: (Pelligrino)* I think your results indicate that despite the relative paucity of nNOS-positive neurons in the cortex (1–2% of neurons) that surface vessels like the pial arterioles are quite sensitive to nNOS activation. This suggests that NO diffusion is rather extensive within brain tissue and/or that nNOS neurons have an extensive distribution arising from neuronal processes connected to these cells.

Answer: (Busija) You are correct on both points. We believe that NO produced by NMDA application is able to diffuse up to 500 μm through cortex and dilate surface arterioles. Further, based upon the intensity of nNOS staining and the extensive branching of these neurons, we believe that the total potentiation for NO production in cortex is quite substantial.

3.1.7.7.2. *Question: (Hamel)* NO neurons have cell bodies deep in cortex, but this may be misleading as dendorites or terminals project widely in cortex; thus, NMDA receptors may be located not on cell bodies only, but also on projections.

Answer: (Busija) Indeed, in our original paper, we pointed out the extensive ramifications and projections of the nNOS-containing neurons in the cortex. We believe that the amount and locations of nNOS with respect to the vasculature is able to support our suggestion that enough NO is produced during NMDA receptor activation to account for the arteriolar dilator responses observed.

3.1.7.7.3. *Question: (Benyó)* Your results demonstrate that K^+ channel openers prevent the reduction of NMDA-induced pial arteriolar dilations after ischemia. Activation of K^+ channels by increased $[Ca^{2+}]_i$ could, therefore, also act as a protective mechanism during and after ischemia. Did you try if K^+ channel blockers augment the ischemia-induced reduction of the NMDA response?

Answer: (Busija) We have not done these experiments yet.

3.1.7.7.4. *Question: (Traystman)* Does NMDA placed on the surface of brain of NOS KO animals have any effect on V.D. of vessels?

Answer: (Busija) We have not done these experiments yet.

Acknowledgements

Supported by grants HL-30260, HL-46558, and HL-50587 from the National Institutes of Health and grant-in-aid #9951272U from the American Heart Association.

References

[1] W. Meng, J.R. Tobin, D.W. Busija, Glutamate-induced cerebral vasodilation is mediated by nitric oxide through *N*-methyl-D-aspartate receptors, Stroke 26 (1995) 857–863.

[2] W.M. Armstead, R. Mirro, S. Zuckerman, D.W. Busija, C.W. Leffler, The influence of opioids on local cerebral glucose utilization in the newborn pig, Brain Res. 571 (1992) 97–102.

[3] F.M. Faraci, K.R. Breese, Nitric oxide mediates vasodilation in response to activation of *N*-methyl-D-aspartate receptors in brain, Circ. Res. 72 (1993) 476–480.

[4] F. Bari, C.R. Thore, T.M. Louis, D.W. Busija, Inhibitory effects of hypoxia and adenosine on *N*-methyl-D-aspartate-induced pial arteriolar dilation in piglets, Brain Res. 780 (1998) 237–244.

[5] A. Bhardwaj, F.J. Northington, J.R. Carhuapoma, J.R. Falck, D.R. Harder, R.J. Traystman, R.C. Koehler, P-450 epoxygenase and NO synthase inhibitors reduce cerebral blood flow response to *N*-methyl-D-aspartate, Am. J. Physiol. 279 (2000) H1616–H1624.

[6] D.W. Busija, W. Meng, Altered cerebrovascular responsiveness to *N*-methyl-D-aspartate after asphyxia in piglets, Am. J. Physiol. 265 (1993) H389–H394.

[7] D.W. Busija, W. Meng, F. Bari, P.S. McGough, R.A. Errico, J.R. Tobin, T.M. Louis, Effects of ischemia on cerebrovascular responses to *N*-methyl-D-aspartate in piglets, Am. J. Physiol. 270 (1996) H1225–H1230.

[8] D.J. Hoffman, J.E. McGowan, P.J. Marro, O.P. Mishra, M. Delivoria-Papadopoulos, Hypoxia-induced modification of the *N*-methyl-D-aspartate receptor in the brain of the newborn piglet, Neurosci. Lett. 167 (1994) 156–160.

[9] F. Bari, R.A. Errico, T.M. Louis, D.W. Busija, Differential effects of short-term hypoxia and hypercapnia on *N*-methyl-D-aspartate-induced cerebral vasodilatation in piglets, Stroke 27 (1996) 1634–1640.

[10] R. Veltkamp, F. Domoki, F. Bari, D.W. Busija, Potassium channel activators protect the *N*-methyl-D-aspartate-induced cerebral vascular dilation after combined hypoxia and ischemia in piglets, Stroke 29 (1998) 837–843.

[11] F. Domoki, J.V. Perciaccante, R. Veltkamp, F. Bari, D.W. Busija, Mitochondrial potassium channel opener diazoxide preserves neuronal-vascular function after cerebral ischemia in newborn pigs, Stroke 30 (1999) 2713–2719.

[12] G.J. Gross, R. Fryer, Sarcolemmal versus mitochondrial ATP-sensitive K^+ channels and myocardial pre-conditioning, Circ. Res. 84 (1999) 973–979.

[13] D.W. Busija, C.W. Leffler, Dilator effects of amino acid neurotransmitters on piglet pial arterioles, Am. J. Physiol. 257 (1989) H1200–H1203.

[14] F. Bari, R.S. Errico, T.M. Louis, D.W. Busija, Interaction between ATP-sensitive K^+ channels and nitric oxide on pial arterioles in piglets, J. Cereb. Blood Flow Metab. 16 (1996) 1158–1164.

[15] D. Domoki, F. Bari, J. Perciaccante, M. Puskar, D.W. Busija, *N*-methyl-D-aspartate-induced vasodilation is mediated by endothelium-independent nitric oxide release in piglets, FASEB J. 15 (2001) A126, abstract.

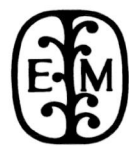

International Congress Series 1235 (2002) 313–324

The metabotropic glutamate receptor system: a novel pathway for the molecular protection against microvascular programmed cell death

Kenneth Maiese [a,b,c,d,*], Shi-Hua Lin [a], Zhao Zhong Chong [a]

[a]*Division of Cellular and Molecular Cerebral Ischemia, Wayne State University School of Medicine, Detroit, MI 48201, USA*
[b]*Departments of Neurology and Anatomy and Cell Biology, Wayne State University School of Medicine, Detroit, MI 48201, USA*
[c]*Center for Molecular Medicine and Genetics, Wayne State University School of Medicine, Detroit, MI 48201, USA*
[d]*Center for Molecular and Cellular Toxicology, Wayne State University School of Medicine, Detroit, MI 48201, USA*

Abstract

Specific metabotropic glutamate receptor (mGluR) subtypes can prevent neuronal programmed cell death (PCD), but the role of the mGluR subtypes in the cerebrovascular endothelial cell (EC) system is not known. EC degeneration may be dependent upon the generation of the free radical nitric oxide (NO) and the subsequent induction of programmed cell death (PCD). In rat cerebrovascular ECs, we examined the modulation of Group I mGluR subtypes during NO toxicity. Cell injury was determined through trypan blue dye exclusion, DNA fragmentation, membrane phosphatidylserine (PS) exposure, and cysteine protease activity following treatment with the NO generators SNP (1000 μM) or NOC-9 (1000 μM). NO-induced EC injury was principally linked to the induction of PCD and was dependent upon both caspase 1- and caspase 3-like activities. Activation of the Group I mGluR system with (S)-3,5-dihydroxyphenylglycine (DHPG, 750 μM), but not antagonism, significantly decreased EC DNA fragmentation, membrane PS exposure, and relied on the specific downregulation of caspase 1- and caspase 3-like activities. The ability of Group I mGluR system to protect cerebrovascular ECs from NO-induced PCD may have important therapeutic implications for disorders that tightly integrate both neuronal and vascular pathways.
© 2002 Elsevier Science B.V. All rights reserved.

Keywords: Apoptosis; Endothelial cells; Cysteine proteases; Metabotropic glutamate receptors; Phosphatidylserine

* Corresponding author. Department of Neurology, 8C-1 UHC, Wayne State University School of Medicine, 4201 St. Antoine, Detroit, MI 48201, USA. Tel.: +1-313-966-0833; fax: +1-313-966-0486.
E-mail address: kmaiese@med.wayne.edu (K. Maiese).

0531-5131/02 © 2002 Elsevier Science B.V. All rights reserved.
PII: S 0 5 3 1 - 5 1 3 1 (0 2) 0 0 2 0 0 - 5

1. Introduction

Endothelial cell (EC) injury can be initiated by several different stimuli that ultimately lead to apoptosis or programmed cell death (PCD). PCD consists of two distinct components that involve DNA degradation and the loss of membrane asymmetry with exposure of membrane phosphatidylserine (PS) residues [1,2]. The cleavage of genomic DNA into fragments can occur once a cell has been committed to die. In contrast to DNA fragmentation, the redistribution of membrane PS residues from the inside of plasma membrane to the cell surface can occur early in the process of PCD [3]. Exposure of membrane PS residues can subsequently function to initiate both phagocytosis [4] and a hypercoagulable state in ECs [5].

Central to the mechanisms that contribute to EC injury is the generation of the free radical nitric oxide (NO) during toxic insults. In a positive light, NO has a significant role in the inhibition of platelet aggregation and the modulation of inflammatory cell adhesion [6,7]. Yet, NO is also an important contributor during ischemic injury and reperfusion insults [8,9]. As a result, injury to vascular ECs by NO can lead to the development of several disease states such as atherosclerosis and intravascular coagulation [10,11].

Recent work has suggested that the metabotropic glutamate receptor (mGluR) system may offer a novel alternative for the prevention of vascular EC injury. Although activation of specific subtypes of mGluRs has been shown to prevent neuronal injury during anoxia [12], glutamate toxicity [13], and free radical NO exposure [14,15], the role of the mGluR system in ECs remains to be defined. In the present study, we examined the role of the Group I mGluR system in rat cerebrovascular ECs during NO toxicity. Our work illustrates that Group I mGluR receptors are present in vascular ECs. The work is also the first to illustrate that EC protection by the Group I mGluR system prevents both the progression of NO-induced DNA degradation and membrane PS exposure. The ability of the mGluR system to prevent PCD in ECs is mediated through the direct modulation of caspase 1- and caspase 3-like activities and may provide significant protection against thrombotic and ischemic injury.

2. Materials and methods

2.1. EC cultures

Vascular ECs were isolated from Sprague–Dawley adult rat brains. Briefly, the cerebrum was suspended in a dissociation medium containing 1 mg/ml collagenase/dispase (Roche, Mannheim, Germany) in M199E with 0.5% antibiotic–antimycotic solution for 2 h at 37 °C. The slurry was homogenized, initially centrifuged at $4000 \times g$ for 20 min at 4 °C, and then resuspended and centrifuged at $20,000 \times g$ for 20 min at 10 °C. The pellet was then resuspended in culture media consisting of M199E with 20% heat-inactivated fetal bovine serum, 2 mM L-glutamine, 90 µg/ml heparin, and 20 µg/ml EC growth supplement (ICN Biomedicals, Aurora, OH). Cultures were maintained at 37 °C in a humidified atmosphere of 5% CO_2 and 95% room air with cells from the third passage. Cells were identified as endothelial by a cobblestone appearance with phase contrast microscopy, were negative for GFAP staining, and were positive for direct immunocytochemistry for factor VIII-related antigen. For each experimental paradigm, four to five Petri dishes (35 mm) of ECs were employed.

2.2. Immunocytochemistry for Group I mGluR 5/1

Following fixation in 4% paraformaldehyde and treatment with 0.3% H_2O_2, cells were incubated with the primary rabbit anti-mGluR 5/1 antibody (1:1000) (NOVUS Biologicals, CO) overnight at 4 °C. The detection was performed by Elite ABC kit (Vector Laboratories, Burlingame, CA) with the use of biotinylated goat anti-rabbit IgG (1:400) (Vector Laboratories).

2.3. Western blot analysis for Group I mGluR 5/1

Antibodies for the primary rabbit anti-mGluR 5/1 antibody (NOVUS Biologicals) were commercially obtained. Cells were homogenized with ice-cold buffer containing 20 mM Tris–HCl, pH 7.5, 1 mM EDTA, 5 mM $MgCl_2$, 1 mM DTT, 10 μg/ml PMSF, 1 μg/ml aprotinin, 1 μg/ml leupeptin. Each sample (30 μg/lane) was subjected to 7.5% SDS-polyacrylamide gel electrophoresis followed by a transfer onto a nitrocellulose membrane at high-field position. After blocking overnight at 4 °C with 5% skim milk, membranes were incubated for 2 h at room temperature with the primary rabbit anti-mGluR 5/1 antibody (1:1000). Subsequently, membranes were incubated with horseradish peroxidase conjugated secondary antibody (goat anti-rabbit IgG 1:2000, Pierce, Rockford, IL). The antibody-reactive bands were revealed by enhanced chemiluminescence detection on Hyperfilm (Amersham Pharmacia Biotech, Piscataway, NJ).

2.4. NO application and Group I metabotropic glutamate receptor modulation

NO administration was performed by replacing the culture media with media containing 6-(2-hydroxy-1-methyl-2-nitrosohydrazino)-N-methyl-l-hexanamine (NOC-9) (1000 μM) (Calbiochem, San Diego, CA) or sodium nitroprusside (SNP) (1000 μM) (Sigma, St. Louis, MO). Ligands for the metabotropic glutamate receptor subtypes (S)-3,5-dihydroxyphenylglycine (DHPG) and methylphenylethynylpyridine (MPEP) were obtained from Tocris Cookson (St. Louis, MO) and applied 1 h prior to NO exposure.

2.5. EC survival assays

EC injury was determined by bright field microscopy using a 0.4% trypan blue dye exclusion assay 24 h following treatment with the NO donors. For trypan blue dye exclusion, the mean survival was determined by counting eight randomly selected nonoverlapping fields with each containing approximately 10–20 cells (viable + nonviable).

2.6. Assessment of DNA fragmentation

Genomic DNA fragmentation was determined by the terminal deoxynucleotidyl transferase nick end labeling (TUNEL) assay. Briefly, cells were fixed in 4% paraformaldehyde/0.2% picric acid/0.05% glutaraldehyde in phosphate buffered saline solution (PBS: 10 mM KH_2PO_4, 37 mM Na_2HPO_4, 87 mM NaCl, 53 mM KCl, pH 7.4). Cells were permeabilized using 0.1% Triton X-100, then endogenous peroxidase was blocked using 0.3% H_2O_2 in methanol. The 3′-hydroxy ends of cut DNA were labeled with biotinylated dUTP (Promega, Madison, WI) using the enzyme terminal deoxytransferase (Promega). Incorporation of the label was detected using streptavidin–peroxidase (Sigma) and visualized with 3,3′-diaminobenzidine (Vector Laboratories).

2.7. Reversible membrane PS residue assay

Per our prior protocols [2], annexin V conjugated to phycoerythrin (PE) (R&D Systems, Minneapolis, MN) was prepared as a 30-µg/ml stock solution and diluted directly before use to 3 µg/ml in warmed (37 °C) binding buffer (10 mM HEPES, pH 7.5, 150 mM NaCl, 5 mM KCl, 1 mM $MgCl_2$, 1.8 mM $CaCl_2$). Plates were incubated with the annexin V conjugate at 37 °C in a humidified atmosphere in the dark for 10 min, then rinsed twice using fresh binding buffer. The ECs were examined using a Leitz DMIRB microscope (Leica, McHenry, IL) and Oncor Image 2.0 imaging software (Oncor, Gaithersburg, MD). Images were acquired using both transmitted light, as well as fluorescent single excitation light at 490 nm and detected emission at 585 nm.

2.8. Statistical analysis

For each experiment involving assessment of endothelial survival, DNA degradation, and membrane PS exposure, differences between groups were statistically analyzed by means of analysis of variance (ANOVA) with the post hoc Student's *t*-test. Statistical significance was considered at $p<0.05$.

3. Results

3.1. Expression of Group I mGluRs in ECs

Prior to the assessment of the biological role the Group I mGluR system may offer in ECs, we investigated whether the Group I mGluR was expressed in untreated ECs. Fig. 1A(1) illustrates untreated ECs that were not exposed to the anti-mGluR 5/1 antibody. In contrast, untreated ECs that are exposed to the anti-mGluR 5/1 antibody reveal the presence of the Group I mGluR system in primary rat ECs (Fig. 1A(2)). Following the detection of the Group I mGluR system through immunocytochemistry, we next assessed Group I mGluR 5/1 protein expression through Western analysis. Our work demonstrated the constitutive expression of a 145- and 44-kD segment of the Group I mGluR 5/1 proteins in ECs (Fig. 1B).

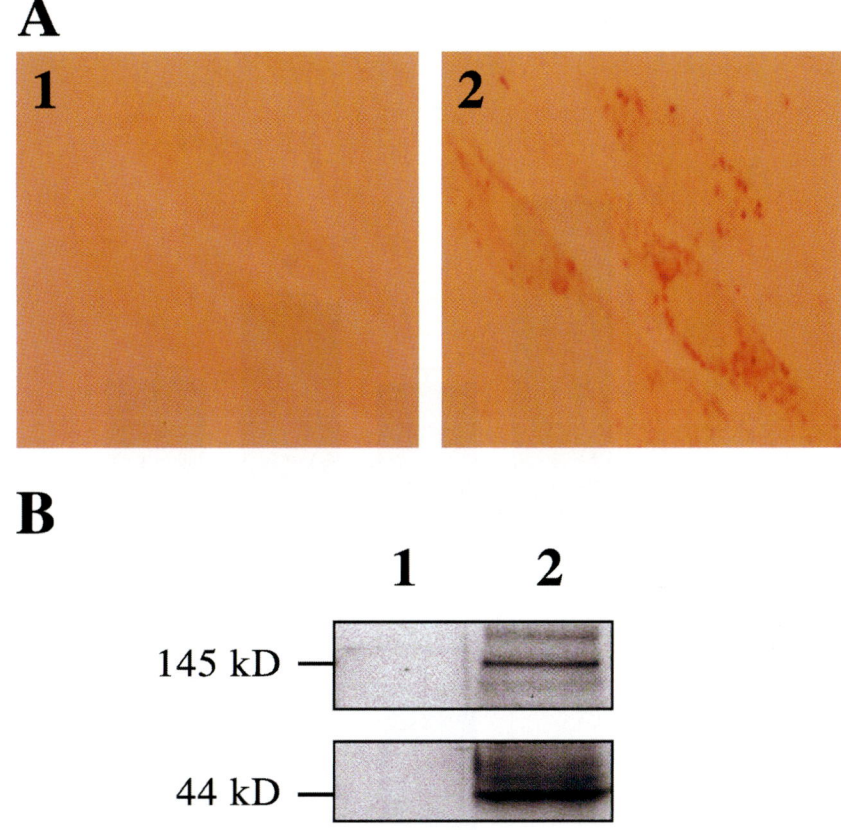

Fig. 1. Group I mGluRs are expressed in ECs. In (A), representative fields of ECs illustrate the constitutive presence of the Group I mGluR system following either no exposure to the anti-mGluR 5/1 antibody (A(1)) or with exposure to the anti-mGluR 5/1 antibody (1:1000) (A(2)). Detection was performed with the use of biotinylated goat anti-rabbit IgG (1:400). In (B), representative Western blots are illustrated for untreated ECs not exposed to the anti-mGluR 5/1 antibody (1) and for untreated ECs exposed to the anti-mGluR 5/1 antibody (2). Data presented are taken from one of the three individual experiments for each experimental group yielding similar results. All lanes received equal amounts of EC protein extracts (30 μg/lane).

3.2. Activation of Group I mGluRs prevents NO-induced toxicity in ECs

A NO-donor concentration of 1000 μM significantly decreased EC viability during a 24-h period (Fig. 2A). Activation of Group I mGluRs during NO exposure significantly increased EC survival with a concentration of 750 μM. For example, a 1-h pretreatment with the Group I agonist DHPG (750 μM) prior to NO exposure increased neuronal survival from approximately 39% (NO) to a plateau survival of 66% (Fig. 2A). Yet, application of the antagonist MPEP (100 μM), a selective and potent Group I mGluR antagonist, did not protect against NO injury (Fig. 2A), supporting the premise that only specific activation of the Group I mGluRs offers cytoprotection in ECs.

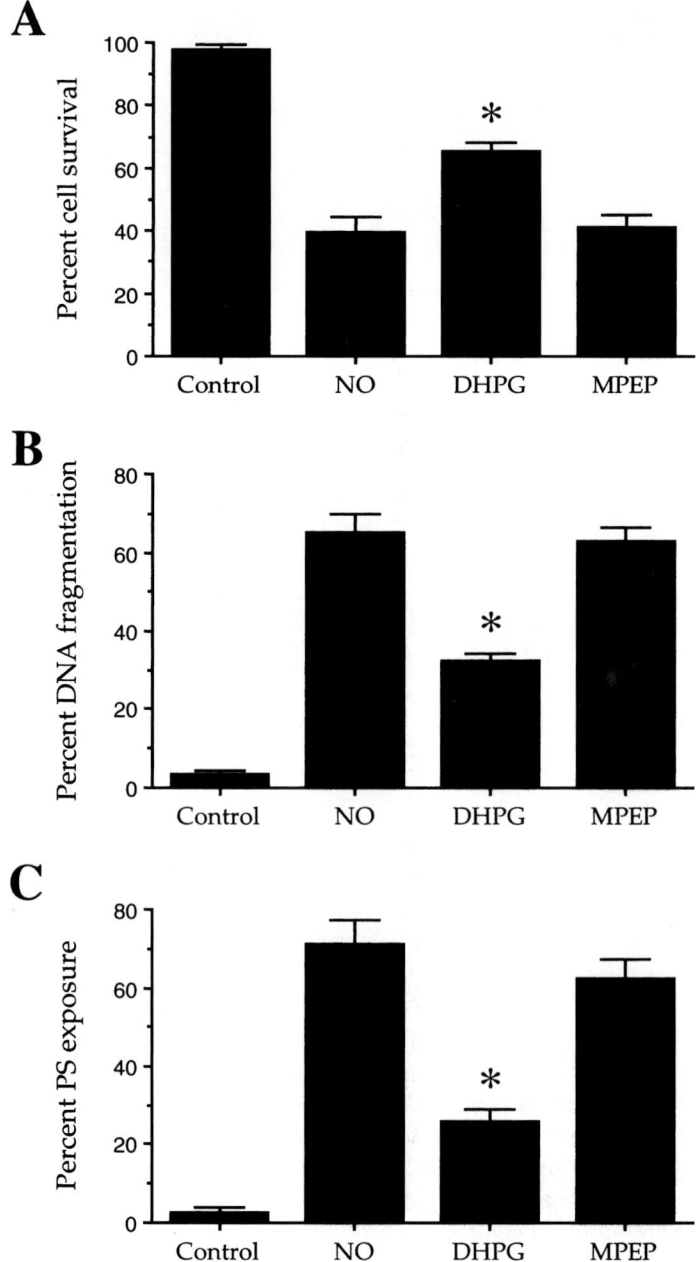

3.3. Group I mGluR activation prevents genomic DNA degradation and membrane PS exposure

Activation of the Group I mGluRs in the presence of NO also results in the prevention of DNA degradation. Application of DHPG (750 µM) 1 h prior to NO exposure significantly reduced DNA fragmentation from $65\pm5\%$ (NO only) to $32\pm2\%$ (DHPG/ NO) (Fig. 2B). Antagonism of the Group I mGluR system with MPEP did not significantly alter DNA degradation when compared to ECs treated only with NO (Fig. 2B). We next employed a reversible assay to detect membrane PS residue exposure over time in living cells [2] during modulation of the Group I mGluR system. A progressive increase in the percent of membrane PS residue exposure was observed over a 24-h period during NO administration alone (Fig. 2C). Activation of the Group I mGluR system with DHPG (750 µM, 1 h prior to NO) significantly prevented NO-induced externalization of membrane PS residues over a 24-h period. Antagonism of the Group I mGluR system with MPEP (100 µM) did not prevent membrane PS exposure following NO administration.

3.4. Activation of the mGluR system prevents the induction of caspase 1- and caspase 3-like activities following NO administration

Since activation of the Group I mGluR system can increase EC survival, decrease DNA fragmentation, and inhibit membrane PS exposure in the presence of NO, we further examined whether protection by the Group I mGluR system is dependent upon the modulation of caspase 1- and caspase 3-like activities. During activation and inhibition of the Group I mGluR system, we assessed caspase 1- and caspase 3-like activities 12 h following NO exposure (1000 µM). The 12-h time point was selected since this represents maximum caspase 1- and caspase 3-like activities following NO application [16]. Activation of Group I mGluR subtypes significantly prevented the induction of both caspase 1- and caspase 3-like activities following NO exposure (Fig. 3A and B). Administration of DHPG (750 µM) decreased caspase 1-like activity from 0.60 ± 0.10

Fig. 2. Activation of Group I mGluRs prevents NO-induced toxicity, DNA degradation, membrane PS exposure in ECs. In (A), EC viability was assessed in cultures with and without a 1-h pretreatment with the mGluR agonist DHPG (750 µM) and the mGluR antagonist MPEP (100 µM) during NO exposure (NOC-9, 1000 µM or SNP, 1000 µM). The mean survival was determined by counting eight randomly selected nonoverlapping fields containing 10–20 cells. To simplify the figure, the results for the two NO donors were combined. Data represent the mean and S.E. In (B), EC DNA fragmentation was assessed in cultures with and without a 1-h pretreatment with the mGluR agonist DHPG (750 µM) and the mGluR antagonist MPEP (100 µM) during NO exposure (NOC-9, 1000 µM or SNP, 1000 µM). The mean TUNEL-positive cells were determined by counting eight randomly selected nonoverlapping fields containing 10–20 cells. To simplify the figure, the results for the two NO donors were combined. Data represent the mean and S.E. (*p<0.05, NO exposure only versus mGluR ligand). In (C), EC membrane PS residue exposure was assessed with annexin V labeling in cultures with and without a 1-h pretreatment with the mGluR agonist DHPG (750 µM) and the mGluR antagonist MPEP (100 µM) during NO exposure (NOC-9, 1000 µM or SNP, 1000 µM). The percentage of annexin V-labeled cells was counted in 5–10 discrete fields with 5–20 cells in each field at each indicated time point following NO application. To simplify the figure, the results for the two NO donors were combined. Data represent the mean and S.E. (*p<0.01, NO exposure only versus untreated control; †p<0.01, NO exposure only versus mGluR ligand).

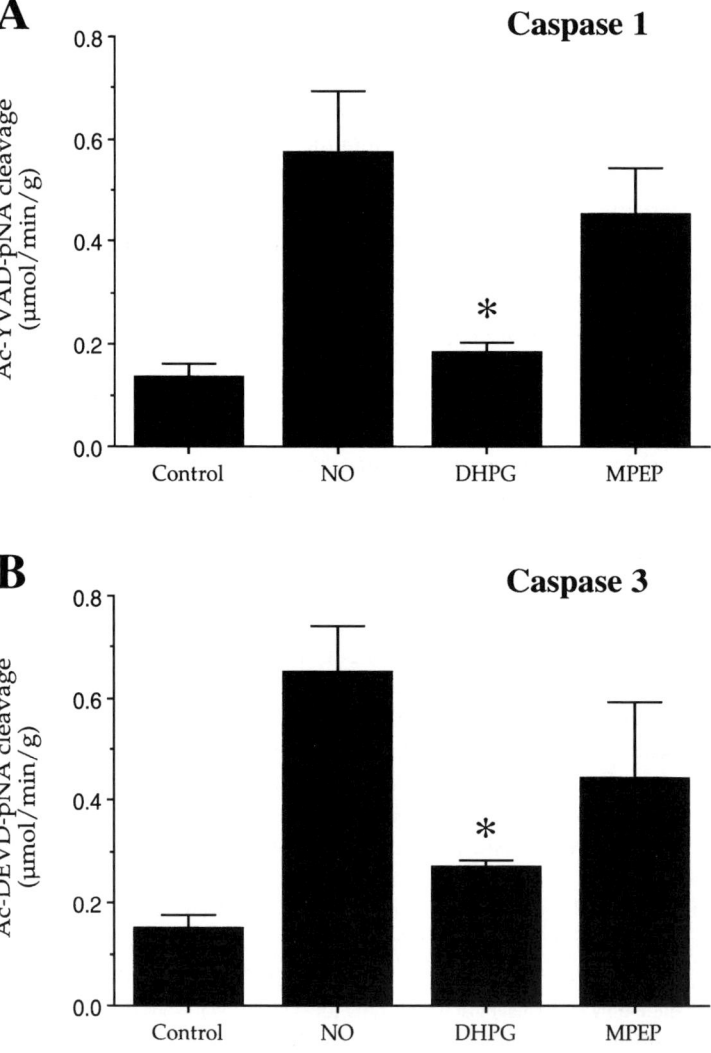

Fig. 3. Activation of the mGluR system prevents the induction of caspase 1- and caspase 3-like activities following NO exposure. The mGluR agonist DHPG (750 μM) and the mGluR antagonist MPEP (100 μM) were applied 1 h prior to NO treatment (NOC-9, 1000 μM or SNP, 1000 μM). (A) Caspase 1-like activity was determined by measuring the cleavage of Ac-YVAD-pNA at 12 h following NO exposure. Pretreatment with DHPG prevented the induction of caspase 1-like activity induced by NO. Pretreatment with MPEP did not significantly alter NO-induced increase in caspase 1-like activity. (B) Caspase 3-like activity was determined by measuring the cleavage of Ac-DEVD-pNA at 12 h following NO exposure (NOC-9, 1000 μM or SNP, 1000 μM). Pretreatment with DHPG prevented the induction of caspase 3-like activity induced by NO. Pretreatment with MPEP did not significantly alter caspase 3-like activity. To simplify the figures (A and B), the results for the two NO donors were combined. Data represent the mean and S.E. with each experiment replicated independently four times using different cultures (*$p < 0.05$, NO exposure only versus mGluR ligand).

μmol/min/g (NO only) to 0.18±0.02 μmol/min/g (DHPG/NO), and decreased caspase 3-like activity from 0.65±0.09 μmol/min/g (NO only) to 0.27±0.01 μmol/min/g (DHPG/ NO). Antagonism of the Group I mGluR system with MPEP (100 μM) did not significantly alter caspase 1- and caspase 3-like activities when compared to ECs treated with NO only (Fig. 3A and B).

4. Discussion

The cerebral vascular system plays a crucial function in the maintenance of an anti-thrombotic state and the homeostasis of the brain. Since vascular ECs are primary cellular targets for a variety of insults such as ischemic injury, a clear understanding of the mechanisms that mediate free radical EC injury may contribute to the development of safe and efficacious therapeutic regiments. In this respect, the mGluR system in ECs becomes an attractive candidate to offer treatment for vascular-based disease entities. Prior work has illustrated that activation of the Group I mGluR system in neurons can protect against epileptic neuronal sclerosis, ischemic neuronal injury, and NO-induced PCD [15,17–19]. Yet, the role of the mGluR system in ECs has not been investigated.

Our work begins to lay the initial foundation for the role of the Group I mGluR in cerebrovascular ECs during NO-induced injury. In the present study, we initially show that Group I mGluR receptors are expressed in rat ECs. Although prior studies have demonstrated the existence of the mGluR system in the rat heart and in ECs with reverse transcriptase-polymerase chain reaction [20,21], we have extended this work through the direct demonstration of the Group I mGluR receptor system in cerebral ECs through the use of both Western analysis and immunocytochemistry. These results are crucial for future investigations that investigate a physiologic role for Group I mGluR system during vascular injury paradigms.

We further demonstrate that the Group I mGluR system serves as an important protectant against EC injury. Activation of Group I mGluRs significantly increased EC survival during free-radical NO exposure. Yet, inhibition of the Group I mGluR system did not prevent NO-induced EC toxicity. These results illustrate a significant cytoprotective effect of the Group I mGluR system in ECs. The Group I mGluR system also provides a unique advantage for the vascular system. Activation of the Group I mGluRs in ECs addresses two distinct pathways of PCD [2]. Agonism of the Group I mGluRs prevents the destruction of genomic DNA and maintains EC membrane asymmetry by inhibiting the early exposure of membrane PS residues. In essence, this degree of cytoprotection by the Group I mGluRs offers both immediate cellular protection through the preservation of intact genomic DNA as well as prolonged cellular protection through the maintenance of membrane asymmetry that prevents EC destruction by phagocytes [4]. Preservation of membrane PS asymmetry can also maintain the anticoagulant state of ECs and prevents the development of atherosclerosis [5].

The downstream cellular pathways that mediate the protective effects of the mGluR system in ECs appear to be closely linked to the modulation of cysteine protease activity. Activation of the Group I mGluR system mediates protection against PCD in neurons [15,22] and now in ECs through the direct inhibition of both caspase 1- and caspase 3-like activities. Caspase 1 has been linked to the modulation of membrane PS residues through cytoskeletal proteins such as fodrin [23] and caspase 3 can lead to the direct degradation of DNA through the enhancement of DNase activity [24]. As a result, the Group I mGluR system may maintain both genomic DNA integrity and membrane PS asymmetry through the inhibition of cysteine protease activity. Yet, it is conceivable that several additional pathways may play a significant role by the Group I mGluR system for the intact maintenance of the EC environment, such as the signal transduction pathways of protein kinase C and protein kinase A [12,25], intracellular calcium [26], intracellular pH [15], endonuclease activity [15], and mitogen-activated protein kinase activity [27]. Further investigations into the ability of the Group I mGluR system to prevent NO-generated PCD in ECs may open new therapeutic foundations for the treatment of circulatory disease.

3.1.8.7. On-Site Discussion

3.1.8.7.1. *Question: (Nemoto)* In vivo endothelial cell damage occurs with much shorter period of ischemia or arterial hypertension. Can you relate your observations to the in vivo situation?

Answer: (Maiese) Our work has begun to investigate the underlying cellular and molecular mechanisms that may mediate endothelial cell injury as well as examine the novel role of the metabotropic glutamate system in the cerebrovasculature. Our in vitro system has defined two independent pathways of endothelial programmed cell death that consist of nuclear genomic DNA degradation and membrane phosphatidylserine (PS) exposure (K. Maiese, A.M. Vincent, J. Neurosci. Res., 55 (4) (2000) 472). Destruction of genomic DNA usually occurs during the late stages of endothelial injury. Yet, as you suggest, endothelial cell damage also consists of an early phase. We have demonstrated that this early phase of endothelial cell damage is consistent with the exposure of membrane PS residues (S.H. Lin, K. Maiese, J. Cereb. Blood Flow Metab., 21 (2001) 262). Exposure of membrane PS residues can subsequently lead to both the phagocytosis of endothelial cells as well as the development of thrombosis. As a result, these "acute" mechanisms of endothelial cell injury may account for the primary debilitating effects of ischemia or arterial hypertension.

Acknowledgements

This research was supported by the following grants to K.M.: American Heart Association (National), Boehringer Ingelheim Training Grant Award, Janssen Neuroscience Award, Johnson and Johnson Focused Investigator Award, and the NIH NIEHS.

References

[1] K. Maiese, The dynamics of cellular injury: transformation into neuronal and vascular protection, Histol. Histopathol. 16 (2) (2001) 633–644.

[2] K. Maiese, A.M. Vincent, Membrane asymmetry and DNA degradation: functionally distinct determinants of neuronal programmed cell death, J. Neurosci. Res. 59 (4) (2000) 568–580.

[3] G. Rimon, C.E. Bazenet, K.L. Philpott, L.L. Rubin, Increased surface phosphatidylserine is an early marker of neuronal apoptosis, J. Neurosci. Res. 48 (6) (1997) 563–570.

[4] J. Savill, Recognition and phagocytosis of cells undergoing apoptosis, Br. Med. Bull. 53 (3) (1997) 491–508.

[5] T. Bombeli, A. Karsan, J.F. Tait, J.M. Harlan, Apoptotic vascular endothelial cells become procoagulant, Blood 89 (7) (1997) 2429–2442.

[6] H. Li, U. Forstermann, Nitric oxide in the pathogenesis of vascular disease, J. Pathol. 190 (3) (2000) 244–254.

[7] M. Suematsu, T. Tamatani, F.A. Delano, M. Miyasaka, M. Forrest, H. Suzuki, G.W. Schmid-Schonbein, Microvascular oxidative stress preceding leukocyte activation elicited by in vivo nitric oxide suppression, Am. J. Physiol. 266 (6 Pt. 2) (1994) H2410–H2415.

[8] K. Bhagat, P. Vallance, Effects of cytokines on nitric oxide pathways in human vasculature, Curr. Opin. Nephrol. Hypertens. 8 (1) (1999) 89–96.

[9] S. Moncada, R.M. Palmer, E.A. Higgs, Nitric oxide: physiology, pathophysiology, and pharmacology, Pharmacol. Rev. 43 (2) (1991) 109–142.

[10] P. Grammas, T.R. Botchlet, P. Moore, P.H. Weigel, Production of neurotoxic factors by brain endothelium in Alzheimer's disease, Ann. N. Y. Acad. Sci. 826 (1997) 47–55.

[11] I. Kurose, R. Wolf, M.B. Grisham, D.N. Granger, Modulation of ischemia/reperfusion-induced microvascular dysfunction by nitric oxide, Circ. Res. 74 (3) (1994) 376–382.

[12] K. Maiese, M. Swiriduk, M. TenBroeke, Cellular mechanisms of protection by metabotropic glutamate receptors during anoxia and nitric oxide toxicity, J. Neurochem. 66 (6) (1996) 2419–2428.

[13] V. Bruno, A. Copani, L. Bonanno, T. Knoepfel, R. Kuhn, P.J. Roberts, F. Nicoletti, Activation of group III metabotropic receptors is neuroprotective in cortical cultures, Eur. J. Pharmacol. 310 (1996) 61–66.

[14] K. Maiese, A. Vincent, S.H. Lin, T. Shaw, Group I and Group III metabotropic glutamate receptor subtypes provide enhanced neuroprotection, J. Neurosci. Res. 62 (2) (2000) 257–272.

[15] A.M. Vincent, M. TenBroeke, K. Maiese, Metabotropic glutamate receptors prevent programmed cell death through the modulation of neuronal endonuclease activity and intracellular pH, Exp. Neurol. 155 (1) (1999) 79–94.

[16] S.H. Lin, K. Maiese, The metabotropic glutamate receptor system protects against ischemic free radical programmed cell death in rat brain endothelial cells, J. Cereb. Blood Flow Metab. 21 (3) (2001) 262–275.

[17] F. Bordi, A. Ugolini, Group I metabotropic glutamate receptors: implications for brain diseases, Prog. Neurobiol. 59 (1) (1999) 55–79.

[18] K. Maiese, A.M. Vincent, Group I metabotropic receptors down-regulate nitric oxide induced caspase-3 activity in rat hippocampal neurons, Neurosci. Lett. 264 (1–3) (1999) 17–20.

[19] U.H. Schroder, T. Opitz, T. Jager, C.F. Sabelhaus, J. Breder, K.G. Reymann, Protective effect of group I metabotropic glutamate receptor activation against hypoxic/hypoglycemic injury in rat hippocampal slices: timing and involvement of protein kinase C, Neuropharmacology 38 (2) (1999) 209–216.

[20] S.S. Gill, O.M. Pulido, R.W. Mueller, P.F. McGuire, Immunochemical localization of the metabotropic glutamate receptors in the rat heart, Brain Res. Bull. 48 (2) (1999) 143–146.

[21] I.A. Krizbai, M.A. Deli, A. Pestenacz, L. Siklos, C.A. Szabo, I. Andras, F. Joo, Expression of glutamate receptors on cultured cerebral endothelial cells, J. Neurosci. Res. 54 (6) (1998) 814–819.

[22] A.M. Vincent, Y. Mohammad, I. Ahmad, R. Greenberg, K. Maiese, Metabotropic glutamate receptors prevent nitric oxide induced programmed cell death, J. Neurosci. Res. 50 (1997) 549–564.

[23] V.L. Cryns, L. Bergeron, H. Zhu, H. Li, J. Yuan, Specific cleavage of alpha-fodrin during Fas- and tumor necrosis factor-induced apoptosis is mediated by an interleukin-1 beta-converting enzyme/Ced-3 protease distinct from the poly(ADP-ribose) polymerase protease, J. Biol. Chem. 271 (49) (1996) 31277–31282.

[24] M. Enari, H. Sakahira, H. Yokoyama, K. Okawa, A. Iwamatsu, S. Nagata, A caspase-activated DNase that degrades DNA during apoptosis, and its inhibitor ICAD [see comments]. Nature 391 (6662) (1998) 43–50.

[25] M.A. Abdul-Ghani, T.A. Valiante, P.L. Carlen, P.S. Pennefather, Metabotropic glutamate receptors coupled

to IP3 production mediate inhibition of IAHP in rat dentate granule neurons, J. Neurophysiol. 76 (4) (1996) 2691–2700.

[26] K. Maiese, I. Ahmad, M. TenBroeke, J. Gallant, Metabotropic glutamate receptor subtypes independently modulate neuronal intracellular calcium, J. Neurosci. Res. 55 (1999) 472–485.

[27] S.H. Lin, K. Maiese, Group I metabotropic glutamate receptors prevent endothelial programmed cell death independent from MAP kinase p38 activation in rat, Neurosci. Lett. 298 (3) (2001) 207–211.

Neural and endothelial mediators

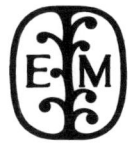

International Congress Series 1235 (2002) 325–335

The Roy–Sherrington hypothesis: facts and surmises

Péter Sándor*, Zoltán Benyó, Benedek Erdös,
Zsombor Lacza, Katalin Komjáti

Institute of Human Physiology and Clinical Experimental Research, Faculty of Medicine, Semmelweis University, Üllöi út 78/A, 1082 Budapest, Hungary

Abstract

The 110-year-old metabolic hypothesis of Roy and Sherrington cannot fully explain the increases of cerebral blood flow (CBF) during increased functional activity of the central neurons. CBF may increase (a) much faster than the accumulation of the metabolic end products, (b) out of proportion to metabolic demands, (c) without significant change in local metabolism. The tight coupling of neuronal activity and blood flow in the brain is demonstrated by a large amount of data. Perivascular nerve endings were identified in the outer smooth muscle layer of the pial and intraparenchymal vessels. Their axon terminals contain a large variety of neurotransmitters, often co-localized in synaptic vesicles. Stimulation of the nerves results in a release of transmitters into the 80–100-nm neuromuscular synaptic clefts, and their specific receptors were identified in the vessel wall. There is ample evidence to suggest that neurogenic stimuli via perivascular nerve endings may act as rapid initiators, inducing a moment-to-moment dynamic adjustment of CBF to the metabolic demands, and further maintenance of these adjusted parameters is ensured by the metabolic and chemical factors. The significance of the perivascular nerves in the regulation of the cerebral blood flow, however, is either underestimated or completely neglected in the majority of textbooks for both medical students and clinicians. Since the regulatory role of the nervous system in the cerebrovascular bed has been fully appreciated among investigators in the last decades, revision of this antiquated view of the common medical knowledge is urgent. © 2002 Elsevier Science B.V. All rights reserved.

Keywords: Cerebral blood flow; Metabolic regulation; Neural regulation; Perivascular nerves; Neurotransmission

1. Introduction

Since the hypothesis of Roy and Sherrington [1] was published in 1890, there has always been a general agreement among investigators that *products of cerebral tissue metabolism* and *chemical stimuli* are among the key factors that affect the resistance of the cerebral

---

* Corresponding author. Tel.: +36-1-210-0306; fax: +36-1-334-3162.
  E-mail address: sandor@elet2.sote.hu (P. Sándor).

0531-5131/02 © 2002 Elsevier Science B.V. All rights reserved.
PII: S 0 5 3 1 - 5 1 3 1 (0 2) 0 0 2 0 1 - 7

vessels, and as a consequence, the local blood flow of the brain. However, contribution of another group of regulatory components, *neural stimuli*, to the control of the brain blood supply has been controversial ever since the first description of the perivascular nerve fibers in the walls of cerebral vessels.

In spite of the slow advancement in this topic, a substantial part of the questions causing doubt has been answered in the last 20 years. A clear-cut, detailed definition of the role of the cerebral perivascular nerves has still not been obtained [2]. However, extensive review of the literature relating to nervous control of cerebral blood flow (CBF) shows clearly that the basic question: importance of the nervous control of the cerebral circulation has been fully appreciated among investigators [3].

Textbooks of physiology, pathophysiology or neurology are too slow to incorporate convincing new facts into the already existing body of evidences, and to reflect the changed views on the role of nervous regulation of the cerebrovascular bed. In spite of a number of highly informative publications on this subject [2–16], the significance of nervous regulation of the cerebral blood flow is still underestimated. Statements such as "the role of these nerves remains a matter of debate" or "the importance of neural regulation of the cerebral circulation is controversial" are typical in the majority of the textbooks for graduate and postgraduate medical studies. As a result, students as well as experienced clinicians handle the role of the neural control as either a non-existing or, at best, a negligible component of CBF regulation.

The aim of this paper was to provide a concise overview about some of the major advances in the last decades that make it necessary to revise false views about the importance of nervous regulation of the cerebral vessels.

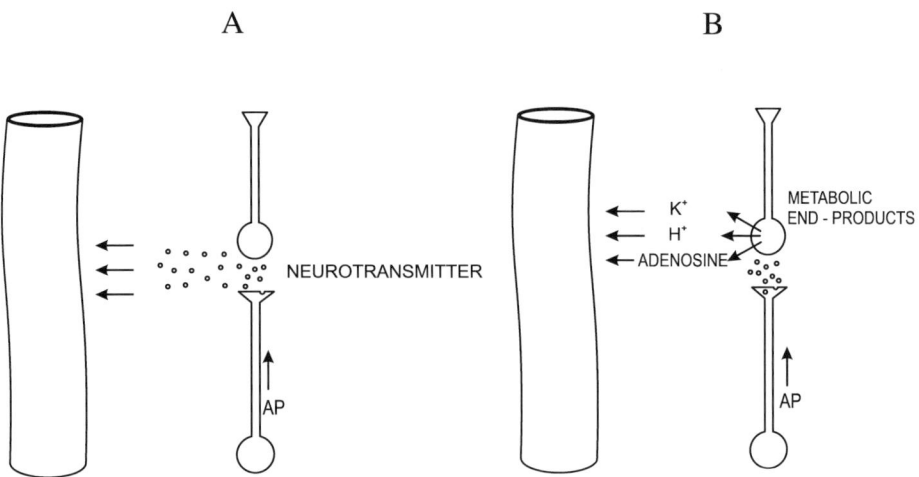

Fig. 1. Interactions between intracerebral, non-perivascular neurons and intracerebral vessels. (A) Neurotransmitters may have access to cerebrovascular smooth muscle after escaping into the extracellular fluid from neuron-neuronal or neuron-glial synapses. Transmitter levels near cerebral resistance vessels may reach or exceed threshold values in extracellular fluid for vascular effects. In this mechanism, vasodilation is induced by neurotransmitters, instead of vasoactive end products of the cellular metabolism, as shown on panel (B).

2. The Roy–Sherrington hypothesis: questions related to a hundred-year-old theory

The chemical products of cerebral metabolism contained in the lymph, which bathes the walls of the arterioles of the brain, can cause variations in the caliber of the cerebral vessels. In this reaction, the brain possesses an intrinsic mechanism by which its vascular supply can be varied locally in correspondence with local variations of functional activity [1]. Since this hypothesis was formulated, it is generally accepted that increased activity of the central neurons results in increased production of vasodilatory end products (H^+, K^+, adenosine) of the neuronal metabolism, which in turn, results in increased cerebral blood flow (Fig. 1B).

Contrary to the assumptions in much of the work to date, however, the association of oxidative metabolism and cerebral blood flow does not prove that oxidative metabolism is the only determinant of the flow in the brain. The metabolic homeostasis hypothesis of Roy and Sherrington does not fully explain the increases in regional cerebral blood flow (rCBF) accompanying increased metabolic activity, because rCBF (a) may increase much faster than the accumulation of metabolic end products, (b) may increase out of proportion to metabolic demands, and (c) may increase without significant change in local metabolism.

3. Perivascular nerve fibers of the cerebrovascular bed: possible initiators of rapid cerebral flow changes

H^+, K^+, and adenosine are principal metabolic candidates for causing local vasodilation and increased local blood flow during increased local cerebral neuronal activity. However, these metabolites may be important for the maintenance of flow and metabolism levels after they have been set at a higher level by a common, rapid initiator factor. The perivascular innervation is a primary candidate for such a common determinant [2].

4. Nervous regulation of the cerebral blood flow: its history and the causes of confusion on its role in the medical literature

Thomas Willis [17] has already demonstrated the perivascular nerve fibers in human cerebral arteries in 1664. The sympathetic origin of part of these nerves was demonstrated 200 years later [18–20]. In 1932, Penfield [21] showed that the nerves not only supplied the extracortical pial vessels, but also followed both the intracortical arteries and veins into the cerebral parenchyma. The histological evidences of the innervation of the cerebral vessels with peripheral adrenergic and cholinergic axon terminals resulted in a great enthusiasm among physiologists. These early studies strongly suggested that perivascular nerves, which innervate cerebral vessels, are likely to be involved in the moment-to-moment dynamic adjustment of cerebral tissue perfusion due to the metabolic demand of the central neurons.

The early enthusiasm evoked by the anatomical and physiological [22,23] observations, however, was soon followed by disappointment since (a) α-adrenoceptor antagonists were unable to alter the pial arteriolar diameter [24,25], and (b) section of the sympathetic nerves resulted either in minimal or no effect at all on the cerebral blood flow [26–28]. It became evident that the resting sympathetic tone, which is present in other vascular beds, is minimal or non-existent in cerebral circulation. Leading investigators obtained different, often contradictory results in connection with the role of the cerebral perivascular nerves (see Refs. [29,30]). This resulted in confusion and in a generalized false conclusion: nervous control of the cerebrovascular bed (in general) is uncertain, and perhaps, non-existent.

The main reason for the contradictory results was the lack of basic methodical information, which was not considered at the time of the disappointments. For instance, the density of the sympathetic innervation and the density of the sympathetic α and β receptors are different in the different cerebral regions [24,31]. The constrictor response of noradrenaline is pH sensitive and it is inhibited by alkalosis [32]. Prostanoids, nitric oxide, and histamine can counteract constrictor effects of noradrenaline [33]. The degree of blood–brain barrier permeability for the different neurotransmitters can be variable in the different experimental models [34,35]. Segmental resistance of the upstream pial vessels may be different from that of the downstream vessels during sympathetic stimulation [28]. The effect of sympathetic stimulation depends on the actual arterial pressure [36].

5. Facts supporting the significance of the nervous control of the cerebral blood flow

Perivascular nerves form a highly complex network around the brain blood vessels, which contains all the elements of an active neuroregulatory system that were studied. The perivascular nerve endings were identified in close proximity to the smooth muscle layer of the cerebral vessels. The axon terminals of these nerves contain an astonishing variety of neurotransmitters, stored (and often co-localized) in synaptic vesicles. Section of the nerves reduces their transmitter content, and stimulation of the nerves results in a release of the transmitter molecules into the narrow synaptic clefts between the axon terminals and the vascular smooth muscle. Specific receptors were identified in the cerebral vessel wall to capture the released transmitter molecules. Taking into account all of the data, it would be illogical to presume that all these elements of neuroregulation are just silent "decorations" around the vessel wall without any function [37].

6. Major advances in the last decades that make it necessary to revise false views about nervous regulation of the cerebral vessels

The current view of the role of nervous regulation of the cerebrovascular bed is based partly on neuroanatomical, and partly on neurochemical considerations.

6.1. Neuroanatomical considerations

(1) Peripheral and central origins [38–40] and the main pathways of the innervation of the intracranial vessels were identified. (2) Vessel types (pial arterioles, veins, intra-parenchymal vessels) innervated by the perivascular nerves were determined. (3) Location

of the axon terminals within the cerebral vessel wall and the size of the neuromuscular synaptic cleft were determined. (4) A transmitter containing synaptic vesicles was found in the axon terminals. (5) Enzymes for the synthesis, release, and breakdown of the neurotransmitters in the perivascular nerves were identified. (6) Receptors were identified in the cerebral vessel wall to capture the transmitter molecules (for details, see Ref. [37]).

6.2. Neurochemical considerations

Perivascular nerves in the cerebrovascular bed were classified for a long time according to their peripheral or central anatomical origin, and according to their sympathetic or parasympathetic character. Identification of new neurotransmitters (especially neuropeptides and nitric oxide) in the central nervous system in the last decades resulted in a new way of classification of the cerebral perivascular nerves, according to their neurotransmitters. The terms peptidergic innervation and nitric oxidergic innervation (besides the well-established terms of adrenergic, cholinergic, serotonergic, histaminergic innervation) of the cerebral vessels gained general acceptance in the literature since peptide-containing nerves [41–43] and NO-releasing nerves [44] were identified around the cerebral vessels. Edvinsson et al. [2] emphasized that the cerebrovascular peptidergic fibers do not appear to provide the very same function as sub served by the sympathetic and parasympathetic systems: "Neuropeptides do not merely provide greater variety in the chemical signals that are employed to initiate one of two possible responses, vasoconstriction or vasodilatation, rather, many neuropeptides are implicated in a diversity of responses distinct from being the initiator of vasomotor responses in an autonomic neuronal circuit." Sir Henry Dale's "one neuron one transmitter" theory was overruled; neuropeptides are generally co-localized in the cerebrovascular nerve fibers with other neuropeptides and/or classical neurotransmitters (Fig. 3A, for details see Ref. [2], for a concise summary see Ref. [3]).

7. New aspects of the neural regulation in the cerebrovascular bed

(1) Neurotransmitters, derived from non-perivascular nerves, can exert an effect upon the cerebral vessels when these neurons are activated [3]. In the cerebral circulation, many neurotransmitters have access to cerebrovascular smooth muscle (and to other cells as well) after escaping into the extracellular fluid from neuron-neuronal, neuron-glial synapses or, from the non-synaptic varicosities of the extensive terminal-branching fibers along the cerebral vessels (Fig. 1A). Thus, under baseline conditions, but more commonly under stressed conditions, neurotransmitter levels near cerebral resistance vessels may reach or exceed threshold values in extracellular fluid for vascular effects. The levels of brain extracellular fluid increase into vasoactive range for opioids [45], for dopamine [46], for excitatory amino acids [47–49], for acetylcholine [50,51], and probably also for serotonin [52].

(2) Ascending neuronal systems, originating in the brainstem, may provide direct innervation of the cortical vessels either with their axon terminals or with their serotonine-

containing collateral fibers (Fig. 2A). The different segments of the same intracortical vessel may receive innervations from different neurons, with different neurotransmitters in the different layers of the cortex (Fig. 2B) [2,53].

(3) Since neurotransmitters in the extracellular fluid have access not only to vascular muscle, to other varicosities [54,55], but to other cells as well, the potential exists for these neurotransmitters to cause synthesis and release of other vasoactive substances such as prostanoids. Dilator prostanoids, released from neurons and astroglia, appear to mediate the effects on the cerebral arterioles of histamine, leu- and met-enkephalin and oxytocin in piglets, and they can counteract constrictor effects on the cerebral arterioles of dynorphin, β-endorphin, noradrenaline and vasopressin [3,45,56–60].

(4) Another aspect is the mobile varicosities in terminal-branching fibers to vascular smooth muscle cells. Since the early 1960s, major advances have been made that make it necessary to revise our thinking about the mechanisms of autonomic transmission. "In broad terms, these new concepts shift the earlier emphasis on central control mechanisms toward greater consideration of the sophisticated local peripheral control mechanisms" [54,61]. Autonomic neuromuscular junction is not a "synapse" in the usual sense of the term where there is a fixed junction with both pre- and postjunctional specialization, but rather that the transmitter is released from mobile, non-synaptic varicosities [54,55,62,63] in extensive terminal-branching fibers at variable distances from effector cells or bundles of the cerebral vascular smooth muscle cells (Fig. 3B). The smooth muscle cells are in

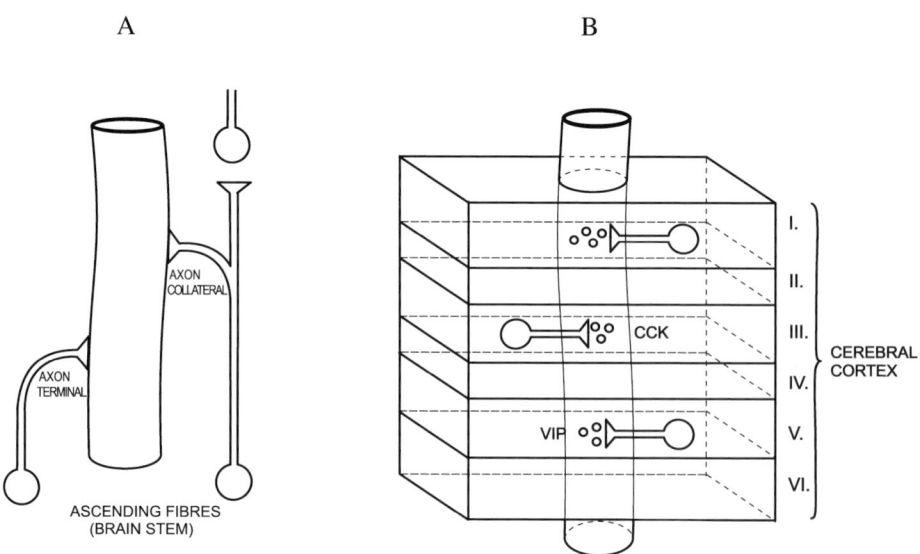

Fig. 2. Interactions between intracerebral, non-perivascular neurons and intracerebral vessels. (A) Ascending neuronal systems may provide direct innervation of the cortical vessels with either axon terminals or collateral fibers. (B) The different segments of the same intracortical vessel may receive innervations from different neurons, with different neurotransmitters in the different layers of the cerebral cortex.

A   B

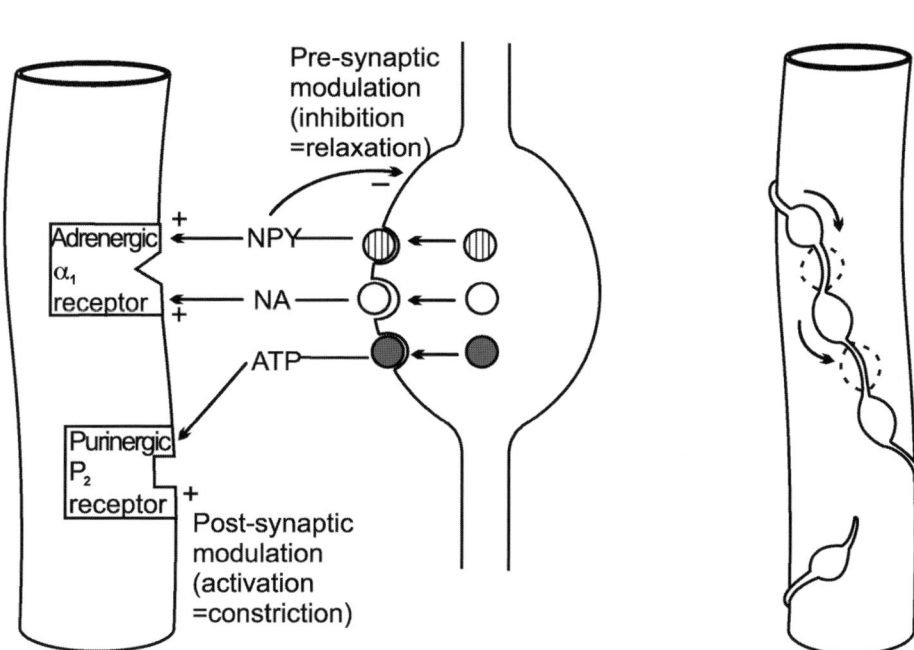

Fig. 3. Interactions between intracerebral, non-perivascular neurons and intracerebral vessels. (A) Transmitters are often co-localized with other transmitters in the synaptic vesicles of the autonomic perivascular nerves. Some transmitters (in this example, NPY) may induce opposite effects presynaptically than postsynaptically. (B) Autonomic neuromuscular junction is not a synapse in the usual sense of the term where there is a fixed presynaptic and postsynaptic junction. The transmitters are released from mobile, non-synaptic varicosities.

electrical contact with each other and they have a diffuse distribution of receptors [64,65].

(5) Noradrenergic varicosities of the sympathetic perivascular nerve fibers are equipped with $\alpha 2$ adrenoceptors [66–68], whose stimulation by noradrenaline results in a reduction of the transmitter release (negative feedback mechanism).

(6) Serotonin may act as a "false neurotransmitter" in the cerebral circulation. It is known that serotonin has a direct constrictor effect in cerebral vessels [3]. It is less well known, however, that sympathetic nerve terminals are able to take up serotonin from the extracellular fluid, store it and release the serotonin when depolarized [69,70]. This way, serotonin may act as a "false neurotransmitter" associated with sympathetic nerve terminals in the cerebral circulation. Neurally released serotonin can interact with sympathetic nerve fibers by either limiting the release of noradrenaline from nerve terminals [71] or by potentiation of the vasoconstrictor effects of noradrenaline [72].

3.2.1.10. On-Site Discussion

3.2.1.10.1. **Question: (Gaehtgens)** Related to the last sentence of your presentation: In views of the very little space that textbook authors are given to cover the subject, would it still be reasonable to write, as Gannong did, that the topic is still a matter of debate?

Answer: (Sándor) I do not believe that it would be enough today. It is true that nervous regulation of the cerebral blood flow was, it still is, and it will be a matter of debate for awaiting future. It does not mean, however, that our knowledge is not increasing in the mean time. In this symposium, we are discussing already the details of the nervous regulation of the cerebral vessel calibre at the time, when even the role of the cerebral perivascular nerves is not yet acknowledged by the text book authors. It is time to write more about the tremendous amount of new data we gained in the last two decades in connection with the role of nervous regulation of cerebral blood flow. It is our responsibility to encourage the text book authors to realize the fact.

3.2.1.10.2. **Question: (Paulson)** You mentioned several interesting mechanisms which might be involved in the mediation of signals from the activated neurons to the vessels, e.g., released neurotransmitters and direct signals from the neurons. Should we not add possible influence of the astrocyte as well as of increased concentration of the ions K^+ and H^+?

Answer: (Sándor) Yes, I quite agree, these factors may all be of major importance. Time limitation, however, let me focus on the other factors in my presentation.

Acknowledgements

The authors are grateful to Mrs. Maria Harvich-Velkei for her excellent technical assistance and for typing the manuscript. Original studies by the author's research group that are mentioned in this review were supported by Hungarian foundations (Széchenyi Professor Fellowship, National Science Fund OTKA T-029169, T037885, T037386, F-029801, and Ministry of Health ETT 218/2001), by The Netherlands Organization for Pure Research (ZWO), by the NIH of the US (NS 10939-20) and by the JSPS of Japan (58480230). The authors are indebted to the Eisai, Japan, for a travel grant to the Satellite Symposium of BRAIN 01 "Brain Activation and CBF Control" in Tokyo, 2001.

References

[1] C.S. Roy, C.S. Sherrington, On the regulation of the blood supply of the brain, Journal of Physiology 11 (1890) 85–108.

[2] L. Edvinsson, E.T. MacKenzie, J. McCulloch (Eds.), Cerebral Blood Flow and Metabolism, Raven Press, New York, 1993, pp. 57–84.

[3] D.W. Busija, Nervous control of the cerebral circulation, in: T. Bennett, S.M. Gardiner (Eds.), Nervous Control of Blood Vessels, Autonomic Nervous System, vol. 8, Harwood Academic Publishers, UK, 1996, pp. 177–205.

[4] L. Edvinsson, C. Owman, B. Siesjö, Physiological role of cerebrovascular sympathetic nerves in the autoregulation of cerebral blood flow, Brain Research 117 (1976) 519–523.

[5] C. Owman, L. Edvinsson (Eds.), Neurogenic Control of the Brain Circulation, Pergamon, Oxford, 1977.

[6] W. Kuschinsky, M. Wahl, Local chemical and neurogenic regulation of cerebral vascular resistance, Physiological Reviews 58 (1978) 656–689.

[7] D.J. Reis, Nervous control of the cerebral blood flow in normal health and in relationship to cerebrovascular disease, in: P. Castaigne, F. Lhermitte, J.C. Gautier, A. Moriniére (Eds.), Maladies Vasculaires Cérebrales: Deuxiéme Conférence de la Salpetriére, Bailliére-Tindall, Paris, 1979, pp. 197–224.

[8] T.A. McCalden, Sympathetic control of the cerebral circulation, Journal of Autonomic Pharmacology 1 (1981) 421–431.

[9] D.D. Heistad, D.W. Busija, M.L. Marcus, Neural effects on cerebral vessels: alteration of pressure–flow relationship, Federation Proceedings 40 (1981) 2317–2321.

[10] H.A. Kontos, Regulation of the cerebral circulation, Annual Review of Physiology 43 (1981) 397–407.

[11] L. Edvinsson, Sympathetic control of cerebral circulation, Trends in Neurosciences 5 (1982) 425–428.

[12] D.D. Heistad, M.L. Marcus (Eds.), Cerebral Blood Flow: Effect of Nerves and Neurotransmitters, Elsevier, New York, 1982.

[13] C. Owman, J.E. Hardebo (Eds.), Neural Regulation of Brain Circulation, Elsevier, Amsterdam, 1986.

[14] E.T. MacKenzie, B. Scatton, Cerebral circulatory and metabolic effect of perivascular neurotransmitters, Critical Review in Clinical Neurobiology 2 (1987) 367–419.

[15] E. Hamel, L. Edvinsson, E.T. MacKenzie, Heterogeneous vasomotor responses of anatomically distinct feline cerebral arteries, British Journal of Pharmacology 94 (1988) 423–436.

[16] U. Dirnagl, Metabolic aspects of neurovascular coupling, Advances in Experimental Medicine and Biology 413 (1997) 149–153.

[17] T. Willis, Cerebri anatome, cui accessit nervorum, descriptio et usus, Flesher J., London, 1664.

[18] M. Benedikt, Über die Innervation des Plexus Chorioideus Inferior, Virchows Archiv fuer Pathologische Anatomie und Physiologie und fuer Klinische Medizin 59 (1874) 395–400.

[19] H. Aronson, Über Nerven und Nervendigungen in der Pia Mater, Zeitschrift für Medizinisce Wissenschaft 28 (1890) 594–595.

[20] G.C. Hüber, Observations on the innervation of intracranial vessels, Journal of Comparative Neurology 9 (1899) 1–34.

[21] W. Penfield, Intracerebral vascular nerves, Archives of Neurology and Psychiatry 27 (1932) 30–44.

[22] S. Cobb, Cerebral circulation: a critical discussion of the symposium, Research Publication—Association for Research in Nervous and Mental Disease 18 (1938) 719–752.

[23] M.J. Purves, The Physiology of the Cerebral Circulation, Cambridge Univ. Press, Cambridge, UK, 1972.

[24] W. Kuschinsky, M. Wahl, α-Receptor stimulation by endogenous and exogenous noradrenaline and blockade by phentolamine in pial arteries in cats. A microapplication study, Circulation Research 37 (1975) 168–174.

[25] D.W. Busija, C.W. Leffler, Postjunctional a2-adrenoceptors in pial arteries of anaesthetized newborn pigs, Developmental Pharmacology and Therapeutics 10 (1987) 36–46.

[26] S.M. Mueller, D.D. Heistad, M.L. Marcus, Total and regional cerebral blood flow during hypotension, hypertension and hypocapnia: effect of sympathetic denervation in dogs, Circulation Research 41 (1977) 350–356.

[27] D.D. Heistad, M.L. Marcus, S. Sandberg, F.M. Abbouod, Effect of sympathetic nerve stimulation on cerebral blood flow and on large cerebral arteries of dogs, Circulation Research 41 (1977) 342–350.

[28] D.W. Busija, M.L. Marcus, D.D. Heistad, Pial artery diameter and blood flow velocity during sympathetic stimulation in cats, Journal of Cerebral Blood Flow and Metabolism 2 (1982) 363–367.

[29] M.J. Purves, Do vasomotor nerves significantly regulate cerebral blood flow? Circulation Research 43 (1978) 485–495.

[30] D.D. Heistad, M.L. Marcus, Evidence that the neural mechanisms do not have important effects on cerebral blood flow, Circulation Research 42 (1978) 295–302.

[31] L. Edvinsson, C. Owman, Sympathetic innervations and adrenergic receptors in intraparenchymal cerebral arteries of baboon, in: D.H. Ingvar, N.A. Lassen (Eds.), Proceedings of the 8th International Symposium on Cerebral Function, Metabolism and Circulation, Munksgaard, Copenhagen, 1977, pp. 403–405.

[32] R. Navari, E.P. Wei, H.A. Kontos, J.L. Patterson Jr., Comparation of the open skull and cranial window preparations is the study of the cerebral microcirculation, Microvascular Research 16 (1978) 304–315.

[33] P.M. Gross, A.M. Harper, G.M. Teasdale, Interaction of histamine with noradrenergic constrictory mech-

anisms in cat cerebral arteries and veins, Canadian Journal of Physiology and Pharmacology 61 (1983) 756–763.

[34] E.T. MacKenzie, S. Strandgaard, D.I. Graham, J.V. Jones, A.M. Harper, J.K. Farrar, Effects of acutely induced hypertension in cats on pial arteriolar caliber, local cerebral blood flow and the blood–brain barrier, Circulation Research 39 (1976) 33–41.

[35] L. Dahlgren, O. Lindvall, T. Sakabe, U. Steneni, B.K. Siasjö, Cerebral blood flow and oxygen consumption in rat brain after lesions of the noradrenergic locus coeruleus system, Brain Research 209 (1981) 11–23.

[36] A.G.B. Kovach, P. Sandor, Cerebral blood flow and brain function during hypotension and shock, Annual Review of Physiology 39 (1976) 571–596.

[37] P. Sándor, Nervous control of the cerebrovascular system: doubts and facts. Invited review, Neurochemistry International 35 (1999) 237–259.

[38] L. Molnár, J. Szántó, The effect of electrical stimulation of the bulbar vasomotor centre on the cerebral blood flow, Quarterly Journal of Experimental Physiology 49 (1964) 184–190.

[39] M.E. Raichle, B.K. Hartman, J.O. Eichling, L.G. Sharpe, Central noradrenergic regulation of cerebral blood flow and vascular permeability, Proceedings of the National Academy of Sciences of the United States of America 72 (1975) pp. 3726–3730.

[40] C. Iadecola, D.J. Reis, Continuous monitoring of cerebrocortical blood flow during stimulation of the cerebellar fastigial nucleus: a study by laser-doppler flowmetry, Journal of Cerebral Blood Flow and Metabolism 10 (1990) 608–617.

[41] L.I. Larson, L. Edvinsson, J. Fahrenkrug, R. Hakanson, Ch. Owman, O.B. Schaffalitzky de Muckadel, et al., Immunohistochemical localization of a vasodilatory polypeptide (VIP) in cerebrovascular nerves, Brain Research 113 (1976) 400–404.

[42] V. Chan-Palay, Innervation of cerebral blood vessels by norepinephrine, indoleamine, substance P and neurotensin fibers and the leptomeningeal indoleamine axons: their roles in vasomotor activity and local alteration of brain blood composition, in: C. Owman, L. Edvinson (Eds.), Neurogenic Control of the Brain Circulation, Pergamon, Oxford, 1977, pp. 39–53.

[43] L. Edvinsson, J. McCulloch, R. Uddman, Substance P: immunohistochemical localization and effect upon cat pial arteries in vitro and in situ, Journal of Physiology (London) 318 (1981) 251–258.

[44] F.M. Faraci, J.E. Brian, Nitric oxide and the cerebral circulation, Stroke 25 (1994) 692–703.

[45] W.M. Armstead, R. Mirro, D.W. Busija, D.M. Desiderio, C.W. Leffler, Opioids in cerebrospinal fluid in hypotensive newborn pigs, Circulation Research 68 (1991) 922–929.

[46] D. Bentue-Ferrer, J.M. Reymann, H. Bagot, J. Van den Driesche, J. de Certaines, H. Allain, Aminergic neurotransmitter and water content changes in rats after transient forebrain ischaemia, Journal of Neurochemistry 47 (1986) 1672–1677.

[47] H. Hagberg, P. Andersson, I. Kjellmer, K. Thiringer, M. Thordstein, Extracellular overflow of glutamate, aspartate, GABA and taurine in the cortex and basal ganglia of fetal lambs during hypoxia-ischemia, Neuroscience Letters 78 (1987) 311–317.

[48] N. Nakakita, K. Hiroyuki, K. Kogure, Effects of repeated cerebral ischemia on extracellular amino acid concentration measured with intracerebral microdialysis in the gerbil hyppocampus, Stroke 24 (1993) 458–464.

[49] K.M. Kendrick, E.B. Keverne, C. Chapman, B.A. Baldwin, Microdialysis measurement of oxytocin, aspartate, D-amino-butyric acid and glutamate release from the olfactory bulb of the sheep during vaginocervical stimulation, Brain Research 442 (1988) 171–174.

[50] S.P. Arneric, C. Iadecola, M.D. Underwood, D.J. Reis, Local cholinergic mechanisms participate in the increase in cortical cerebral blood flow elicited by electrical stimulation of the fastigial nucleus in rat, Brain Research 411 (1987) 212–225.

[51] M. Kurosawa, A. Sato, Y. Sato, Well maintained responses of acetylcholine release and blood flow in the cerebral cortex to local electrical stimulation of the nucleus basalis Meynert in the aged rats, Neuroscience Letters 100 (1989) 198–202.

[52] J.F. Reinhard Jr., J.E. Liebmann, A.J. Schlossberg, M.A. Moskowitz, Serotonine neurons project to small blood vessels in the brain, Science 206 (1979) 85–87.

[53] H.C. Lou, L. Edvinsson, E.T. MacKenzie, The concept of coupling blood flow to brain function: revision required? Annals of Neurology 22 (1987) 29–297.

[54] E.S. Vizi, Non-Synaptic Interactions Between Neurons: Modulation of Neurochemical Transmission. Pharmacological and Clinical Aspects, Wiley, Chicester, 1984.

[55] E.S. Vizi, E. Lábos, Non-synaptic interactions at presynaptic level, Progress in Neurobiology 37 (1991) 145–163.

[56] D.W. Busija, C.W. Leffler, Eicosanoid synthesis elicited by norepinephrine in piglet parietal cortex, Brain Research 403 (1987) 243–248.

[57] D.W. Busija, C.W. Leffler, Dilator effects of amino acid neurotransmitters on piglet pial arterioles, American Journal of Physiology 26 (1989) H1200–H1203.

[58] W.M. Armstead, R.C. Mirro, D.W. Busija, C.W. Leffler, Permissible role of prostanoids in acetylcholine-induced cerebral vasoconstriction, Journal of Pharmacology and Experimental Therapeutics 251 (1989) 1012–1019.

[59] W.M. Armstead, R. Mirro, C.W. Leffler, D.W. Busija, Vascular responses to vasopressin are tone-dependent in the cerebral circulation of the newborn pig, Circulation Research 64 (1989) 136–144.

[60] R. Mirro, D.W. Busija, W.M. Armstead, C.W. Leffler, Histamine dilates the pial arterioles of newborn pigs through prostanoid production, American Journal of Physiology 23 (1988) H1023–H1026.

[61] G. Burnstock, Historical and conceptual perspective of the autonomic nervous system book series, in: T. Bennett, S.M. Gardiner (Eds.), Nervous Control of Blood Vessels, The Autonomic Nervous System, vol. 8, Harwood Academic Publishers, UK, 1996, pp. vii–xii.

[62] E.S. Vizi, Non-synaptic modulation of transmitter release: pharmacological implication, Trends in Pharmacological Sciences 2 (1980) 172–175.

[63] E.S. Vizi, J. Kiss, Neurochemistry and pharmacology of the major hippocampal transmitter systems: synaptic and nonsynaptic interactions, Hippocampus 8 (1998) 566–607.

[64] N.-A. Hillarp, The construction and functional organisation of the autonomic innervation apparatus, Acta Physiologica Scandinavica 46 (Suppl. 157) (1959) 1–38.

[65] G. Burnstock, Autonomic neuromuscular junctions: current developments and future directions, Journal of Anatomy 146 (1986) 1–30.

[66] E.S. Vizi, Presynaptic modulation of neurochemical transmission, Progress in Neurobiology 12 (1979) 181–290.

[67] E.S. Vizi, J. Kiss, I.J. Elenkov, Presynaptic modulation of cholinergic and noradrenergic neurotransmission: interaction between them, News in Physiological Sciences 6 (1991) 119–123.

[68] E. Schlicker, K. Fink, M. Kathmann, G.J. Molderings, M. Gothert, Effects of imidazolines on noradrenaline release in brain: an investigation into their relationship to imidazoline, alpha 2 and H3 receptors, 30 (1) (1997) 73–83.

[69] T.J. Verbeuren, F.H. Jordaens, A.G. Herman, Accumulation and release of (^{3}H)-5-hydroxytryptamine in saphenous vein and cerebral arteries of the dog, Journal of Pharmacology and Experimental Therapeutics 226 (1983) 579–588.

[70] J.Y. Chang, E. Ekblad, P. Kannisto, C. Owman, Sertotonin uptake into cerebrovascular nerve fibers of rat, visualization by immunohistochemistry, disappearance following sympathectomy and release during electrical stimulation, Brain Research 492 (1989) 79–88.

[71] M.A. McGrath, 5-Hydroxytryptamine and neurotransmitter release in canine blood vessels, Circulation Research 41 (1977) 428–435.

[72] I.S. Lande, V.A. Cannell, J.G. Waterson, The interaction of serotonin and noradrenaline on the perfused artery, British Journal of Pharmacology 28 (1966) 255–272.

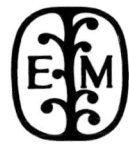

International Congress Series 1235 (2002) 337–345

Adrenergic and cholinergic modulation of cerebrovascular nitrergic vasodilation

Tony J.F. Lee

Department of Pharmacology, Southern Illinois University School of Medicine,
Springfield, IL 62794-9629, USA

Abstract

Large cerebral arteries at the base of the brain from several species are innervated by dense sympathetic adrenergic nerves, and parasympathetic cholinergic and nitrergic nerves. Norepinephrine (NE) and acetylcholine (ACh) released from the respective nerves are not the primary postsynaptic transmitters for vasoconstriction and dilation. Evidence has been presented to indicate that nitric oxide (NO) is the predominant transmitter for cerebral vasodilation. NE and ACh act as presynaptic transmitters in modulating NO release and therefore cerebral vascular tone. This transmitter mechanism in the large cerebral arteries appears to be different from that in the smaller vessels. © 2002 Elsevier Science B.V. All rights reserved.

Keywords: Adrenergic, cholinergic, and nitrergic innervation; Nitric oxide; β_2-Adrenoceptor; Muscarinic M_2 receptor; α_7-Nicotinic receptor; Neurogenic vasodilation; Cerebral vascular tone

1. Cholinergic innervation

The presence of cholinergic innervation in large cerebral arteries is well established [2,4,6,9,20,25]. The cholinergic innervation decreases in smaller arteries, and is usually not present in pial vessels that still receive sympathetic innervation [25]. Based on physiological studies, acetylcholine (ACh) released from the cholinergic nerves innervating cerebral blood vessels was originally thought to be the vasodilator transmitter [2,6,9]. Pharmacological studies using isolated cerebral arterial rings without endothelial cells, however, have demonstrated that ACh (0.1 μM–1 mM) induces constriction exclusively, while transmural nerve stimulation (TNS) induces relaxation in the same preparation [8].

E-mail address: TLEE@wpsmtp.siumed.edu (T.J.F. Lee).

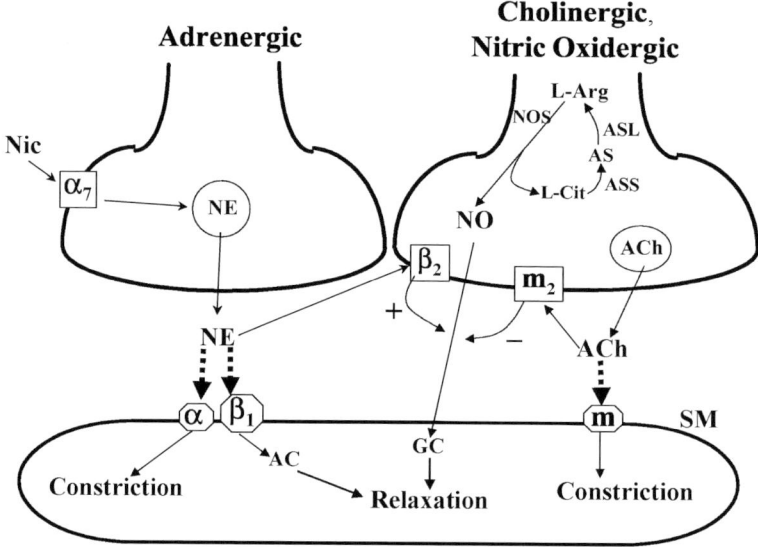

Fig. 1. A diagram showing close apposition of adrenergic and cholinergic–nitric oxidergic nerve terminals in large cerebral arteries at the base of the brain. Nicotine (Nic) acts on presynaptic α_7-nicotinic receptors on adrenergic nerve terminal, causing release of norepinephrine (NE) that then acts on presynaptic β_2-adrenoceptors on the adjacent nitrergic nerve terminal. This effect of NE results in release (+) of NO, which activates guanylate cyclase (GC), increases cGMP contents and relaxes the smooth muscle (SM). NE released from the sympathetic nerve usually does not affect the post-synaptic α or β adrenergic receptors to induce a response. NO, which is not stored in vesicles is co-localized and co-released with ACh that is stored in the vesicles in cholinergic–nitric oxidergic nerves. NO is synthesized from L-arginine (L-Arg) in the presence of nitric oxide synthase (NOS). L-Citrulline (L-Cit), the by-product of NO synthesis, is converted to form argininosuccinate (AS) in the presence of ASS (argininosuccinate synthase), and is further converted to L-Arg, catalyzed by argininosuccinate lyase (ASL). This L-Cit–L-Arg cycle indicates the neuronal synthesis and release of NO. ACh released from cholinergic–nitric oxidergic nerves acts on presynaptic m_2 (muscarinic M_2 receptors), resulting in inhibition (−) of NO release and relaxation. Endogenous ACh does not exhibit direct effect on the smooth muscle tone.

Atropine blocks ACh-induced constriction but does not block TNS-induced vasodilation [14]. These results provide convincing evidence that ACh is not the dilator transmitter at the terminal synapses in these arteries [9], and have led to the suggestion that ACh is co-released with a potent nonadrenergic, noncholinergic (NANC) vasodilator transmitter substance in cerebral blood vessels [10] (Fig. 1).

2. Nitric oxidergic (nitrergic) innervation

Cerebral arteries from all species examined have been shown to receive dense nitric oxide synthase immunoreactive (NOS-I) fibers [9] of multiple origins [5,7], providing direct evidence for the presence of NO synthesizing enzymes in the nitrergic vasodilator nerves in cerebral circulation. Furthermore, biochemical and pharmacological studies have demonstrated that cerebral perivascular nerves can recycle L-citrulline, the by-product of NO synthesis, to L-arginine for synthesizing NO [16] (Fig. 1). All necessary enzymes for recycling L-citrulline to L-arginine (argininosuccinate synthase and argininosuccinate lyase) and for synthesizing NO (NOS) are axoplasmic enzymes and are co-stored in the same neurons (Fig. 1), providing most direct evidence that NO is synthesized and released in perivascular nerves. Results from pharmacological studies in isolated ring preparations further indicate that NO mediates a major component (>90%) of TNS-elicited cerebral neurogenic vasodilation [9].

3. Cholinergic–nitrergic innervation in cerebral circulation

NOS and choline acetyltransferase (ChAT) have been found to coexist in the para-sympathetic ganglion and perivascular nerves in cerebral blood vessels of several species [7] (Fig. 1). Since NO mediates the major component of the neurogenic vasodilator response [9], while endogenous ACh exhibits no direct effect on the smooth muscle in cerebral arteries [8,14], the cholinergic–nitrergic vasodilator nerves in cerebral blood vessels has been proposed [7]. This finding supports the hypothesis that the endogenous ACh plays a modulatory role [10] on NO release from the same perivascular nerves [16]. Evidence has been presented in the porcine [19] and bovine cerebral arteries [1] to indicate that ACh inhibits NO release by acting on presynaptic muscarinic M_2 receptors. This inhibition appears to be due to a negative coupling of muscarinic M_2 receptors to N-type Ca^{2+} channels [19] (Fig. 1).

4. N-type Ca^{2+} channels on cholinergic–nitrergic nerves

The relaxation of porcine basilar arteries induced by TNS at different frequencies was significantly decreased by ω-conotoxin (CTX), suggesting that Ca^{2+} influx via N-type Ca^{2+} channels plays a significant role in activating NOS and therefore NO release in perivascular nerves [19]. The residual relaxation may be due to activation of NOS by other sources of Ca^{2+}, such as Ca^{2+} influx from L-type channels or release of intracellular Ca^{2+}. In the presence of CTX, the residual relaxation in porcine basilar arteries elicited by TNS was no longer affected by either atropine or muscarinic M_2 agonists. These findings suggest that muscarinic M_2-receptor-mediated inhibition of TNS-elicited nitrergic vaso-dilation was due exclusively to a negative coupling of muscarinic M_2 receptors to Ca^{2+} influx via N-type Ca^{2+} channels (Fig. 1).

The presence of N-type Ca^{2+} channels on cerebral perivascular nitrergic nerves is further demonstrated in a single fiber of the cultured sphenopalatine ganglion (SPG, Ref. [18]), a source of cerebral nitrergic innervation [5,7]. Both soma and neurites of these cells were immunoreactive for N-type Ca^{2+} channels and transmitter synthesizing enzymes (i.e., ChAT and NOS). N-type Ca^{2+} channels were found to be completely colocalized with NOS immunoreactivities [18]. In current clamp recordings of the cultured SPG, injection of a small depolarizing current caused action potential firing. In voltage clamp recordings, the fast inward currents were blocked by tetrodotoxin and outward currents blocked by tetraethylammonium, which is typical for neurons. Most Ca^{2+} currents isolated by blockade of sodium and potassium currents were blocked by ω-conotoxin but were not affected by nifedipine, indicating that N-type Ca^{2+} channels are the dominant voltage-dependent Ca^{2+} channels in regulating Ca^{2+} influx during membrane depolarization of SPG neurons. Our preliminary data indicated that the Ca^{2+} current was inhibited by ACh and muscarinic M_2 receptor agonists in a concentration-dependent manner. The inhibition was reversed by atropine and methoctramine (an M_2-receptor antagonist). These results, together with previous pharmacological findings that cerebral neurogenic vasodilation is largely inhibited by ω-conotoxin [19], suggest that N-type Ca^{2+} channels on the para-sympathetic nerves in cerebral blood vessels play an important role in releasing neuro-transmitters from these nerves, thereby regulating cerebral circulation.

5. Adrenergic innervation

Cerebral arteries and veins receive a dense unilateral supply of sympathetic, adrenergic nerves of superior cervical ganglionic origin [2,6,10]. Small arterioles are sometimes accompanied by few fibers. Most intracerebral vessels appear to lack perivascular adrenergic nerves. The endogenous catecholamines are almost exclusively norepinephrine (NE) [11]. Sympathetic stimulation releases NE from perivascular nerves [3,22].

Results from in vitro tissue bath studies have indicated that isolated cerebral arteries, particularly the basilar arteries of the rabbit and dog, constrict upon TNS. The constriction with few exceptions is not blocked but is potentiated by α-adrenoceptor antagonists [11,13]. Furthermore, in pig cerebral arteries, TNS elicits predominant vasodilation that is not affected by propranolol [15]. These results suggest that the synaptic concentration of NE upon maximum stimulation by TNS is too low (below the threshold concentration) to directly affect the vascular smooth muscle tone in vitro. In addition, cerebral arteries are extremely insensitive to exogenously applied catecholamines [11,13]. These results suggest that NE is not the major transmitter for cerebral vasoconstriction in large cerebral arteries at the base of the brain.

6. Adrenergic–nitrergic interaction in cerebral arteries

Ultrastructural studies have demonstrated the close apposition of adrenergic nerve terminals and the nonadrenergic nerve terminals in the neuro-effector region [12]. The close apposition of different types of nerve terminals suggests possible functional interaction between them. It is very likely that transmitters or modulators released from one nerve terminal may act on presynaptic receptors of the neighboring nerve terminals to modulate the release of the transmitter substances from these nerves. Since the axon–axonal distance is always found to be much closer than that between the nerve–muscle synaptic cleft, it is logical to assume that axon–axonal transmitter interaction is more efficient than that between the nerve and the postsynaptic muscle. Our recent studies have demonstrated that NE released from the sympathetic nerves modulates NO release from the neighboring nitrergic nerves in porcine and feline cerebral arteries (Fig. 1).

7. β₂-Adrenoceptors mediate NO release in the nitrergic nerves

Using in vitro tissue bath techniques, nicotine (0.1 mM) and TNS induced neurogenic vasodilation in porcine basilar arteries. Vasodilation induced by both nicotine and TNS was abolished by nitro-L-arginine (L-NNA, 30 μM), and the blockade was reversed by L-arginine (0.3 mM). Hexamethonium and mecamylamine (10 μM) abolished the relaxation induced by nicotine, but did not affect that elicited by TNS. Furthermore, relaxation induced by nicotine was diminished by guanethidine (1–10 μM), which did not affect the relaxation induced by TNS, suggesting that guanethidine blockade of nicotine-induced relaxation was not due to its local anesthetic effect [17,23,26]. Similarly, in adrenergically denervated porcine basilar arteries following incubation with 6-hydroxydopamine (6-OHDA) [26] and cat middle cerebral arteries following chronic superior cervical ganglionectomy (our unpublished data), nicotine-induced NO-mediated relaxation was abolished, while the TNS-elicited NO-mediated relaxation was not affected. These results suggest that in large cerebral arteries, nicotine-induced NO-mediated relaxation is dependent on an intact adrenergic innervation. Nicotine appears to act on nicotinic receptors on the presynaptic adrenergic nerve terminals to release NE, which then stimulates β₂-adrenoceptors located on the neighboring nitrergic nerves resulting in NO release and vasodilation (Refs. [17,26], Fig. 1).

8. α₇-nAChRs mediate nicotine-induced nitrergic neurogenic vasodilation

The mecamylamine- and hexamethonium-sensitive relaxation of isolated porcine cerebral arterial rings induced by nicotine (100 μM) was blocked by preferential α₇-nAChR antagonists (methyllycaconitine and α-bungarotoxin) in a concentration-dependent manner, but was not affected by dihydro-β-erythroidine (DHβE, a preferential α₄-nAChR antagonist) [23,26]. These nAChR antagonists did not affect relaxation elicited by TNS (8 Hz) or that by sodium nitroprusside and NE. Results from double-labeling immunohistochemical studies in whole-mount porcine basilar and middle cerebral arteries and in cultured neuronal cells of the porcine superior cervical ganglia (SCG) indicated that α₇-nAChR- and tyrosine hydroxylase-immunoreactivities were colocalized in same nerve fibers [23]. These results suggest the presence of functional α₇-nAChRs on postganglionic sympathetic adrenergic nerve terminals of SCG origin, which mediate nicotine-induced neurogenic nitrergic vasodilation.

9. Summary and discussion

Dense adrenergic, cholinergic and nitrergic innervations are demonstrated in large cerebral arteries at the base of the brain in several species. The endogenously released ACh and NE do not exhibit significant direct effect on postsynaptic smooth muscle cells in these arteries. These two classical transmitters act as presynaptic transmitters in modulating NO release from nitrergic nerves and therefore vasodilation. Nicotine, acting on α₇-nAChRs on presynaptic sympathetic nerve terminals, releases NE which then acts on presynaptic β_2-adrenoceptors located on the neighboring nitrergic nerve terminals, resulting in release of NO and dilation of cerebral arteries (Fig. 1). This mode of action of NE in large arteries at the base of the brain may be quite different from that released in adrenergic nerves innervating small blood vessels that do not receive nitrergic innervation. Regional variations in sympathetic control of cerebral vessel tone appear to be related to the presence or absence of axo-axonal interaction. It is very likely that stimulation of sympathetic nerves may result in vasodilation of large arteries at the base of the brain and constriction of smaller arteries. Evidence has also been presented that ACh and NO are co-released from cholinergic–nitrergic nerves. ACh via binding to presynaptic muscarinic M_2 receptors inhibits cerebral nitrergic neurogenic vasodilation. This inhibition is due to a Gi-protein-mediated suppression of Ca^{2+} influx via voltage-dependent N-type Ca^{2+} channels on perivascular nitrergic nerves. This finding on the role of muscarinic cholinergic receptors in mediating inhibition of neurogenic vasodilation in large cerebral arteries at the base of the brain is different from that found in the cortical microvascular circulation. Electrical stimulation of a central cholinergic system originating in the nucleus basalis of Meynert (NBM) and substantia innominata (SI) has been shown to contribute to the cortical vasodilator response via activation of muscarinic cholinergic receptors [21], while nicotinic cholinergic receptors have been shown to mediate vasodilator response in both cortical circulation and large arteries at the base of the brain [21,24]. These findings on the regional differences in adrenergic and cholinergic mechanisms in vascular tone regulation are important for a complete elucidation of the physiological role of neurogenic control of cerebral circulation.

3.2.2.12. On-Site Discussion

3.2.2.12.1. *Question: (Pelligrino)* Last year, we published a paper in the American Journal of Physiology that may represent a physiologic manifestation of what you have proposed here. In the study, we found that hypoglycemia induced cerebral arteriolar dilation was repressed only in the presence of combined β-adrenoceptor blockade and neuronal NOS blockade, but not when each inhibition was presented alone. We surmised that β-adrenoceptor activation was important to nNOS-derived NO generation during hypogly-cemia, which is consistant with your findings. However, our data also suggested that NO might have some influence on the release (or action) of norepinephrine. Have you looked at the possibility that NO might have a "feedback" effect on norepinephrine release action?

Answer: (Lee) It is interesting to know that hypoglycemia induced arteriolar dilation is repressed only in the presence of combined β-adrenoceptor blockade and neuronal nNOS blockade. This suggests, based on our findings and hypothesis, that hypoglycemia activates release of not only NO but also transmitters such as norepinephrine which may act on β-adrenoceptors on nitrergic nerves to release NO or on non-nitrergic nerves to release non-NO vasodilators. It is logical to predict that NO can also modify the release of other transmitters such as norepinephrine. However, our preliminary results failed to demonstrate such an effect of NO in cerebral arteries of the pig, while we did demonstrate that norepinephrine release is partially dependent on NO release in the mesenteric arterial preparations (Yamamoto et al., Am J Physiol 1997; 272: H207).

3.2.2.12.2. **Question: (Maiese)** Dr. Lee, your presentation on the role of NOS during adrenegic cerebrovascular vasodilation describes a dependence on calcium, suggesting a primary role for constitutive NOS. Have you examined whether your system involves inducible NOS expression?

Answer: (Lee) There is no evidence of the presence of iNOS in normal cerebral arterial preparations we used in our experiments. iNOS is expressed only in cerebral arteries preincubated with lipopolysaccharides (Ueno and Lee, J Cereb Blood Flow Metab 1993; 13: 712).

3.2.2.12.3. **Comment: (Harder)** NADPH is not specific only for NOS!!

3.2.2.12.4. **Question: (Suzuki)** Vasoactive intestinal polypeptide (VIP) has been shown to co-localized with acetylcholine and nitric oxide synthase in the cholinergic–nitroxydergic nerve terminals. So how does VIP concern to such Ach–NOS system in the cholinergic–nitroxydergic nerve terminals?

Answer: (Lee) VIP and NO as well as ACh and NO are colocalized in the same axons in cerebral perivascular nerves in many species. The sphenopalatine ganglion (SPG) is a major origin of cerebral perivascular cholinergic, VIPergic, and NOergic nerves. Most VIP-immunoreactive and ChAT-immunoreactive fibers, however, are not found to be coincident fibers in cerebral arteries (Miao and Lee, J Cereb Blood Flow Metab 1990; 10: 32; Yu et al., Brain Res 1998; 801: 78). This result raises an important possibility that neurotransmitter and modulator colocalized within the same nerve cell body can distribute totally independently and differently at the terminal level. Ample evidence from pharmacological studies have indicated that NO is the predominant substance mediating neurogenic vasodilator response while ACh and VIP do not exhibit a significant direct effect on vascular smooth muscle (Lee, J Biomed Sci 2000; 7: 16–26) in isolated cerebral arteries. Recent studies, however, have indicated that ACh acts on the presynaptic muscarinic receptors to mediate an inhibition of NO release in bovine and porcine cerebral arteries. A presynaptic modulatory role of VIP on NO release from the bovine cerebral arteries has also been proposed, except that VIP in contrast to ACh causes an increase in NO release from the nitrergic nerves (Gonzalez et al., J Cereb Blood Flow Metab 1997; 17: 977). Thus, from a functional point of view in cerebral perivascular nerves, colocalization of VIP and NO in axons which are separate from those containing NO plus ACh could account for an efficient modulation of release of the main transmitter, NO. This would be the result of ACh and VIP being concurrently released from either cholinergic–nitrergic nerves or VIPergic–nitrergic nerves (Yu et al., Brain Res 1998; 801: 78). The finding of the segregation of cholinergic–nitrergic innervation and VIPergic–nitrergic innervation will be important for an understanding of the exact transmitter mechanisms which regulate cerebral neurogenic vasodilation.

3.2.2.12.5. **Question: (Paulson)** You mentioned that stimulation of β-adrenergic receptors was responsible for NO release in the brain. Could this be a mechanism responsible for flow increase and uncoupling of flow, oxygen and glucose metabolism during functional activation?

Answer: (Lee) Yes, it is possible. But this is just a beginning, and it needs to be carefully examined.

3.2.2.12.6. *Question: (Gaehtgens)* You indicated that the complex interplay between Ach and NA with the NO system is different between the basilar arteries which you presented and the smaller cortical arteries. 1) What are the major differences? 2) Can you give us a speculation under which physiological circumstance this difference becomes relevant?

Answer: (Lee) The major difference is that ACh inhibits NO release, causing less vasodilation in basilar arteries. ACh, on the other hand, causes vasodilation in cortical blood vessels based on reports by others, while nicotine consistently induces dilation in both preparations. It is very clear from our findings that cholinergic mechanisms in modulating cerebral circulation are regionally different. 2) The importance of this difference seems dependent on the balance between peripheral cholinergic neurons and central cholinergic neurons. I believe that there are physiological circumstances this difference may become relevant. This needs to be explored.

Acknowledgements

This work was supported by NIH HL 27763 and HL 47574, AHA/IHA (9807871), and SIU-CRC/EAM. We thank Jean Long for preparing the manuscript.

References

[1] K. Ayajiki, T. Okamoto, N. Toda, Nitric oxide mediates, and acetylcholine modulates, neurally induced relaxation of bovine cerebral arteries, Neuroscience 54 (1993) 819–825.

[2] D.W. Busija, D.D. Heistad, Factors involved in the physiological regulation of cerebral circulation, Rev. Physiol., Biochem. Pharmacol. 101 (1984) 161–211.

[3] S.P. Duckles, R. Rapoport, Release of endogenous norepinephrine from a rabbit cerebral artery, J. Pharmacol. Exp. Ther. 211 (1979) 219–224.

[4] S.P. Duckles, Evidence for a functional cholinergic innervation of cerebral arteries, J. Pharmacol. Exp. Ther. 217 (1981) 544–548.

[5] L. Edvinsson, T. Elsas, N. Suzuki, T. Shimiza, T.J.F. Lee, Origin and colocalization of nitric oxide synthase, CGRP, PACAP, and VIP in the cerebral circulation of the rat, Microsc. Res. Tech. 53 (2001) 221–228.

[6] L. Edvinsson, E.T. Mackenzie, J. McCulloch, Cerebral Blood Flow and Metabolism, Raven Press, New York, 1993.

[7] T. Kimura, J.G. Yu, L. Edvinsson, T.J.F. Lee, Cholinergic, nitric oxidergic innervation in cerebral arteries of the cat, Brain Res. 773 (1997) 117–124.

[8] T.J.F. Lee, Direct evidence against acetylcholine as the dilator transmitter in the cat cerebral arteries, Eur. J. Pharmacol. 68 (1980) 393–394.

[9] T.J.F. Lee, Putative transmitters in cerebral neurogenic vasodilation, in: J.A. Bevan, R.D. Bevan, C.L. Walters (Eds.), The Human Brain Circulation: Functional Changes in Disease, Humana Press, Totowa, NJ, 1994, pp. 73–91.

[10] T.J.F. Lee, Sympathetic and nonsympathetic transmitter mechanisms in cerebral vasodilation and constriction, in: T.J.F. Owman, J.E. Hardebo (Eds.), Neural Regulation of Brain Circulation, Elsevier, Oxford, New York, Toronto, Sydney, Paris, Frankfurt, 1986, pp. 285–296.

[11] T.J.F. Lee, Synaptic transmission of vasoconstrictor nerves in rabbit basilar artery, Eur. J. Pharmacol. 61 (1980) 55–70.

[12] T.J.F. Lee, Ultrastructural distribution of vasodilator and constrictor nerves in cat cerebral arteries, Circ. Res. 49 (1981) 971–979.

[13] T.J.F. Lee, C. Su, J.A. Bevan, Neurogenic vasoconstriction of the rabbit basilar artery, Circ. Res. 39 (1976) 120–126.

[14] T.J.F. Lee, C. Su, J.A. Bevan, Nonsympathetic dilator innervation of cat cerebral arteries, Experientia 31 (1875) 1424–1425.

[15] T.J.F. Lee, L. Kinkead, S. Sarwinski, Transmitter role of norepinephrine and acetylcholine in pig cerebral arteries, J. Cereb. Blood Flow Metab. 2 (1982) 439–450.

[16] T.J.F. Lee, J. Liu, M.S. Evans, Cholinergic–nitrergic transmitter mechanisms in the cerebral circulation, Microsc. Res. Tech. 53 (2001) 119–128.

[17] T.J.F. Lee, W. Zhang, S. Sarwinski, Presynaptic beta2-adrenoceptors mediate nicotine-induced NOergic neurogenic vasodilation in the pig cerebral arteries, Am. J. Physiol.: Heart Circ. Physiol. 279 (2) (2000) H808–H816.

[18] J. Liu, M.S. Evans, G.J. Brewer, T.J.F. Lee, N-type Ca^{2+}-channels in cultured rat sphenopalatine ganglion neurons: an immunohistochemical and electrophysiological study, J. Cereb. Blood Flow Metab. 20 (2000) 183–191.

[19] J. Liu, T.J.F. Lee, Mechanism of prejunctional muscarinic receptor-mediated inhibition of neurogenic vaso-dilation in cerebral arteries, Am. J. Physiol. 276 (1999) H194–H204.

[20] A. Saito, J.Y. Wu, T.J.F. Lee, Evidence for the presence of cholinergic nerves in cerebral artery. An immunohistochemical demonstration of choline acetyltransferase, J. Cereb. Blood Flow Metab. 5 (1985) 327–334.

[21] A. Sato, Y. Sato, Cholinergic neural regulation of regional cerebral blood flow, Alzheimer Dis. Assoc. Disord. 9 (1995) 28–38.

[22] E. Satoh, M. Nishimura, T.J.F. Lee, Comparison of ability to release norepinephrine from four portions of porcine cerebral arteries, Jpn. J. Pharmacol. 73 (Suppl. 1) (1997) 268P.

[23] M.L. Si, T.J.F. Lee, Presynaptic α_7-nicotinic acetylcholine receptors mediate nicotine-induced NOergic neurogenic vasodilation in porcine basilar arteries, J. Pharmacol. Exp. Ther. 298 (2001) 122–128.

[24] S. Uchida, F. Kagitani, H. Nakayama, A. Sato, Effect of stimulation of nicotinic cholinergic receptors on cortical cerebral blood flow and changes in the effect during aging in anesthetized rats, Neurosci. Lett. 228 (1997) 203–206.

[25] J.G. Yu, J.Y. Wu, T.J.F. Lee, Choline acetyltransferase-immunoreactivities in cerebral blood vessels, Chin. J. Pharmacol. Toxicol. 6 (1992) 28–35.

[26] W. Zhang, L. Edvinsson, T.J.F. Lee, Mechanism of nicotine-induced relaxation in the porcine basilar artery, J. Pharmacol. Exp. Ther. 284 (1998) 790–797.

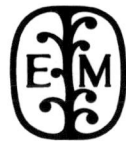

International Congress Series 1235 (2002) 347–355

Endothelium-derived hyperpolarizing factor in the cerebral circulation

Robert M. Bryan Jr. [a,b,c,*], Junping You [a],
Sean P. Marrelli [a], Elke M. Golding [a,d]

[a] *Department of Anesthesiology, Baylor College of Medicine, Houston, TX 77030, USA*
[b] *Department of Molecular Physiology and Biophysics, Baylor College of Medicine, Houston, TX 77030, USA*
[c] *Department of Medicine (Section of Cardiovascular Sciences), Baylor College of Medicine, Houston, TX 77030, USA*
[d] *Department of Neurosurgery, Baylor College of Medicine, Houston, TX 77030, USA*

Abstract

In cerebral vessels, there is at least one factor or mechanism not involving nitric oxide/endothelium-derived relaxing factor (NO/EDRF) or prostacyclin that is responsible for dilations when endothelial receptors are stimulated. This factor or mechanism is termed endothelium-derived hyperpolarizing factor (EDHF). In rat middle cerebral arteries, branches of the middle cerebral arteries and penetrating arterioles, ATP or UTP elicits the release of EDHF through stimulation of $P2Y_2$ receptors on the endothelium. The dilations are characterized by the involvement of calcium-activated potassium channels (K_{Ca}) and hyperpolarizations in vascular smooth muscle. In smaller arteries and in arterioles, EDHF appears to be more important than in larger cerebral arteries. Finally, the EDHF response is upregulated 24 h following mild traumatic brain injury (TBI). EDHF may play an important role in the regulation of cerebral blood flow during normal physiological conditions and an even greater role following pathological conditions such as TBI. © 2002 Elsevier Science B.V. All rights reserved.

Keywords: Cerebral circulation; Endothelium-derived hyperpolarizating factor (EDHF); Cerebral microcirculation; Traumatic brain injury; Endothelium; Vascular smooth muscle; Nitric oxide; P2Y receptors

* Corresponding author. Department of Anesthesiology, Room 434D, Baylor College of Medicine, One Baylor Plaza, Houston, TX 77030, USA. Tel.: +1-713-798-7720; fax: +1-713-798-7644.
E-mail address: rbryan@bcm.tmc.edu (R.M. Bryan Jr.).

0531-5131/02 © 2002 Elsevier Science B.V. All rights reserved.
PII: S0531-5131(02)00206-6

1. Introduction

In the mid- to late 1980s, evidence began to emerge that at least one factor or mechanism not involving nitric oxide/endothelium-derived relaxing factor (NO/EDRF) or prostacyclin could be responsible for dilations when endothelial receptors were stimulated [1–5]. Based on the fact that this newly emerging process involved hyperpolarization of the vascular smooth muscle and based on the assumption that a "factor" must be involved, it was termed endothelium-derived hyperpolarizing factor (EDHF). While the defining criteria for EDHF varies, it can be characterized by the following: (a) it requires endothelium; (b) it is distinct from either NO/EDRF or prostacyclin; (c) it relaxes by hyperpolarizing the vascular smooth muscle; (d) it involves calcium-activated potassium channels (K_{Ca}) [2–5].

Although the mechanism of the EDHF response has been hotly debated over the past decade, there is presently no general consensus as to its identity or mechanism of action. Presently, there are three major candidates for EDHF or the EDHF process. Substantial evidence supports the idea that epoxyeicosatrienoic acids (or EETs), metabolites of arachidonic acid through P450-epoxygenase pathways, are EDHF [6–8]. Upon stimulation of endothelial receptors, EETs would be either synthesized or released from stored pools in the endothelium. Once released, the EETS would diffuse to the vascular smooth muscle, open K_{Ca} and hyperpolarize the vascular smooth muscle.

A second hypothesis implicates the potassium ion, K^+, as EDHF [9]. In this scenario, stimulation of endothelial receptors would open K_{Ca} on the endothelium. When open, K^+ would move from the cytoplasmic space in the endothelium to the extracellular space adjacent to the vascular smooth muscle. An increase in extracellular K^+ (from 3 to 10 mM) would activate inwardly rectifying potassium channels (K_{ir}) and the sodium pump on the vascular smooth muscle resulting in hyperpolarization and relaxation of the vascular smooth muscle.

The third, major hypothesis for EDHF involves gap junctions [10]. Stimulation of endothelial receptors would hyperpolarize vascular smooth muscle through the opening of myoendothelial gap junctions. The gap junctions would allow for EDHF to move from the endothelium to the vascular smooth muscle or would hyperpolarize vascular smooth muscle by allowing the movement of cations into the endothelium. If cations (or current) move through the gap junction to hyperpolarize the vascular smooth muscle, then "EDHF" does not involve a factor per se but rather a process of current movement. Given the preceding, the process would be best described as "endothelium-dependent hyperpolarizations". Other mechanisms have been considered but they have not been substantiated or have not been as closely scrutinized. In all likelihood several EDHFs and/or EDHF-like processes exist and are dependent on the vascular bed, species, or physiological state.

Although it was previously known that cerebrovascular smooth muscle could be hyperpolarized by endothelial mechanisms [11], it was not until 1995 that evidence began to emerge for the existence of EDHF in cerebral vessels. ATP, UTP, substance P, A23187 (Ca ionophore) and acetylcholine have been reported to elicit dilations through the release of EDHF in addition to NO [12–24]. EDHF mediates dilations in arteries and arterioles by hyperpolarizing the cerebrovascular smooth muscle by approximately 14 mV and the dilation can be blocked by inhibitors of K_{Ca} channels [15,19,23]. The identification of

EDHF or the mechanism of endothelium-dependent hyperpolarizations in cerebral vessels is in its infancy.

The purpose of the present investigation was threefold: (1) to determine whether ATP (agonist for P2Y$_2$ receptors) elicits dilations in cerebral vessels; (2) to determine the relative importance of EDHF in ATP mediated dilations in larger and smaller cerebral vessels in the rat; and (3) to determine whether mild traumatic brain injury alters the EDHF-mediated dilations in small cerebral arteries.

2. Materials and methods

Male Long–Evans rats (250–350 g) were anesthetized with 3% isoflurane, decapitated, and the brains were removed. Middle cerebral arteries (MCAs), third- and fourth-order branches of the middle artery (bMCAs) and penetrating arterioles (PAs) were carefully removed and mounted on micropipettes as previously described [25]. MCAs were pressurized to 85 mm Hg; bMCAs and PAs were pressurized to 60 mm Hg. Vessels were luminally perfused with physiological saline solution (PSS) at a rate that produced a shear stress between 20 and 30 dyn/cm^2. Each vessel was magnified and the image was displayed on a video screen. Outside diameters were measured manually from the video screen and continuously measured using image analysis software. ATP was added to the luminal perfusate to elicit dilations of the vessels [15,23,26]. Dilations of cerebral vessels are presented as either outside diameter in μm or as percent maximum diameter, where:

$$\% \text{ maximum diameter} = [(D_{agonist} - D_{base})/(D_{max} - D_{base})] \times 100$$

where $D_{agonist}$ is the diameter after luminal administration of ATP, D_{base} is the baseline diameter before addition of ATP and D_{max} is the maximum diameter (measured using calcium-free PSS).

In some vessels, the endothelium was removed by passing air through the lumen [25]. Mild traumatic brain injury (TBI) was accomplished using controlled cortical impact injury as previously described [27,28]. Twenty-four hours following the injury, bMCAs at the injury site were isolated and mounted as described above.

3. Results and discussion

Additions of ATP to the luminal perfusate caused rat PAs to dilate from 87 ± 6 μm ($n=6$) to 112 ± 6 μm ($p=0.002$) (control response in Fig. 1A). Removal of the endothelium abolished this dilation to ATP. The presence of 10^{-5} M L-NAME and 10^{-5} M indomethacin (indo), blockers of NO synthase and cyclooxygenase respectively, had no effect on the dilations to 10^{-5} M ATP. However, L-NAME and indo did block dilations at 10^{-6} M ATP (data not shown). The addition of charybdotoxin (CHTX, 100 nM), an inhibitor of K$_{Ca}$, in the presence of L-NAME and indo completely blocked the dilation to

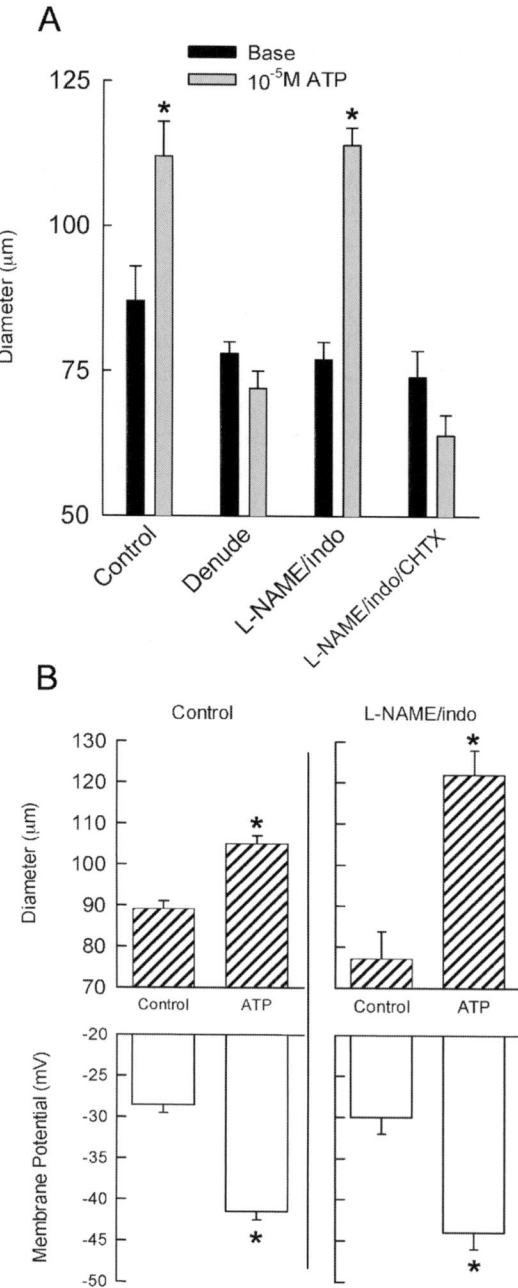

Fig. 1. (A) The effects of luminally applied ATP (10^{-5} M) on outside diameter in rat penetrating arterioles. (B) Simultaneous measurement of membrane potential in vascular smooth muscle and diameter after luminally applied ATP (10^{-5} M) in rat penetrating arterioles.

ATP. Fig. 1B demonstrates that 10^{-5} M ATP dilated PAs and significantly hyperpolarized the vascular smooth muscle by approximately 13 mV in the absence (control) or in the presence of L-NAME and indomethacin. Thus, ATP fulfills the criteria for EDHF as defined in the Introduction. We conclude that EDHF-mediated dilations exist in the cerebral circulation.

Fig. 2 shows the effects of luminally administered ATP to rat MCAs (226 ± 5, $n=10$), bMCAs (96 ± 4, $n=6$) and PAs (87 ± 6, $n=6$). The presence of L-NAME and indo significantly shifted the concentration response curve for ATP to the right in MCAs but had lesser effect or no significant effect in the bMCAs and PAs, respectively. The L-NAME/indo-resistant component of the dilation for the MCAs, bMCAs, and PAs fulfilled the criteria for EDHF as described in Section 1. That is, the L-NAME/indo-resistant dilations in all three vessel groups, were dependent on endothelium, could be blocked by CHTX and hyperpolarized the vascular smooth muscle (data not shown). Since the EDHF component of the dilation contributed to a greater degree to the overall dilation in more distal and smaller cerebral vessels, EDHF must be more prevalent and have a greater importance in smaller vessels than in larger cerebral vessels (Fig. 2).

Fig. 3 shows that the EDHF response 24 h following mild traumatic brain injury was enhanced in bMCAs (129 ± 7 μm, $n=6$) compared to those isolated from sham-injured rats (138 ± 5 μm, $n=6$). Dilations to ATP in bMCAs from the injured area were

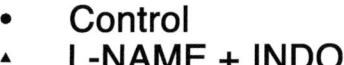

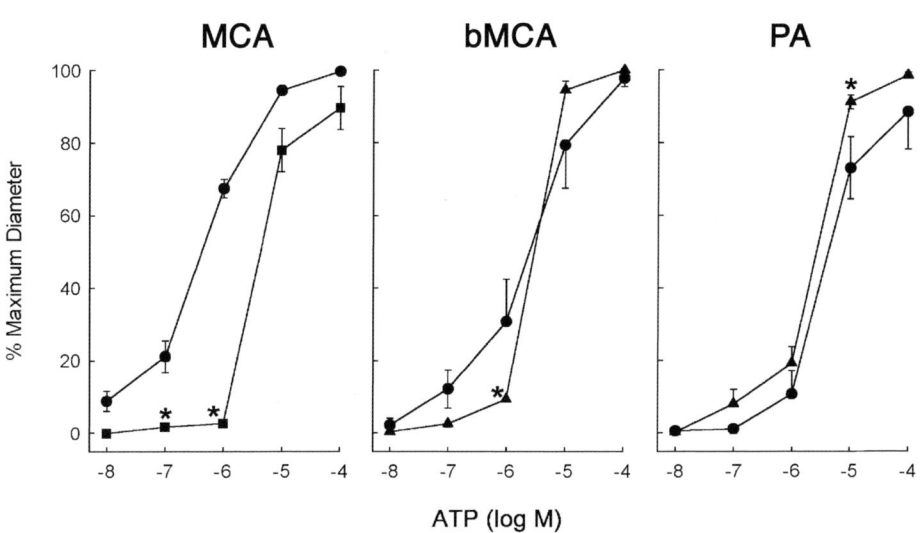

Fig. 2. Dilations to luminally applied ATP in rat middle cerebral arteries (MCA, 226 ± 5 μm, $n=10$), third- and fourth-order branches of the MCA (bMCA, 96 ± 4 μm, $n=6$) and penetrating arterioles (PA, 87 ± 6 μm, $n=6$) of the rat.

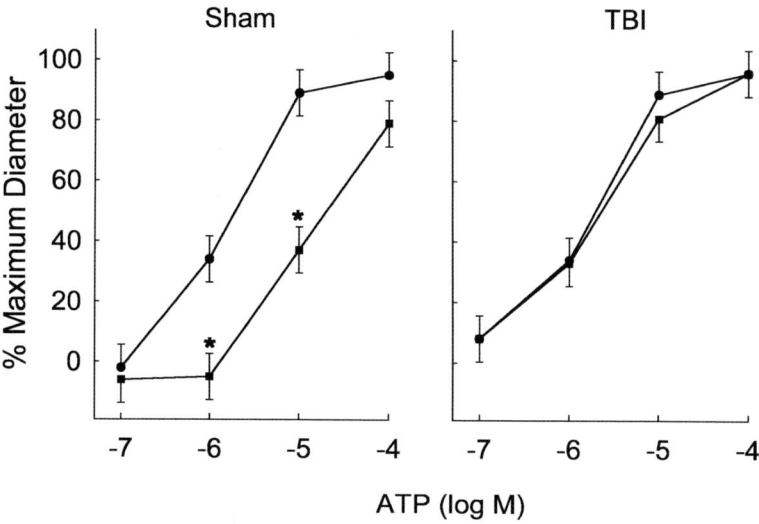

Fig. 3. The effects of mild traumatic brain injury (TBI) on ATP-mediated dilations in branches of the rat middle cerebral artery.

insensitive to L-NAME/indo. Dilations in the presence of L-NAME/indo from sham-injured ($n=3$) or TBI arteries ($n=3$) could be further blocked by the K_{Ca} inhibitor, CHTX ($p<0.05$, data not shown).

We conclude that endothelial dependent dilations that fit the criteria for EDHF occur in cerebral vessels. Furthermore, EDHF is more prominent in smaller cerebral arteries and arterioles than in the larger arteries. We hypothesize that EDHF has a major role in regulation of arteriolar tone and, thus, is an important regulator of cerebral blood flow in vivo. However, our hypothesis cannot be fully tested until the mechanism of action for EDHF is understood. Presently, the only way in which EDHF can be studied is following inhibition of both NO and PGI_2. Only when the mechanism of EDHF-mediated dilations is elucidated can it be studied in the presence of NO and PGI_2, and only then can its relative importance in cerebral vessels during normal physiological conditions be determined.

Finally we report that EDHF is upregulated 24 h following mild TBI. This finding is consistent with our previous results showing that EDHF is upregulated 24 h following ischemia/reperfusion [22,24]. Although the role of EDHF in pathological conditions is not presently known, we speculate that it is an adaptive mechanism offering cerebral protection. The next several years will be critical in determining the mechanism and nature of EDHF in brain. It is possible that protection afforded by EDHF (or the endothelium-dependent hyperpolarizing process) will be considered clinically relevant during pathological conditions.

3.2.3.6. On-Site Discussion

3.2.3.6.1. Question: (Busija) You haven't discussed the nature of EDHF. Would you care to speculate on what EDHF is? Is it a p450 metabolite such as an EET?

Answer: (Bryan) Its identity has been illusive, likely due to the fact that it might be more than one process involved. However, after stating this, we do have evidence that arachidonic acid has a role in the process.

3.2.3.6.2. Question: (Pelligrino) Is there cross-regulation between the NO and EDHF systems? Could such cross-regulation explain the findings of your lab which showed that estrogen depletion which reduces endothelial NO generation was associated with an increase in the contributions from EDHF to ATP-induced dilations in rat MCA's?

Answer: (Bryan) Good question! Although the EDHF is upregulated during conditions when NO is downregulated; however, there is no evidence in cerebral vessels that NO directly regulates EDHF.

3.2.3.6.3. Question: (Ances) Under the pathophysiological condition of cortical unjury could the results be a loss of NO instead of an upregulation of EDHF?

Answer: (Bryan) There is an idea that there is an equipoise between NO and EDHF. In situations where NO is diminished, such as pathological condition, EDHF is often upregulated; however, there is no evidence for a cause and effect relationship in brain.

3.2.3.6.4. Question: (Kempski) (1) Does spreading depression have any effect on the EDHF response? (2) Is CO involved in EDHF action?

Answer: (Bryan) (1) We do not know the effects of spreading depression on the EDHF response. (2) EDHF is regulated during conditions when hemeoxygenase, the enzyme responsible for generating CO, is also upregulated. However, CO may not be involved with the EDHF response.

Acknowledgements

These studies were supported by NIH grants NS 27616 and NS 37250.

References

[1] J.V. Mombouli, P.M. Vanhoutte, Endothelium-derived hyperpolarizing factor(s): updating the unknown, Trends Pharmacol. Sci. 18 (1997) 252–256.

[2] R.A. Cohen, P.M. Vanhoutte, Endothelium-dependent hyperpolarization—beyond nitric oxide and cyclic GMP, Circulation 92 (1995) 3337–3349.

[3] M. Feletou, P.M. Vanhoutte, The third pathway: endothelium-dependent hyperpolarization, J. Physiol. Pharmacol. 50 (1999) 525–534.

[4] C.J. Garland, F. Plane, B.K. Kemp, T.M. Cocks, Endothelium-dependent hyperpolarization: a role in the control of vascular tone, Trends Pharmacol. Sci. 16 (1995) 23–30.

[5] J.V. Mombouli, P.M. Vanhoutte, Endothelial dysfunction: from physiology to therapy, J. Mol. Cell. Cardiol. 31 (1999) 61–74.

[6] W.B. Campbell, D. Gebremedhin, P.F. Pratt, D.R. Harder, Identification of epoxyeicosatrienoic acids as endothelium-derived hyperpolarizing factors, Circ. Res. 78 (1996) 415–423.

[7] S.S. Bolz, B. Fisslthaler, S. Pieperhoff, C. De Wit, I. Fleming, R. Busse, U. Pohl, Antisense oligonucleotides against cytochrome P450 2C8 attenuate EDHF-mediated Ca(2+) changes and dilation in isolated resistance arteries, FASEB J. 14 (2000) 255–260.

[8] B. Fisslthaler, R. Popp, L. Kiss, M. Potente, D.R. Harder, I. Fleming, R. Busse, Cytochrome P450 2C is an EDHF synthase in coronary arteries, Nature 401 (1999) 493–497.

[9] G. Edwards, K.A. Dora, M.J. Gardener, C.J. Garland, A.H. Weston, K^+ is an endothelium-derived hyperpolarizing factor in rat arteries, Nature 396 (1998) 269–272.

[10] A.T. Chaytor, W.H. Evans, T.M. Griffith, Central role of heterocellular gap junctional communication in endothelium-dependent relaxations of rabbit arteries, J. Physiol. (London) 508 (Pt 2) (1998) 561–573.

[11] J.E. Brayden, G.C. Wellman, Endothelium-dependent dilation of feline cerebral arteries: role of membrane potential and cyclic nucleotides, J. Cereb. Blood Flow Metab. 9 (1989) 256–263.

[12] H. Dong, Y. Jiang, W.C. Cole, C.R. Triggle, Comparison of the pharmacological properties of EDHF-mediated vasorelaxation in guinea-pig cerebral and mesenteric resistance vessels, Br. J. Pharmacol. 130 (2000) 1983–1991.

[13] J. Petersson, P.M. Zygmunt, E.D. Hogestatt, Characterization of the potassium channels involved in EDHF-mediated relaxation in cerebral arteries, Br. J. Pharmacol. 120 (1997) 1344–1350.

[14] C.R. Triggle, H. Dong, G.J. Waldron, W.C. Cole, Endothelium-derived hyperpolarizing factor(s): species and tissue heterogeneity, Clin. Exp. Pharmacol. Physiol. 26 (1999) 176–179.

[15] J. You, T.D. Johnson, S.P. Marrelli, R.M. Bryan Jr., Functional heterogeneity of endothelial P2 purinoceptors in the cerebrovascular tree of the rat, Am. J. Physiol. 277 (1999) H893–H900.

[16] N. Yamakawa, M. Ohhashi, S. Waga, T. Itoh, Role of endothelium in regulation of smooth muscle membrane potential and tone in the rabbit middle cerebral artery, Br. J. Pharmacol. 121 (1997) 1315–1322.

[17] J. Petersson, P.M. Zygmunt, L. Brandt, E.D. Högestätt, Substance P-induced relaxation and hyperpolarization in human cerebral arteries, Br. J. Pharmacol. 115 (1995) 889–894.

[18] J. Petersson, P.M. Zygmunt, P. Jonsson, E.D. Hogestatt, Characterization of endothelium-dependent relaxation in guinea pig basilar artery—effect of hypoxia and role of cytochrome P450 mono-oxygenase, J. Vasc. Res. 35 (1998) 285–294.

[19] P.M. Zygmunt, M. Sorgard, J. Petersson, R. Johansson, E.D. Hogestatt, Differential actions of anandamide, potassium ions and endothelium-derived hyperpolarizing factor in guinea-pig basilar artery, Naunyn-Schmiedeberg's Arch. Pharmacol. 361 (2000) 535–542.

[20] E.M. Golding, J. You, C.S. Robertson, R.M. Bryan Jr., Potentiated EDHF-mediated dilations in cerebral arteries following mild head injury, J. Neurotrauma 18 (2001) 691–697.

[21] S.P. Marrelli, Mechanisms of endothelial P2Y(1)- and P2Y(2)-mediated vasodilatation involve differential $[Ca^{2+}]i$ responses, Am. J. Physiol. Heart Circ. Physiol. 281 (2001) H1759–H1766.

[22] S.P. Marrelli, A. Khorovets, T.D. Johnson, W.F. Childres, R.M. Bryan Jr., P2 purinoceptor-mediated dilations in the rat middle cerebral artery after ischemia/reperfusion, Am. J. Physiol. 276 (1999) H33–H41.

[23] J.P. You, T.D. Johnson, S.P. Marrelli, J.V. Mombouli, W.F. Childres, R.M. Bryan Jr., P2u-receptor mediated release of endothelium-derived relaxing factor/nitric oxide and endothelium-derived hyperpolarizing factor from cerebrovascular endothelium in rats, Stroke 30 (1999) 1125–1133.

[24] S.P. Marrelli, W.F. Childres, J. Goddard-Finegold, R.M. Bryan Jr., Potentiated EDHF-mediated dilations in the rat middle cerebral artery following ischemia/reperfusion, in: P.M. Vanhoutte (Ed.), EDHF 2000, Taylor & Francis, New York, 2001.

[25] R.M. Bryan Jr., M.Y. Eichler, M.W.G. Swafford, T.D. Johnson, M.S. Suresh, W.F. Childres, Stimulation of α_2 adrenoceptors dilates the rat middle cerebral artery, Anesthesiology 85 (1996) 82–90.

[26] J.P. You, T.D. Johnson, W.F. Childres, R.M. Bryan Jr., Endothelial-mediated dilations of rat middle cerebral arteries by ATP and ADP, Am. J. Physiol. 273 (1997) H1472–H1477.

[27] E.M. Golding, M.L. Steenberg, C.F. Contant Jr., I.K. Krishnappa, C.S. Robertson, R.M. Bryan Jr., Cerebrovascular reactivity to CO_2 and hypotension after mild cortical impact injury, Am. J. Physiol.: Heart Circ. Physiol. 277 (1999) 1457–1466.

[28] E.M. Golding, C.S. Robertson, R.M. Bryan Jr., L-arginine partially restores the diminished CO_2 reactivity after mild controlled cortical impact injury in the adult rat, J. Cereb. Blood Flow Metab. 20 (2000) 820–828.

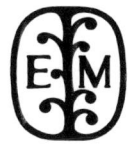

International Congress Series 1235 (2002) 357–368

Variations in CBF during hypotension and in cortical eNOS in rats

Stephen C. Jones [a,*], Alexander Kharlamov [a], D. Kyle Kim [b], Kirk A. Easley [c], Laurie Machen [a]

[a]*Department of Anesthesiology, Allegheny General Hospital, 320 East North Avenue, Pittsburgh, PA 15212-4772, USA*
[b]*Department of Neurosurgery, Allegheny General Hospital, 320 East North Avenue, Pittsburgh, PA 15212, USA*
[c]*Department of Biostatistics, Cleveland Clinic Foundation, 9500 Euclid Avenue, Cleveland, OH 44195, USA*

Abstract

Variations in the height of the autoregulatory curve near the lower limit present the intriguing suggestion that there are local differences in cortical vascular regulation. We suspect that these variations are related to local variations in the amount of cortical eNOS, $[eNOS]_{br}$. Laser Doppler flowmetry (LDF) monitoring of CBF in rat cortex during hemorrhagic hypotension revealed that the CBF at a mean arterial pressure of 70 mmHg ($\%CBF_{70}$) was highly variable and distributed normally. Both paradoxical rises in CBF and pressure-passive CBF were common during moderate hypotension. In other experiments, similar variations in the concentration of eNOS, $[eNOS]_{br}$, were observed in brain samples of similar volume to the volume sensed by LDF and differences in $\%CBF_{70}$ were noted in different regions of the same animal's cortex. These observations suggest the surprising possibility that cortical variations in the amount of eNOS protein, not its regulation, relate to variations in the CBF response to moderate hypotension. © 2002 Elsevier Science B.V. All rights reserved.

Keywords: Autoregulation; Cerebral blood flow; Hypotension; Nitric oxide; Cerebrovascular regulation; Cerebral blood flow autoregulation; Western analysis; eNOS

Abbreviations: CBF, Cerebral blood flow; eNOS, endothelial nitric oxide synthase; LDF, laser Doppler flowmetry; ACh, acetylcholine; ADP, adenosine diphosphate; aCSF, artificial cerebrospinal fluid; MABP, mean arterial blood pressure; $\%CBF_{70}$, cerebral blood flow at a mean arterial blood pressure of 70 mmHg as percent of control CBF at 100 mmHg.

* Corresponding author. Tel.: +1-412-359-4919; fax: +1-412-359-3986.
E-mail address: sjones@wpahs.org (S.C. Jones).

1. Introduction

Parameters relating to cerebrovascular regulation show heterogeneity during both normal conditions (brain pO_2 [1]) and when the limit of brain integrity is threatened by ischemia, moderate hypotension [2,3] or hypoxia. The source of this heterogeneity is possibly due to inherent microvascular factors. Here, we investigate the heterogeneity of CBF during moderate hypotension using laser Doppler flowmetry (LDF) with a detection volume of ~ 2 mg, and of the amount of brain cortex eNOS protein, $[eNOS]_{br}$ using Western analysis in brain samples of similar weight. Since autoregulatory responses during hypotension have been associated with nitric oxide [2,4], we hypothesize that the heterogeneity of the height of the CBF response to moderate hypotension is related to the heterogeneity of $[eNOS]_{br}$.

2. Methods

2.1. Animal preparation

Male Sprague–Dawley rats weighing between 250 and 350 g were induced with 2.5% isoflurane or halothane, tracheotomized or entubated, and femoral arteries and veins were cannulated with PE-50 polyethylene catheters under 1.8–2.0% isoflurane or halothane, all with 70% N_2O balance O_2 administered via mechanical ventilation. The concentration of isoflurane or halothane was adjusted to remove the response of blood pressure, visualized on the polygraph, to tail pinch. Animals were immobilized with 4 mg/kg pancuronium bromide or gallamine triethiodide (10 mg/kg/h), and heparinized (100 IU/kg). Body temperature was maintained at 37°C with a servo-controlled heating lamp and a rectal thermistor. One femoral artery was used for the monitoring of blood pressure with a strain gauge transducer. Mean arterial blood pressure (MABP) and end-tidal CO_2, as determined with an infrared CO_2 analyzer, were recorded on a polygraph. Animals were stabilized at PaO_2 of >90 mmHg. $PaCO_2$ was maintained between 33 and 37 mmHg by adjusting the respirator rate. After surgery and for maintenance during the experimental procedure, 0.8–1% isoflurane or halothane, supplemented by 70% N_2O in O_2, was used. Animals were not studied until 30 min had elapsed since isoflurane or halothane had been lowered to the maintenance concentration. An ABL3 (Radiometer) or IL1620 (Instrumentation Laboratory, MA) blood gas analyzer was used to measure arterial blood gases (PaO_2, $PaCO_2$) and pH.

Three groups of rats were used. In Group I ($n=65$), the CBF response to moderate hypotension was studied. In Group II ($n=2$), differences in the autoregulatory curve between different regions of cortex were studied. In Group III ($n=3$ for 41 brain samples), variations in eNOS were analyzed.

2.2. Groups I and II

Sixty-five rats under halothane anesthesia [3] (Group I) and two rats under isoflurane anesthesia (Group II) were subjected to graded hypotension while %CBF was monitored with LDF, with 100%CBF defined as the LDF value at a mean arterial pressure of 100 mmHg (see Fig. 1). The %CBF at an arterial pressure of 70 mmHg, %CBF$_{70}$, was determined for each individual curve.

2.3. Laser Doppler flowmetry (LDF) monitoring

For Group I, we used the superfused closed cranial window preparation, including a thermocouple for monitoring window temperature, continuous monitoring of intracranial pressure and inflow and outflow ports [2]. Artificial cerebrospinal fluid was bubbled through 6% CO_2, 10% O_2 balance N_2 at 37°C. CBF was continuously monitored (time constant 1 s) using LDF (Model BMP-403A, Vasamedics, MN) through the superfused cranial window. The 0.8-mm diameter LDF probe was positioned just above the cranial window over a relatively avascular area using a micromanipulator attached to the stereotaxic frame. Both the position of the probe and the integrity of the vasculature were tested using the CBF response to hypercapnia [5] and to superfused 10^{-4} M adenosine diphosphate or 10^{-5} M acetylcholine (ACh).

For Group II, we used the bone window method and laser Doppler flowmetry with a Perimed laser Doppler flowmeter (Periflux 4001) with two laser Doppler probes. The probes were placed 1.5 mm behind bregma and 1.5 mm lateral from midline (BZ region) and 1.5 behind bregma and 3.5–4 mm (MCA region) in holes drilled in the skull leaving a thin bone window. CO_2 reactivity and endothelium dependent reactivity to the intravenously administered blood–brain barrier (BBB) permeant muscarinic agonist oxotremorine (1 μg/kg/min) were tested before a graded blood withdrawal. To minimize the systemic effect of oxotremorine, the muscarinic antagonist atropine methyl bromide (0.5 mg/kg, i.p.), that does not cross the BBB, was injected 15 min before oxotremorine

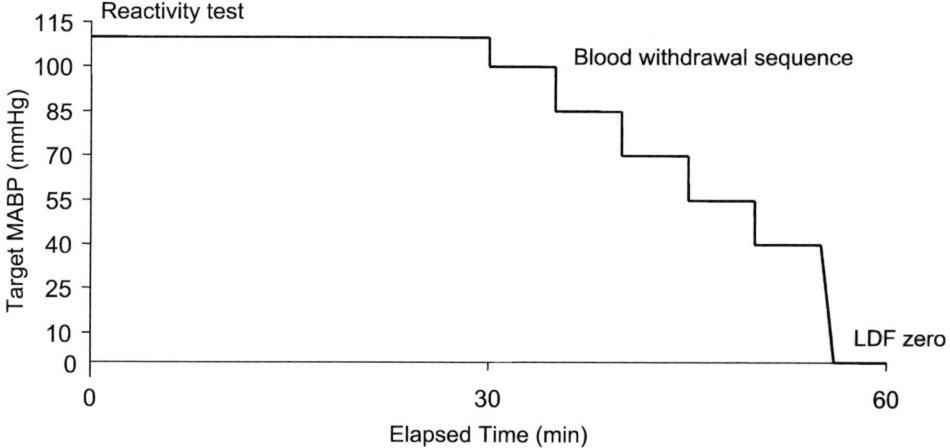

Fig. 1. The blood-withdrawal protocol is depicted in schematic form, showing the time progression from the initial assessment of vascular reactivity, the sequence of hemorrhagic hypotension to the target MABPs and the LDF biological zero.

infusion. Graded hemorrhagic hypotension was performed 40 min after oxotremorine infusion.

For both Groups I and II, the flow signal obtained at the end of each experiment after the animal was sacrificed (LDF zero) was used to confirm that the laser Doppler flowmeter was properly zeroed. The vascular reactivities to CO_2, ADP, ATP and oxotremorine were calculated after the end of the experiment using the LDF zero value. If the CO_2, ADP, ATP and oxotremorine reactivities were less than 1%/mmHg, 10%/mmHg, 15%/mmHg or 10%/mmHg, respectively, the animal was excluded.

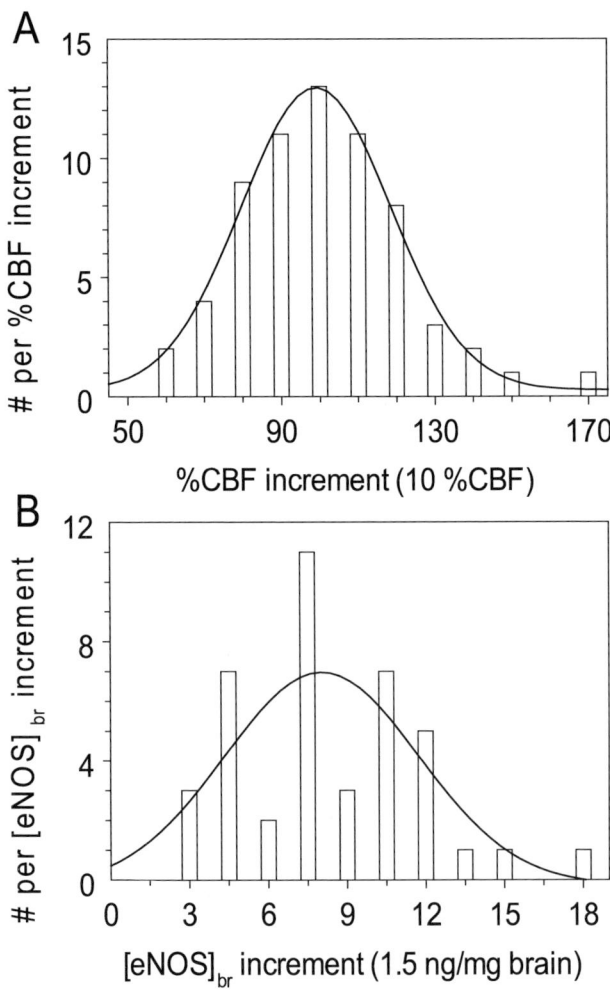

Fig. 2. Frequency histograms and Gaussian fits of %CBF$_{70}$ (with permission from Ref. [3]) (Panel A) and [eNOS]$_{br}$ (Panel B).

2.4. Group III—eNOS immunoblotting

For Group III, 41 cortical brain samples were collected from three rats under isoflurane (in 30% O_2, 70% N_2O) anesthesia. The brain samples were weighted, flash frozen in liquid N_2, sonicated for 2×5 s (50% pulse) in extraction buffer, analyzed for protein concen-

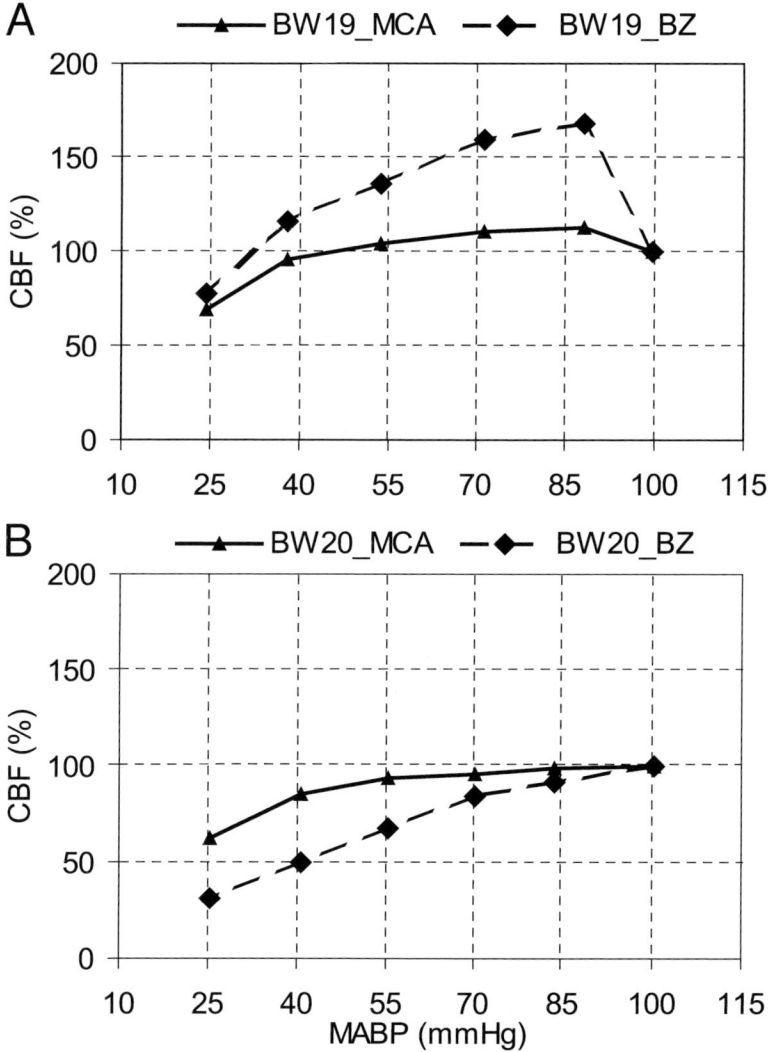

Fig. 3. Panel A shows two autoregulatory curves from the same sequence of hemorrhagic hypotension in animal BW19. Panel B shows two curves in animal BW20. The solid line and triangles refer to %CBF and MABP pairs from the LDF probe over the MCA territory (MCA region). The dashed line and diamonds refer to data pairs from the second LDF place over the border zone, BZ, region. It is clear that the autoregulatory curves are dramatically different in the different regions in both animals.

Table 1
Cortical heterogeneity of autoregulation

Animal no.	CBF_{70} (mmHg)	
	Region	
	MCA	BS
BW19	110	158
BW20	96	84

tration and run in duplicate on different gels with an eNOS standard (Transduction Laboratories). Immunoreactive bands at 140 kDa to eNOS Ab (Transduction Laboratory) were recorded with ECL, digitized and quantitated in reference to the eNOS standard (1 µg/µl total protein with an assumed 0.1 ng eNOS/µl).

3. Results

Only 51% of the $\%CBF_{70}$ values were near the 100% expected for an autoregulatory curve that was a simple plateau followed by a fall at the lower limit of 70 mmHg [3]. The wide distribution of $\%CBF_{70}$ values included many that increased (32%) to over 115%CBF and decreased (17%) to less than 85%CBF at a MABP of 70 mmHg.

The mean ($\pm$S.E.M.) sample weight was 4.6 ± 0.6 mg for the 41 brain cortex samples. Mean $[eNOS]_{br}$ was 9.1 ± 0.5 ng/mg brain or 0.10 ± 0.006 ng/µg total protein (TP). There was no correlation between sample weight and $[eNOS]_{br}$, nor were there differences in $[eNOS]_{br}$ between animals. The frequency histograms and fitted Gaussian distributions of $\%CBF_{70}$ and $[eNOS]_{br}$ are shown in Fig. 2. Both the $[eNOS]_{br}$ and $\%CBF_{70}$ frequency distributions are normally distributed ($p>0.25$, $p>0.25$, Anderson–Darling test).

3.1. Dual laser Doppler flowmetry after hemorrhagic hypotension

As shown in Fig. 3 and Table 1, the autoregulatory curves were different in the MCA and the BZ areas, the region of shared blood supply between the MCA and ACA, for both animals. In both areas of BW19, the first MABP drop from 100 to 85 mmHg caused an increase of CBF, with a much more substantial rise in the BZ region ($\%CBF_{70}=158\%CBF$) than in the MCA region ($CBF_{70}=110\%CBF$). In animal BW20, CBF remained stable down to a MABP of 55 mmHg in the MCA region, but in the BZ region, CBF constantly decreased starting at a MABP of 100 mmHg.

4. Discussion

Previous work indicates that the lower limit of autoregulation is increased [2] and $\%CBF_{70}$ is decreased (unpublished data), by cortical nitric oxide synthase inhibition, and there is suggestive evidence that eNOS is the responsible NOS isoform for these effects [6]. We suspected that the heterogeneity of $\%CBF_{70}$ would be related to the regulation of eNOS activity by many factors, including its association with caveolin-1 [7] or its dependence on O_2 as a substrate [8]. The similarity of the Gaussian distributions of %CBF_{70} and [eNOS]$_{br}$ observed here suggest that variations in [eNOS]$_{br}$ itself could be responsible, and that an [eNOS]$_{br}$ of 9 ng/mg (based on an assumed eNOS/TP weight fraction of 10^{-4}) supports the vasodilation necessary for a normal response to hypotension of 70 mmHg.

4.1. Regional variations in the height of the autoregulatory response [3]

The presence of different shapes of autoregulatory curves in the same animal in different cortical locations, as shown in Fig. 3, suggests that this heterogeneity of autoregulation is due to regional variations in some aspect of cerebrovascular regulatory control during hypotension. Although regional differences in the lower limit have been well characterized between cortex and brain stem [9], we show that variations in %CBF_{70} also exist within the cortex. Does the fraction of large and small vessels, and arterioles and venules, near the LDF probe account for the different patterns of autoregulation? For instance, a large %CBF_{70} might occur because the LDF probe was situated near a large vessel. Although for our observation of the heterogeneity of %CBF_{70}, the probe was positioned far from large vessels in a relatively avascular region of the cortex, the sensitive region measured by the LDF probe approaches the 1–2-mm spacing observed in O_2 heterogeneity in normal cat cortex by Wilson et al. [1]. This distance approaches the spacing between approximately two of Bär's medium vascular nodules of 300–700 μm [10]. The recent work by Lübbers and Baumgartl [11] shows O_2 heterogeneity of the same spacing. So there is reason to believe that the net distance of the LDF probe from the nearest penetrating arterioles influences the patterns. From this point of view, this heterogeneity is a property dependent on the vascular architecture.

4.2. Summary

We have observed wide variations between animals in the pattern of autoregulation that cannot be explained by damaged vessels or nonphysiological factors [2,3], and similar variations in [eNOS]$_{br}$ in cortical samples of similar volume. The regional heterogeneity of %CBF_{70} in the same animal that we observed suggests that there are substantial regional variations in cerebrovascular control during moderate hypotension.

3.2.4.7. On-Site Discussion

3.2.4.7.1. *Question: (Iadecola)* I was intrigued by the fact that a long superfusion time for N^{ω}-nitro-L-arginine (LNNA) was needed in order to observe the effects on autoregulation. If, as you suggest, eNOS is the target enzyme inhibited in LNNA, eNOS inhibition can be achieved with a much shorter time by superfusion in cranial window preparations. The requirement for a long superfusion period (105 min) raises the possibility that LNNA may act through non-eNOS-mediated mechanisms.

Answer: (Jones) Data from our previous work (Jones et al., Am. J. Physiol. Heart Circ. Physiol., 1999, 276: H1253) showed an effect for 105 min of LNNA superfusion on the lower limit of autoregulation, but not for 35 min of superfusion. In this previous work, we consider ourselves lucky to have found that lengthy superfusion was effective, but not shorter superfusion. We ascribe the lack of this lengthy superfusion to be why some workers did not find an effect of NOS inhibition on autoregulation (Shin et al., Am. J. Physiol., 2000, 278: H339). The ineffectiveness of the shorter suffusion of 35 min of NOS inhibitor compared to the 105-min suffusion period suggested that the inhibited NOS was diffusionally distant. Our data indicate that 35 min of suffusion was not long enough to permit LNNA to inhibit the NOS that is the source of nitric oxide that mediates the vasodilation near the lower limit, but that 105 min of LNNA exposure did allow inhibition of this NOS source. Diffusional barriers to suffused agents have been reported in the pial circulation (Regidor et al., NeuroReport, 1993, 4(1): 112), and are probably even more important for intra-parenchymal arteries such as penetrator arterioles. The lack of change in lower limit with 35 min suffusion of LNNA is consistent with the lack of effect until 60 min of LNNA suffusion in some parameters used to assess functional activation (Irikura et al., J. Cereb. Blood Flow Metab., 1994, 14: 45) and CBF and pial artery diameter response to CO_2 (Irikura et al., Am. J. Physiol., 1994, 267: H837), although changes in other parameters were noticeable after shorter periods of LNNA suffusion. Even 60 min after topical administration of LNNA, NOS activity was still decreasing (Irikura et al., J. Cereb. Blood Flow Metab., 1994, 14: 45; Irikura et al., Am. J. Physiol., 1994, 267: H837). In contrast, Fabricius et al. (Am. J. Physiol., 1996, 271: H2035) showed rapid decreases in NOS activity and in CO_2 reactivity within 5–15 and 30–45 min, respectively, after cortical LNNA suffusion. However, the timing of the effect of NOS inhibition on the CO_2 reactivity, cGMP, or functional activation, or even NOS activity assayed by the ex vivo NOS assay, might be different from the timing for its influence on the lower limit. Different and multiple anatomical and cellular locations of either or both of the constitutive isoforms of NOS contribute to this issue.

Consider that the NOS in the tissue volume sensed by the laser Doppler probe must be fully inhibited before a change in CBF can be detected. If our laser Doppler probe illuminates to a median depth of 1 mm, LNNA must diffuse and inhibit NOS to at least this depth. Our data showing that 105 min of LNNA suffusion did, and 35 min did not, affect the lower limit is consistent with autoradiographic observations using ^{14}C-LNNA that 1 mM LNNA suffused for 2 h gives a concentration of 0.25 mM and for 30 min, of 0.10 mM, at a depth of 1 mm (Greenberg et al., Neurosci. Lett., 1997, 229: 1).

3.2.4.7.2 **Question: (Golanov)** Could the "peak" groups increase in CBF in response to hyperfusion relate to EEG changes as we observed in some animals in response to blood pressure drugs?

Answer: (Jones) We did not measure EEG in our experiments, so it is hard to formulate an answer to your question, because we have no comparable data.

3.2.4.7.3. **Question: (Kuschinsky)** The heterogeneity of autoregulatory reaction patterns is a general phenomenon in the brain. Using the iodoantipyrine technique, we could demonstrate different patterns of autoregulatory reactions in different brain structures. These reactions were reproducible for each structure, but differed between structures.

Answer: (Jones) Yes, one of your studies (Waschke et al., Intensive Care Med., 1996, 22: 1026) shows similar characteristics of the autoregulatory patterns in conscious animals using a different CBF technique than the one used by ourselves. This correspondence of findings lends support to both works.

3.2.4.7.4. *Question: (Gaehtgens)* The stimulus for the autoregulatory response is the distensing pressure in the arterial microvessels, not arterial pressure. Therefore, and particularly in view of the differential innervation of larger conduits and cortical vessels, one might speculate that your three different types of autoregulatory response might be related to a variation of large vessel resistance. In other words, would the three types also be present, if small vessel pressure rather than MABP had been measured? Have such studies been made?

Answer: (Jones) It is very reasonable to assume that conduit arteries and pre-capillary vessels would show different responses to hemorrhagic hypotension, not only because the pressure at each portion of the circulation differs from systemic arterial pressure, but also because of differences in innervation and local environmental influences. However, the data of Toyoda et al. (J. Cereb. Blood Flow Metab., 1997, 17: 1089) indicate that both larger intermediate and small arteries dilate in response to hypotension in the brain stem of the rat. Although in these studies and in ours the pressure was not determined at arterioles, such measurements would not have changed our results or the results Toyoda et al. (J. Cereb. Blood Flow Metab., 1997, 17: 1089).

3.2.4.7.5. *Question: (Krause)* Were your studies done in male or female animals? Since there are high levels of eNOS in cerebral vessels from females, it would be interesting to try these studies using female animals.

Answer: (Jones) All our studies were done in male animals. It would be interesting to see if these patterns differed between ovariectomized female and estrogen repleted females. The working hypothesis would be that estrogen promotes the peak autoregulatory response.

3.2.4.7.6 *Question: (Benyó)* (1) Superfusion of L-NAME probably constricted cerebral arteries and decreased resting blood flow in your experiments. Changing of resting vascular resistance and blood flow may influence autoregulation by itself (Paulson et al., Cerebrovasc. Brain Metab. Rev., 1990, 2: 161–192). Did you consider this possibility in your study? (2) Hemorrhage may significantly influence arterial CO_2 tensions with marked individual differences. Is it possible that the different autoregulatory patterns observed in your experiments are induced by changes at arterial CO_2 tensions?

Answer: (Jones) In answer to your first query: we did not see a statistically significant change in CBF in response to LNNA superfusion, even though we expected to see a decrease, as you suggest. This result is in contrast to the usual effect of NOS inhibition of a slight decrease in cortical flow: flow decreased to 71% with topical 1 mM LNNA (Dirnagl et al., Neurosci. Lett., 1993, 149: 43), although other workers have noted no changes in pial artery diameter (Pelligrino et al., Brain Res., 1995, 704: 61) or CBF (Fabricius et al., Am. J. Physiol., 1994, 266: H1457; Fabricius et al., Am. J. Physiol., 1996, 271: H2035) after topical NOS inhibition for 45 min.

In answer to your second query: We noted that during hypotension, $PaCO_2$ fell, so we compensated for this fall by decreasing the respirator rate by changing the ventilator settings. Even with this compensation, $PaCO_2$ was depressed as a result of hemorrhagic hypotension, but these changes occurred equally in all groups, as evidenced by the lack of group-by-time interactions in the ANOVA. The changes in $PaCO_2$, from 36 to 33 mmHg from the start of the drop in MABP at 100 mmHg to the final MABP of 40 mmHg would decrease CBF at 40 mmHg by approximately 10% using the normal $PaCO_2$ reactivity of 2.5% $mmHg^{-1}$ (Jones et al., Am. J. Physiol., 1989, 257: H473) although this is maximal estimate since $PaCO_2$ reactivity is depressed at low arterial pressures (Harper and Glass, J. Neurol. Neurosurg. Psychiatry, 1965, 28: 449). Thus, the magnitude of the estimated depression in CBF by this drop in $PaCO_2$ is of little significance for our conclusions.

3.2.4.7.7 ***Question: (Paulson)*** I have a few questions. (1) In our study using global CBF measurements, we essentially only see the classical autoregulatory response. When you see the three types of responses, do you think it represents differences between animals or regional differences in the brain? (2) Fog observed in the 1930s "pressure passive" response in what he called "bad animals". Could the "pressure passive" response represent problems with the technical preparation of the experimental animal? (3) We previously observed that systemic L-arginine did not influence autoregulation in contrast to a reduction of the CO_2 response. What are your comments?

Answer: (Jones) (1) We think that these patterns represent differences between regions in the same animal. In one of the slides, using double LDF probes, we showed one animal with both classical and none patterns, and another with peak and classical patterns, during the same sequence of hemorrhage hypotension. (2) For various reasons, we strongly feel that these "none" patterns are not related to the technical preparation of the animal. Although if you are using a global CBF technique, the "none" pattern could well be interpreted as a damaged preparation, but we feel that using a highly regional method such as LDF, the "none" pattern is a normal autoregulatory response. Surgical trauma is not present because the cranial window surgery was performed the previous day in our animals. Our requirement for acceptable vascular reactivities to inhaled CO_2 and super-fused ACh and the presence of normal brain temperature and cranial window pressure ensured that the cerebral circulation was "healthy" in our animals.

(3) Your previous results showing that NOS inhibition did not influence autoregulation (Wang et al., Acta Physiol. Scand., 1992, 145: 297) used intravenous NOS inhibition and global CBF measurements. Global assessments of CBF combine brain regions that react differently to arterial pressure decreases and are known to have different lower limits (McPherson et al., Am. J. Physiol., 1988, 255: H1516; Tanaka et al., NeuroReport, 1993, 4: 267). It is well accepted that the deeper, more archaic cytoarchitectural structures are protected against ischemia and hypotension (Chen et al., Stroke, 1984, 15: 343): these structures possess (Tanaka et al., NeuroReport, 1993, 4: 267) a lower limit of CBF-pressure autoregulation that is less than that of the telencephalon. Intravenous NOS administration causes systemic vasoconstriction by blocking tonic release of nitric oxide from endothelium, leading to moderate hypertension. When intravenous NOS inhibition is used to evaluate autoregulation, a rise in arterial pressure occurs that does not occur in the

control group. Comparison of a normotensive control group with a hypertensive NOS inhibited group is a problematic experimental design for assessment of the lower limit. The hypertensive effect of intravenous NOS inhibition may be controlled by one of two strategies: (1) the control group may be made hypertensive, pharmacologically, to the same degree as the NOS inhibited group; or (2) the NOS inhibited group may be made normotensive, using hemorrhage or a pharmacological agent. Neither of these strategies is ideal. Either one of these strategies produce equivalent starting MABP in the control and treated groups, so the lower limit can be compared from an equivalent starting point. Our restriction of NOS inhibition to the brain avoids these potential complications.

3.2.4.7.8. *Question: (Pearce)* Traditional studies of autoregulation plot arterial pressure against cerebral blood flow after a variable volume hemorrhage. Interestingly, the volume of hemorrhage required to obtain a given decrease in arterial pressure can be largely variable. Thus, whole body systemic responses to hemorrhage can add significant variability to circulatory status for any post-hemorrhage blood pressure. To what extent does this variability contribute to the heterogeneity in autoregulatory responses you observe? Did the volume of hemorrhage necessary to lower arterial pressure vary significantly among animals? Would your autoregulatory variability be improved or worsened if you plotted CBF against hemorrhage volume (normalized as % blood volume)?

Answer: (Jones) There were no differences in the volume of blood withdrawn to reach a mean arterial pressure of 40 mmHg (4.3 ± 0.2 ml) between the three autoregulatory patterns.

Acknowledgements

Support is gratefully acknowledged from an American Heart Association-Bugher, Stroke Grant.

References

[1] D.F. Wilson, S. Gomi, A. Pastuszko, J.H. Greenberg, Microvascular damage in the cortex of cat brain from middle cerebral artery occlusion and reperfusion, J. Appl. Physiol. 74 (1993) 580–589.

[2] S.C. Jones, C.R. Radinsky, A.J. Furlan, D. Chyatte, A.D. Perez-Trepichio, Cortical NOS inhibition raises the lower limit of cerebral blood flow–arterial pressure autoregulation, Am. J. Physiol.: Heart Circ. Physiol. 276 (4 Part 2) (1999) H1253–H1262.

[3] S.C. Jones, C.R. Radinsky, A.J. Furlan, D. Chyatte, Y. Qu, K.A. Easley, et al., Variability in the magnitude of the cerebral blood flow response and the shape of the cerebral blood flow–pressure autoregulation curve during hypotension in normal rats, Anesthesiology (2002). In press.

[4] K. Toyoda, K. Fujii, S. Ibayashi, T. Nagao, T. Kitazono, M. Fujishima, Role of nitric oxide in regulation of brain stem circulation during hypotension, J. Cereb. Blood Flow Metab. 17 (10) (1997) 1089–1096.

[5] S.C. Jones, B. Bose, A.J. Furlan, H.T. Friel, K.A. Easley, M.P. Meredith, et al., CO_2 reactivity and heterogeneity of cerebral blood flow in ischemic, border zone, and normal cortex, Am. J. Physiol.: Heart Circ. Physiol. 257 (2 Part 2) (1989) H473–H482.

[6] S.C. Jones, A. Kharlamov, C.R. Radinsky, Y. Qu, K.A. Easley, Role of nitric oxide in variations of the response of cerebral blood flow to hypotension and focal ischemia, in: Y. Fukuuchi, M. Tomita, A. Koto (Eds.), Ischemic Blood Flow in the Brain, Springer Verlag, Tokyo, 2000, pp. 265–281.

[7] T. Michel, O. Feron, Nitric oxide synthases: which, where, how, and why? J. Clin. Invest. 100 (1997) 2146–2152.

[8] M. Toporsian, K. Govindaraju, M. Nagi, D. Eidelman, G. Thibault, M.E. Ward, Downregulation of endothelial nitric oxide synthase in rat aorta after prolonged hypoxia in vivo, Circ. Res. 86 (6) (2000) 671–675.

[9] G.L. Baumbach, D.D. Heistad, Regional, segmental, and temporal heterogeneity of cerebral vascular autoregulation, Ann. Biomed. Eng. 13 (3–4) (1985) 303–310.

[10] T. Bär, Distribution of radially penetrating arteries and veins in the neocortex of rat, in: J. Cervós-Navarro, E. Fritschka (Eds.), Cerebral Microcirculation and Metabolism, Raven Press, New York, 1981, pp. 1–8.

[11] D.W. Lübbers, H. Baumgartl, Heterogeneities and profiles of oxygen pressure in brain and kidney as examples of the pO_2 distribution in the living tissue, Kidney Int. 51 (2) (1997) 372–380.

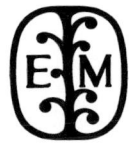

International Congress Series 1235 (2002) 369–377

Neuronal nitric oxide synthase in the cerebrovascular endothelium

Zoltán Benyó [a,b,*], Zsombor Lacza [a,b], Tibor Hortobágyi [a],
Christoph Görlach [a], Péter Sándor [b], Michael Wahl [a]

[a]*Department of Physiology, Ludwig-Maximilians University, Pettenkoferstr. 12, D-80336 Munich, Germany*
[b]*Institute of Human Physiology and Clinical Experimental Research, Semmelweis University,*
POB 448, H-1446 Budapest, Hungary

Abstract

The presence of the neuronal isoform of nitric oxide synthase (nNOS) in astrocytes and neurons as well as in the perivascular nerves and cerebrovascular endothelium is well documented. The role of the nNOS, however, is not yet understood. In the present study, the function of cerebrovascular nNOS was investigated by comparing the effects of the specific nNOS blocker 7-nitro indazole monosodium salt (7-NINA) to that of the general NOS inhibitor N^G-nitro-L-arginine (L-NA) in isolated rat basilar arteries (BAs). 7-NINA had no significant effect on the resting tone of the vessels, while L-NA induced strong contraction. The relaxant effect of bradykinin was attenuated in the presence of L-NA but was not changed by 7-NINA. In contrast, 7-NINA markedly reduced the acetylcholine-induced, endothelium-dependent relaxation. These results demonstrate that nNOS contributes significantly to the relaxant effect of acetylcholine, indicating the functional importance of this isoenzyme in the cerebrovascular endothelium. © 2002 Elsevier Science B.V. All rights reserved.

Keywords: Rat basilar artery; Neuronal nitric oxide synthase; Endothelium; Acetylcholine; Bradykinin

1. Introduction

Although the role of the endothelium-derived relaxing factor nitric oxide (NO) in the cerebral circulation has been studied extensively for more than 20 years, several important

---

* Corresponding author. Institute of Human Physiology and Clinical Experimental Research, Semmelweis University, POB 448, H-1446 Budapest, Hungary. Tel.: +36-1-2100306; fax: +36-1-3343162.
E-mail address: benyo@elet2.sote.hu (Z. Benyó).

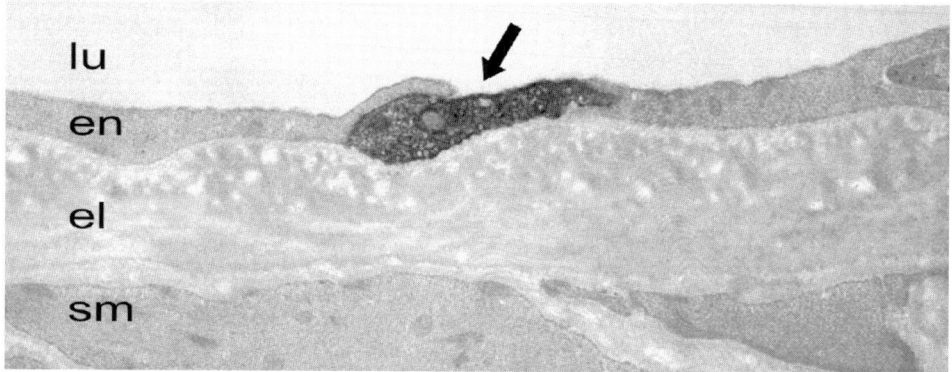

Fig. 1. Rat basilar artery labeled for nNOS. Arrow indicates NOS-positive process of an endothelial cell (showing "black" cytoplasmic labeling) between two NOS negative cells. Abbreviations: lu, lumen; en, endothelial cell layer; el, elastic lamina; sm, smooth muscle. (Courtesy of Loesch et al. [4].)

questions have still not been answered. Neuronal nitric oxide synthase (nNOS)-derived NO has been implicated in a wide range of physiological actions in the cerebral circulation, including the maintenance of the resting blood flow, cerebrovascular CO_2 reactivity, neurogenic and excitatory amino acid induced vasodilation and flow-metabolism coupling (for review, see Ref. [1]). Excessive NO release by nNOS during and after cerebral ischemia may also contribute to the development of neuronal damage and its consequences (for review, see Ref. [2]). The presence of nNOS in the brain has been described in neurons, glial cells and perivascular nerves [1]. Several recent studies indicate, however, that nNOS is also present in the endothelium of the cerebral vasculature (for review, see Ref. [3]). The functional importance of the cerebrovascular nNOS, however, has not yet been established.

Our study was designed to investigate the possible contribution of nNOS to resting and agonist-induced NO release in isolated rat basilar arteries (BAs), by comparing the effect of the specific nNOS blocker 7-nitro indazole monosodium salt (7-NINA) to that of the general NOS inhibitor N^G-nitro-L-arginine (L-NA). We chose this particular cerebral artery because it reportedly expresses nNOS in the endothelium [4–7] (Fig. 1), and its reactivity can be studied by conventional methods of isometric tension recording. Resting NO production was determined by the evaluation of the contraction developing after the NOS blockade, while agonist-induced NO release was evaluated by the endothelium-dependent relaxant effects of acetylcholine (Ach) and bradykinin (BK) after pre-contraction of the vessels.

2. Methods

Adult male Wistar rats were rapidly exsanguinated under deep ether anesthesia. Ring segments of the BA were prepared for measurement of the isometric force as described [8,9]. Special care was taken to preserve the endothelium during the preparation of the artery. The segments were transferred into 5 ml organ baths filled with a modified Krebs solution of the following composition (mM): NaCl, 119; KCl, 4.6; NaH_2PO_4, 1.2; $CaCl_2 \cdot 2H_2O$, 1.5; $MgCl_2 \cdot 6H_2O$, 1.2; $NaHCO_3$, 15; glucose, 10. The bath solution was bubbled continuously with a humidified gas mixture (90% O_2/10% CO_2) to maintain a pH of 7.25–7.3. The ring segments were mounted on two L-shaped stainless steel wires (70 μm diameter), one of which was attached rigidly to the bath and the other was connected to a force transducer for measuring the isometric force.

The vessels were allowed a 90-min equilibration period during which they were warmed to 37 °C and washed repeatedly every 20–25 min. The resting tension was adjusted to 2.5–3.5 mN. After the equilibration period, the segments were pre-contracted with 2 μM 5-hydroxytryptamine (5-HT) and the concentration–effect curves (CECs) for Ach (0.01–10 μM) or BK (0.01–10 μM) were constructed before and after the general NOS blockade induced by 10 μM L-NA, or the selective inhibition of the nNOS by 100 μM 7-NINA [10]. The maximal response (E_{max}) values were calculated for the individual CECs. In the control segments, the effects of Ach or BK during the first and second applications were compared without NOS inhibition. At the end of the experiment, each segment was exposed to a 124 mM K^+ Krebs solution to obtain a reference contraction. The effects of L-NA and 7-NINA on the basal tone of the segments were expressed as the percentage of the reference contraction, while the dilator actions of Ach and BK were expressed as a percentage of the pre-contraction. Only segments in which Ach induced at least 30% or BK at least 15% relaxation were considered to have functionally intact endothelium and were therefore used in this study.

All the values are presented as mean ± SEM, and the number of BA segments studied is expressed by n. The results were analyzed statistically using one-way ANOVA followed by Fisher's protected least-significant difference test or Student's unpaired t-test. $P < 0.05$ was considered significant.

3. Results and discussion

The resting tension of the BA segments increased after the administration of L-NA, however, the segments were not influenced by the 7-NINA (Fig. 2). These effects were similar to those observed previously in isolated rat middle cerebral arteries (MCAs) with the same method [11] (Fig. 2).

Both Ach and BK induced relaxation after pre-contraction of the BA segments with 5-HT. These relaxant effects were not significantly different in the different experimental groups during the first application of the respective drugs, and remained unchanged during the second application in the control vessels (Figs. 3 and 4). 7-NINA inhibited the vaso-dilatory action of Ach (Fig. 3), however, did not significantly influence that of BK (Fig. 4). In contrast, L-NA markedly attenuated both the Ach- and BK-induced relaxations (Figs. 3 and 4). The relaxant effect of Ach was more strongly attenuated after L-NA than after 7-NINA (E_{max}: 44.6 ± 6.0% vs. 30.2 ± 3.2%, $P < 0.05$).

Taken together, 7-NINA did not influence the resting tone or the BK-induced dilatation, but significantly attenuated the relaxant effect of Ach in isolated rat BAs. In contrast, L-NA induced vasoconstriction and reduced both BK- and Ach-induced relaxations.

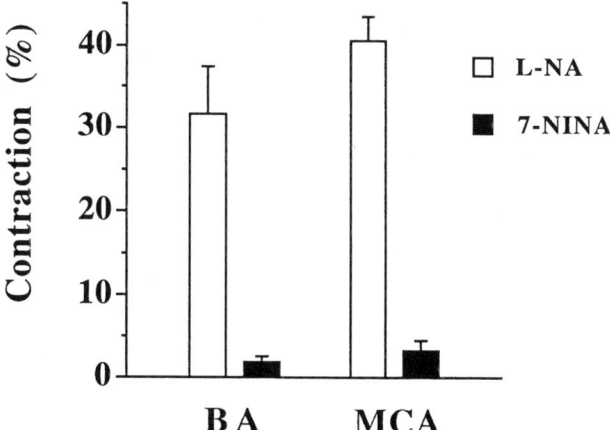

Fig. 2. The effects of L-NA (open bars) and 7-NINA (solid bars) on the resting tension of rat basilar (BA) and middle cerebral artery (MCA) segments. Values (mean ± SEM) are expressed as the percentage of the reference contraction induced by 124 mM K$^+$ Krebs solution. Note that 7-NINA, in contrast to L-NA, did not significantly influence the resting tension of the vessels.

3.1. Role of nNOS in the maintenance of resting cerebrovascular resistance

Constitutive NO production plays a crucial role in the maintenance of the resting cerebrovascular tone and blood flow [1]. Our observation that 7-NINA fails to alter the resting tension of isolated BAs indicates that nNOS is not involved in the maintenance of the resting dilator tone in these vessels. Since ODQ was found to induce similar

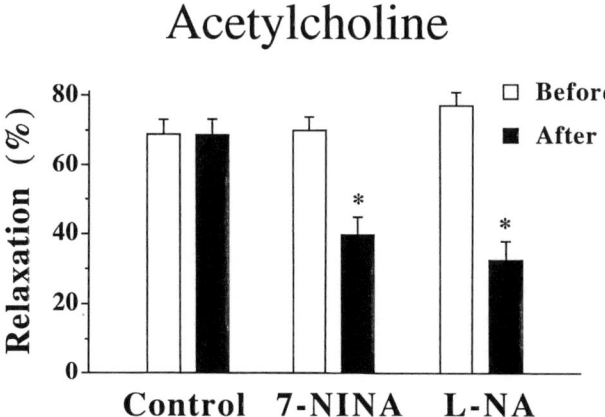

Fig. 3. The E_{max} values of acetylcholine-induced relaxations in pre-contracted rat basilar arteries for two consecutive applications of Ach in the control (untreated) vessels ($n = 21$), as well as before (open bars) and after (solid bars) the administration of 100 μM 7-NINA ($n = 22$) or 10 μM L-NA ($n = 15$). The values are presented as mean (±SEM) percentage of the pre-contraction. *$P < 0.01$ versus the corresponding value before 7-NINA or L-NA.

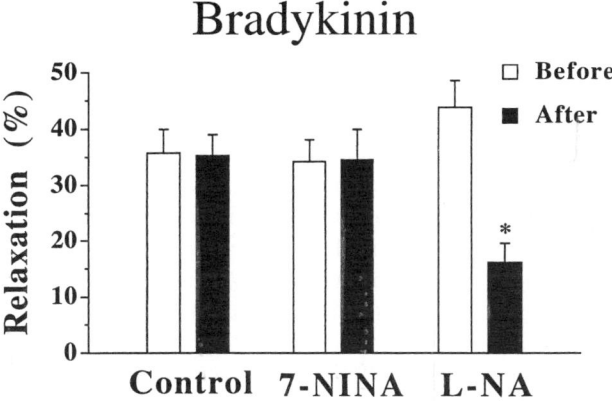

Fig. 4. E_{max} values of bradykinin-induced relaxations in pre-contracted rat basilar arteries for two consecutive applications of BK in the control (untreated) vessels ($n=33$), as well as before (open bars) and after (solid bars) the administration of 100 μM 7-NINA ($n=12$) or 10 μM L-NA ($n=11$). Values are presented as mean ($\pm$ SEM) percentage of the precontraction. *$P<0.01$ versus the corresponding value before L-NA.

contraction in rat BAs as L-NA [12], constitutive NO release by endothelial NOS and the consequent cGMP formation in the smooth muscle appears to be responsible for the maintenance of the resting vasodilation. In vivo inhibition of the nNOS with 7-NI or ARL 17477, however, results in a significant reduction of the cerebral blood flow in rats, indicating that nNOS-derived NO is an important factor in the maintenance of the perfusion rate in steady-state, resting conditions of the brain [13–29]. On the other hand, 7-NI fails to alter the diameter of rat pial vessels in vivo [29–31] or that of the MCAs in vitro [32]. These observations, together with ours demonstrating the absence of nNOS-mediated resting vasodilation in isolated rat MCAs [11,33], indicate that nNOS-derived NO released by neurons and/or glial cells regulates the resting cerebral perfusion rate at the level of microcirculation. The morphological data showing that nitroxidergic nerve fibers are located around the intraparenchymal vessels within the diffusion distance of NO are consistent with this view [34]. The resting activity of nNOS may also have an important modulatory function in the cerebral circulation. In a recent study, it was demonstrated that basal NO release by nNOS in the perivascular nerves is required for the normal pH reactivity of the rat MCA [32].

3.2. Role of nNOS in endothelium-dependent cerebrovascular relaxations

The most interesting finding of this study is the inhibition of the Ach-induced cerebrovascular relaxation by 7-NINA. Although the presence of nNOS in cerebrovascular endothelial cells has been demonstrated in several studies [4–7,35–39], our observation is the first evidence of its functional importance. We can exclude the possibility that Ach stimulates NO release from perivascular nerves, which may also contain nNOS in our preparation, because the removal of the endothelium abolishes the relaxation to Ach of the rat BA [9,40–44]. Therefore, endothelial nNOS may be the only source of the 7-NINA-sensitive NO liberation in our study. Nevertheless, the Ach-induced relaxation was more strongly inhibited by L-NA than by 7-NINA, indicating that Ach stimulates not only the neuronal but also the endothelial isoform of NOS.

Various and contradictory data have been reported regarding the effect of nNOS blockade on the cerebrovascular action of Ach or the specific muscarinic agonist oxotremorine in vivo. Intraperitoneal administration of 7-NI in rats failed to alter the cerebrocortical blood flow increase in response to topical Ach in two studies [23,25], but abolished it in another study under similar experimental conditions [14]. 7-NI has no effect on the intravenous oxotremorine-induced cerebrocortical hyperemia [21] or the vaso-dilation produced by microinjection of Ach into the cerebellar molecular layer of rats [17,22]. Furthermore, topical Ach-induced vasodilation of rat pial arteries is not altered significantly by intraperitoneal 7-NI administration [30,31], which is also the case in mouse pial arterioles after topical 7-NI [45]. Interestingly, antisense oligonucleotide to nNOS inhibited the relaxant effect of Ach in mouse brain surface arterioles [46], while an unchanged [47,48] or even increased [49] cerebrocortical arteriolar Ach reactivity was observed in the nNOS knockout mice. Whilst not attempting to interpret the divergent data obtained in vivo, we would emphasize two important facts that should be considered with respect to our results. First, in the above-mentioned in vivo experimental models there was no indication that the removal of the endothelium abolishes the effect of Ach. In the vicinity of the cerebral blood vessels nitroxidergic neurons express muscarinic Ach receptors [34] and may, therefore, be involved in the NO-mediated effects of topical Ach. In our study, we can state that nNOS-derived NO was released from the endothelium, because endothelial denudation of rat BA abolishes the relaxant effect of Ach (see above). Second, in situ hybridization and immunoelectron microscopy have shown the endothelial nNOS expression to be localized mostly in the extraparenchymal rather than intra-parenchymal cerebral arteries of the rat [38,39]. Similar distribution of nNOS was demonstrated in isolated bovine cerebral arteries by Western blot analysis [50]. Therefore, cerebrovascular endothelial nNOS is probably an important regulatory factor in large arteries, but not at the level of microcirculation.

Bradykinin induces endothelium-dependent NO-mediated relaxation of the rat BA [51,52]. The lack of the effect of 7-NINA on this action indicates that only endothelial NOS is stimulated by BK. Indeed, the maximal relaxation induced by BK was only about half of that induced by Ach, which apparently stimulates both constitutive NOS isoenzymes. Further studies need to be carried out in order to identify the intraendothelial signal transduction mechanisms mediating the different actions of Ach and BK in the cerebral vasculature.

In a recent study, Lindauer et al. [32] reported that 7-NI did not significantly influence the resting diameter of isolated perfused rat MCAs, but attenuated the endothelium-dependent relaxant effect of Ach. Using the same vessels, we have previously reported that 7-NINA did not significantly influence the resting vascular tension or BK-induced relaxations [33]. In our study, however, the effect of Ach could not be tested. Nevertheless, these two studies together show very similar results in the rat MCA to those obtained in the BA, i.e., selective nNOS blockade attenuates the relaxant effect of Ach, however, it fails to change the resting vascular tone or BK-induced relaxation. Therefore, nNOS appears to mediate, at least in part, the relaxant effect of Ach in large cerebral arteries of the rat.

In conclusion, our study demonstrates that nNOS-derived NO contributes significantly to Ach-induced endothelium-dependent vasodilation, however, not to the maintenance of the resting tension or the relaxant effect of BK in rat BAs. The exact physiological role of this isoenzyme in the regulation of the cerebral circulation or blood–brain barrier permeability remains to be clarified.

Acknowledgements

The authors are grateful to Professor Geoffrey Burnstock for providing Fig. 1. This work was supported by grants from the German BMBF, the Hungarian OTKA (F 029801, T 029169, W 015186) and FKFP (0518/2000), the DAAD-MÖB Scientist Exchange Program and the Alexander von Humboldt Foundation. Z.B. was supported by a Bolyai Research Fellowship. Z.L. was supported by a Hungarian National Eötvös Fellowship.

References

[1] F.M. Faraci, D.D. Heistad, Regulation of the cerebral circulation: role of endothelium and potassium channels, Physiol. Rev. 78 (1998) 53–97.

[2] C. Iadecola, Bright and dark sides of nitric oxide in ischemic brain injury, Trends Neurosci. 20 (1997) 132–139.

[3] A. Loesch, G. Burnstock, Immunocytochemistry of vasoactive agents and nitric oxide synthase in vascular endothelial cells with emphasis on the cerebral blood vessels, Cell Vision 3 (5) (1996) 346–357.

[4] A. Loesch, A. Belai, G. Burnstock, An ultrastructural study of NADPH-diaphorase and nitric oxide synthase in the perivascular nerves and vascular endothelium of the rat basilar artery, J. Neurocytol. 23 (1994) 49–59.

[5] A. Loesch, G. Burnstock, Perivascluar nerve fibres and endothelial cells of the rat basilar artery: immuno-gold labelling of antigenic sites for type I and type III nitric oxide synthase, J. Neurocytol. 27 (1998) 197–204.

[6] A. Loesch, G. Burnstock, Ultrastructural study of perivascular nerve fibres and endothelial cells of the rat basilar artery immunolabelled with monoclonal antibodies to neuronal and endothelial nitric oxide synthase, J. Neurocytol. 25 (1996) 525–534.

[7] M. Shochina, A. Loesch, A. Rubino, S. Miah, G. Macdonald, G. Burnstock, Immunoreactivity for nitric oxide synthase and endothelin in the coronary and basilar arteries of renal hypertensive rats, Cell Tissue Res. 288 (1997) 509–516.

[8] G.I. Feger, L. Schilling, H. Ehrenreich, M. Wahl, Endothelin-induced contraction and relaxation of rat isolated basilar artery: effect of BQ-123, J. Cereb. Blood Flow Metab. 14 (1994) 845–852.

[9] G.I. Feger, L. Schilling, H. Ehrenreich, M. Wahl, Endothelium-dependent relaxation counteracting the contractile action of endothelin-1 is partly due to ETB receptor activation, Res. Exp. Med. 196 (1997) 327–337.

[10] M.T. Silva, S. Rose, J.G. Hindmarsh, G. Aislaitner, J.W. Gorrod, P.K. Moore, P. Jenner, C.D. Marsden, Increased striatal dopamine efflux in vivo following inhibition of cerebral nitric oxide synthase by the novel monosodium salt of 7-nitro indazole, Br. J. Pharmacol. 114 (1995) 257–258.

[11] Z. Benyó, C. Görlach, M. Wahl, Interaction between nitric oxide and thromboxane A_2 in the regulation of the resting cerebrovascular tone, Adv. Exp. Med. Biol. 471 (1999) 373–379.

[12] Z. Benyó, Z. Lacza, T. Hortobágyi, C. Görlach, M. Wahl, Functional importance of neuronal nitric oxide synthase in the endothelium of rat basilar arteries, Brain Res. 877 (2000) 79–84.

[13] N. Cholet, J. Seylaz, P. Lacombe, G. Bonvento, Local uncoupling of the cerebrovascular and metabolic responses to somatosensory stimulation after neuronal nitric oxide synthase inhibition, J. Cereb. Blood Flow Metab. 17 (1997) 1191–1201.

[14] M. Fabricius, I. Rubin, M. Bundgaard, M. Lauritzen, NOS activity in brain endothelium: relation to hypercapnic rise of cerebral blood flow in rats, Am. J. Physiol. 271 (1996) H2035–H2044.

[15] G. Heinert, B. Casadei, D.J. Paterson, Hypercapnic cerebral blood flow in spontaneously hypertensive rats, J. Hypertens. 16 (1998) 1491–1498.

[16] A.G. Hudetz, H. Shen, J.P. Kampine, Nitric oxide from neuronal NOS plays critical role in cerebral capillary flow response to hypoxia, Am. J. Physiol. 274 (1998) H982–H989.

[17] C. Iadecola, G. Yang, S. Xu, 7-Nitroindazole attenuates vasodilation from cerebellar parallel fiber stimulation but not acetylcholine, Am. J. Physiol. 270 (1996) R914–R919.

[18] P.A.T. Kelly, I.M. Ritchie, G.W. Arbuthnott, Inhibition of neuronal nitric oxide synthase by 7-nitroindazole: effects upon local cerebral blood flow and glucose use in the rat, J. Cereb. Blood Flow Metab. 15 (1995) 766–773.

[19] C. Montécot, L. Rondi-Reig, V. Springhetti, J. Seylaz, E. Pinard, Inhibition of neuronal (type 1) nitric oxide synthase prevents hyperaemia and hippocampal lesions resulting from kainate-induced seizures, Neuroscience 84 (1998) 791–800.

[20] H. Okamoto, A.G. Hudetz, R.J. Roman, Z.J. Bosnjak, J.P. Kampine, Neuronal NOS-derived NO plays permissive role in cerebral blood flow response to hypercapnia, Am. J. Physiol. 272 (1997) H559–H566.

[21] Q. Wang, D.A. Pelligrino, V.L. Baughman, H.M. Koenig, R.F. Albrecht, The role of neuronal nitric oxide synthase in regulation of cerebral blood flow in normocapnia and hypercapnia in rats, J. Cereb. Blood Flow Metab. 15 (1995) 774–778.

[22] G. Yang, C. Iadecola, Glutamate microinjections in cerebellar cortex reproduce cerebrovascular effects of parallel fiber stimulation, Am. J. Physiol. 271 (1996) R1568–R1575.

[23] S.T. Yang, H.H. Chang, Nitric oxide of neuronal origin mediates NMDA-induced cerebral hyperemia in rats, NeuroReport 9 (1998) 415–418.

[24] Y. Zagvazdin, G. Sancesario, M.E.C. Fitzgerald, A. Reiner, Effects of halothane and urethane-chloralose anaesthesia on the pressor and cerebrovascular responses to 7-nitroindazole, an inhibitor of nitric oxide synthase, Pharmacol. Res. 38 (1998) 339–346.

[25] F. Zhang, S. Xu, C. Iadecola, Role of nitric oxide and acetylcholine in neocortical hyperemia elicited by basal forebrain stimulation: evidence for an involvement of endothelial nitric oxide, Neuroscience 69 (1995) 1195–1204.

[26] Z.G. Zhang, D. Reif, J. Macdonald, W.X. Tang, D.K. Kamp, R.J. Gentile, W.C. Shakespeare, R.J. Murray, M. Chopp, ARL 17477, a potent and selective neuronal NOS inhibitor decreases infarct volume after transient middle cerebral artery occlusion in rats, J. Cereb. Blood Flow Metab. 16 (1996) 599–604.

[27] A.G. Hudetz, J.D. Wood, J.P. Kampine, 7-Nitroindazole impedes erythrocyte flow response to isovolemic hemodilution in the cerebral capillary circulation, J. Cereb. Blood Flow Metab. 20 (2000) 220–224.

[28] P.A.T. Kelly, I.M. Ritchie, D.E. McBean, 7-Nitroindazole reduces cerebral blood flow following chronic nitric oxide synthase inhibition, Brain Res. 885 (2000) 295–297.

[29] E. Pinard, N. Engrand, J. Seylaz, Dynamic cerebral microcirculatory changes in transient forebrain ischemia in rats: involvement of type I nitric oxide synthase, J. Cereb. Blood Flow Metab. 20 (2000) 1648–1658.

[30] F.M. Faraci, J.E. Brian, 7-Nitroindazole inhibits brain nitric oxide synthase and cerebral vasodilatation in response to N-methyl-D-aspartate, Stroke 26 (1995) 2172–2176.

[31] T. Yoshida, V. Limmroth, K. Irikura, M.A. Moskowitz, The NOS inhibitor, 7-nitroindazole, decreases focal infarct volume but not the response to topical acetylcholine in pial vessels, J. Cereb. Blood Flow Metab. 14 (1994) 924–929.

[32] U. Lindauer, A. Kunz, S. Schuh-Hofer, J. Vogt, J.P. Dreier, U. Dirnagl, Nitric oxide from perivascular nerves modulates cerebral arteriolar pH reactivity, Am. J. Physiol., (2001) 1353–1363.

[33] Z. Benyó, Z. Lacza, C. Görlach, M. Wahl, Selective inhibition of neuronal nitric oxide synthase fails to alter the resting tension and the relaxant effect of bradykinin in isolated rat middle cerebral arteries, Acta Physiol. Hung. 86 (2) (1999) 161–165.

[34] V. Moro, J. Badaut, V. Springhetti, L. Edvinsson, J. Seylaz, F. Lasbennes, Regional study of the co-localization of neuronal nitric oxide synthase with muscarinic receptors in the rat cerebral cortex, Neuroscience 69 (1995) 797–805.

[35] D.S. Bredt, P.M. Hwang, S.H. Snyder, Localization of nitric oxide synthase indicating a neural role for nitric oxide, Nature 347 (1990) 768–770.

[36] E. Gorelova, A. Loesch, P. Bodin, L. Chadwick, P.J. Hamlyn, G. Burnstock, Localisation of immunoreactive factor VIII, nitric oxide synthase, substance P, endothelin-1 and 5-hydroxytryptamine in human postmortem middle cerebral artery, J. Anat. 188 (1996) 97–107.

[37] K. Nozaki, M.A. Moskowitz, K.I. Maynard, N. Koketsu, T.M. Dawson, D.S. Bredt, S.H. Snyder, Possible origins and distribution of immunoreactive nitric oxide synthase-containing nerve fibers in cerebral arteries, J. Cereb. Blood Flow Metab. 13 (1993) 70–79.

[38] B. Seidel, A. Stanarius, G. Wolf, Differential expression of neuronal and endothelial nitric oxide synthase in blood vessels of the rat brain, Neurosci. Lett. 239 (1997) 109–112.

[39] A. Stanarius, B. Seidel, G. Wolf, Neuronal nitric oxide synthase in the vasculature of the rat brain: an immunocytochemical study using the tyramide signal amplification technique, J. Neurocytol. 27 (1998) 731–736.

[40] M.V. Conde, J. Marín, G. Balfagón, Superoxide anion and K^+ channels mediate electrical stimulation-induced relaxation in the rat basilar artery, Eur. J. Pharmacol. 372 (1999) 179–186.

[41] K. Kamata, H. Kondoh, Impairment of endothelium-dependent relaxation of the isolated basilar artery from streptozotocin-induced diabetic rats, Res. Commun. Mol. Pathol. Pharmacol. 94 (1996) 239–249.

[42] F.M. Lai, A. Cobuzzi, C. Shepherd, T. Tanikella, A. Hoffman, P. Cervoni, Endothelium-dependent basilar and aortic vascular responses in normotensive and coarctation hypertensive rats, Life Sci. 45 (1989) 607–614.

[43] L. Schilling, G.I. Feger, H. Ehrenreich, M. Wahl, Endothelin-3-induced relaxation of isolated rat basilar artery is mediated by an endothelial ET_B-type endothelin receptor, J. Cereb. Blood Flow Metab. 15 (1995) 699–705.

[44] J.P. You, Q. Wang, W. Zhang, I. Jansen-Olesen, O.B. Paulson, N.A. Lassen, L. Edvinsson, Hypercapnic vasodilatation in isolated rat basilar arteries is exerted via low pH and does not involve nitric oxide synthase stimulation or cyclic GMP production, Acta Physiol. Scand. 152 (1994) 391–397.

[45] W. Meng, C. Ayata, C. Waeber, P.L. Huang, M.A. Moskowitz, Neuronal NOS-cGMP-dependent ACh-induced relaxation in pial arterioles of endothelial NOS knockout mice, Am. J. Physiol. 274 (1998) H411–H415.

[46] W.I. Rosenblum, S. Murata, Antisense evidence for two functionally active forms of nitric oxide synthase in brain microvascular endothelium, Biochem. Biophys. Res. Commun. 224 (1996) 535–543.

[47] K. Irikura, P.L. Huang, J. Ma, W.S. Lee, T. Dalkara, M.C. Fishman, T.M. Dawson, S.H. Snyder, M.A. Moskowitz, Cerebrovascular alterations in mice lacking neuronal nitric oxide synthase expression, Proc. Natl. Acad. Sci. U. S. A. 92 (1995) 6823–6827.

[48] J. Ma, C. Ayata, P.L. Huang, M.C. Fishman, M.A. Moskowitz, Regional cerebral blood flow response to vibrissal stimulation in mice lacking type I NOS gene expression, Am. J. Physiol. 270 (1996) H1085–H1090.

[49] W. Meng, J. Ma, C. Ayata, H. Hara, P.L. Huang, M.C. Fishman, M.A. Moskowitz, ACh dilates pial arterioles in endothelial and neuronal NOS knockout mice by NO-dependent mechanisms, Am. J. Physiol. 271 (1996) H1145–H1150.

[50] R.E. Catalán, A.M. Martínez, M.D. Aragonés, F. Hernández, Identification of nitric oxide synthases in isolated bovine brain vessels, Neurosci. Res. 25 (1996) 195–199.

[51] S.M. Arribas, E. Vila, J.C. McGrath, Impairment of vasodilator function in basilar arteries from aged rats, Stroke 28 (1997) 1812–1820.

[52] W.G. Mayhan, Impairment of endothelium-dependent dilatation of basilar artery during chronic hypertension, Am. J. Physiol. 259 (1990) H1455–H1462.

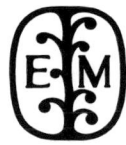

International Congress Series 1235 (2002) 379–393

Mechanisms of cGMP-induced cerebral vasodilatation: contractile agonist and developmental age make a difference

William J. Pearce*, Surya M. Nauli

*Center for Perinatal Biology, Departments of Physiology and Pharmacology,
Loma Linda University School of Medicine, Loma Linda, CA 92350, USA*

Abstract

In light of observations that maturation dramatically influences cerebrovascular metabolism of cGMP, the present study examines the hypothesis that the ability of cGMP to produce cerebral vasodilatation changes during maturation. Specifically, these experiments explore age-related changes in cGMP's ability to depress cytosolic calcium concentration and attenuate myofilament calcium sensitivity. The results obtained in α-toxin-permeabilized and Fura-2-loaded ovine basilar arteries demonstrate that cGMP produces relaxation by attenuating both the cytosolic calcium concentration and myofilament calcium sensitivity in ovine basilar arteries. More importantly, these findings reveal that the vasorelaxant potency and efficacy of cGMP are much greater in immature than in mature cerebral arteries. Together with the elevated levels of the cGMP characteristic of immature cerebral arteries, these data implicate cGMP as a major regulator of cerebrovascular tone in the immature cerebral circulation. © 2002 Elsevier Science B.V. All rights reserved.

Keywords: 8-(4-Chlorophenylthio)-3′, 5′-cyclic monophosphate; Cerebrovascular circulation; Guanosine 3′, 5′-cyclic monophosphate; Guanylate cyclase; Rp 8-(4-Chlorophenylthio)-3′, 5′-cyclic monophosphorothioate

1. Introduction

The transition from fetal to adult life exacts many changes in cerebrovascular function [1]. Compared to mature cerebral arteries, fetal cerebral arteries exhibit reduced force development, greater sensitivity to most contractile agonists, greater myofilament calcium

---

Abbreviations: cGMP, cyclic guanosine monophosphate; PKG, protein kinase G.
* Corresponding author. Tel.: +1-909-558-4325; fax: +1-909-558-4029.
E-mail address: wpearce@som.llu.edu (W.J. Pearce).

sensitivity, and altered patterns of calcium mobilization and distribution [1–7]. Cerebrovascular maturation also alters patterns of cerebrovascular relaxation, including elevated basal concentrations of cGMP and greater rates of cGMP synthesis in response to either endogenous or exogenous nitric oxide (NO) [8,9]. Expression of soluble guanylate cyclase, the enzyme responsible for cGMP synthesis, is also greater in fetal than in adult arteries [9–11], as are the rates of cGMP hydrolysis [12,13]. Despite the enhanced ability of immature cerebral arteries to increase cytosolic cGMP concentrations, the ability of endothelium-dependent vasodilators to relax cerebral arteries is depressed in fetal compared to adult cerebral arteries. One possible explanation of this finding is that the ability of cGMP to mediate vasorelaxation is down regulated in immature arteries. The present series of experiments was designed to evaluate this hypothesis.

Given that the relaxant effects of cGMP involve both mechanisms which decrease cytosolic calcium and mechanisms which decrease myofilament calcium sensitivity, we examined cGMP-induced changes in both cytosolic calcium and myofilament calcium sensitivity in these experiments. Given that regulation of contractile tone varies considerably for depolarization-induced (receptor-independent) and agonist-induced (receptor-dependent) contractions, we examined the effects of cGMP on both potassium- and serotonin-induced contractile tone. In addition, comparing responses in the arteries from term-fetal lambs and nonpregnant adult sheep assessed the effects of maturation.

2. Effects of 8-pCPT-cGMP on K$^+$ and 5HT-induced tone

Our first approach was to examine the concentration-related effects of a non-metabolizable cell-permeant cGMP analogue, 8-pCPT-cGMP, on contractile tone in fetal and

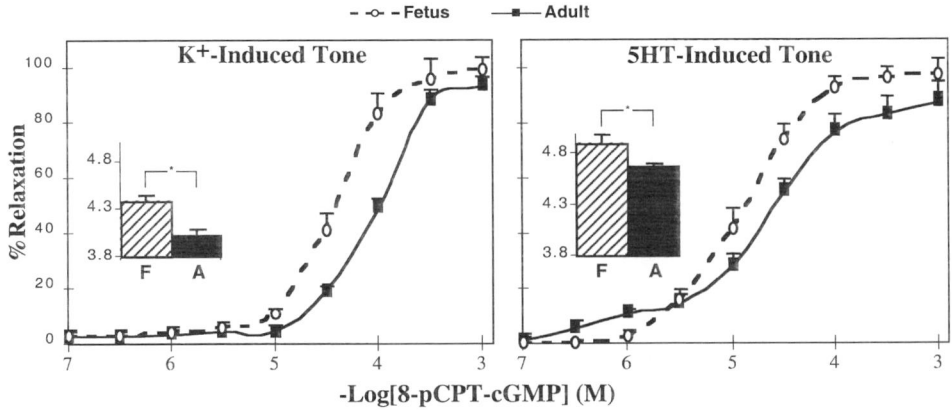

Fig. 1. Concentration–response curves for 8-pCPT-cGMP in basilar arteries contracted with potassium and 5HT. In arteries precontracted with 5HT, the pD_2 (= – log [EC$_{50}$]) averages (inset bar graphs) of the concentration–response relations for 8-pCPT-cGMP were significantly greater in fetal than adult basilars. In arteries precontracted with potassium, the pD_2 averages were also significantly greater in fetal than adult basilars. These findings suggest that the fetal arteries are more sensitive to cGMP than the corresponding adult arteries. Vertical error bars indicate standard errors for $n = 5$ in all groups, and asterisks indicate significant differences via ANOVA at $P < 0.05$.

adult basilar arteries. In these experiments, artery segments were contracted with the age-specific EC_{50} and EC_{95} concentrations for 5HT and potassium, respectively. Once the initial contractile tensions were stable, 8-pCPT-cGMP was added in cumulative half-log concentrations from 1 nM to 1 mM [14]. As shown in Fig. 1, 8-pCPT-cGMP significantly inhibited the contractile tone produced by both potassium and 5HT. In addition, sensitivity to 8-pCPT-cGMP was significantly greater in fetal compared to adult arteries, as indicated by the obtained pD_2 ($-\log EC_{50}$) values of the concentration–response curves.

To further examine the age-related differences in sensitivity to cGMP, we carried out concentration–response experiments for 5HT in the control arteries, and in arteries pretreated with the EC_{30} concentration of 8-pCPT-cGMP for 5HT contractions (6 μM), as determined in the experiments shown in Fig. 1. In these experiments, pretreatment with 8-pCPT-cGMP right-shifted the concentration–response relations for 5HT; however, this shift was significant only in the fetal arteries (Fig. 2). Similarly, pretreatment with the EC_{30} concentration of 8-pCPT-cGMP for potassium contractions (25 μM) right-shifted the

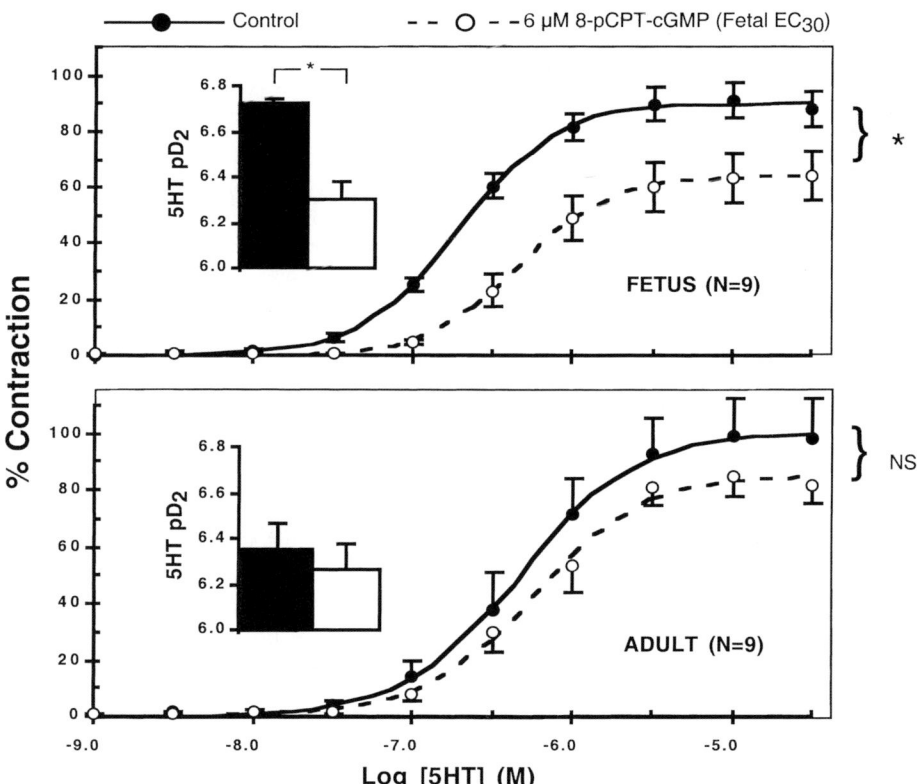

Fig. 2. Effects of 8-pCPT-cGMP on concentration–response curves for 5HT. Pretreatment with 6 μM 8-pCPT-cGMP (the fetal EC_{30} concentration for 5HT contractions) significantly right-shifted the concentration–response relation for 5HT in fetal but not adult basilar arteries, as indicated by changes in the pD_2 values (inset bar graphs). Vertical error bars indicate standard errors for $n = 9$ in all groups, and asterisks indicate significant differences via ANOVA at $P < 0.05$.

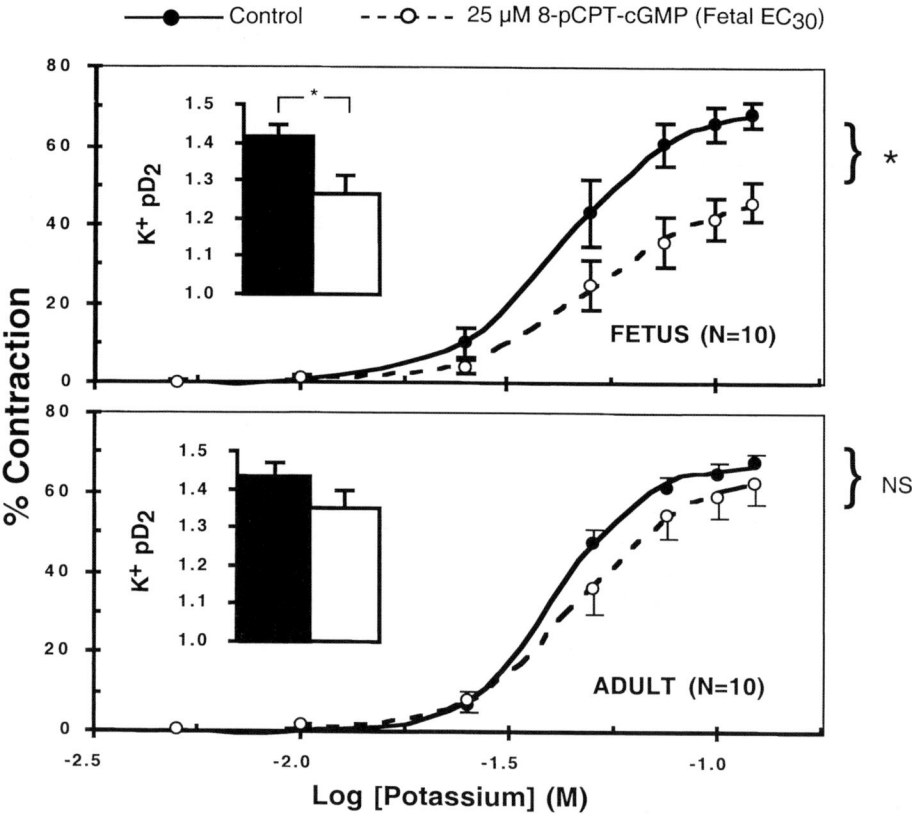

Fig. 3. Effects of 8-pCPT-cGMP on concentration–response curves for potassium. Pretreatment with 25 μM 8-pCPT-cGMP (the fetal EC_{30} concentration for potassium contractions) significantly right-shifted the concentration–response relation for potassium in fetal but not adult basilar arteries, as indicated by changes in the pD_2 values (inset bar graphs). Vertical error bars indicate standard errors for $n = 10$ in all groups, and asterisks indicate significant differences via ANOVA at $P < 0.05$.

concentration–response relations for potassium, but again, this shift was significant only in fetal arteries (Fig. 3).

Altogether, the concentration–response experiments demonstrate that the reduced endothelial vasodilator capacity in immature arteries cannot be explained by attenuated cGMP efficacy, and thus, must be due to the reduced release of endothelial NO and/or other relaxant factors. In turn, the enhanced reactivity to cGMP in immature arteries may be attributable to an increased ability to reduce cytosolic calcium through inhibition of either release or entry and/or stimulation of either extrusion or sequestration.

3. Effects of 8-pCPT-cGMP on K^+ and 5HT-induced increases in cytosolic calcium

To explore the possible age-related differences in the ability of cGMP to influence cytosolic calcium concentrations, we loaded basilar artery segments with the calcium-sensitive fluorescent dye Fura-2AM (5 μM), and then washed and mounted the arteries in a fluorometer (CAF-110, Japan Spectroscopic) as previously described [14,15]. The artery segments were then pretreated with the fetal EC_{30} concentration of 8-pCPT-cGMP for 5HT contractions (6 μM), and exposed to half-log increments in 5HT concentration. In these experiments, 8-pCPT-cGMP depressed the ability of 5HT to elevate cytosolic calcium in the fetal arteries, as indicated by a significant reduction in the pD_2 values for 5HT (Fig. 4). In contrast, no such depression was evident in the adult arteries treated with 8-pCPT-cGMP. In similar experiments using potassium to contract the arteries, however, 8-pCPT-

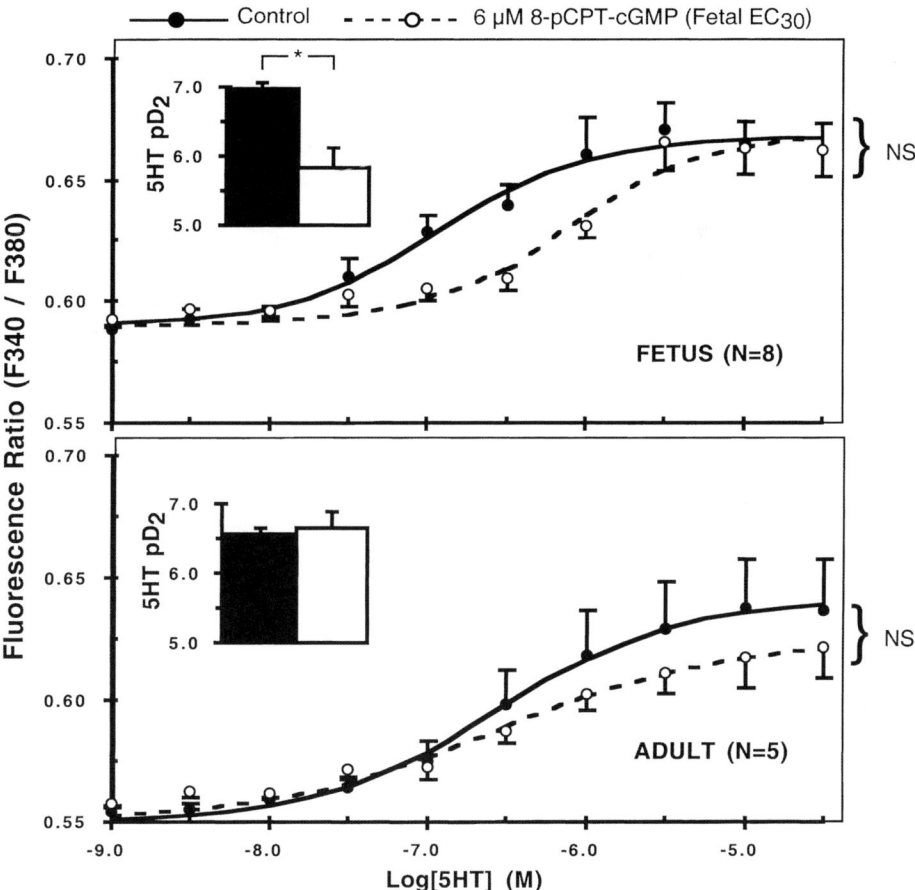

Fig. 4. Effects of 8-pCPT-cGMP on calcium concentration–response curves for 5HT. Pretreatment with 6 μM 8-pCPT-cGMP (the fetal EC_{30} concentration for 5HT contractions) significantly right-shifted the calcium concentration–response relation for 5HT in fetal but not adult basilar arteries, as indicated by changes in pD_2 values (inset bar graphs). Vertical error bars indicate standard errors for eight fetal and five adult arteries. Asterisks indicate significant differences via ANOVA at $P<0.05$.

cGMP had no effect on the ability of potassium to elevate cytosolic calcium in either fetal or adult arteries (Fig. 5).

In light of the marked differences in the ability of 8-pCPT-cGMP to influence 5HT- and potassium-induced increases in cytosolic calcium, we examined the near-maximal effects of 8-pCPT-cGMP on the responses of cytosolic calcium to both potassium and 5HT. In these experiments, the arteries were contracted with the EC_{50} or EC_{95} concentrations of 5HT or potassium, then returned to the baseline and incubated for 40 min with the age- and agonist-specific EC_{90} concentrations of 8-pCPT-cGMP. Separate time control experiments in which no 8-pCPT-cGMP was added during the incubation period were also carried out. After the incubation period, responses to 5HT and potassium were again obtained. As previously observed, even the EC_{90} concentrations of 8-pCPT-cGMP had no significant effects on the responses of cytosolic calcium concentration to potassium in either fetal or

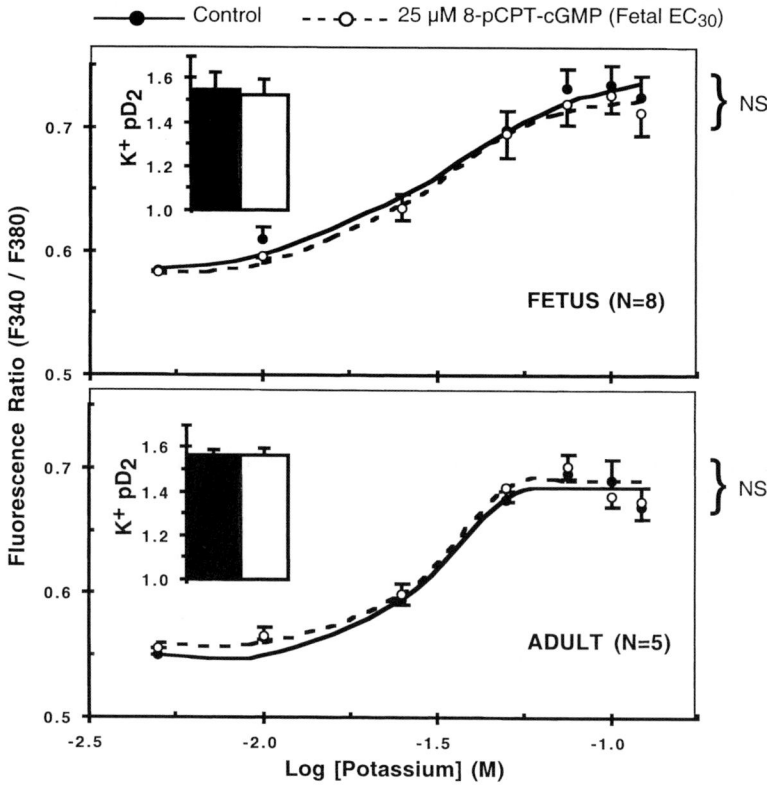

Fig. 5. Effects of 8-pCPT-cGMP on calcium concentration–response curves for potassium. Pretreatment with 25 µM 8-pCPT-cGMP (the fetal EC_{30} concentration for potassium contractions) had no significant effect on the calcium concentration–response relation for potassium in either fetal or adult basilar arteries. Vertical error bars indicate standard errors for eight fetal and five adult arteries.

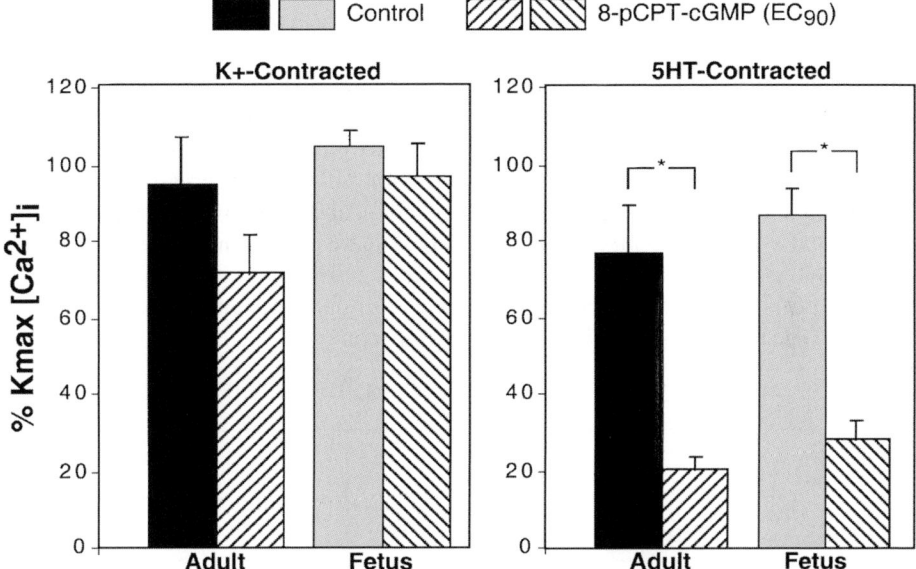

Fig. 6. Effects of EC_{90} concentrations of 8-pCPT-cGMP on K- and 5HT-induced increases in cytosolic Ca^{2+} concentration. Pretreatment with age- and agonist-specific EC_{90} concentrations of 8-pCPT-cGMP had no significant effect on the ability of the EC_{95} concentration of potassium to increase cytosolic calcium concentration. In contrast, the EC_{90} concentrations of 8-pCPT-cGMP significantly attenuated the ability of the EC_{50} concentration of 5HT to increase cytosolic calcium concentration. Vertical error bars indicate standard errors and asterisks indicate significant differences via ANOVA at $P<0.05$.

adult arteries (Fig. 6). In contrast, the EC_{90} concentrations of 8-pCPT-cGMP significantly depressed the ability of 5HT to increase cytosolic calcium in both fetal and adult arteries.

4. Effects of 8-pCPT-cGMP on K^+ and 5HT-induced increases in myofilament calcium sensitivity

Given that 8-pCPT-cGMP relaxed the potassium-induced tone (Fig. 1) without altering the ability of potassium to increase cytosolic calcium (Fig. 5), it follows that 8-pCPT-cGMP must relax the potassium-induced tone by attenuating myofilament calcium sensitivity. In addition, because 8-pCPT-cGMP inhibited potassium-induced tone more in fetal than adult arteries (Fig. 1), it also follows that the effect of 8-pCPT-cGMP on calcium sensitivity must be greater in fetal than in adult basilar arteries. In order to explore these possibilities, we again used Fura-2-loaded basilar arteries and simultaneously measured the cytosolic calcium concentration and contractile force in the presence and absence of 8-pCPT-cGMP. The myofilament calcium sensitivity was estimated as the ratio of the change in tension divided by the corresponding change in cytosolic calcium concentration, as previously described [14]. In one group of such arteries, we monitored tension and calcium concentrations during exposure to graded concentrations of 5HT in the presence and absence of 6 μM 8-pCPT-cGMP (the fetal EC_{30} for 5HT contractions). All of the arteries were incubated with either 8-pCPT-cGMP or vehicle for 30 min prior to exposure of the first 5HT concentration. In the fetal arteries, 8-pCPT-cGMP attenuated the ability of 5HT to increase myofilament calcium sensitivity, as indicated by a significant decrease in the pD_2 values for 5HT in the treated arteries (Fig. 7). Treatment with 8-pCPT-cGMP also significantly decreased the maximum efficacy of 5HT toward calcium sensitivity in the fetal arteries. In contrast, 8-pCPT-cGMP had no significant effect on the calcium sensitivity responses to 5HT in the adult basilar arteries.

In an additional group of arteries, we monitored tension and calcium concentrations during exposure to graded concentrations of potassium in the presence and absence of 25 μM 8-pCPT-cGMP (the fetal EC_{30} for potassium contractions). Again, 8-pCPT-cGMP

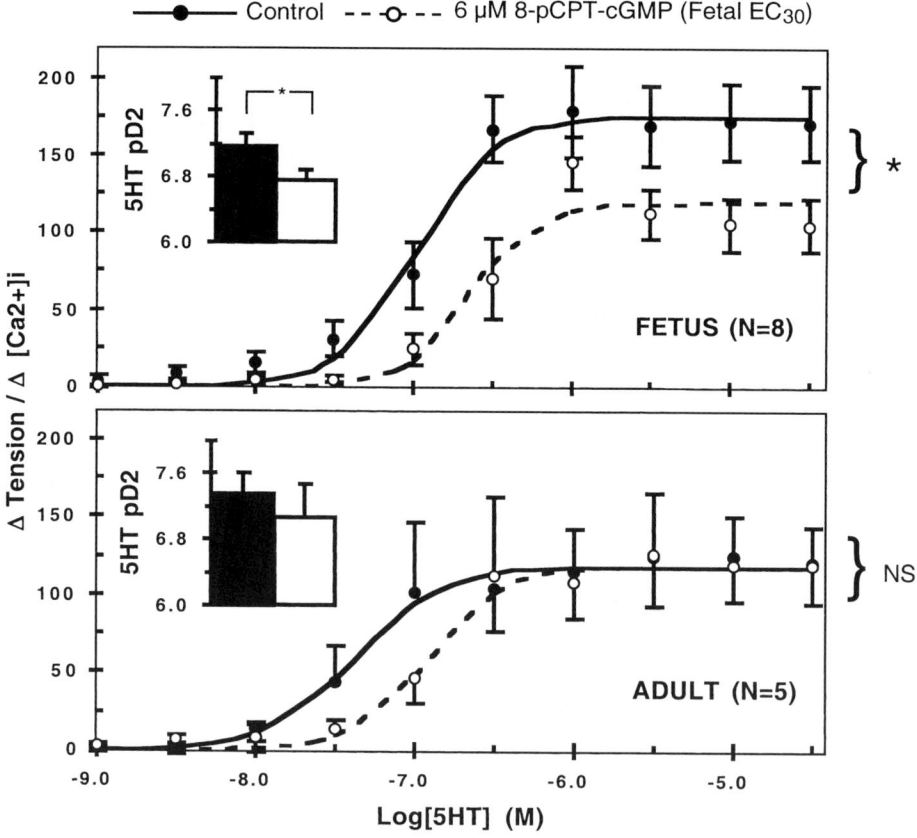

Fig. 7. 8-pCPT-cGMP can attenuate 5HT-induced increases in Ca-sensitivity. Basilar arteries were loaded with Fura-2AM, then incubated 30 min with either 6 μM 8-pCPT-cGMP (the fetal EC_{30} concentration for 5HT contractions) or vehicle, and then exposed to graded concentrations of 5HT. The resulting changes in tension were divided by corresponding increases in cytosolic calcium concentration to estimate changes in myofilament calcium sensitivity. The ability of 5HT to enhance calcium sensitivity was depressed by 8-pCPT-cGMP as reflected by change in both the potency (inset bar graphs) and efficacy of 5HT. Vertical error bars indicate standard errors and asterisks indicate significant differences via ANOVA at $P < 0.05$.

depressed both the potency and efficacy of the potassium-induced changes in myofilament calcium sensitivity in the fetal arteries, but was without significant effect in the adult arteries (Fig. 8), at least at the fetal EC$_{30}$ concentration of 8-pCPT-cGMP.

To confirm the ability of 8-pCPT-cGMP to influence myofilament calcium sensitivity, we examined calcium concentration–response relations in permeabilized basilar arteries. The arteries were permeabilized with α-toxin at 10 μg/ml as previously described [3,14], and exposed to graded concentrations of buffered calcium in the presence and absence of

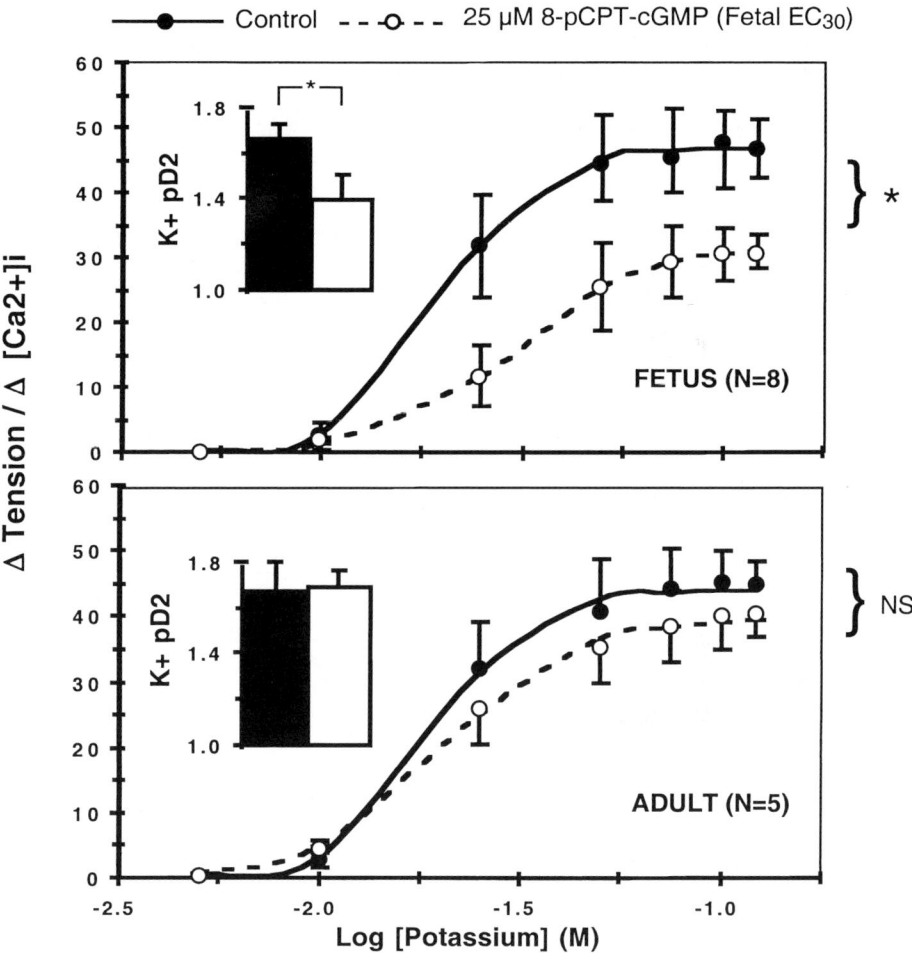

Fig. 8. 8-pCPT-cGMP can attenuate potassium-induced increases in Ca-sensitivity. The effects of 8-pCPT-cGMP on potassium-induced changes in myofilament calcium sensitivity were determined as described in Fig. 7, with the exception that 25 μM 8-pCPT-cGMP (the fetal EC$_{30}$ concentration for potassium contractions) was used, and concentration–response relations were determined for potassium. The ability of potassium to enhance calcium sensitivity was depressed by 8-pCPT-cGMP as reflected by change in both the potency (inset bar graphs) and efficacy of 5HT. Vertical error bars indicate standard errors and asterisks indicate significant differences via ANOVA at $P < 0.05$.

25 μM 8-pCPT-cGMP (the fetal EC_{30} for potassium contractions). Under these conditions, 8-pCPT-cGMP significantly reduced the myofilament calcium sensitivity in the fetal arteries, as indicated by a significant reduction in the pD_2 concentration for calcium (Fig. 9). Treatment with 8-pCPT-cGMP, however, had no significant effect on the calcium–force relation in the adult arteries. These data demonstrate that basal myofilament calcium sensitivity is more potently attenuated by 8-pCPT-cGMP in fetal than in adult basilar arteries.

Because myofilament calcium sensitivity is often dramatically enhanced by heterotrimeric G-protein receptor activation [3,16], it is possible that cGMP-mediated influences on calcium sensitivity may differ under basal and agonist-stimulated conditions. In order to explore this idea, we contracted permeabilized arteries with their EC_{30} concentration of calcium, and then added the non-metabolizable G-protein activator, GTPγS, to baths in

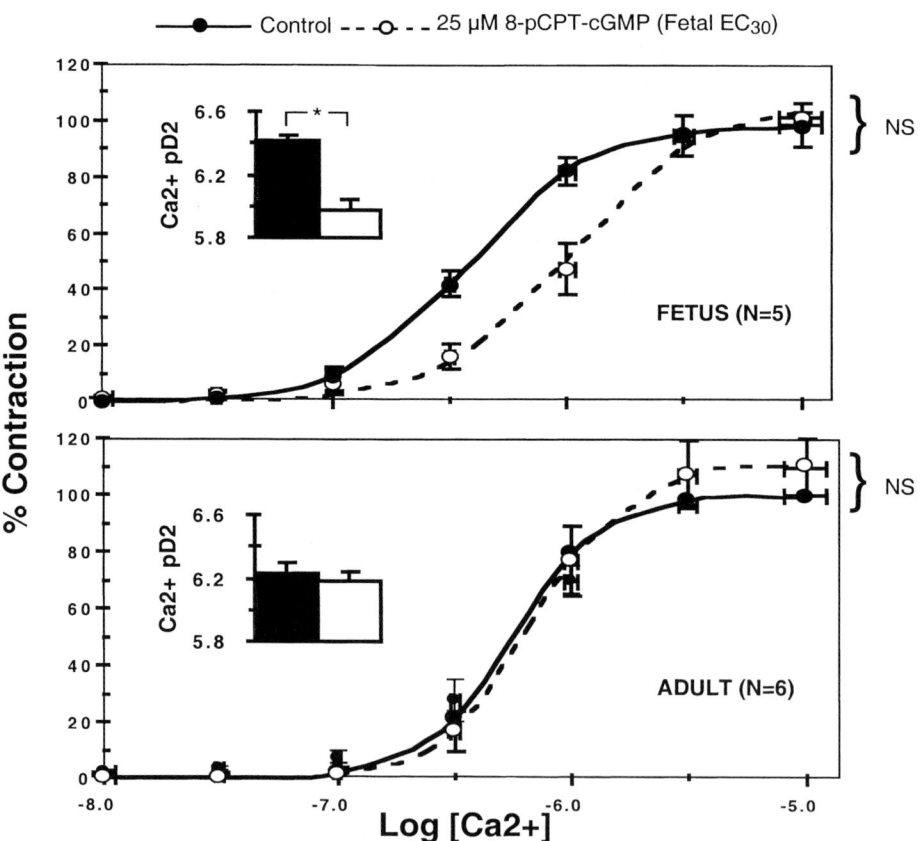

Fig. 9. 8-pCPT-cGMP shifts the basal Ca–force concentration–response relation. Pretreatment with 25 μM 8-pCPT-cGMP (the fetal EC_{30} concentration for potassium contractions) significantly right-shifted the basal calcium–force concentration–response relations obtained in permeabilized fetal basilar arteries, as indicated by a significant reduction in the pD_2 concentration of calcium (inset). In contrast, pretreatment with 25 μM 8-pCPT-cGMP had no significant effect on basal calcium–force concentration–response relations in adult basilar arteries. Vertical error bars indicate standard errors and asterisks indicate significant differences via ANOVA at $P < 0.05$.

stepwise cumulative increments. As previously reported [16], the addition of GTPγS produced a concentration-related increase in myofilament calcium sensitivity. Pre-equilibration with the age-dependent EC_{90} concentrations of 8-pCPT-cGMP (fetal $EC_{90} = 172$ μM; adult $EC_{90} = 410$ μM) significantly reduced sensitivity to GTPγS in both age groups, indicating that cGMP influences not only basal, but also agonist-enhanced myofilament

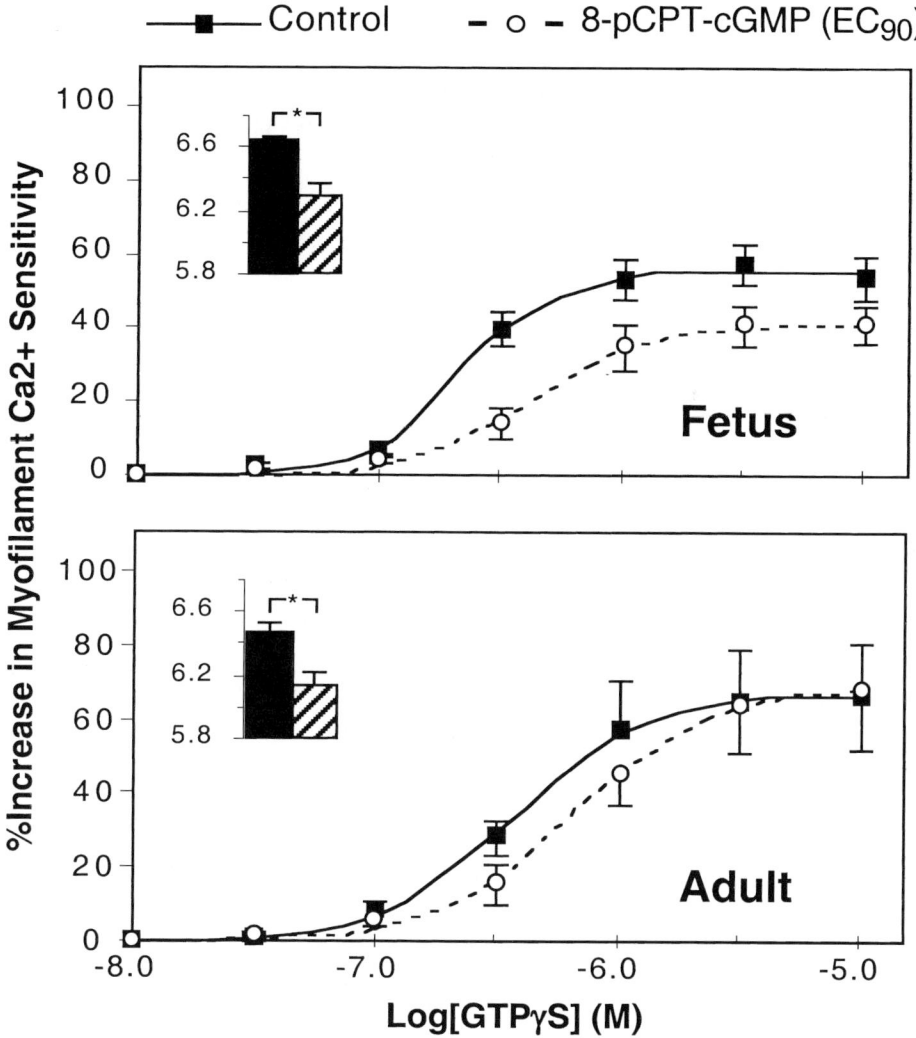

Fig. 10. 8-pCPT-cGMP attenuates the ability of GTPγS to enhance Ca-sensitivity. Permeabilized basilar arteries were precontracted with their EC_{30} concentration of calcium, and then exposed to graded cumulative concentrations of GTPγS, a non-metabolizable activator of G-proteins. GTPγS increased the myofilament calcium sensitivity in a concentration-dependent manner, and these increases were attenuated by pretreatment with the EC_{90} concentrations of 8-pCPT-cGMP in both fetal (172 μM) and adult (410 μM) arteries. Vertical error bars indicate standard errors and asterisks indicate significant differences via ANOVA at $P < 0.05$.

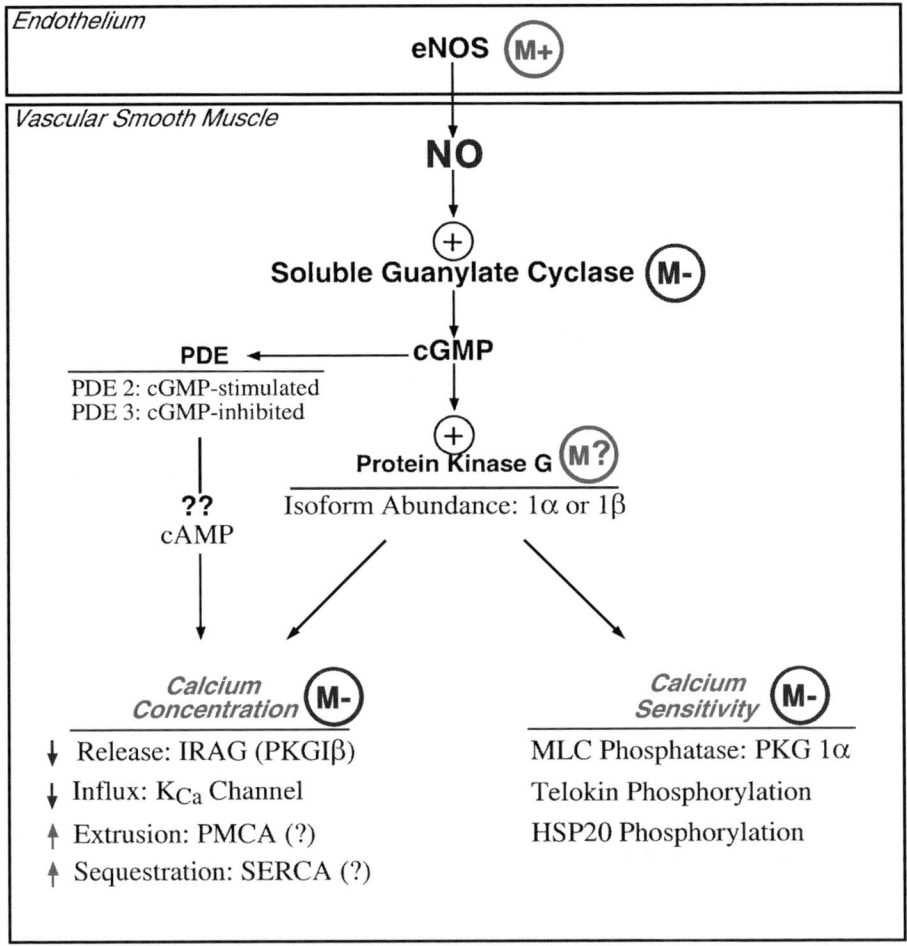

Fig. 11. Effects of maturation on mechanisms of cGMP-dependent vasodilatation. In the above diagram, a circled M with a plus sign indicates enhancement by maturation, whereas a circled M with a minus sign indicates reduced activity or expression during maturation. Compared to the adult arteries, immature cerebral arteries typically exhibit a reduced eNOS abundance and capacity for endothelial NO release [17], which is partially offset by an increased abundance and activity of soluble guanylate cyclase [18]. Levels of cGMP are elevated in fetal compared to adult cerebral arteries, and this can produce changes in cAMP levels through actions on cGMP-sensitive phosphodiesterases [19]. The predominant effect of cGMP on vascular tone, however, is mediated through activation of protein kinase G, which exists in at least two isoforms [20]. The effect of maturation on the abundance and activity of PKG isoforms in cerebral arteries is, at present, unknown. PKG can potentially lower calcium concentration through inhibition of release through phosphorylation of IRAG, a specialized protein in the sarcoplasmic reticulum [25]. By increasing the activity of calcium-sensitive potassium channels, PKG can also hyperpolarize the sarcolemma and further limit calcium entry [26]. PKG may also stimulate extrusion and sequestration directly [27,28]. Regarding the calcium sensitivity, PKG might phosphorylate proteins such as telokin [29,30], myosin light chain phosphatase [30,31], Rho kinase [32], SM22-α [33], and possibly even HSP-20 [34].

calcium sensitivity (Fig. 10). Because similar reductions in sensitivity to GTPγS were achieved with much lower concentrations of 8-pCPT-cGMP in fetal (172 μM) than in the adult arteries (410 μM), these data also demonstrate that agonist-enhanced calcium sensitivity is more sensitive to cGMP in fetal than in adult arteries.

5. Overview

Whereas it is well established that immature cerebral arteries exhibit a depressed capacity for endothelial NO production [17] that is offset in part by an increased abundance of soluble guanylate cyclase [18], the present results further suggest that increased reactivity to cGMP is also characteristic of the immature cerebral arteries. Certainly, increased basal cGMP concentrations [8,9,11] can have important effects by modulating cGMP-sensitive phosphodiesterases [19], but the predominant vasoactive effects of cGMP are probably mediated by protein kinase G [20]. Correspondingly, it is reasonable to postulate that the greater sensitivity to cGMP typical of the immature arteries is simply a consequence of the greater abundance of PKG in the fetal compared to the adult cerebral arteries, as it is in fetal compared to adult hearts [21]. Similarly, the predominant isoform of PKG [20] may also vary with developmental age.

Downstream from PKG, numerous different proteins could mediate PKG's effects on calcium concentration and myofilament calcium sensitivity (Fig. 11). PKG can phosphorylate membrane channels and ion pumps to inhibit calcium influx, inhibit calcium release from the sarcoplasmic reticulum (SR), and thereby decrease cytosolic calcium concentrations [22–26]. PKG can also increase calcium efflux and calcium uptake into the SR [27,28]. As regards to the possible inhibitory effects on the myofilament calcium sensitivity, PKG might phosphorylate proteins such as telokin [29,30], myosin light chain phosphatase [30,31], Rho kinase [32], SM22-α [33], and possibly even HSP-20 [34]. Without doubt, there are many possibilities to explore, particularly because developmental differences in the relative abundance and activity of almost all of these proteins are largely unknown. Nonetheless, the present data clearly indicate that cerebrovascular sensitivity to cGMP is elevated in immature cerebral arteries, a factor that undoubtedly contributes to the lower resting cerebrovascular resistance characteristic of neonates, particularly when combined with the elevated levels of cGMP also typical in this age group.

Acknowledgements

USPHS Grants HL54120, HL64867 and HD31266, and the Loma Linda University School of Medicine supported the work reported here. The authors extend their sincere appreciation to James Williams for his excellent technical support of this project.

References

[1] W.J. Pearce, A.D. Hull, D.M. Long, L.D. Longo, Developmental changes in ovine cerebral artery composition and reactivity, Am. J. Physiol. 261 (2 Pt. 2) (1991) R458–R465.

[2] C.F. Elliott, W.J. Pearce, Effects of maturation on cell water, protein, and DNA content in ovine cerebral arteries, J. Appl. Physiol. 79 (3) (1995) 831–837.

[3] S.E. Akopov, L. Zhang, W.J. Pearce, Physiological variations in ovine cerebrovascular calcium sensitivity, Am. J. Physiol. 272 (5 Pt. 2) (1997) H2271–H2281.

[4] S.E. Akopov, L. Zhang, W.J. Pearce, Maturation alters the contractile role of calcium in ovine basilar arteries, Pediatr. Res. 44 (2) (1998) 154–160.

[5] S. Hayashi, M.K. Park, T.J. Kuehl, Higher sensitivity of cerebral arteries isolated from premature and newborn baboons to adrenergic and cholinergic stimulation, Life Sci. 35 (3) (1984) 253–260.

[6] J. Marin, Age-related changes in vascular responses: a review, Mech. Ageing Dev. 79 (2–3) (1995) 71–114.

[7] S.D. Zurcher, W.J. Pearce, Maturation modulates serotonin- and potassium-induced calcium-45 uptake in ovine carotid and cerebral arteries, Pediatr. Res. 38 (4) (1995) 493–500.

[8] W.J. Pearce, A.D. Hull, D.M. Long, C.R. White, Effects of maturation on cyclic GMP-dependent vaso-dilation in ovine basilar and carotid arteries, Pediatr. Res. 36 (1 Pt. 1) (1994) 25–33.

[9] C.R. White, W.J. Pearce, Effects of maturation on cyclic GMP metabolism in ovine carotid arteries, Pediatr. Res. 39 (1) (1996) 25–31.

[10] K.D. Bloch, G. Filippov, L.S. Sanchez, M. Nakane, S.M. de la Monte, Pulmonary soluble guanylate cyclase, a nitric oxide receptor, is increased during the perinatal period, Am. J. Physiol. 272 (3 Pt. 1) (1997) L400–L406.

[11] C.R. White, X. Hao, W.J. Pearce, Maturational differences in soluble guanylate cyclase activity in ovine carotid and cerebral arteries, Pediatr. Res. 47 (3) (2000) 369–375.

[12] R.E. White, J.P. Kryman, A.M. El-Mowafy, G. Han, G.O. Carrier, cAMP-dependent vasodilators cross-activate the cGMP-dependent protein kinase to stimulate BK(Ca) channel activity in coronary artery smooth muscle cells, Circ. Res. 86 (8) (2000) 897–905.

[13] M. Chalimoniuk, J.B. Strosznajder, Aging modulates nitric oxide synthesis and cGMP levels in hippo-campus and cerebellum. Effects of amyloid beta peptide, Mol. Chem. Neuropathol. 35 (1–3) (1998) 77–95.

[14] S.M. Nauli, L. Zhang, W.J. Pearce, Maturation depresses cGMP-mediated decreases in [Ca2+]i and Ca2+ sensitivity in ovine cranial arteries, Am. J. Physiol.: Heart Circ. Physiol. 280 (3) (2001) H1019–H1028.

[15] S.E. Akopov, L. Zhang, W.J. Pearce, Developmental changes in the calcium sensitivity of rabbit cranial arteries, Biol. Neonate 74 (1) (1998) 60–71.

[16] S.E. Akopov, L. Zhang, W.J. Pearce, Regulation of Ca2+ sensitization by PKC and rho proteins in ovine cerebral arteries: effects of artery size and age, Am. J. Physiol. 275 (3 Pt. 2) (1998) H930–H939.

[17] H. Parfenova, V. Massie, C.W. Leffler, Developmental changes in endothelium-derived vasorelaxant factors in cerebral circulation, Am. J. Physiol.: Heart Circ. Physiol. 278 (3) (2000) H780–H788.

[18] C.R. White, X. Hao, W.J. Pearce, Maturational differences in soluble guanylate cyclase activity in ovine carotid and cerebral arteries, Pediatr. Res. 47 (3) (2000) 369–375.

[19] D.A. Pelligrino, Q. Wang, Cyclic nucleotide crosstalk and the regulation of cerebral vasodilation, Prog. Neurobiol. 56 (1) (1998) 1–18.

[20] F. Hofmann, A. Ammendola, J. Schlossmann, Rising behind NO: cGMP-dependent protein kinases, J. Cell Sci. 113 (Pt. 10) (2000) 1671–1676.

[21] R. Kumar, R.W. Joyner, P. Komalavilas, T.M. Lincoln, Analysis of expression of cGMP-dependent protein kinase in rabbit heart cells, J. Pharmacol. Exp. Ther. 291 (3) (1999) 967–975.

[22] D.J. Darkow, L. Lu, R.E. White, Estrogen relaxation of coronary artery smooth muscle is mediated by nitric oxide and cGMP, Am. J. Physiol. 272 (6 Pt. 2) (1997) H2765–H2773.

[23] Z. Xiong, N. Sperelakis, Regulation of L-type calcium channels of vascular smooth muscle cells, J. Mol. Cell. Cardiol. 27 (1) (1995) 75–91.

[24] L.S. Haug, V. Jensen, O. Hvalby, S.I. Walaas, A.C. Ostvold, Phosphorylation of the inositol 1,4,5-tri-sphosphate receptor by cyclic nucleotide-dependent kinases in vitro and in rat cerebellar slices in situ, J. Biol. Chem. 274 (11) (1999) 7467–7473.

[25] A. Ammendola, A. Geiselhoringer, F. Hofmann, J. Schlossmann, Molecular determinants of the interaction between the inositol 1,4,5-trisphosphate receptor-associated cGMP kinase substrate (IRAG) and cGMP kinase ibeta, J. Biol. Chem. 276 (26) (2001) 24153–24159.

[26] R.D. Swayze, A.P. Braun, A catalytically inactive mutant of type I cGMP-dependent protein kinase prevents

enhancement of large conductance, calcium-sensitive K+ channels by sodium nitroprusside and cGMP, J. Biol. Chem. 276 (23) (2001) 19729–19737.

[27] J. Colyer, Phosphorylation states of phospholamban, Ann. N. Y. Acad. Sci. 853 (1998) 79–91.

[28] Y. Yoshida, A. Toyosato, M.O. Islam, T. Koga, S. Fujita, S. Imai, Stimulation of plasma membrane Ca2+-pump ATPase of vascular smooth muscle by cGMP-dependent protein kinase: functional reconstitution with purified proteins, Mol. Cell. Biochem. 190 (1–2) (1999) 157–167.

[29] J.A. MacDonald, L.A. Walker, R.K. Nakamotom, et al., Phosphorylation of telokin by cyclic nucleotide kinases and the identification of in vivo phosphorylation sites in smooth muscle, FEBS Lett. 479 (3) (2000) 83–88.

[30] X. Wu, A.V. Somlyo, A.P. Somlyo, Cyclic GMP-dependent stimulation reverses G-protein-coupled inhibition of smooth muscle myosin light chain phosphate, Biochem. Biophys. Res. Commun. 220 (3) (1996) 658–663.

[31] G. Torrecillas, M.L. Diez-Marques, C. Garcia-Escribano, R.J. Bosch, D. Rodriguez-Puyol, M. Rodriguez-Puyol, Mechanisms of cGMP-dependent mesangial-cell relaxation: a role for myosin light-chain phosphatase activation, Biochem. J. 346 (Pt. 1) (2000) 217–222.

[32] V. Sauzeau, H. Le Jeune, C. Cario-Toumaniantz, et al., Cyclic GMP-dependent protein kinase signaling pathway inhibits RhoA-induced Ca2+ sensitization of contraction in vascular smooth muscle, J. Biol. Chem. 275 (28) (2000) 21722–21729.

[33] U.S. Schmidt, M. Troschka, G. Pfitzer, The variable coupling between force and myosin light chain phosphorylation in Triton-skinned chicken gizzard fibre bundles: role of myosin light chain phosphatase, Pfluegers Arch. 429 (5) (1995) 708–715.

[34] A. Beall, D. Bagwell, D. Woodrum, et al., The small heat shock-related protein, HSP20, is phosphorylated on serine 16 during cyclic nucleotide-dependent relaxation, J. Biol. Chem. 274 (16) (1999) 11344–11351.

Hormonal regulation

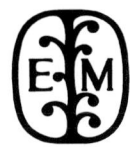

International Congress Series 1235 (2002) 395–399

Impact of hormones on the regulation of cerebral vascular tone

Diana N. Krause*, Greg G. Geary, Anne Marie McNeill, Jose Ospina, Sue P. Duckles

Department of Pharmacology, College of Medicine, University of California, Irvine, CA 92697-4625, USA

Abstract

A number of circulating hormones affect cerebral vascular function. Using isolated blood vessels from rodent models, we have found that the gonadal hormones estrogen and testosterone and the pineal hormone melatonin modify cerebral vascular tone. Melatonin directly constricted vascular smooth muscle, whereas prior in vivo treatment with gonadal steroids altered endothelial function. Endothelium-dependent dilation in pressurized cerebral arteries was decreased by testosterone but enhanced by estrogen. In vivo estrogen treatment also increased nitric oxide synthase (NOS) activity, as well as protein levels of endothelial NOS (eNOS), cyclooxygenase-1 (COX-1) and prostacyclin synthase in cerebral blood vessels. In vitro overnight incubation of isolated brain vessels with estrogen alone and with estrogen receptor blockers confirmed that estrogen is acting directly on vascular estrogen receptors to increase levels of eNOS. Western blot analysis also indicated the presence of estrogen receptors in cerebral vessels. When using mice deficient in the alpha estrogen receptor (ERKO mice), effects of estrogen on cerebral vascular tone and protein levels of eNOS and COX-1 were not observed. Together, these studies indicate that vascular function in the brain may vary with time of day (melatonin) or gender (estrogen/testosterone) and underscore the important impact that circulating hormones have on the cerebral circulation. © 2002 Elsevier Science B.V. All rights reserved.

Keywords: Estrogen; Testosterone; Melatonin; Nitric oxide; Prostacyclin; Endothelium

1. Introduction

Control of cerebral blood flow is well known to involve a multitude of influences (Fig. 1). As discussed elsewhere in this volume, metabolic factors from the tissue surrounding

---

* Corresponding author. Tel.: +1-949-824-5040; fax: +1-949-824-4855.
E-mail addresses: dnkrause@uci.edu (D.N. Krause), spduckle@uci.edu (S.P. Duckles).

0531-5131/02 © 2002 Elsevier Science B.V. All rights reserved.
PII: S 0 5 3 1 - 5 1 3 1 (0 2) 0 0 2 1 1 - X

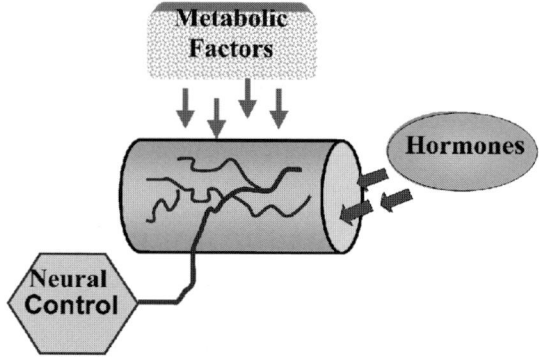

Fig. 1. Factors controlling cerebral blood flow.

intraparenchymal blood vessels are thought to help couple blood flow to the activity of neurons and possibly astrocytes. Neurotransmitters released from perivascular nerves clearly modulate pial vessel reactivity and also appear to locally affect intracerebral vessels. Overlaying these influences is the circulating hormonal milieu; a variety of hormones directly alter cerebrovascular function to impact cerebral blood flow.

Using rodent models, we have focussed on two different hormonal influences: the pineal hormone melatonin and the gonadal steroids estrogen and testosterone. Our interest in these hormones stems from clinical observations that risk of cerebrovascular disease varies with time of day, gender and levels of reproductive hormones [1–4]. As discussed below, we have found that melatonin acutely constricts vascular smooth muscle [5,6], whereas prior treatment with gonadal steroids alters endothelial function [7–10]. We have further investigated underlying mechanisms of estrogen action with biochemical analyses of isolated vessels and use of genetically altered mice. Our findings indicate that estrogen acts on cerebrovascular receptors to increase the synthetic machinery for both nitric oxide (NO) and prostacyclin.

2. Impact of melatonin

Melatonin is considered the hormonal output of the circadian clock; it is only released from the pineal gland during the hours of darkness [11]. The cerebral vasculature has been identified as one of the targets of melatonin, beginning with the initial observation of ^{125}I-melatonin binding to the smooth muscle layer of large cerebral arteries [12]. We investigated functional consequences of these receptors using isolated segments of rat middle cerebral artery, pressurized in vitro [5]. Application of nanomolar concentrations of melatonin acutely constrict the artery with an EC_{50} of 3 nM. This effect is blocked by the competitive antagonist luzindole and by pertussis toxin pretreatment, consistent with the action of $G_{i/o}$-coupled melatonin receptors. The magnitude of the constrictor response to melatonin is similar to that of blockers of K_{Ca} channels and, in fact, constrictor effects of melatonin are prevented by prior inhibition of K_{Ca} channels with either tetraethylammonium or charybdotoxin [5]. We have hypothesized that melatonin-induced constriction involves closure of K_{Ca} channels, possibly via inhibition of the cyclic AMP-protein kinase A pathway [5]. In smaller branches of the middle cerebral artery, we have also seen constriction, and occasionally dilation [6], to melatonin. These observations may reflect the presence in cerebral arteries of multiple melatonin receptor subtypes, similar to what we have found in peripheral arteries, i.e., a constrictor MT_1 receptor and a dilator MT_2 receptor [6]. However, the distribution of specific melatonin receptors throughout the cerebral vasculature has yet to be determined.

At this point, not much is known regarding the physiological consequence of nightly stimulation of cerebrovascular melatonin receptors. Because of its lipophilicity, plasma melatonin would be expected to have access to the medial layer of the cerebral arteries and influence tone. One role of melatonin may be to adjust the autoregulatory range to a lower limit, as shown in a rat study of hemorrhage-induced hypotension [13].

3. Impact of estrogen

Because of growing interest in possible benefits of estrogen for reducing stroke risk and morbidity [3,4,14], we have been investigating how estrogen may influence the cerebral circulation. Contractile effects were studied in isolated, pressurized segments of cerebral arteries from gonadectomized rats and mice, either with or without one month of estrogen treatment. In addition, blood vessels were isolated from brain parenchyma for Western blot analysis and biochemical measurements.

In vivo estrogen treatment of female animals increased nitric oxide synthase (NOS) activity as well as protein levels of endothelial NOS (eNOS), cyclooxygenase-1 (COX-1) and prostacyclin synthase in isolated cerebral vessels [8,15]. Estrogen treatment of male rats also increased levels of cerebrovascular eNOS protein [8]. These findings correlated with functional studies showing less tone in pressurized cerebral arteries from estrogen-treated rats and mice [7,9,10]. The decrease in tone was the result of increased endothelium-dependent dilation as revealed by inhibiting NOS, COX and removal of the endothelium [7,9,10].

In vitro overnight incubation of isolated brain vessels with estrogen alone and with estrogen receptor blockers confirmed that estrogen is acting on vascular estrogen receptors to increase levels of eNOS [16]. Western blot analysis also indicated the presence of estrogen receptors in the vascular fraction [17]. In cerebral vessels from mice deficient in the alpha estrogen receptor (ER alpha), effects of estrogen on cerebral vascular tone and protein levels of eNOS and COX-1 were not observed [18], suggesting that estrogen normally acts via the alpha receptor subtype. Together, these data suggest that plasma estrogen directly impacts the cerebral circulation by altering levels of endothelial vasodilators. Evidence from animal models of stroke indicates that estrogen provides protective effects [14]. We hypothesize that increased production of endothelial NO and prostacyclin in cerebral blood vessels is an important neuroprotective action of estrogen.

4. Impact of testosterone

Testosterone also modulates cerebrovascular tone in an endothelium-dependent manner [10]. Middle cerebral arteries were isolated from male rats that were either intact, orchiectomized, or orchiectomized with testosterone replacement for one month. In all arteries, the amount of tone increased with increasing transmural pressure. However, at all pressures (20–80 mm Hg), the level of tone was less in arteries from orchiectomized as compared to intact animals. Testosterone treatment restored the level of tone to that observed in arteries from intact male rats. The differences between orchiectomized and testosterone-treated rats was abolished by removal of the endothelium but unaffected by the NOS inhibitor L-NAME (N^G-nitro-L-arginine-methyl ester). Levels of cerebrovascular eNOS protein also were unaffected by testosterone [8]. The mechanisms by which testosterone enhances the tone of cerebral arteries remains to be determined, but may involve increased release of endothelial vasoconstrictors [10].

5. Conclusions

Evidence is presented for direct effects of three different circulating hormones on cerebral blood vessels. Melatonin acts acutely and thus might be expected to increase vascular smooth muscle tone at night when levels of this hormone are elevated in the blood. The gonadal steroids estrogen and testosterone both affect the endothelium, however with opposite functional results. Vascular tone is decreased by estrogen but increased by testosterone. Thus cerebrovascular function would be expected to differ with gender and reproductive status. Thus, the impact of hormones is an important consideration for understanding the control of cerebral blood flow.

3.3.1.8. On-Site Discussion

3.3.1.8.1. **Question: (Maiese)** Dr. Krause, melatonin has been demonstrated to be neuroprotective in some models of cerebral ischemia. Based on your initial results that melatonin may be a vasoconstrictor, do you believe that melatonin exerts its protective effects through direct neuronal or vascular interaction?

Answer: (Krause) At this point, this is purely speculative, but it seems that the cerebrovascular effects of melatonin could certainly contribute to neuroprotective effects of this hormone. It has been shown that melatonin can extend the lower limit of autoregulation which is protective during systemic hypotension. There is still much to be learned regarding cerebrovascular effects of melatonin. We also have preliminary evidence that melatonin can dilate as well as constrict cerebral vessels, perhaps via two different receptor subtypes.

3.3.1.8.2. **Question: (Kalaria)** If chronic estrogen decreased cerebrovascular tone would this explain HRT being ineffective for dementia, particularly in Alzheimer's disease trials?

Answer: (Krause) At this time it is difficult to make conclusions from the currently available clinical data. Studies of both Alzheimer's and cardiovascular disease were conducted in women with preexisting disease. Clearly estrogen has been shown to be protective in animal models of stroke; we don't know about preventive effects on Alzheimer's. It is possible that the decrease in tone with estrogen results in increased cerebral blood flow and that effect may be neuroprotective.

3.3.1.8.3. **Question: (Pelligrino)** Does castration increase estrogen receptor expression in males?

Answer: (Krause) No one has looked at this, so we don't know.

Acknowledgements

This work was supported by Grant RO1 HL-50775 from the National Heart, Lung and Blood Institute, NIH, USA.

References

[1] M. Kelly-Hayes, P.A. Wolf, C.S. Kase, F.N. Brand, J.M. McGuirk, R.B. D'Agostino, Temporal patterns of stroke onset. The Framingham Study, Stroke 26 (1995) 1343–1347.

[2] M. Gallerani, R. Manfredini, L. Ricci, A. Cocurullo, C. Goldoni, M. Bigoni, C. Fersini, Chronobiological aspects of acute cerebrovascular diseases, Acta Neurol. Scand. 87 (1993) 482–487.

[3] C.S. Hayward, R.P. Kelly, P. Collins, The roles of gender, the menopause and hormone replacement on cardiovascular function, Cardiovasc. Res. 46 (2000) 28–49.

[4] M. Prencipe, C. Ferretti, A.R. Casini, M. Santini, F. Giubilei, F. Culasso, Stroke, disability, and dementia: results of a population survey, Stroke 28 (1997) 531–536.

[5] G.G. Geary, D.N. Krause, S.P. Duckles, Melatonin directly constricts cerebral arteries through modulation of potassium channels, Am. J. Physiol. 273 (1997) H1530–H1536.

[6] D.N. Krause, G.G. Geary, S. Doolen, S.P. Duckles, Melatonin and cardiovascular function, In: J. Olcese (Ed.), Melatonin After Four Decades: An Assessment of its Potential, New York: Kluwer Academic/Plenum Press, 2000, 7 pp. 299–310.

[7] G.G. Geary, D.N. Krause, S.P. Duckles, Estrogen reduces myogenic tone through a nitric oxide-dependent mechanism in rat cerebral arteries, Am. J. Physiol. 275 (1998) H292–H300.

[8] A.M. McNeill, N. Kim, S.P. Duckles, D.N. Krause, Chronic estrogen treatment increases levels of endothelial nitric oxide synthase protein in rat cerebral microvessels, Stroke 30 (1999) 2186–2190.

[9] G.G. Geary, D.N. Krause, S.P. Duckles, Estrogen reduces mouse cerebral artery tone through endothelial NOS- and cyclooxygenase-dependent mechanisms, Am. J. Physiol. 279 (2000) H511–H519.

[10] G.G. Geary, D.N. Krause, S.P. Duckles, Gonadal hormones affect diameter of male rat cerebral arteries through endothelium-dependent mechanisms, Am. J. Physiol. 279 (2000) H610–H618.

[11] D.N. Krause, M.L. Dubocovich, Regulatory sites in the melatonin system of mammals, Trends Neurosci. 13 (1990) 464–470.

[12] M. Viswanathan, J.T. Laitinen, J.M. Saavedra, Expression of melatonin receptors in arteries involved in thermoregulation, Proc. Natl. Acad. Sci. U. S. A. 87 (1990) 6200–6203.

[13] O. Regrigny, P. Delagrange, E. Scalbert, J. Atkinson, I. Lartaud-Idjouadiene, Melatonin improves cerebral circulation security margin in rats. Am. J. Physiol. 275:H139–H144.

[14] P.D. Hurn, I.M. Macrae, Estrogen as a neuroprotectant in stroke, J. Cereb. Blood Flow Metab. 20 (2000) 631–652.

[15] J.A. Ospina, D.N. Krause, S.P. Duckles, 17β-estradiol increases rat cerebrovascular prostacyclin synthesis by elevating cyclooxygenase-1 and prostacyclin synthase, Stroke 33 (2002) 600–605.

[16] A.M. McNeill, D.N. Krause, S.P. Duckles, Estrogen directly increases levels of endothelial nitric oxide synthase in rat cerebral microvessels, FASEB J. 14 (2000) A32.

[17] D.N. Krause, A.M. McNeill, S. Shah, S.P. Duckles, Estrogen receptors in rat cerebral microvessels, FASEB J. 14 (2000) A1340.

[18] G.G. Geary, A.M. McNeill, J.A. Ospina, D.N. Krause, K.S. Korach, S.P. Duckles, Cerebrovascular nitric oxide synthase and cyclooxygenase are unaffected by estrogen in mice lacking estrogen receptor alpha, J. Appl. Physiol. 91 (2001) 2391–2399.

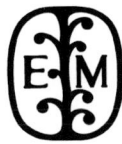

International Congress Series 1235 (2002) 401–411

Unique aspects of NO-related cerebrovascular regulation: influence of estrogen and caveolin-1

Dale A. Pelligrino*, Hao-Liang Xu,
Roberto A. Santizo, Elena Galea

*Neuroanesthesia Research Laboratory, Molecular Biology Research Building (M/C 513),
University of Illinois at Chicago, 900 S. Ashland Ave., Chicago, IL 60607, USA*

Abstract

The endothelial isoform of nitric oxide synthase (eNOS) has been found to be an important neuroprotective enzyme. NO produced in the endothelium is ideally positioned to defend the brain by a variety of mechanisms, including vasodilation, thereby improving perfusion, and via anti-inflammatory actions. Estrogen depletion, which is known to increase the risk for brain damage in experimental stroke models, has been linked to a marked repression of eNOS function in both cerebral and non-cerebral blood vessels. Those changes can be reversed with chronic 17β-estradiol (E_2) supplementation. Current information would suggest that E_2 potentiation of eNOS-derived NO-generating capacity goes beyond simply modulating eNOS protein abundance, and seems to involve a reduction in the expression of the endogenous eNOS inhibitor, caveolin-1 (CAV-1). We endeavored to establish a link between these correlative findings by independently manipulating eNOS and CAV-1 expression (via chronic simvastatin treatment and topical antisense oligonucleotide applications, respectively), while monitoring two indicators of eNOS functional activity—acetylcholine (ACh)-induced pial arteriolar dilation and pial venular leukocyte adhesion. We found, in ovariectomized rats, that, *individually*, neither the upregulation of eNOS, nor the downregulation of CAV-1, in vivo is capable of restoring eNOS functional activity (i.e., recovery of ACh reactivity and reduced leukocyte adhesion) in pial vessels. Only when eNOS upregulation *and* CAV-1 downregulation are combined is activity normalized. These results show that changes in CAV-1 expression can have a profound effect on eNOS function in vivo, and establish the existence of a mechanistic link between changes in the abundance of CAV-1 and eNOS protein and eNOS functional activity in cerebral vessels. © 2002 Elsevier Science B.V. All rights reserved.

Keywords: Endothelial nitric oxide synthase; Leukocyte adhesion; 17β-estradiol; Pial; Simvastatin

* Corresponding author. Tel.: +1-312-355-1666; fax: +1-815-333-1493.
E-mail address: dpell@uic.edu (D.A. Pelligrino).

0531-5131/02 © 2002 Elsevier Science B.V. All rights reserved.
PII: S0531-5131(02)00202-9

It is well established that the incidence of cardiovascular disease, including stroke, and related mortality are lower in females before menopause, when compared to males and post-menopausal females. It is quite likely that the protection in pre-menopausal females relates to higher levels of circulating estrogens, principally 17β-estradiol (E_2). The identification of the specific mechanisms involved in E_2-related cardiovascular defense has been the objective of numerous experimental studies, as summarized in recent excellent reviews [1,2]. The results of such investigations have uncovered a wide variety of E_2 effects with apparent cardiovascular benefit, some of the best-known actions being vasodilation, anti-atherogenesis, diminished post-ischemic inflammation, and anti-oxidant effects.

The endothelial isoform of nitric oxide synthase (eNOS) has been found to be an important neuroprotective enzyme. NO produced in the endothelium is ideally positioned to defend the brain by a variety of mechanisms, including vasodilation and improved perfusion. A number of non-hemodynamic mechanisms have been offered as candidates for eNOS-related neuroprotection. Principal among these is restriction of leukocyte adhesion and endothelial transmigration [3]. Estrogen depletion, which is known to increase the risk for brain damage in experimental stroke models, has been linked to a marked repression of eNOS expression and function in both cerebral and non-cerebral blood vessels [2,4,5]. Those changes can be reversed with chronic 17β-estradiol (E_2) supplementation. Current information would suggest that E_2 potentiation of eNOS-derived NO-generating capacity goes beyond simply modulating eNOS protein abundance, and seems to involve a reduction in the expression of the endogenous eNOS inhibitor, caveolin-1 (CAV-1) [4]. We endeavored to establish a mechanistic link between these correlative findings by independently increasing eNOS and reducing CAV-1 expression (via chronic simvastatin treatment and topical antisense oligonucleotide applications, respectively), while monitoring two indicators of eNOS functional activity—acetylcholine (ACh)-induced pial arteriolar dilation and a low level or absence of pial venular leukocyte adhesion. The former reflects agonist-induced eNOS activation, while the latter provides an indication of agonist-independent basal eNOS function.

The basic hypothesis tested in this investigation of pial vessels in vivo was that, in OVX females, normalization of eNOS expression, in the absence of any attempt to reduce CAV-1 expression, would not be sufficient for restoring eNOS functional activity. The proper testing of that hypothesis, in estrogen-depleted rats, required the implementation of two key experimental manipulations: (1) upregulation of eNOS without altering CAV-1 expression; and (2) an eNOS-independent specific downregulation of CAV-1. For the first, we used chronic 3-hydroxy-3-methylglutaryl-coenzyme A (HMG-CoA) reductase inhibitor (simvastatin [SIM]) treatments [6]. In the second case, we used topical applications of a CAV-1 antisense oligonucleotide. The ACh reactivities of pial arterioles *or* pial venular leukocyte

Fig. 1. Comparisons of eNOS (A) or CAV-1 (B) expression in tissue harvested from intact, untreated ovariectomized (OVX), and 17β-estradiol (E_2)-treated OVX (OVX+E_2) females. Comparisons of eNOS (C) or CAV-1 (D) expression in pial tissue from intact, OVX, and simvastatin (SIM)-treated OVX females. For each protein analysis, a single band was seen (~ 140 kDa for eNOS; 22–24 kDa for CAV-1). Similar findings were obtained in three to four additional sets of evaluations, as depicted quantitatively in the bar graphs. The data represent the means±S.D. of three to four separate experiments. The band intensities (integrated optical densities) are expressed relative to a standard (HUVEC extract). *$p<0.05$ vs. OVX; †$p<0.05$ vs. intact.

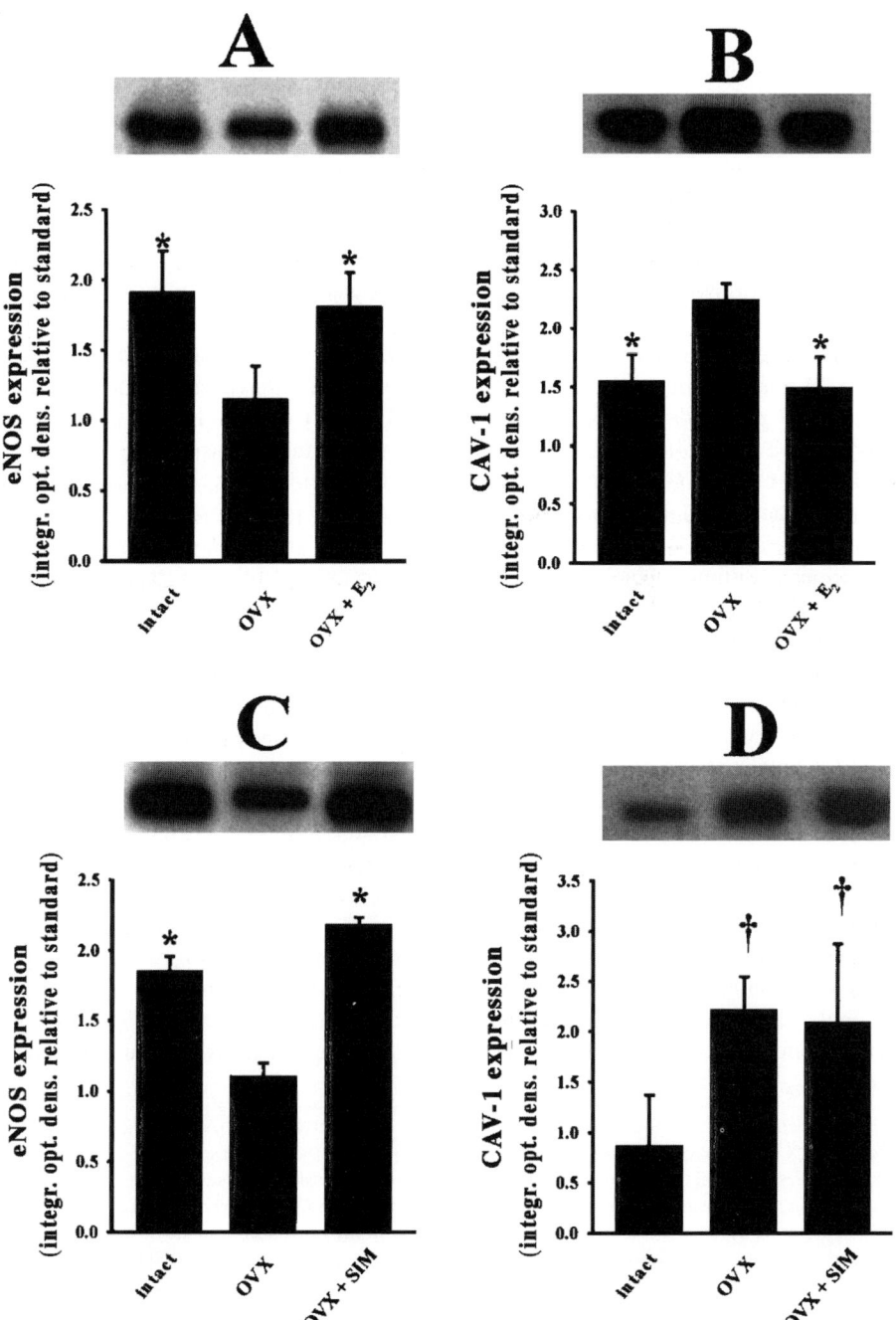

adhesion were compared in six groups of female rats. Those were, (1) SIM-treated OVX; (2) SIM plus CAV-1 antisense-treated OVX; (3) SIM plus CAV-1 missense-treated OVX; (4) CAV-1 missense-treated OVX; (5) CAV-1 antisense-treated OVX; and (6) vehicle-treated OVX, intact, or E_2-supplemented OVX.

1. Methods

Ovariectomized, 300–350 g female Sprague–Dawley rats (4–6 weeks post-ovariectomy at the time of study) were used in most experiments. The only exception was vehicle [artificial cerebrospinal fluid (aCSF)]-injected females, where intact and chronically E_2-treated (0.1 mg/kg/day, ip, for 1 week) OVX females were compared to E_2-depleted OVX rats.

All rats were prepared with closed cranial windows under N_2O/halothane anesthesia. In the SIM-treated groups (1, 2, and 3), SIM was administered subcutaneously for 2 weeks, at 20 mg/kg/day. CAV-1 antisense (5′-**TTTACCCCCAGACAT**-3′), complementary to the initiation sequence of rat CAV-1 (GenBank accession no. Z46614), or missense (5′-**CAATCGGCTAACCTA**-3′) oligonucleotide, was introduced into the space under the cranial window (10 or 25 μg in 200–300 μl of aCSF) immediately after window preparation, 24 h preceding arteriolar reactivity or leukocyte adhesion assessments. In an additional vehicle-treated control group, 300 μl of aCSF was injected into the space under the cranial window. One day after window placement, the animals were reanesthetized (fentanyl/N_2O) and pial arteriolar diameter changes to topical applications of ACh [4], or the extent of pial venular leukocyte adhesion during resting conditions [7,8], were compared. After an initial assessment of CO_2 reactivity, ACh was suffused (in aCSF) at 10 then 100 μM. Diameter changes of 25–50 μm pial arterioles were expressed as a percentage increase from the baseline value measured just before introduction of ACh (or increased CO_2). In separate experiments, adherent Rhodamine-6G-labeled leukocytes were viewed under resting conditions through the closed cranial window using intravital microscopy [7,8]. Experiments were videotaped for subsequent analysis of the percentage of the venular area occupied by adherent leukocytes. To obtain some indication of the importance of pial venular eNOS in the resistance to leukocyte adhesion under basal conditions, pilot studies were conducted using application of a non-selective (N^G-nitro-L-arginine) or a neuronal NOS selective (ARR-17477) inhibitor. We found that pial venular leukocyte adhesion was increased when total NOS activity, but not nNOS activity alone, was blocked. The increased leukocyte adhesion in the presence of

Fig. 2. The recovery of eNOS-dependent, agonist-activated (i.e. acetylcholine [ACh]-induced) vasodilating function in OVX females requires *both* an increase in eNOS expression *and* a decrease in CAV-1 expression. The results are expressed as the percentage increase in diameter from the baseline value (means±S.D., n=4–5 for each group). (A) Demonstration that neither eNOS upregulation nor CAV-1 downregulation individually is capable of restoring eNOS function (along with the absence of any non-specific oligonucleotide effects. (B) Recovery of eNOS-dependent vasodilating function in OVX females requires combined eNOS upregulation and CAV-1 downregulation. The absence of non-specific oligonucleotide effects was demonstrated in animals given CAV-1 missense in the place of the antisense oligonucleotide. $^†p$<0.05 vs. OVX+simvastatin+CAV-1 antisense [10 μg]; *p<0.05 vs. OVX+simvastatin+CAV-1 antisense [25 μg]).

(A)

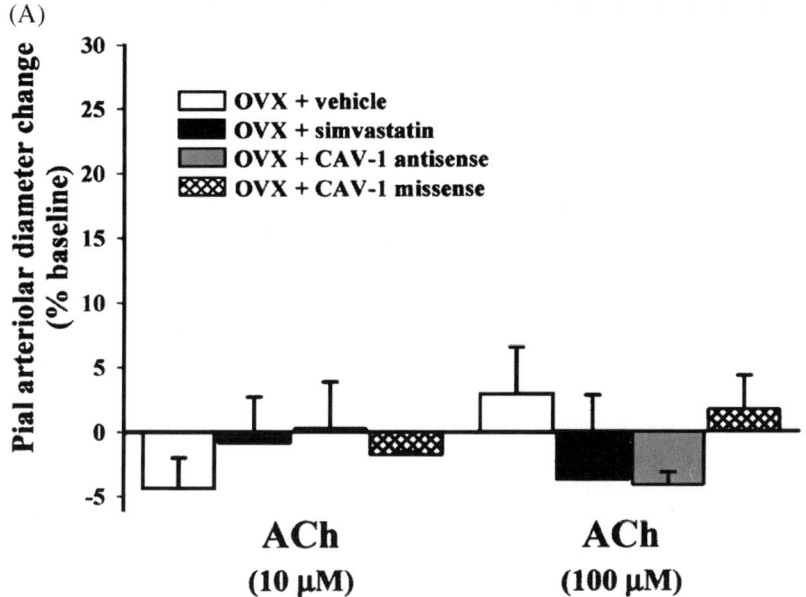

(B)

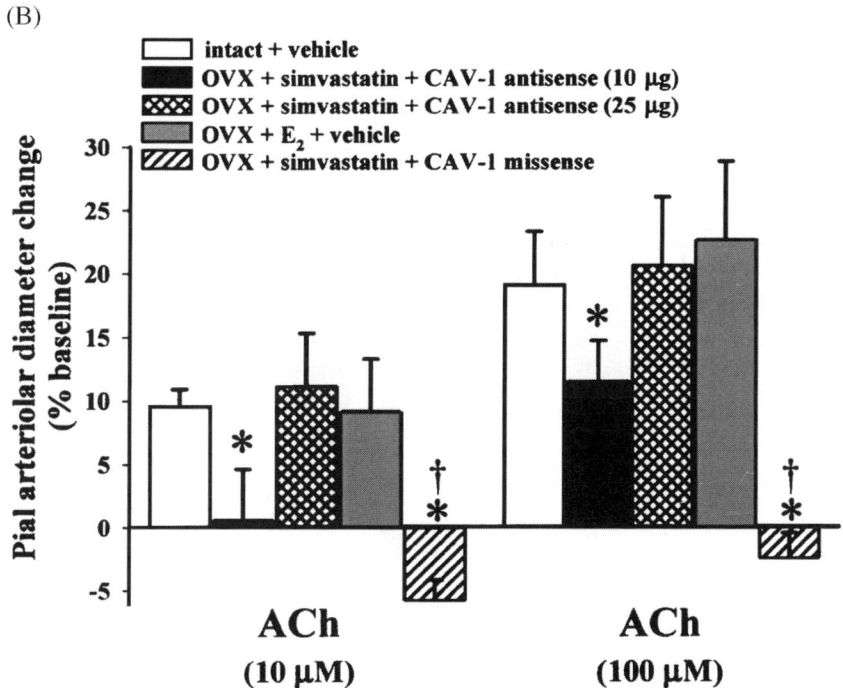

repressed eNOS function is consistent with previous findings [9]. In several rats from each group, pial tissue from under the cranial window was removed and CAV-1 and eNOS protein were assessed via Western immunoblotting.

2. Results

Consistent with previous results from our laboratory, using immunofluorescence techniques [4], Western immunoblots of pial tissue obtained from group 6 (aCSF vehicle-injected) rats indicated that eNOS expression was lower (Fig. 1A) and CAV-1 expression (Fig. 1B) higher in samples from OVX vs. intact females. Treatment of OVX rats with 17β-estradiol (E_2) was accompanied by a restoration of eNOS and CAV-1 expression to levels observed in intact females (Fig. 1A,B). On the other hand, simvastatin treatment of OVX females was associated with a greater eNOS expression (Fig. 1C) than that seen in the untreated OVX group, but CAV-1 expression remained elevated (Fig. 1D, see also Fig. 4).

Moderate or no appreciable differences in CO_2 reactivities were noted among the groups (data not shown). As shown in Fig. 2A, in confirmation of earlier data published by us [4], ACh reactivity was completely lost in OVX females at 24 h following window placement and introduction of aCSF vehicle. No recovery of ACh-induced pial arteriolar dilations was observed in OVX rats where, individually, either eNOS was upregulated (via

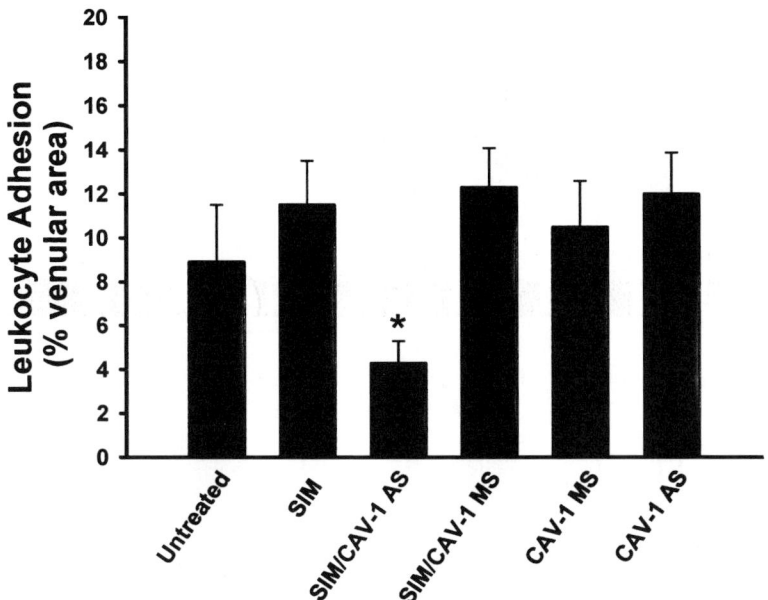

Fig. 3. Basal leukocyte adhesion, measured as the percentage of venular area occupied by adherent leukocytes, was attenuated (by ~ 50%) only in the presence of combined SIM plus CAV-1 antisense (AS, 25 μg) treatment. There were no differences among the remaining groups, including rats given SIM plus CAV-1 missense (MS). Means±S.D. *p<0.05 vs. all other groups.

2 weeks SIM treatment) or CAV-1 was downregulated (via 25 µg of CAV-1 given topically 24 h before study—Fig. 2A). Only in the presence of combined SIM and CAV-1 antisense treatments was any improvement in pial arteriolar ACh reactivity seen (Fig. 2B). Furthermore, the recovery in ACh responsivity, with respect to the antisense, was dose-dependent—to the extent that the higher dose (25 µg) was associated with a level of pial arteriolar dilation identical to that seen in intact and E_2-treated OVX females (Fig. 2B). Thus, combined eNOS upregulation and CAV-1 downregulation, in OVX rats, appears to have the same effect as E_2 supplementation. The specificity of the antisense oligonucleotide action was confirmed by findings showing a lack of any influence of a missense oligonucleotide given in the place of the CAV-1 antisense (Fig. 2A,B). Basal leukocyte adhesion, measured as the percentage of venular area occupied by adherent leukocytes (see Refs. [7,8]), was attenuated (by ~ 50%) only in the presence of combined SIM plus CAV-

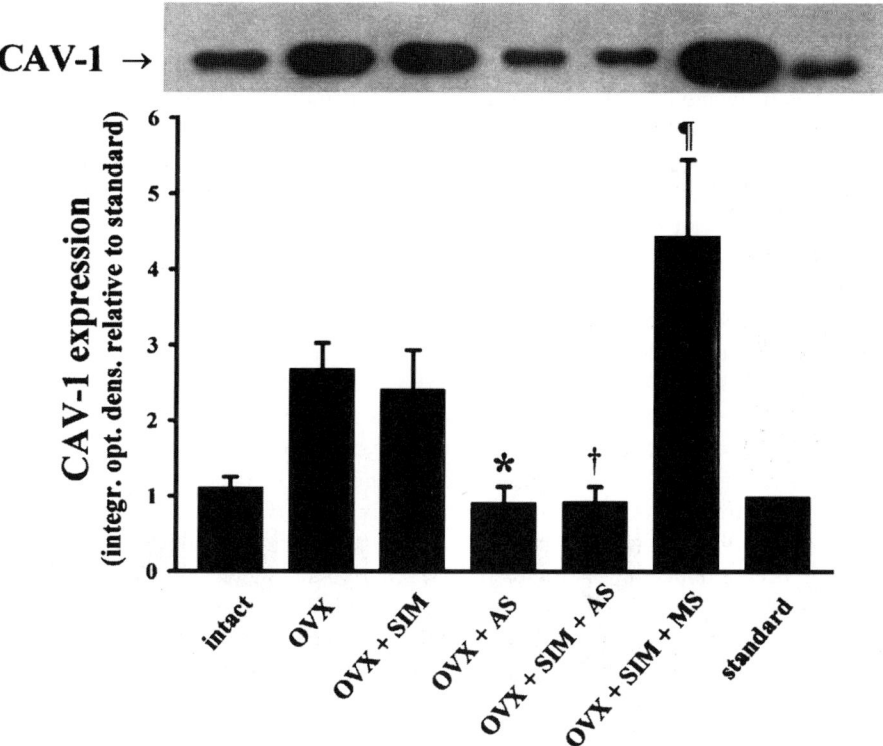

Fig. 4. The expression of CAV-1 protein in pial tissue harvested from the space under the cranial windows in intact females; untreated OVX females; and OVX females given chronic simvastatin treatment (OVX+SIM), 25 µg of CAV-1 antisense oligonucleotide (OVX+AS), chronic simvastatin plus 25 µg of CAV-1 antisense (OVX+SIM+AS); or chronic simvastatin plus 25 µg of CAV-1 missense (OVX+SIM+MS). For comparison, a HUVEC standard is also shown. Similar results were obtained in three separate sets of experiments, as summarized in the bar graph. The data represent the means±S.D. of three separate experiments. The band intensities (integrated optical densities) are expressed relative to a standard (HUVEC extract). *$p<0.05$ vs. OVX; †$p<0.05$ vs. OVX+SIM; ¶$p<0.05$ vs. OVX+SIM+AS.

1 AS treatment (Fig. 3). There were no differences among the remaining groups. The effectiveness of the CAV-1 antisense treatments was confirmed by the finding of a substantially lower CAV-1 expression in OVX rat pial tissue exposed to the CAV-1 antisense oligonucleotide compared to tissue from OVX rats given the missense or treated only with SIM (Fig. 4).

3. Discussion

Originally used in the clinical setting for their cholesterol-lowering capabilities, the 3-hydroxy-3-methyl-coenzyme A (HMG-CoA) reductase inhibitors (statins) have attracted additional interest due to actions seemingly unrelated to cholesterol lowering. A major cholesterol-independent effect of statins is to increase eNOS expression. The product of the HMG-CoA reductase reaction, mevalonate, is a precursor for the isoprenoid, geranylgeranyl pyrophosphate—a substance that can effect post-translational modifications of small GTP-binding proteins such as Rho [10]. Geranylgeranylation of Rho leads to the translocation and anchoring of Rho to the cell membrane. This process is prevented by statins, leading to stabilization of eNOS mRNA [10–12]. Statins can specifically increase eNOS (but not nNOS or iNOS) expression and function in the rodent brain and provide neuroprotection [6,13]. A further demonstration of the eNOS-specific actions of statins in the brain can be taken from the observation that the physiologic and neuroprotective effects of statins are not seen in eNOS knockout mice [6].

Caveolin-1 is a 22- to 24-kDa membrane-associated protein (which, in the brain, is concentrated in vascular endothelial cells) that is capable of binding other proteins, like eNOS, via interactions between a selected amino acid sequence on the CAV-1 molecule (the "scaffolding domain"—a.a. 82–101) and a specific binding motif on eNOS [14]. That particular interaction, which appears to be largely localized to plasma membrane structures called caveolae, results in loss of enzyme function. Upon Ca^{2+}-stimulated calmodulin binding, CAV-1 is displaced and enhanced NO generation ensues. There is remarkable little information in the literature regarding the effects of a primary increase or decrease in CAV-1 expression, by itself, on eNOS function in endothelial cells. Nevertheless, in a recent publication, Feron et al. [15] reported that increasing CAV-1 expression (over 24 h) diminished eNOS activity in cultured aortic endothelial cells.

Although evidence strongly supports a statin-induced increase in eNOS expression as a principal mechanism in the enhancement of eNOS activity accompanying statin treatment, the capacity for HMG-CoA reductase inhibitors to potentiate eNOS function may involve mechanisms separate from simply elevating the levels of eNOS protein. There is published evidence to suggest that statins, at least in the periphery, may enhance eNOS function through increasing Akt-mediated phosphorylation of eNOS [16]—an event known to stimulate eNOS activity independently from increases in Ca^{2+} [17]. Statins may also enhance the recruitment and binding of proteins linked to eNOS activation. One such eNOS-associated protein is heat shock protein 90 (hsp90) [18]. Results from a recent study also provided some evidence indicating that statins can increase eNOS activity, in isolated bovine aortic endothelial cells, via reductions in the levels of CAV-1 and its binding to eNOS [19]. However, the possibility that these potential eNOS-stimulatory effects of statins might have influenced the results of the present study seems rather unlikely, since simvastatin treatment by itself provided no improvement in indices of agonist-stimulated and basal eNOS function. Furthermore, the lack of any simvastatin effect on CAV-1 expression would seem to obviate any direct statin influence on CAV-1. This apparent incongruence between present and previous findings may simply be a reflection of vascular bed, species, and/or model (i.e., in vivo vs. in vitro)-related differences in statin actions and eNOS/CAV-1 interactions in endothelial cells.

The findings of this study have revealed a clinically relevant circumstance where statin-induced upregulation of eNOS is *not* accompanied by an increase in eNOS function—that is, ovariectomy ("surgical" menopause)-induced estrogen depletion. Thus, although chronic statin treatment was able to normalize the diminished expression of brain eNOS seen in ovariectomized rats [4,5,20], eNOS activity remained depressed. This included both agonist-stimulated and basal eNOS activity, as reflected in a maintained repression of ACh-mediated pial arteriolar vasodilation and heightened pial venular leukocyte adhesion, respectively. The likely explanation for these findings relates to the observation that statin treatment did not alter the ovariectomy-associated increased expression of the endogenous eNOS inhibitor, CAV-1 in pial microvessels. The importance of CAV-1 in the ovariec-tomy-induced repression of eNOS function was further underscored by the observation that statin administration increased eNOS activity only when accompanied by specific reductions in cerebrovascular CAV-1 abundance. Moreover, reducing CAV-1 expression in OVX rats, in the absence of eNOS upregulation (via statin treatment), was ineffectual in restoring eNOS function. This implies that a sufficient level of eNOS protein must be present for reductions in CAV-1 to effect an increase in eNOS activity. The significance of combined eNOS upregulation and CAV-1 downregulation, in the recovery of eNOS function, may be exemplified in ovariectomized females given chronic estrogen replace-ment therapy. This treatment raises eNOS expression in pial microvessels, while reducing CAV-1 expression, and restores eNOS function, as indicated by a normalization of ACh reactivity [4] and greatly reduced basal leukocyte adhesion [7].

3.3.2.7. On-Site Discussion

3.3.2.7.1. *Question: (Bryan)* Do you think that part of the effects seen is due changing the affinity of CAV-1 for eNOS?

Answer: (Pelligrino) That is a distinct possibility.

3.3.2.7.2. *Question: (Iadecola)* I was surprised that ovariectomy blocked the ACh response in female rats. Yet males rats have good reactivity to Ach. How do you explain this discrepancy?

Answer: (Pelligrino) Estrogen is a potent transcriptional regulator. That transcriptional activity is initiated by estrogen's interaction with its receptor. Males and females have very different estrogen/estrogen receptor levels. Males seem to have developed other mecha-nisms for regulating eNOS expression (or CAV-1) in the absence of appreciable estrogen transcriptional regulation. In females, on the other hand, eNOS/CAV-1 transcriptional regulation seems to be very dependent upon estrogen, to the extent that when estrogen is removed, there are no good alternative mechanisms to support eNOS.

Acknowledgements

The authors thank Susan Anderson, Dennis Riley, and Shu-Hua Ye for expert technical assistance. Supported by HL 56162 and HL 52594 from the NIH.

References

[1] P.D. Hurn, I.M. Macrae, Estrogen as a neuroprotectant in stroke, J. Cereb. Blood Flow Metab. 20 (2000) 631–652.

[2] M.E. Mendelsohn, R.H. Karas, The protective effects of estrogen on the cardiovascular system, N. Engl. J. Med. 340 (1999) 1801–1811.

[3] S. Sethi, M. Dikshit, Modulation of polymorphonuclear leukocytes function by nitric oxide, Thromb. Res. 100 (2000) 223–247.

[4] D.A. Pelligrino, S. Ye, F. Tan, R.A. Santizo, D.L. Feinstein, Q. Wang, Nitric-oxide-dependent pial arteriolar dilation in the female rat: effects of chronic estrogen depletion and repletion, Biochem. Biophys. Res. Commun. 269 (2000) 165–171.

[5] A.M. Mcneill, N. Kim, S.P. Duckles, D.N. Krause, Chronic estrogen treatment increases levels of endothelial nitric oxide synthase protein in rat cerebral microvessels, Stroke 30 (1999) 2186–2190.

[6] M. Endres, U. Laufs, Z.H. Huang, T. Nakamura, P. Huang, M.A. Moskowitz, J.K. Liao, Stroke protection by 3-hydroxy-3-methylglutaryl (HMG)-CoA reductase inhibitors mediated by endothelial nitric oxide synthase, Proc. Natl. Acad. Sci. U. S. A. 95 (1998) 8880–8885.

[7] R. Santizo, D.A. Pelligrino, Estrogen reduces leukocyte adhesion in the cerebral circulation of female rats, J. Cereb. Blood Flow Metab. 19 (1999) 1061–1065.

[8] R.A. Santizo, H.M. Koenig, D.A. Pelligrino, Estrogen and leukocyte adhesion following transient forebrain ischemia in rats, Stroke 31 (2000) 2231–2235.

[9] A.G. Hudetz, J.D. Wood, J.P. Kampine, Nitric oxide synthase inhibitor augments post-ischemic leukocyte adhesion in the cerebral microcirculation in vivo, Neurol. Res. 21 (1999) 378–384.

[10] U. Laufs, J.K. Liao, Post-transcriptional regulation of endothelial nitric oxide synthase mRNA stability by Rho GTPase, J. Biol. Chem. 273 (1998) 24266–24271.

[11] U. Laufs, V.L. Fata, J.K. Liao, Inhibition of 3-hydroxy-3-methylglutaryl (HMG)-CoA reductase blocks hypoxia-mediated down-regulation of endothelial nitric oxide synthase, J. Biol. Chem. 272 (1997) 31725–31729.

[12] U. Laufs, V. LaFata, J. Plutzky, J.K. Liao, Upregulation of endothelial nitric oxide synthase by HMG CoA reductase inhibitors, Circulation 97 (1998) 1129–1135.

[13] M. Yamada, Z. Huang, T. Dalkara, M. Endres, U. Laufs, C. Waeber, P.L. Huang, J.K. Liao, M.A. Moskowitz, Endothelial nitric oxide synthase-dependent cerebral blood flow augmentation by L-arginine after chronic statin treatment, J. Cereb. Blood Flow Metab. 20 (2000) 709–717.

[14] E.J. Smart, G.A. Graf, M.A. McNiven, W.C. Sessa, J.A. Engelman, P.E. Scherer, T. Okamoto, M.P. Lisanti, Caveolins, liquid-ordered domains, and signal transduction, Mol. Cell Biol. 19 (1999) 7289–7304.

[15] O. Feron, C. Dessy, S. Moniotte, J.P. Desager, J.L. Balligand, Hypercholesterolemia decreases nitric oxide production by promoting the interaction of caveolin and endothelial nitric oxide synthase, J. Clin. Invest. 103 (1999) 897–905.

[16] Y. Kureishi, Z. Luo, I. Shiojima, A. Bialik, D. Fulton, D.J. Lefer, W.C. Sessa, K. Walsh, The HMG-CoA reductase inhibitor simvastatin activates the protein kinase Akt and promotes angiogenesis in normocholesterolemic animals, Nat. Med. 6 (2000) 1004–1010.

[17] D. Fulton, J.P. Gratton, T.J. McCabe, J. Fontana, Y. Fujio, K. Walsh, T.F. Franke, A. Papapetropoulos, W.C. Sessa, Regulation of endothelium-derived nitric oxide production by the protein kinase Akt, Nature 399 (1999) 597–601.

[18] G. Garcia-Cardena, R. Fan, V. Shah, R. Sorrentino, G. Cirino, A. Papapetropoulos, W.C. Sessa, Dynamic activation of endothelial nitric oxide synthase by Hsp90, Nature 392 (1998) 821–824.

[19] O. Feron, C. Dessy, J.P. Desager, J.L. Balligand, Hydroxy-methylglutaryl-coenzyme A reductase inhibition

promotes endothelial nitric oxide synthase activation through a decrease in caveolin abundance, Circulation 103 (2001) 113–118.

[20] H.L. Xu, R.A. Santizo, D.A. Pelligrino, Simvastatin-induced upregulation of brain enos expression and function exhibits regional selectivity in ovariectomized (OVX) rats, Soc. Neurosci. Abst. 26 (2000) 1034.

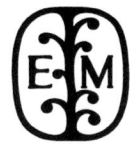

International Congress Series 1235 (2002) 413–418

Effects of estrogen on the microcirculation and thrombus formation in pial vessels of the rat

Yasuto Sasaki [a,*], Hiroaki Ono [a], Junji Seki [b],
John C. Giddings [c], Junichiro Yamamoto [a]

[a]Laboratory of Physiology, Faculty of Nutrition, Kobe Gakuin University, 518 Arise Ikawadani-Cho,
Nishi-Ku, Kobe, 651-2180, Japan
[b]Department of Biomedical Engineering, National Cardiovascular Center Research Institute, Suita,
565-8565, Japan
[c]Department of Haematology, University of Wales College of Medicine, CF4 4XN, Cardiff, UK

Abstract

Female Wistar/ST rats were ovariectomized at 14 weeks of age. Ethynylestradiol, 17β-estradiol ($E_2\beta$), medroxyprogesterone acetate (MPA) and 4-hydroxy-tamoxifen were administered subcutaneously every other day for 3 weeks from 1 week after ovariectomy. Closed cranial windows were created and the thrombotic potential was measured using the He–Ne laser-induced thrombosis method. The mean red cell velocity was measured with a fiber-optic laser-Doppler anemometer microscope. The plasma concentrations of nitrite/nitrate (nitric oxide (NO) metabolites) were determined using the Griess reagent. The diameters mean red cell velocity and blood flow in pial arterioles were reduced after ovariectomy, however, the thrombotic tendency was increased after ovariectomy. These parameters were reversed after $E_2\beta$ treatment. In contrast, MPA had the opposite effects. The plasma concentrations of nitrite/nitrate were significantly decreased following ovariectomy and were increased after treatment with $E_2\beta$. MPA did not affect the concentration of NO metabolites. These results strongly indicated that estrogen in the female rat mediated beneficial effects on the cerebral microcirculation and moderated cerebral thrombotic mechanisms by enhancing the plasma levels of NO. The findings suggest that increased blood flow and inhibition of thrombosis might contribute to the prevention of cerebrovascular disease in a normal female. © 2002 Elsevier Science B.V. All rights reserved.

Keywords: Estrogen; Progesterone; NO; Thrombosis; Microcirculation

* Corresponding author. Tel.: +81-78-974-1551; fax: +81-78-974-5689.
E-mail address: sasakiya@nutr.kobegakuin.ac.jp (Y. Sasaki).

0531-5131/02 © 2002 Elsevier Science B.V. All rights reserved.
PII: S 0 5 3 1 - 5 1 3 1 (0 2) 0 0 2 0 3 - 0

1. Introduction

Estrogen is believed to contribute to the reduced incidence of cardiovascular disease and the lower risk of cerebrovascular disease seen in females compared with males [1]. Estrogen is widely acknowledged to be beneficial to arterial wall function. Estrogen increases the production of prostacyclin and nitric oxide (NO) by enhancing endothelial NO synthase (eNOS) activity. Prostacyclin and NO are known to be potent vasodilators and strong inhibitors of platelet aggregation [2]. Infusion of L-arginine and nitroprusside reduced ischemic brain damage after middle cerebral artery ligation, probably by increasing the cerebral blood flow, and 17β-estradiol assisted recovery of the postischemic cerebral blood flow after an experimental stroke in the rat [3]. Moreover, NO donors inhibited thrombus formation induced by He–Ne laser irradiation in pial vessels, and treatments that increased NO synthesis, such as ingestion of L-arginine and exercise, reduced the incidence of stroke and cerebral thrombosis in stroke-prone spontaneously hypertensive rats (SHRSP) [4]. In addition, estrogen has been reported to moderate the development of atherosclerosis by changing lipoprotein profiles in plasma [5]. The precise role of estrogen in the cerebrovascular circulation and the mechanisms by which estrogen mediates the beneficial effects remain to be fully clarified. It seems likely, therefore, that the NO produced in response to estrogen alters the intravascular physical properties and moderates the thrombotic mechanisms in the cerebral blood vessels. Several steroid hormones, such as ethynylestradiol, medroxyprogesterone acetate (Depo-provera) and others, alone or in combination, are used widely in hormone replacement therapy (HRT) in post-menopausal women. It is generally believed that progesterone antagonizes the beneficial effects of estrogen. The purpose of the present study was to clarify the mechanisms of action of these hormones on the microcirculation and thrombosis in cerebral vessels.

2. Materials and methods

2.1. Ovariectomy and hormones

Ovaries were surgically removed from female Wistar/ST rats at 14 weeks of age. 17α-Ethynylestradiol (EE; 1.0 mg/kg), 17β-estradiol 3-benzoate (E$_2$β; 1.0 mg/kg), medroxyprogesterone acetate (MPA; 1.0 mg/kg) and 4-hydroxy-tamoxifen (TAM; 5.0 mg/kg) were dissolved in ethanol, diluted in sesame oil and administered subcutaneously every other day in the back of the animal for 3 weeks from 1 week after ovariectomy. The blood pressure was measured by the tail-cuff method. Body weights, blood pressures and blood flow parameters were measured once a week.

2.2. Measurement of thrombotic potential assessed by the He–Ne laser-induced thrombus formation method

Animals were anesthetized with sodium pentobarbital and were artificially ventilated. Blood samples were obtained from one of the femoral arteries for the measurement of blood gases and pH. The other femoral artery was used for the measurement of the mean arterial blood pressure. Rates of respiration and the stroke volume of the respirator were adjusted to maintain constant levels of arterial blood gases and pH. The animals were immobilized in a stereotaxic frame, and a craniotomy was performed using a hand drill to form a cranial window with 5 mm in diameter in the center of right parietal bone [6]. Artificial cerebrospinal fluid was continuously infused within the cranial window, and the intracranial pressure was adjusted to 3–5 mm Hg to avoid brain herniation. The animal was placed on the stage of a microscope and the cerebral vessels were monitored with a CCD camera. Images were recorded continuously on videotape. A He–Ne laser beam was focused on the center of the selected arterioles, and thrombi were formed by repeated irradiation. The number of laser pulses needed to form an occlusive thrombus was used as an index of thrombotic potential [4,7].

2.3. Measurements of mean red cell velocity and calculation of blood flow

The mean red cell velocity in the cerebral arterioles was measured with a fiber-optic laser-Doppler anemometer microscope (FLDAM) [8]. Wall shear rates were calculated according to the equation, $8 \times$ mean red cell velocity/inner diameter of the blood vessel. The mean blood flow of each arteriole was calculated from the mean red cell velocity and the diameter.

2.4. Measurements of arteriolar vessel diameter

The diameter of the branch of the middle cerebral artery was measured from video images, captured on a personal computer. The arterioles were delineated from the branch of the middle cerebral artery, which was outlined as a large Y shape in the same position at the right side of the cranial window. The diameters of the arterioles were measured initially in pixels and then converted to micrometers.

2.5. Measurement of regional cerebral blood flow (rCBF)

The regional cerebral blood flow was measured using a laser-Doppler flow meter (ALF-21; Advance Tokyo) with a needle type probe (0.55 mm diameter). The probe was positioned over the surface of the parietal cortex and cortical blood flow in the parietal lobe was measured continuously. The signals of ALF-21 were analyzed by a personal computer.

2.6. Measurement of plasma concentrations of nitrite/nitrate

Blood samples were collected from the femoral artery and centrifuged at $1500 \times g$ for 15 min. The plasma was stored at -70 °C until assayed. The concentrations of nitrite/nitrate and the metabolites of NO were determined using the Griess reagent (Assay kit-C; Dojindo Laboratory, Kumamoto, Japan).

2.7. Measurement of serum concentrations of estradiol (E2) and progesterone

The plasma samples were prepared and stored at -70 °C as described above. The serum concentrations of E_2 and progesterone were determined by radioimmunoassay.

3. Results

3.1. Effects of hormones on various parameters

The body weights and systolic blood pressures of the control rats (sesame oil) were 292 ± 4 g and 128 ± 3 mm Hg, respectively. Treatment with MPA did not change the body weights and blood pressures but EE and $E_2\beta$ decreased these parameters (Table 1). On the other hand, the body weights were increased up to 2 weeks after treatment with TAM but were depressed after this time.

3.2. Changes in uterine wet weight after treatment with hormones

The mean uterine wet weight in the control animals given sesame oil was 222 ± 10 mg. MPA and TAM did not affect this (Table 1). Treatment with EE and $E_2\beta$ increased the uterine wet weight significantly.

3.3. Changes in serum concentrations of estradiol, progesterone and NO metabolites

Serum concentrations of estradiol (E_2) were increased significantly after $E_2\beta$ treatment. Treatment with other hormones, however, did not affect the serum concentrations of E_2. The serum concentrations of progesterone were increased after treatment with MPA. Furthermore, metabolites of NO were increased significantly after treatment with EE, $E_2\beta$ and TAM.

Table 1
Changes in parameters after administration of various hormones

Measurements	Sesame oil	EE (1.0 mg/kg)	$E_2\beta$ (1.0 mg/kg)	Progesterone (1.0 mg/kg)	TAM (5.0 mg/kg)
Body weight (g)	292 ± 4 (6)	247 ± 3 (6)*	242 ± 5 (6)*	300 ± 10 (6)	252 ± 3 (6)*
Systolic pressure (mm Hg)	128 ± 3 (6)	108 ± 3 (6)*	103 ± 3 (6)*	132 ± 2 (6)	114 ± 2 (6)
Uterine wet weight (mg)	222 ± 10 (5)	2198 ± 33 (5)**	875 ± 24 (6)**	210 ± 31 (5)	316 ± 43 (5)
Serum estradiol (pg/ml)	10.0 ± 0.9 (4)	8.2 ± 2.0 (4)	946.6 ± 29.5 (4)**	8.8 ± 0.3 (4)	11 ± 2.5 (4)
Serum progesterone (ng/ml)	17.7 ± 2.5 (4)	18.0 ± 3.0 (4)	13.2 ± 5.0 (4)	27.3 ± 2.7 (4)*	13.2 ± 4.4 (4)
Nitrite/nitrate (μmol/l)	14.2 ± 0.5 (6)	27.4 ± 2.6 (6)*	34.8 ± 2.6 (6)**	14.9 ± 1.0 (6)	23.3 ± 3.1 (6)*
Number of laser pulses	7.7 ± 0.4 (6)	10.1 ± 0.7 (6)**	10.8 ± 0.5 (6)**	5.4 ± 0.2 (4)**	9.7 ± 0.3 (5)**

Mean$\pm$S.E.M. (N).
* $p<0.05$ vs. sesame oil.
** $p<0.01$ vs. sesame oil.

3.4. Effects of hormones on thrombotic potential in pial arterioles

The thrombotic potential was assessed by the He–Ne laser method. The number of laser pulses needed to occlude pial arterioles was used as an index of thrombotic potential. The number of laser pulses needed to occlude the vessel was increased in rats treated with EE, $E_2\beta$, TAM, but was decreased by the MPA treatment. These findings indicated that treatment with EE, $E_2\beta$ and TAM decreased the thrombotic potential. MPA treatment enhanced the thrombotic mechanisms significantly (Table 1).

3.5. Effects of hormones on cerebral microcirculation

The mean red cell velocities measured by FLDAM increased significantly after treatment with EE, $E_2\beta$ and TAM but decreased after MPA. Similarly, arteriole diameters were significantly increased after treatment with EE and $E_2\beta$, but were significantly decreased after MPA. Wall shear rates and blood flow were calculated from red cell velocity. The arteriole diameters were measured from video images. The blood flow was increased significantly after treatment with EE (6.3 ± 0.9 ($N=6$) nl/s; $p<0.05$) and $E_2\beta$ (12.7 ± 1.0 ($N=6$) nl/s; $p<0.01$), compared with sesame oil (4.2 ± 0.3 ($N=6$) nl/s), however, MPA significantly decreased the blood flow (2.9 ± 0.3 ($N=6$) nl/s; $p<0.05$). Laser Doppler measurement (ALF-21), after treatment with hormones, indicated that the cortical blood flow increased significantly after EE, $E_2\beta$ and TAM, but reduced significantly after MPA ($p<0.05$).

4. Discussion

In the current study, the effects of hormones on the cerebral microcirculation and thrombotic potential were studied. The thrombotic potential decreased after treatment with EE, $E_2\beta$ and TAM, but was enhanced by MPA. The plasma concentration of the NO metabolites was significantly increased in rats treated with EE, $E_2\beta$ and TAM, but was unchanged in animals given MPA. Rosselli et al. [9] found that the administration of estrogen alone to post-menopausal women increased the concentration of NO metabolites, whereas the combined progestin/17β-estradiol preparation was not found to increase nitrite/nitrate levels. In the present study, the diameters of pial vessels, red cell velocities and blood flow were increased significantly in rats treated with EE, $E_2\beta$ and TAM. These effects of the hormones might be due to increased plasma NO levels. We found that the treatment, which increased plasma NO levels in the present study, was similar to those seen previously in spontaneously hypertensive rats (SHRSP/Izm) [4]. In contrast, the opposite effect of MPA might be due to decreased levels of plasma NO. The thrombotic potential, assessed by the He–Ne laser method, was decreased by treatment with EE, $E_2\beta$ and TAM, but was increased by MPA. We have previously demonstrated that NO donors increased plasma NO levels and decreased the thrombotic potential in normal rats and SHRSP [4,7]. The increased plasma levels of NO, therefore, seem to contribute at least in part to the beneficial effects of hormones. Moreover, progesterone has been reported to antagonize estrogen binding to the estrogen receptor in nuclei [10]. In HRT, combined estrogen and progesterone preparations are used widely to reduce the risk of carcinoma of the endometrium and breast. It appears that the beneficial effects of estrogen might be moderated by progesterone.

Further studies are required to assess the use of these hormones in the prevention of cerebral vascular diseases.

References

[1] E. Barrett-Connor, T.L. Bush, Estrogen and coronary heart disease in women [see comments], JAMA, J. Am. Med. Assoc. 265 (1991) 1861–1867.

[2] S. Moncada, The 1991 Ulf von Euler Lecture. The L-arginine: nitric oxide pathway, Acta Physiol. Scand. 145 (1992) 201–227.

[3] N.J. Alkayed, I. Harukuni, A.S. Kimes, E.D. London, R.J. Traystman, P.D. Hurn, Gender-linked brain injury in experimental stroke, Stroke 29 (1998) 159–165, discussion 166.

[4] T. Noguchi, Y. Sasaki, J. Seki, J.C. Giddings, J. Yamamoto, Effects of voluntary exercise and L-arginine on thrombogenesis and microcirculation in stroke-prone spontaneously hypertensive rats, Clin. Exp. Pharmacol. Physiol. 26 (1999) 330–335.

[5] X. Zhu, B. Bonet, H. Gillenwater, R.H. Knopp, Opposing effects of estrogen and progestins on LDL oxidation and vascular wall cytotoxicity: implications for atherogenesis, Proc. Soc. Exp. Biol. Med. 222 (1999) 214–221.

[6] S. Morii, A.C. Ngai, H.R. Winn, Reactivity of rat pial arterioles and venules to adenosine and carbon dioxide: with detailed description of the closed cranial window technique in rats, J. Cereb. Blood Flow Metab. 6 (1986) 34–41.

[7] Y. Sasaki, J. Seki, J.C. Giddings, J. Yamamoto, Effects of NO-donors on thrombus formation and microcirculation in cerebral vessels of the rat, Thromb. Haemostasis 76 (1996) 111–117.

[8] J. Seki, Y. Sasaki, T. Oyama, J. Yamamoto, Fiber-optic laser-Doppler anemometer microscope applied to the cerebral microcirculation in rats, Biorheology 33 (1996) 463–470.

[9] M. Rosselli, B. Imthurn, P.J. Keller, E.K. Jackson, R.K. Dubey, Circulating nitric oxide (nitrite/nitrate) levels in postmenopausal women substituted with 17 beta-estradiol and norethisterone acetate. A two-year follow-up study, Hypertension 25 (4 Pt 2) (1995) 848–853.

[10] P. Colburn, V. Buonassisi, Estrogen-binding sites in endothelial cell cultures, Science 201 (1978) 817–819.

Microcirculation

Spreading depression and microcirculation

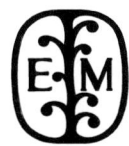

International Congress Series 1235 (2002) 421–437

Imaging and preventing spreading depression independent of cerebral blood flow

R. David Andrew*, T.R. Anderson, A.J. Biedermann, C.R. Jarvis

Department of Anatomy and Cell Biology, Queen's University, Kingston, Ontario, Canada K7L-3N6

Abstract

A moving cortical inactivation termed spreading depression (SD) is considered the physiological event responsible for migraine aura. SD is a mass depolarization of neurons and glia lasting a minute or more. It arises focally and migrates as a wave across gray matter at 2–5 mm/min. SD is generated by a sudden increase in cell membrane permeability to small ions in neurons and glia. This neurogenic origin does not preclude SD being initiated by local vascular change. However, the brain slice preparation does permit the study of SD independent of changes to blood flow or the microvasculature. When arising under near-normoxic conditions, the SD of aura dissipates within 30 min and causes no neuronal damage. In contrast, during the first 3–4 h following stroke, the combined metabolic stress of recurring SD and energy deprivation exacerbates ischemic injury to neurons in the penumbra. *Purpose*: To image and pharmacologically block SD under normoxic and stroke-like conditions in slices of rodent cerebral hemisphere where blood flow is not a modulating factor. *Methods*: Coronal brain slices are submerged in flowing artificial cerebrospinal fluid (aCSF). Normoxic SD is induced by briefly raising $[K^+]_o$. An ischemic version of SD, the anoxic depolarization (AD), is induced by removing O_2/glucose from the aCSF for 10 min. Intrinsic optical signals (IOSs) represent change in the way tissue scatters light. Light transmittance (LT), essentially unscattered light, is imaged using a charge-coupled device (CCD) to measure second-by-second regional ΔLT during periods of 1 h or more. The front of the propagating SD or AD event is imaged as an elevated LT, caused by cell swelling. A negative voltage shift, the electrophysiological signature of SD, is simultaneously recorded extracellularly. In the wake of the AD, the LT increase is overridden by a reduction in LT. This is caused by dendritic beading which efficiently scatters light, thereby revealing neuronal damage not seen following classic SD. *Results*: Normoxic SD evoked by elevated bath K^+ arises multifocally in neocortical layer II/III and migrates as a wave at 2–5 mm/min. It can be elicited repeatedly with no dendritic beading or loss of evoked electrical activity. The AD also initiates multifocally in neocortical gray (and 1–3 min later, in striatum or hippocampus); in its wake, dendritic beading develops and evoked electrical activity is permanently lost. Potentially useful therapeutics can be assessed in terms of whether they block the SD or reduce damage

* Corresponding author. Tel.: +1-613-533-2860; fax: +1-613-533-2566.
E-mail address: andrewd@post.queensu.ca (R.D. Andrew).

0531-5131/02 © 2002 Elsevier Science B.V. All rights reserved.
PII: S 0 5 3 1 - 5 1 3 1 (0 2) 0 0 2 0 5 - 4

following AD. Glutamate receptor antagonists do not block the AD or resultant damage. However, sigma$_1$ receptor (σ_1R) ligands such as $10-100$ μM dextromethorphan, carbetapentane, or 4-IBP block the AD and resultant damage. Normoxic SD is also blocked. σ_1R antagonists oppose AD or SD blockade by these ligands. *Conclusions*: Recurring SD is innocuous in normoxic slices. However, the metabolic stress of O$_2$/glucose deprivation (OGD) for 10 min and a single ischemic SD event (the AD) induces acute neuronal damage in slices. We propose that damage in the ischemic core is difficult to prevent because the AD arises upon stroke onset and normally resists pharmacological blockade. By dissociating the mass depolarization of AD from the ischemia, σ_1R ligands offer a possible way to reduce early stroke damage. © 2002 Elsevier Science B.V. All rights reserved.

Keywords: NMDA; Intrinsic optical signals; Neocortex; Hippocampus; Imaging; Glutamate; Cell volume; Anoxic depolarization; Ischemia; Spreading depression; Sigma receptors

1. Introduction

Classic spreading depression (SD) is a migrating inactivation of gray matter first described by Leao [22] that can be focally induced by mechanical, electrical, or chemical stimulation under normal metabolic conditions. The propagating wave of depolarization and associated electrical silence traverses the cerebral cortex at $2-5$ mm/min. SD is responsible for migraine aura, commonly a marching visual or somatosensory deficit that may precede migraine pain [25]. Although SD involves the mass depolarization of neurons and glia for a minute or longer, no neuronal damage results [30].

Leao [23] also observed that a propagating depolarization similar to normoxic SD arises in the cerebral cortex following $2-5$ min of global ischemia, the depolarization lasting as long as the ischemic period. Electrophysiologists commonly use the term 'anoxic' or 'hypoxic' depolarization although this downplays what Leao originally described as a spreading event. In the hippocampal slice preparation, which is globally deprived of O$_2$ and glucose for $5-10$ min, we imaged a SD-like wave of depolarization, which could arise multifocally. We previously termed it 'ischemic' SD [34] and it is now apparent that it represents the anoxic depolarization (AD).

One approach to the future management of stroke or trauma is the use of neuro-protectants to limit damage to the brain tissue and improve outcome. More effective therapeutic interventions require an understanding of how neurons and glia respond to the first crucial minutes of ischemia or trauma. The initial pathophysiological processes include energy failure, loss of ion homeostasis, mass depolarization, and water influx. Because the prime suspect in the initiation of ischemic damage has been excess glutamate release, much research has focused on glutamate receptor antagonists as neuroprotectants. The therapeutic results have been disappointing and the central role of glutamate in causing acute ischemic damage is increasingly questioned [17,35–37].

In this paper, we review the advantages of the cortical slice preparation for imaging population-wide events such as SD and AD without confounding regional differences in blood flow. The slice preparation also affords the ability to delineate acute neuronal damage and to quickly apply and wash on and off potentially neuroprotective drugs.

1.1. The brain slice and blood flow

Since McIlwan et al. [28] first used the brain slice for neurochemical studies, it has become a versatile neurophysiological preparation. Unlike in vivo, the brain tissue is free of movement associated with heartbeat and respiration. The slice also retains the local synaptic circuitry and endogenous electrical properties of neurons and glia, unlike culture models. The hippocampus and neocortex exhibit a laminar structure easily discerned at low magnification. The ability to recognize anatomical landmarks allows accurate place-ment of electrodes to stimulate and record from specific areas. The brain slice also allows fine manipulation of temperature, oxygen level, ion concentrations, pH, and hormonal levels. The lack of a blood–brain barrier provides a direct route for drug administration. The tissue is isolated from endocrine feedback loops and changes in vascular flow. General anesthetics can be avoided.

In terms of imaging, changes in regional CBF or $CMRO_2$ generate narrow-band signals originating from altered hemoglobin or cytochrome levels, which are detected as small but specific intrinsic optical signals (IOSs). Obviously, these are not generated in slices of brain tissue. However, substantial IOSs are generated across the visible and near infrared spectrum as a result of changes to cellular conformation, in particular to cell swelling. In submerged slices, cell swelling evokes increases in light transmittance (LT) and con-versely, osmotic shrinkage decreases LT [3]. Such signals are large, wide band and complex in their cellular origin (Fig. 1). However, imaging transmitted light avoids the optical complexity inherent in measuring reflected light (see below) and slice submersion eliminates the air–tissue boundary that can further complicate the light path.

The brain slice preparation also has some disadvantages. These include the inability to directly measure vascular changes involved with neuronal activation, the lost influence of neuromodulators or hormones and the significantly less afferent synaptic input to neurons. Also, during the dissection and slicing procedure, the tissue may undergo a period of brief hypoxia. This can be counteracted by cooling the head in ice within seconds of decapitation. Finally, the brain slice is healthiest for only a span of several hours.

1.2. Imaging intrinsic optical signals (IOSs)

IOSs are generated in living biological tissue by changes in light scattering (through refraction and reflection) or by changes in light absorption. IOSs are detected by collecting light that is either reflected from brain tissue or transmitted through a brain slice. The collected light is detected using a photodiode array or a charged-coupled device (CCD) for imaging IOSs or using a spectrometer for analysing spectral content. Changes to the light path are 'intrinsic' in that they result from the endogenous biological properties of the tissue. IOSs have been used to investigate cortical activity [8,13,42] where several distinct signal components are associated with altered blood flow, hemoglobin oxidation, cyto-chrome reduction, or cell swelling. In submerged brain slices, cell swelling is a predominant IOS source and is associated with elevated light transmittance (LT) [3,6,21,26], whereas cell shrinkage induced by hyperosmotic agents reduces LT. For tissue slices a few hundred microns thick, LT varies inversely with both the light scattering coefficient and the absorption coefficient. Light reflectance (LR) from the brain slice can also be collected

Cell swelling increases light transmittance

particle
size

H_2O

membrane
configuration

H_2O

refractive
index

H_2O

increasing
volume/surface area

H_2O

Beading of dendrites <u>de</u>creases light transmittance

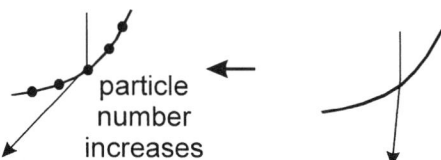

particle
number
increases

but does not probe the entire thickness of the slice. Moreover, minor changes in light scattering properties can cause variations in reflectance at small angles from the normal tissue surface. These variations in reflectance are a function of the incidence angle such that LR can have preferred reflectance angles. Thus, LR becomes strongly dependent on the alignment of the optical detection system. For all of these reasons, LT then is more easily imaged and analysed than LR.

Increased light transmittance is generated by change to subcellular structure that reduces light scattering during cell swelling (Fig. 1). However, in responsive dendritic regions, the initial LT elevation caused by cell swelling is overridden by the formation of dendritic beads, a conformation that increases light scattering (thereby reducing LT) [35,39] even as the tissue continues to swell [17]. Thus, IOS imaging reveals acute somatic and dendritic damage during metabolic stress that can be monitored across slices of brain tissue in real time.

IOS imaging in the hippocampal slice preparation has revealed dynamic changes in light transmittance in both dendritic and cell body regions following exposure to agonists of the excitatory neurotransmitter glutamate [4,38,39] or during oxygen/glucose deprivation [34]. Dramatic changes also occur in neocortical slices following OGD in rat [18] and in mouse [19]. These signals, which are independent of blood flow, are the subject of this study.

2. Methods and materials

2.1. Neocortical slice preparation

Male Sprague–Dawley rats, 21–28 days old, were housed in a controlled environment (25 °C, 12-h light/dark cycle) with food and water available ad libitum. A rat was placed in a rodent restrainer, guillotined, and the brain quickly excised under cold artificial cerebrospinal fluid (aCSF). Coronal slices (350–400 μm) were cut using a vibrating microtome (Leica VT100S) and incubated at 22 °C in oxygenated (95% O_2/5% CO_2) aCSF for at least 1 h before transferring to the imaging chamber. The aCSF contained (in mM): NaCl 120, KCl 3.3, $NaHCO_3$ 26, $MgSO_4$ 1.3, $NaH_2 PO_4$ 1.2, D-glucose 11, and $CaCl_2$ 1.8 (pH 7.3–7.4). Slices were weighted at the edges with silver wire and superfused with oxygenated aCSF at 35–37 °C. The superfusion rate was 1 ml/min but we have found that a higher rate of 3–4 ml/min promotes better recovery from OGD and complete recovery following normoxic spreading depression induced with KCl.

Fig. 1. At least four factors act to increase light transmittance through tissue undergoing cell swelling [17]. First, particles such as mitochondria tend to scatter less light when they swell. Second, cell membranes can be considered a large object with superimposed smaller particles. With swelling, membrane takes a more planar configuration as it unfolds, thereby scattering less light. Third, as water is taken up intracellularly, the refractive index of the cytosol becomes more like the extracellular fluid. This should reduce refraction at all membrane boundaries where the fluids interface. Fourth, as cell bodies (or dendrites) expand, there is less internal scattering of light because the cell volume increases disproportionately to the membrane surface area. On the other hand, dendritic beading opposes the above effects by increasing particle number which promotes light scatter, thereby reducing transmittance.

2.2. Imaging intrinsic optical signals (IOSs)

The imaging hardware is shown in Fig. 2. Video frames were obtained at 30 Hz using a COHU 4910 charge-coupled device (CCD) which was set at high gain and medium black level. With gamma set to 1.0, CCD output was linear with respect to the change in light intensity. CCD sensitivity spanned 690–1000 nm, comprising the far red to near infrared. Frames were averaged and digitized using a frame grabber board (DT3155, Data Translation) in a Pentium computer controlled by Axon Imaging Workbench (AIW) software (Axon Instruments).

Either 128 or 256 frames were acquired at 30 Hz and averaged to a single image. The first averaged image in a series (T_{cont}) was subtracted from each subsequent experimental image (T_{exp}) so the difference image revealed areas in the slice where LT changed over time. To quantify and graphically display data, zones of interest were boxed using the AIW software. The change in LT was expressed as the intensity of the difference image ($T_{exp} - T_{cont}$) divided by the gain set by the AIW software program. This value was expressed as a percentage change of the intensity in the zone of interest by division of the control value of the zone. That is,

$$LT = \frac{(T_{exp} - T_{cont})/\text{gain}}{T_{cont}} \times 100 = \frac{\Delta T}{T}\%.$$

Note that T_{cont} in the denominator served to normalize plotted data across regions differing in transmittance. The control image was displayed using a gray intensity scale and each subtracted image was displayed using a pseudocolor intensity scale. A graphics program (CorelDRAW) was used to arrange and label images. Data were plotted using either Microsoft Excel or SigmaPlot for Windows (Jandel Scientific).

2.3. Electrophysiology

To measure the evoked field potential or the spontaneous negative shift, a micropipette (5–10 MΩ) was pulled from a thin-walled capillary glass, filled with 2 M NaCl and mounted on a 3-D micromanipulator. It was connected by a silver wire coated with AgCl to an amplifier probe whose output was monitored using an online oscilloscope. This extracellular recording electrode was placed in layers II/III of the neocortex and a concentric bipolar electrode (Rhodes Electronics) was placed in layer VI to stimulate the immediately overlying layers. In hippocampal slices, the Schaffer collaterals were stimulated by recording a population spike from the CA1 pyramidal layer. A current pulse (0.1 ms duration; 0.25 Hz) was applied to produce a population spike of near-maximal

Fig. 2. The light paths and hardware for imaging intrinsic optical signals (IOSs). An inverted microscope is used to view a brain slice, which is maintained in a chamber with a cover slip as a base. A voltage-regulated halogen lamp emits broad band light which passes through a NIR pass filter (> 650 nm). The filter is optional because the visible spectrum displays similar scattering properties to NIR light (Fig. 1). The light transmitted through the slice is detected by a CCD and processed using a frame grabber (DT 3155, Data Translation Systems) controlled by Axon Imaging Workbench software.

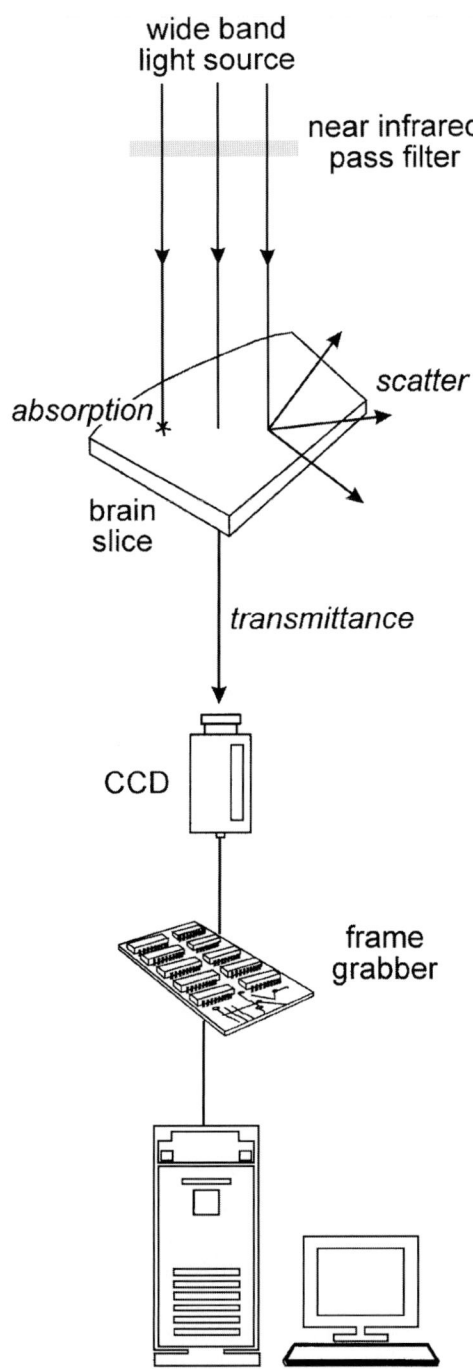

wide band
light source

near infrared
pass filter

scatter

absorption

brain
slice

transmittance

CCD

frame
grabber

amplitude. The amplified signals were digitized (Neuro Data Instruments) and stored on videocassette. Digitized data were signal averaged (six sweeps/trace), displayed, and plotted using pCLAMP software (Axon Instruments).

3. Results/discussion

3.1. Spreading depression under normoxic conditions

Spreading depression in normoxic tissue represents a profound increase in membrane permeability. Potassium and hydrogen ions immediately leave the neurons while Na^+, Ca^{2+}, and Cl^- enter along with water, thereby decreasing the extracellular space [14,33]. Ion concentrations return to near normal within a minute or so where there is no decreased energy supply or neuronal damage [25]. SD can be induced in submerged brain slices by focal [11] or global application of high K^+ aCSF (Fig. 3A). It is crucial to observe a return of the elevated LT signal back to baseline and that several SD events can be evoked to demonstrate that the slice remains healthy despite multiple SD events. It would also be expected that NMDAR antagonists would block SD as in vivo [15,20,24,27,32]. These studies showed that SD in 'normoxic' tissue (induced by focal K^+ or by mechanical or tetanic stimulation) is blocked by NMDAR antagonists (but not by non-NMDAR antagonists). The effects of a series of glutamate receptor antagonists (kynurenate, AP-5, CNQX, and MK-801) were tested upon normoxic SD to confirm NMDAR antagonism of SD in neocortical slices [1]. All except CNQX were effective in blocking SD during normal metabolic conditions. Therefore, with respect to SD repeatability, survivability, and NMDAR antagonist sensitivity, the neocortical slice reflects in vivo characteristics.

3.2. Spreading depression during O_2/glucose deprivation: the anoxic depolarization

Following focal ischemia, peri-infarct depolarizations (PIDs) can arise at the border of the ischemic core and spread into the penumbra. Here, neurons are at risk and recurring PIDs, each more prolonged than SD, exacerbate damage during 3–4 h following stroke onset [7,10,29,31].

We have recently shown that the anoxic depolarization (AD) during O_2/glucose deprivation (OGD) arises multifocally and propagates through gray matter [5,18,19], remarkably similar to SD induced by bath elevation of KCl. We consider the AD as essentially an 'ischemic' SD that is more difficult to block because of bioenergetic failure. This causes loss of the Na^+/K^+ pump resulting in a very strong depolarizing drive. We found that depriving the hemi-brain slice of oxygen/glucose, or inhibiting Na^+/K^+ ATPase with ouabain induced a spreading AD in neocortex and an independent AD event about a minute later in underlying striatum or hippocampus (Fig. 4). A single electrode within cortical gray records the AD, but cannot show the spreading nature of the signal. The correlation in time and space between the negative shift and the LT front confirms that the optical signal represents AD.

Only in areas where AD passed did an irreversible decrease in LT develop within 10 min of the insult. Several lines of evidence indicate that this represents cellular damage. Obeidat

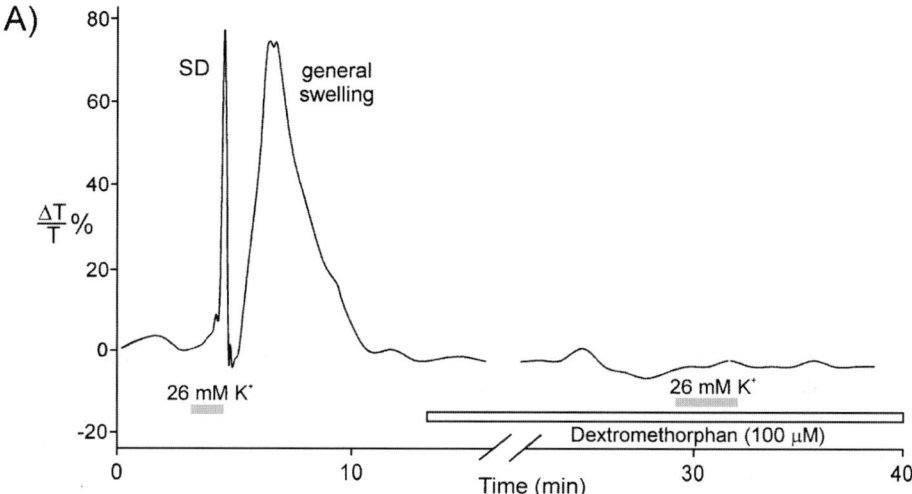

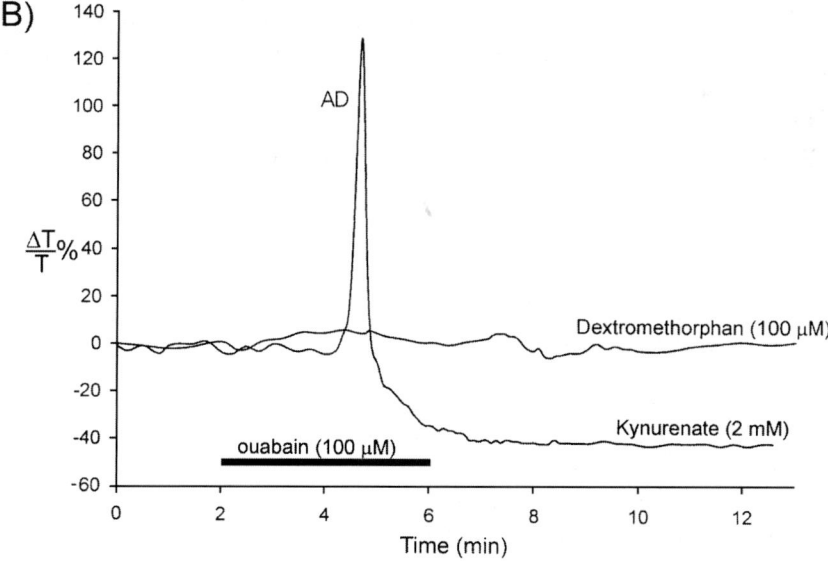

Fig. 3. (A) Spreading depression (SD) evoked by brief bath application of KCl propagates across neocortical gray. Plot from a single region of interest (~ 150 pixels) shows a rapid rise in LT representing the moving SD front. This is followed by a general LT increase that involves cell swelling, a delayed effect caused by the elevated KCl. Subsequent dextromethorphan (100 μM) pretreatment blocks both SD onset and the general swelling. (B) Brief exposure of a neocortical slice to ouabain (or to O_2/glucose deprivation, not shown) evokes a propagating anoxic depolarization (AD). In its wake, a reduced light transmittance develops, representing damage to the tissue (see Fig. 5). The nonspecific GluR antagonist kynurenate does not affect the AD. Dextromethorphan blocks the AD and so protects from post-AD damage.

et al. [35] showed that this LT reduction is associated with damage to pyramidal cell dendrites in the wake of AD. Filling single CA1 neurons with the fluorescent dye lucifer yellow revealed extensive dendritic beading not observed in tissue without O_2/glucose deprivation (Fig. 5). The beading is of an ideal diameter (0.5 μm) to scatter visible or NIR light [17] as shown in Fig. 1. Irreversible decreases in LT occurred only where AD propagated whether in rat neocortex (Fig. 4A and C) or mouse neocortex/hippocampus (Fig. 4B). The evoked field potential was permanently lost in these areas (not shown). Our

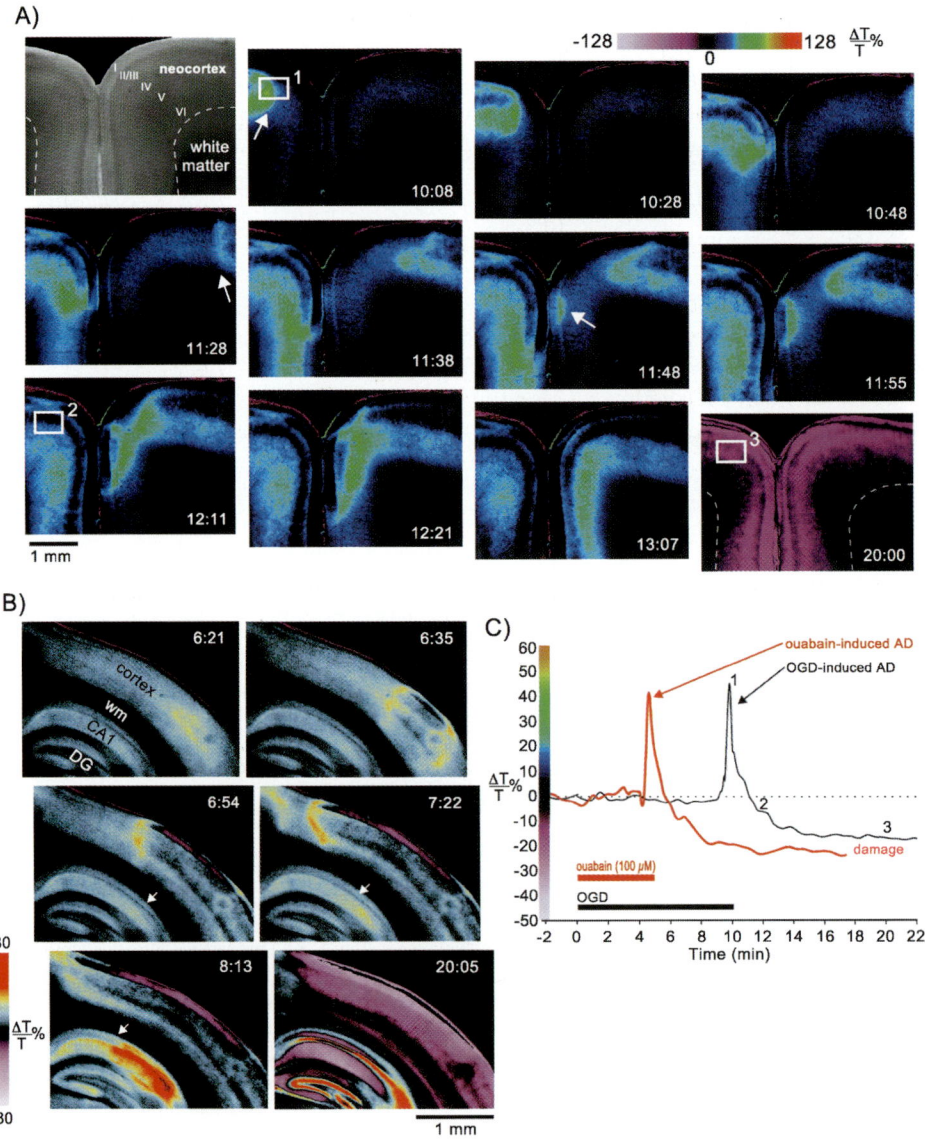

results indicate that acute neuronal swelling and beading is not due to metabolic compromise of OGD alone, but is contingent on the AD occurring concurrently. The combination of OGD and AD greatly increases energy demand and thereby accelerates neuronal damage.

We found no significant difference in the peak LT values at the AD front (representing cell swelling) between control slices and those pretreated with GluR antagonists (Fig. 3A) [18,19,35]. In addition, there was no significant difference in the time of signal onset, propagation rate, or the extent of LT reversal (representing neuronal damage). Kynurenate (2 mM) or 50 μm AP-5 or 50 μm MK-801 was without effect on the AD, despite the fact that these doses block swelling induced by 100 μm NMDA [4]. As noted above, these antagonists are effective in blocking classic SD induced by elevated K^+ in our neocortical slices.

These results are consistent with several electrophysiological studies of intact animals. As noted earlier, competitive and noncompetitive NMDAR antagonists (but not non-NMDAR antagonists) block normoxic SD but not the AD. MK-801 reduces the number of peri-infarct depolarizations (PIDs) and infarct size ([16], but see Ref. [20]), possibly, we propose, by inhibiting PID propagation in tissue away from the core where conditions are less ischemic. The implication is that accumulating extracellular glutamate is not a critical factor in AD genesis and in acute ischemic damage. Recent modeling of the reversal of glutamate uptake mechanisms during ischemia [41] agrees with data reviewed by Obrenovitch and Urenjak [36], and numerous, more recent studies that glutamate starts to accumulate only after the anoxic depolarization and that such accumulation does not drive the AD and PIDs [5] or represent a major cause of ischemic damage [37]. While a cocktail of GluR antagonists blocked AD in young rats [41], the technique is not effective in adult rats where NMDAR levels are lower.

3.3. Sigma$_1$ receptor agonists block SD and AD

The only effective method of neuroprotection from stroke in the clinical setting to date has been to lower temperature which blocks the AD during metabolic stress by reducing energy demand (see Ref. [19]). However, to be as effective as reducing body temperature, a neuroprotective drug would have to uncouple the AD from ischemia during the period of

---

Fig. 4. IOSs generated by O_2/glucose deprivation (OGD) in coronal brain slices. (A) Pseudo-colored images demonstrating light transmittance changes ($\Delta T/T$ %) in a midline coronal slice of rat neocortex in response to a 10-min exposure to OGD (00:00–10:00). Anoxic depolarization (AD) initiated at 10:08 and propagated across the slice followed by an irreversible LT decrease (magenta color). Similar changes were induced by application of ouabain (100 μM) for 5 min (not shown). Boxes represent regions of interest (ROIs) used to generate the OGD plot in (C). The signals propagate independently in each hemisphere. (B) The AD induced by O_2/glucose deprivation (8 min, 35 °C) in a slice of mouse neocortex/hippocampus. The AD initiates first in neocortex (6:21) and propagates bidirectionally along the gray matter (6:35). AD independently initiates later in hippocampus (6:54) and propagates along CA1 (arrow), finally invading the dentate gyrus (DG). By 20:05, dendritic regions display a pronounced opacity (magenta pseudo-coloring) due to dendritic beading (Fig. 5), while hippocampal cell body regions (lacking dendrites) display elevated LT (yellow–red). (C) Time course of mean LT changes in layers II/III of the rat neocortex following exposure to 10 min OGD or to 5 min ouabain (100 μM). The labels 1, 2, and 3 represent the ROIs in (A). The initial increase in LT (1) represents the anoxic depolarization (AD) front followed by a return to baseline (2), and then an irreversible decrease in LT (3).

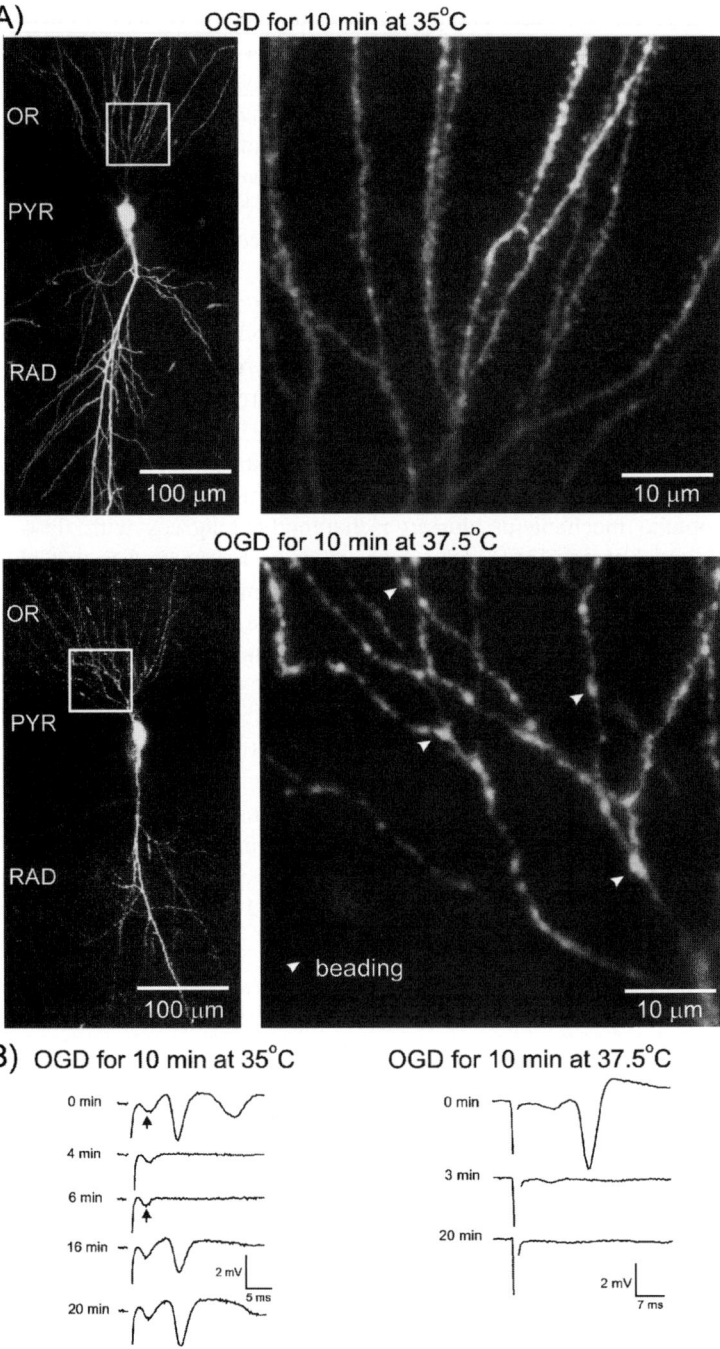

A) OGD for 10 min at 35°C

OGD for 10 min at 37.5°C

B) OGD for 10 min at 35°C   OGD for 10 min at 37.5°C

energy deprivation. In this regard, we are currently testing sigma receptor (σR) ligands. The ability of some σR ligands to reduce ischemic damage in vivo [12,40] and in vitro [9,44] suggests that their neuroprotective action might be through inhibition of the AD that occurs during ischemia. We have recently found that bath application of certain sigma$_1$ receptor (σ_1R) ligands to neocortical slices just prior to OGD blocks the AD [2,5]. These ligands also block classic SD in normoxic slices (Fig. 3A).

We have examined the AD blockade induced by σ_1R ligands (Figs. 3B and 6A) in more detail. As noted above, GluR antagonists such as AP-5 or MK-801 do not affect AD onset or propagation (Fig. 3B), whether induced by OGD or ouabain. In contrast 10–100 μM dextromethorphan or other σ_1R ligands such as carbetapentane and 4-IBP inhibit AD onset (Figs. 3B and 6A). To date, we have also tested two σ_1R antagonists (3-PPP and BD-1063) and found neither effective at 100 μM in blocking AD onset or migration (Fig. 6B). However, pretreatment of slices with either antagonist effectively inhibits blockade by 100 μM DM or CP (Fig. 6C). In other words, σ_1R agonist activity appears to be lost when the σ_1 receptor is occupied by an antagonist. This agonist/antagonist scenario also holds for SD evoked by bath application of 26 mM KCl. The SD is blocked by the σ_1R agonist (Fig. 3A, right) but the activity is lost with σ_1R antagonist pretreatment (not shown).

Most σ_1R ligands possess some NMDAR antagonist activity [9,43] and the neuro-protective effects of dextromethorphan are attributed to this activity. We have no evidence, to date, that these ligands are acting through NMDAR antagonism. First and foremost, NMDAR antagonists themselves do not block the AD [18,19,35].

The finding that σ_1R ligands block classic SD in normoxic slices and AD in ischemic slices [1] suggests that SD and AD initiation share common features. Indeed the AD is SD-like in that it arises suddenly at a focus, propagates across gray matter, and is recorded as a negative voltage shift. We propose that in vivo, the PID is a hybrid of the AD and SD, essentially an AD that can repolarize using the intermediate level of energy stores available in the penumbra. Theoretically then, PIDs should also be blocked by σ_1R ligands. These ligands could prove to be protective if they penetrate the blood–brain barrier and are administered during the first 3 h following stroke when PIDs are recurring.

4.1.1.6. On-Site Discussion

4.1.1.6.1. *Question: (Tomita)* You mentioned membrane depolarization-cell swelling as a possible cause of changes in light transmission through the tissue slice during spreading depression, and I completely agree with this. However, could you speculate on which kind of brain cells is it that swells: neurons or glia?

Fig. 5. Dendritic beading caused by AD is associated with permanent loss of the evoked field potential. (A) In the hippocampal slice, lowering temperature from 37 to 35 °C delays AD onset such that 10 min of OGD does not evoke the AD. As a result, CA1 pyramidal cells injected with lucifer yellow are normal in appearance (top). However, if the CA1 region undergoes AD, the dendrites of the stratium oriens (OR) and stratum radiatum (RAD) are beaded (below, arrowheads). (B) The evoked field potential recorded from CA1 pyramidal is only briefly lost without AD (left) but is permanently lost if AD occurs (right). Thus, the AD causes structural and functional damage.

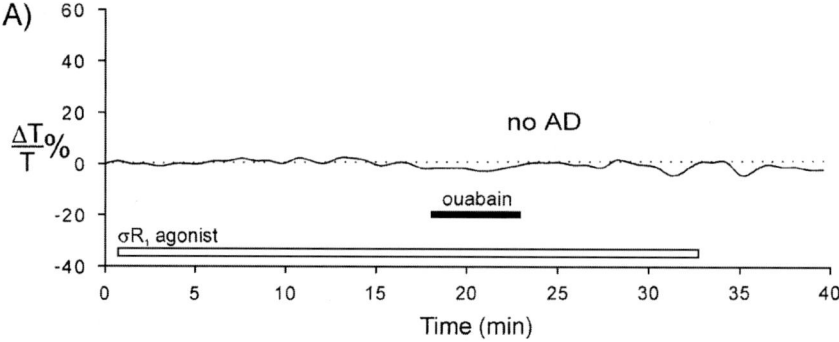

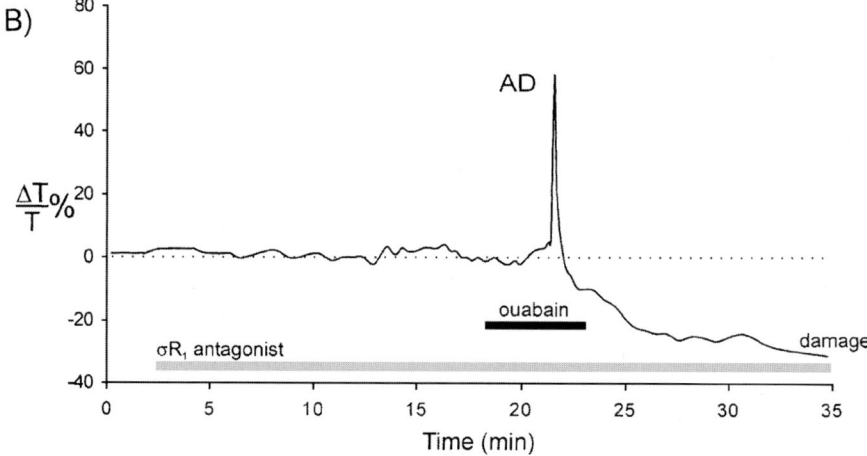

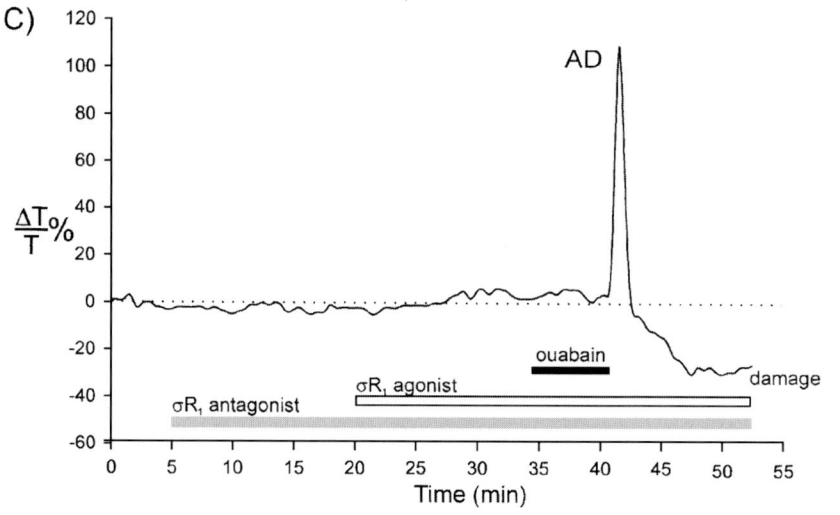

Answer: (Andrew) Since both neurons and glia precipitously depolarize at the onset of AD or SD, it is likely that the swelling of both cell types contributes to the front of elevated light transmittance. However, the damage following AD seems to be primarily neuronal, based on the distinctly laminar appearance observed post-AD in the CA1 and dentate gyrus (Fig. 4B). Specifically, large LT increases remain in cell body regions (swelling) and large decreases remain in dendritic regions (where the swelling signal is swamped by the light scattering properties of dendritic beading) (Obeidat and Andrew, Eur. J. Neurosci. 1998; 10(11): 3451).

4.1.1.6.2. *Question: (Lauritzen)* By definition, anoxic depolarization (AD) is irreversible while spreading depression (SD) is reversible. The DC potential recordings showed reversibility suggesting that the changes induced were an hypoxic-like SD. Therefore, the interpretation that carbetapentane block AD may be subject to some criticism. One question relates to the use of kynureric acid as a glutamate receptor antagonist. The tissue usually adapts to the substance rather fast and it is nonselective with respect to glutamate receptor subtypes: why use it at all?

Answer: (Andrew) Unlike in vivo, return of the DC negative shift to near baseline occurs in the slice preparation several minutes following AD even though O_2/glucose deprivation is maintained. Subsequently, the slice is electrophysiologically silent and appears permanently damaged. The same is true following AD induced by exposure to ouabain or cyanide. This is probably because elevated extracellular K^+ released within the slice is not maintained as in the in vivo ischemic core, but instead is washed out in the superfusate. This probably allows some repolarization particularly by undamaged glia.

Regarding kynurenate, it is an inexpensive and somewhat dirty drug that nonetheless blocks ionotropic glutamate receptors, showing that they are not required for AD generation. The same is true following slice pretreatment with more specific NMDAR antagonists (AP-5 or MK-801) or AMPAR antagonists (CNQX). Either separately or in combination, AD is unaffected by these antagonists (Jarvis et al., 2001; Joshi and Andrew, 2001).

4.1.1.6.3. *Question: (Tamura)* Did you measure the scattering image with changing the geometry between the surface of slice and illuminating light? The angular dependence of scattering gives us the information about the nature of scattering change, cell swelling or the change of internal cell structure such as mitochondria or nucleus.

Answer: (Andrew) To date, we have only concerned ourselves with the large increases in light transmittance (LT). Increased LT delineates the SD or AD front; decreased LT delineates damage to dendrites. In brain slices, measuring broad band reflected light can yield perplexing responses as the cell swelling increases. This can involve biphasic responses and even signal inversions, which we attribute to changes in preferred scattering angle as swelling progresses. Transmitted light, being minimally scattered, is not subject to such vagaries. In addition, the entire thickness of the slice is sampled.

Fig. 6. (A) Pretreatment with the $\sigma_1 R$ agonists dextromethorphan, carbetapentane, or 4-IBP ($10-100\,\mu M$) blocks the anoxic depolarization (AD) induced by ouabain (or OGD, not shown). (B) Pretreatment with the $\sigma_1 R$ antagonists (+) 3-PPP or BD-1063 has no effect on AD generation, propagation or post-AD damage. (C) Pretreatment with an σR_1 antagonist removes the ability of a σR_1 agonist to block the AD and the resultant post-AD damage.

Acknowledgements

This work was supported by the Heart and Stroke Foundation of Ontario (Grant B-4003).

References

[1] T.R. Anderson, C.R. Jarvis, R.D. Andrew, Imaging repetitive spreading depression in submerged neocortical slices, Soc. Neurosci. Abstr. 25 (1999) 293.2.

[2] T.R. Anderson, A.J. Biedermann, R.D. Andrew, Sigma receptor ligands block spreading depression in rat neocortical slices, Soc. Neurosci. Abstr. 26 (2000) 282.15.

[3] R.D. Andrew, B.A. MacVicar, Imaging cell volume changes and neuronal excitation in the hippocampal slice, Neuroscience 62 (1994) 371–383.

[4] R.D. Andrew, J.R. Adams, T.M. Polischuk, Imaging NMDA- and kainate-induced intrinsic optical signals from the hippocampal slice, J. Neurophysiol. 76 (1996) 2707–2717.

[5] R.D. Andrew, T.R. Anderson, A.J. Biedermann, I. Joshi, C.R. Jarvis, Imaging the anoxic depolarization, a multifocal and propagating event, in: J. Krieglstein, S. Klumpp (Eds.), Pharmacology of Cerebral Ischemia, Medpharm Scientific Publishers, Stuttgart, 2000, pp. 75–94.

[6] R.D. Andrew, M.E. Lobinowich, E.P. Osehobo, Evidence against volume regulation by cortical brain cells during acute osmotic stress, Exp. Neurol. 143 (1997) 300–312.

[7] T. Back, M.D. Ginsberg, W.D. Dietrich, B.D. Watson, Induction of spreading depression in the ischemic hemisphere following experimental middle cerebral artery occlusion: effect on infarct morphology, J. Cereb. Blood Flow Metab. 16 (1996) 202–213.

[8] T. Bonhoeffer, Optical imaging of intrinsic signals as a tool to visualize the functional architecture of adult and developing visual cortex, Arzneim.-Forsch. 45 (1995) 351–356.

[9] J. Church, J.A. Shacklock, K.G. Baimbridge, Dextromethorphan and phencyclidine receptor ligands: differential effects on K^+- and NMDA-evoked increases in cytosolic free Ca^{2+} concentration, Neurosci. Lett. 124 (1991) 232–234.

[10] R.M. Dijkhuizen, J.P. Beekwilder, H.B. van der Worp, J.W. Berkelbach van der Sprenkel, K.A. Tulleken, K. Nicolay, Correlation between tissue depolarizations and damage in focal ischemic rat brain, Brain Res. 840 (1999) 194–205.

[11] D.R. Footit, N.R. Newberry, Cortical spreading depression induces an LTP-like effect in rat neocortex in vivo, Brain Res. 781 (1998) 339–342.

[12] C.P. George, M.P. Goldberg, D.W. Choi, G.K. Steinberg, Dextromethorphan reduces neocortical ischemic neuronal damage in vivo, Brain Res. 440 (1988) 375–379.

[13] A. Grinvald, E. Lieke, R.D. Frostig, C.D. Gilbert, T.N. Wiesel, Functional architecture of cortex revealed by optical imaging of intrinsic signals, Nature 324 (1986) 361–364.

[14] A.J. Hansen, Effect of anoxia on ion distribution in the brain, Physiol. Rev. 65 (1985) 101–148.

[15] J. Hernandez-Caceres, R. Macias-Gonzalez, G. Brozek, J. Bures, Systemic ketamine blocks cortical spreading depression but does not delay the onset of terminal anoxic depolarization in rats, Brain Res. 437 (1987) 360–364.

[16] T. Iijima, G. Mies, K.A. Hossmann, Repeated negative DC deflections in rat cortex following middle cerebral artery occlusion are abolished by MK-801: effect on volume of ischemic injury, J. Cereb. Blood Flow Metab. 12 (1992) 727–733.

[17] C.R. Jarvis, L. Lilge, G. Vipond, R.D. Andrew, Interpretation of intrinsic optical signals and calcein fluorescence during excitotoxic insult in the hippocampal slice, NeuroImage 10 (1999) 357–372.

[18] C.R. Jarvis, T.R. Anderson, R.D. Andrew, Anoxic depolarization mediates acute damage independent of glutamate in neocortical brain slices, Cereb. Cortex 11 (2001) 249–259.

[19] I. Joshi, R.D. Andrew, Imaging anoxic depolarization during ischemia-like conditions in the mouse hemibrain slice, J. Neurophysiol. 85 (2001) 414–424.

[20] V.I. Koroleva, O.S. Korolev, E. Loseva, J. Bures, The effect of MK-801 and of brain-derived polypeptides on the development of ischemic lesion induced by photothrombotic occlusion of the distal middle cerebral artery in rats, Brain Res. 786 (1998) 104–114.

[21] N.R. Kreisman, J.C. LaManna, S.C. Liao, E.R. Yeh, J.R. Alcala, Light transmittance as an index of cell volume in hippocampal slices: optical differences of interfaced and submerged positions, Brain Res. 693 (1995) 179–186.

[22] A.A.P. Leao, Spreading depression of activity in the cerebral cortex, J. Neurophysiol. 7 (1944) 359–390.

[23] A.A.P. Leao, Further observations on the spreading depression of activity in the cerebral cortex, J. Neurophysiol. 10 (1947) 409–414.

[24] M. Lauritzen, A.J. Hansen, The effect of glutamate receptor blockade on anoxic depolarization and cortical spreading depression, J. Cereb. Blood Flow Metab. 12 (1992) 223–229.

[25] M. Lauritzen, Pathophysiology of the migraine aura. The spreading depression theory, Brain 117 (Pt. 1) (1994) 199–210.

[26] B.A. MacVicar, D. Hochman, Imaging of synaptically evoked intrinsic optical signals in hippocampal slices, J. Neurosci. 11 (1991) 1458–1469.

[27] R. Marrannes, R. Willems, E. De Prins, A. Wauquier, Evidence for a role of the N-methyl-D-aspartate (NMDA) receptor in cortical spreading depression in the rat, Brain Res. 457 (1988) 226–240.

[28] H. McIlwan, L. Buchel, D. Cheshire, The inorganic phosphate and phosphocreatine especially during metabolism in vitro, J. Biochem. 48 (1951) 12–20.

[29] G. Mies, Blood flow dependent duration of cortical depolarizations in the periphery of focal ischemia of rat brain, Neurosci. Lett. 221 (1997) 165–168.

[30] M. Nedergaard, A.J. Hansen, Spreading depression is not associated with neuronal injury in the normal brain, Brain Res. 449 (1988) 395–398.

[31] M. Nedergaard, A.J. Hansen, Characterization of cortical depolarizations evoked in focal cerebral ischemia, J. Cereb. Blood Flow Metab. 13 (1993) 568–574.

[32] B. Nellgard, T. Wieloch, NMDA-receptor blockers but not NBQX, an AMPA-receptor antagonist, inhibit spreading depression in the rat brain, Acta Physiol. Scand. 146 (1992) 497–503.

[33] C. Nicholson, T.P. Kraig, The behaviour of extracellular ions during spreading depression, in: T. Zeuthen (Ed.), The Application of Ion-Selective Electrodes, Elsevier, Amsterdam, 1981, pp. 217–238.

[34] A.S. Obeidat, R.D. Andrew, Spreading depression determines acute cellular damage in the hippocampal slice during oxygen/glucose deprivation, Eur. J. Neurosci. 10 (1998) 3451–3461.

[35] A.S. Obeidat, C.R. Jarvis, R.D. Andrew, Glutamate does not mediate acute neuronal damage after spreading depression induced by O_2/glucose deprivation in the hippocampal slice, J. Cereb. Blood Flow Metab. 20 (2000) 412–422.

[36] T.P. Obrenovitch, J. Urenjak, Altered glutamatergic transmission in neurological disorders: from high extracellular glutamate to excessive synaptic efficacy, Prog. Neurobiol. 51 (1997) 39–87.

[37] T.P. Obrenovitch, High extracellular glutamate and neuronal death in neurological disorders. Cause, contribution or consequence? Ann. N. Y. Acad. Sci. 890 (1999) 273–286.

[38] T.M. Polischuk, R.D. Andrew, Real-time imaging of intrinsic optical signals during early excitotoxicity evoked by domoic acid in the rat hippocampal slice, Can. J. Physiol. Pharmacol. 74 (1996) 712–722.

[39] T.M. Polischuk, C.R. Jarvis, R.D. Andrew, Intrinsic optical signaling denoting neuronal damage in response to acute excitotoxic insult by domoic acid in the hippocampal slice, Neurobiol. Dis. 4 (1998) 423–437.

[40] D.A. Prince, H.R. Feeser, Dextromethorphan protects against cerebral infarction in a rat model of hypoxia–ischemia, Neurosci. Lett. 85 (1988) 291–296.

[41] D.J. Rossi, T. Oshima, D. Attwell, Glutamate release in severe brain ischemia is mainly by reversed uptake, Nature 403 (1999) 316–321.

[42] A. Villringer, B. Chance, Non-invasive optical spectroscopy and imaging of human brain function, Trends Neurosci. 20 (1997) 435–442.

[43] E.R. Whittemore, V.I. Ilyin, R.M. Woodward, Antagonism of N-methyl-D-aspartate receptors by sigma site ligands: potency, sub-type selectivity and mechanisms of inhibition, J. Pharmacol. Exp. Ther. 282 (1997) 326–338.

[44] B.Y. Wong, D.A. Coulter, D.W. Choi, D.A. Prince, Dextrorphan and dextromethorphan, common antitussives, are antiepileptic and antagonize N-methyl-D-aspartate in brain slices, Neurosci. Lett. 85 (1988) 261–266.

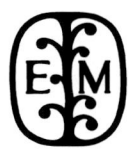

International Congress Series 1235 (2002) 439–447

A time-variable concentric wave-ring increase in light transparency and associated microflow changes during a potassium-induced spreading depression in the rat cerebral cortex

Minoru Tomita [a,*], Istvan Schiszler [a,1], Yasuo Fukuuchi [a],
Takahiro Amano [a], Norio Tanahashi [a], Masahiro Kobari [b],
Hidetaka Takeda [a], Yutaka Tomita [c], Manabu Ohtomo [a], Koji Inoue [a]

[a]*Department of Neurology, School of Medicine, Keio University, Tokyo, Japan*
[b]*Department of Neurology, Tachikawa Hospital, Tokyo, Japan*
[c]*Department of Neurology, Urawa City Hospital, Saitama, Japan*

Abstract

The mechanism of coupling between neurons and the microvasculature continues to remain unclear. This was examined during potassium-induced spreading depression (SD), since SD is thought to be a phenomenon of local neuronal depolarization in association with flow changes. In α-chloralose-urethane anesthetized rats, a new optical method was employed by which both the light transparency (LT) changes of the somatosensory cortex as well as its associated capillary-level flow were measured simultaneously in a region of interest (ROI; 2×2 mm) of the sensorimotor cortex. Microinjection of concentrated potassium chloride solution into the cortex produced spreading depression which was observed as a function of time and space, with attention given to the increase and decrease in wave-rings marked by cortical LT variance. The wave-ring was observed to enlarge at a speed of ca. 2.2 mm/min and approximately 1–2 min later, a new wave-ring appeared. This cycle continued repeatedly for more than 30 min. The study was performed on seven rats, with ring propagation in three, an abortive form in another three, and no rings in one rat. In a 3-D microflow map produced by intracarotid injection of diluted carbon black (CB) (Pelikan Werke, Germany) in Ringer solution, a low-flow ring was approximately collocated at the wave-front ΔLT ring, followed by a flow increase. A close correlation between topographical microflow changes and LT changes indicates that local depolarization of the neurons induces an immediate decrease followed rapidly by

---

* Corresponding author. Postal address: 26 minaminakamachi, Motojuku-cho, Okazaki 444-3505, Japan. Tel.: +81-564-48-2431; fax: +81-564-48-4885.
E-mail address: mtomita@gol.com (M. Tomita).
[1] Present address: Torokbalint, Petofi u. 4, 2045, Hungary.

an increase in microflow, suggesting that the depolarized neurons induced changes in adjacent microvascular (capillary) flow. © 2002 Elsevier Science B.V. All rights reserved.

Keywords: Optical method; Neurovascular coupling; Potassium-induced spreading depression; Cortical light transparency; 3-Dimensional microflow map

1. Introduction

In order to gain an insight into the neurovascular coupling in the cerebral cortex, we examined the topographical changes in cortical tissue blood flow, which occur during propagation of neuronal depolarization (spreading depression).

2. Methods

2.1. General description

As the details of the methods have been reported elsewhere, we briefly describe them in this paper [1,2]. The experiments were carried out on male rats weighing 300–350 g ($n=7$), anesthetized by IV administration of 70 mg/kg α-chloralose and 0.7 g/kg urethane. The animals were placed on a head holder with ear bars, and the calvarium overlying the right parietal region was removed for cortical exposure. The defect was covered with immersion oil and a glass cover slip. The cortical tissue was transilluminated by an optical fiber, which was inserted into the cortex postero-obliquely and affixed at the bony edge with dental cement, so as to keep the light source tip 1 mm below the brain surface and at the center of the region of interest (ROI). The other end of the optical fibre was connected to a halogen lamp (Moritex, Tokyo). Utilizing a Nikon lens with a band pass filter ($\lambda=550 \pm 15$ nm of the width at half maximum) focused on the brain surface, an SIT camera (Hamamatsu photonics) was used to monitor the transmitted light through the ROI (2×2 mm). The camera output was fed into a videotape recorder (Sony) and recorded on digital videotapes continuously at a rate of 30 frames per second. Selected parts were taken ad libitum and inputted into a personal computer through an 8-bit Scion LG-3 frame grabber card, so that the intensity of the transmitted light was continuously stored in the RAM disc. The data acquisition and analysis were the same as those of the original method [1,2]. A period of 1 h was allowed so that the brain could recover from the damage caused by the insertion of the optical fiber. Subsequently, concentrated potassium chloride solution (KCl) was injected into the cortex at the center of the ROI through a glass micropipette, originally made for intracellular injections. Due to technical difficulties in inserting the micropipette into the cortex, the depth of insertion and the amount of solution injected were not consistent.

2.2. Data analysis

After the KCl injections, the images recorded were used for three purposes: (1) microphotographs to evaluate leptomeningeal vessel changes, (2) cortical light transmission changes (ΔLT), and (3) microflow maps calculated from tracer transit times. The first image of the brain surface (control video frame) immediately before K^+ injection was subtracted in a series from each subsequent frame of the experimental image at time t at location x,y, so that changes in LT were revealed in the cerebral cortex ($LT_{t,x,y} - LT_{c,x,y}$ $= \Delta LT_{t,x,y}$), where x,y denote the coordinates on the brain surface. The magnitude in $\Delta LT_{t,x,y}$ was automatically calculated in numerical figures on the Scion 256 grey scale. Because the baseline value was determined by subtraction of the same frame as 128, any changes in LT (t,x,y) were quantitatively expressed in positive (increase) or negative (decrease) figures if they were above or below 128. Sequential subtraction frames were arranged every 3 s to observe the propagation of ΔLT images on the cerebral cortex. Plots of $\Delta LT_{t,x,y}$ were made at a given point $A_{X,Y}$ for 10 min in order to examine an oscillation cycle, and on a horizontal axis passing through the K^+ injection point to determine the speed of changes in light transmission as the solution spreads. To determine the regional MTT, 200 consecutive video frames were acquired before, during, and after injection of 1/30 diluted carbon black (CB) (Pelikan Werke, Germany) in Ringer solution into the carotid artery. CB transit in pixels of a 50×50 matrix in the ROI was grabbed and the hemodilution curves of the individual pixels were analyzed by MATLAB employing a customized algorithm. MTTs were calculated in all 2500 pixels based on the conventional formula MTT $= t LT(t)_{x,y} dt / LT(t)_{x,y} dt$, where $LT(t)_{x,y}$ denotes the intensity of transmitted light at time t at a given pixel (x,y). Since reciprocal MTT (or velocity) was a major factor of flow, we denoted 1/MTT of pixels as microvascular flow or "microflow." The values of the microflow were displayed on a two-dimensional (2-D) map with the help of the MATLAB software. Thus, the spatial resolution of the flow map was 625 microflow elements per 1 mm^2, almost 500 times higher than that of LDF with a 1-mm-diameter flow probe [3]. The flow values were not influenced by the brightness of the location, because the values were based on changes in the intensity of transmitted light due to tracer transit through the pixels. The tracer of 25-μl diluted CB solution was injected into the internal carotid artery through the external carotid artery to produce 2500 hemodilution curves in the ROI.

3. Results

KCl injection into the cerebral cortex immediately elicited a dark spot of ca. 100 μm in diameter at the site of injection (Fig. 1), which was only visible through the microscope. Initially, this was thought to be a small bleeding due to glass pipette insertion. However, the dark spot was transformed, which seemed sometimes to be "boiling" (Fig. 1: 0–21 s). After "boiling" for some time, a corona-like transparent projection, at the edge of the dark spot, started and fused into a concentric ring. The ring gradually increased its diameter propagating peripherally, similar to ripples in a pond. Fig. 1 demonstrates the wave-ring enlargement shown every 3 s after the initiation. The upper graph in Fig. 2 demonstrates a plot profile of $LT(t)_{x,Y=0}$, where $t = 3, 6, 9, 12, 15, 18, 21$, and 24 s, and $x = 2$ mm. It should be noted that the peaks of LT moved slowly every 3 s. The speed was calculated to be 2.2 ± 0.5 mm/min (Fig. 2, upper graph). The bottom graph in Fig. 2 was a trace of $LT(t)_{A_{X,Y}}$. It showed a cyclic fluctuation of ca. 3.5 cycles every 5 min (0.7

Light transparency spread with time

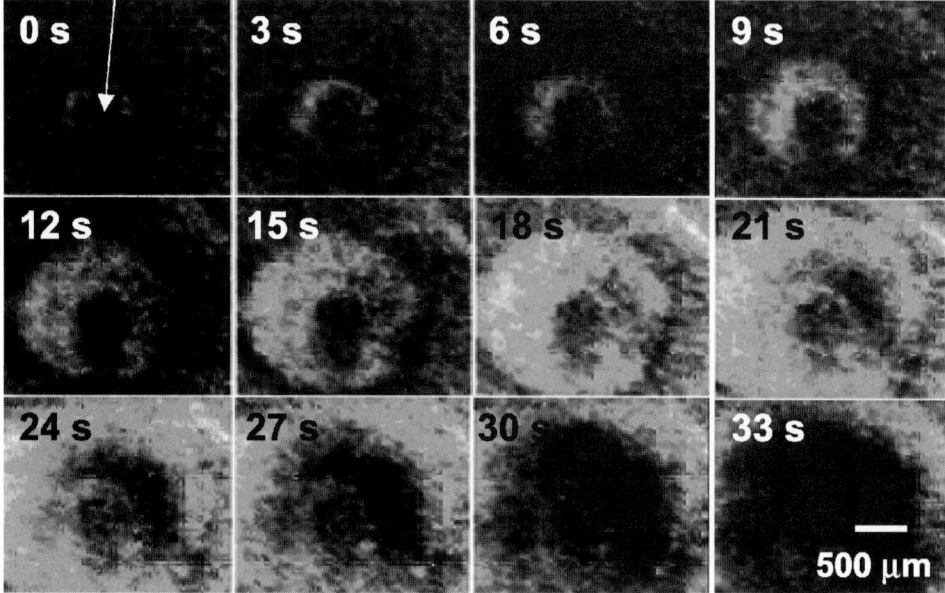

Fig. 1. Rat sensorimotor cortex (2×2 mm) trans-illuminated by a light at a wavelength of 550 nm. KCl injection (arrow) produced a wave-ring of cortical light transparency change, which enlarged after the wave generation. The light transparent (white) ring enlargement is shown in sequential 3-s frames. The white ring was followed by a dark circle, which also spread and tended to occupy the entire measuring area. It should be noted that a second white ring appeared to be initiating in the center. The speed of the white ring spread was ca. 2.2 mm/min in this case.

cpm = 0.01 cps (Hz)). As shown, a new wave-ring appeared approximately 1 min later, and this cycle continued repeatedly for more than 30 min. Such ring generation and propagation occurred in three rats, an abortive form in another three rats, and no wave (but dark spot) generation occurred in one of the rats. Fig. 3 (upper panel, left) depicts the three-dimensional map of microflow produced by carbon black dye injection into the carotid artery, and Fig. 3 (upper panel, right) shows the surface plots of the light transparency during passage of spreading depression. In the wave front of microflow change, there was a low-flow ring belt of approximately 80 μm in width, the flow value of which was ca. 0.3/s or a 50% decrease when compared with the control value of 0.60±0.21/s. The lower panel of Fig. 3 demonstrates select subtraction pictures. It may be of interest to note that the subtraction of the two control sequential frames, LT_1 and LT_2, yielded a picture (top left), which suggested fluctuations of individual microflows during the short interval. From subsequent pictures, the microflow ring was also recognized to be spreading with time. Although the two maps (upper panel of Fig. 3) appeared to be grossly similar, they were different by spot-to-spot comparison. The low-flow ring pre-

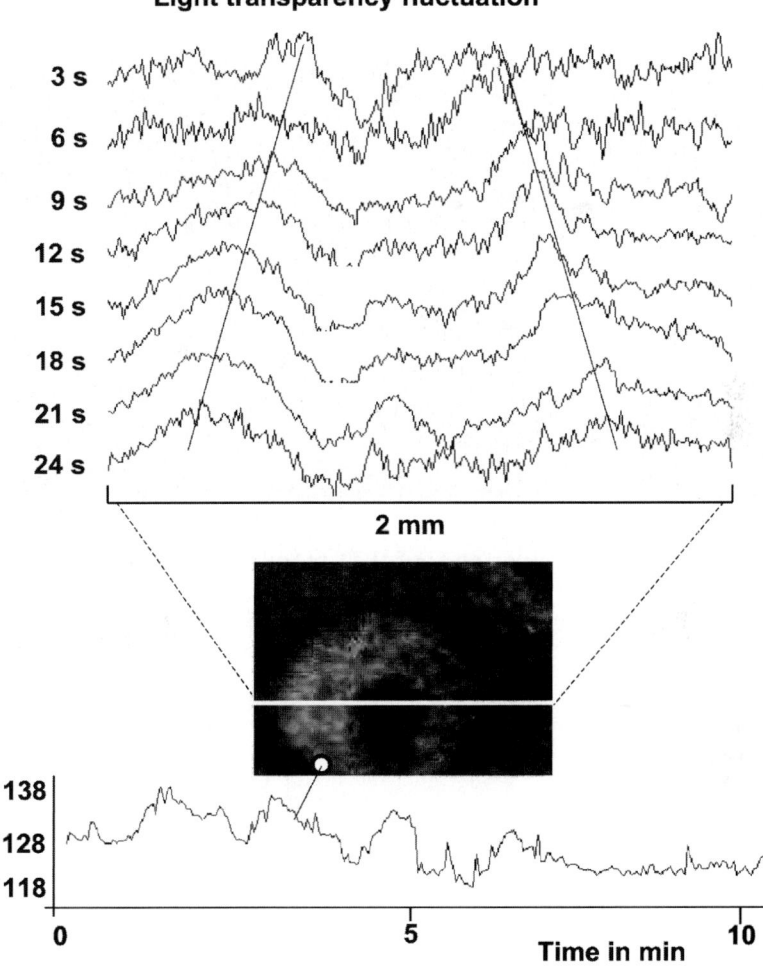

Fig. 2. The upper graph depicts the changes in the light transparency (LT) intensity that was traced along a line across the ROI passing through the site of KCl injection (shown by the white line). Plot profiles of LT were taken every 3 s. Upward deflection indicates an increase in light transparency. Note that peaks of the range moved outwards with time. The lower graph represents a trace of intensity change at a point indicated by the small circle. It showed an oscillation of ca. 3.5 cycles per 5 min.

ceded microflow changes collocated at around the border zone of the concentric ring. The dark spot was shown to be a flow-decreased area (Fig. 3, upper panel), but the subtraction picture revealed that the area seemed to be quite active with ceaseless flow changes dispatching wave-ring signals towards the periphery repeatedly, sometimes for more than 30 min (two cases).

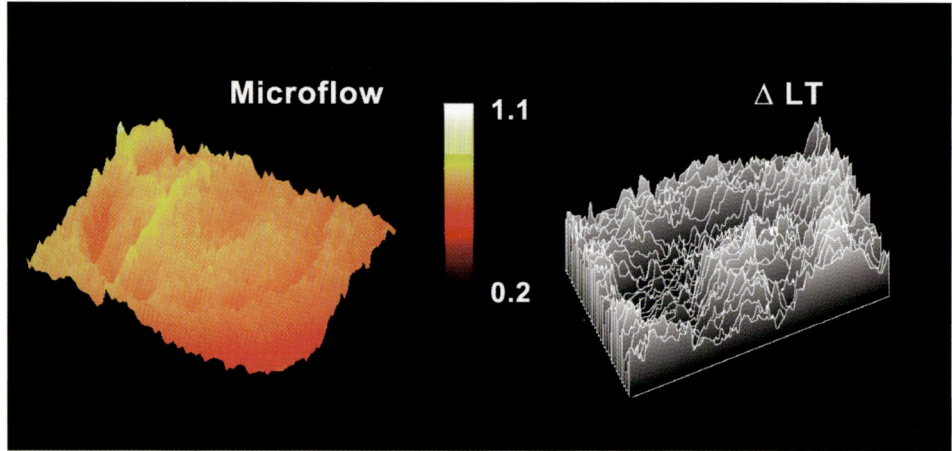

Subtraction pictures of 2-D microflow maps

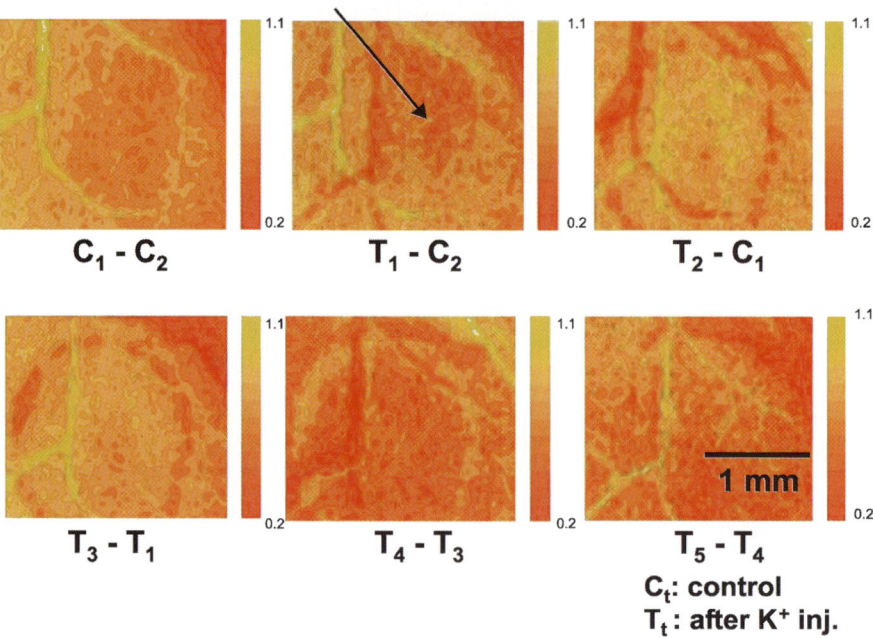

C_t: control
T_t: after K$^+$ inj.

Fig. 3. The upper panel showed the microflow change (left) and the concomitant LT change (right) in three-dimensional maps. They were similar in gross comparison. The calibration bar shows that the yellow areas denote faster flow. Yellow lines corresponded to feeding arterioles whereas dark orange lines to venules. The lower panel is sequential subtraction pictures of 2-D microflow changes during passage of the spreading depression. It was evident that the microflow ring also expanded following spreading depression. Note: the orange ring in T_3-T_1 turned into a yellow ring in T_4-T_3 due to subtraction order.

4. Discussion

Van Harreveld [4] showed that the visual concomitants of spreading depression in the retina consisted of a number of expanding concentric rings of different width and darkness around a mechanically stimulated area. He described that the most peripheral ring consisted of a narrow dark line. A light ring, then a wide dark band, and most centrally, a light area followed this more centrally. If we consider that the reflection of light is a reversal of the transmission of light (increased light transmittance means decreased light reflectance), Van Harreveld's description matches the findings of this experiment. Similar changes in the optical property of the submerged rat neocortical slices during spreading depression have been studied by several investigators [5–8]. After approximately 6 min of anoxic and glycemic deprivation, the depolarization was imaged by Andrew [9] and resulted in a focal increase in light transmittance, which then propagated across the neocortical gray area at approximately 2 mm/min. The value of $\Delta T/T$ seemed to be large in the rat hippocampal interface slices where the optical property was not influenced by the blood component, the maximum chromophore in the tissue in situ. Hansen and Lauritzen [10] summarized that the early increase in K^+, with a negative DC shift, correlated with an initial arrest of neuronal activity and subsequent blood flow changes in SD. However, the blood flow changes were far from conclusive.

According to our research of the literature, our experiment marks the first description of the microflow measured in conjunction with the light transparency of the given cortex. This may lend some insight into the functional organization of the cortical micro-circulation in the brain, and the adaptive features of microflow regulation in response to K^+ stimuli. The optical property changes could be due to either blood volume (CBV) changes or to neuronal depolarization. The mechanism of wave-ring spread is not likely to be of arteriolar origin, since the spread was independent of the location of the arterioles where the flow regulator was placed (Fig. 3). We speculate that a unit of self-perpetuating process outlined as "K^+ increase–neuronal depolarization–cell swelling due to thermo-dynamic energy discharge [11]–compression of the microvasculature-squeezing blood", might be ignited as a chain reaction next to the cerebral cortex as a domino effect. The speed of the ring spread may be limited by various factors such as the time for the adjacent neurons to fire or the refractory stage of the given neurons, which had previously depolarized. The response of microflow to neuronal stimulation is suggested by our findings. If neuronal activation caused depolarization resulting in microflow increases, our theory of adaptive neurovascular coupling would be supported. Whether this is an adaptive increase to assist neuronal recovery or a vascular overcompensation is unknown. In fact, Schiszler et al. [12] reported a microflow increase in the somatosensory cortex even after the cessation of electrical stimulation to the hind leg in rats. Whichever the case, this "reflex" can be a target of future research either as a possible route to augmenting physiologic adaptive mechanisms, or as a way of ascertaining the mismatch response.

In conclusion, K^+-induced spreading depression was observed as a function of time and space with attention given to the increase and decrease in wave-rings, marked by tissue light transmission and its accompanying cyclic microflow fluctuations. The propagation was speculated to be due to a cascade of the thermodynamic discharge, as well as the re-covery of stored potential inherent within the given neurons.

4.1.2.7. On-Site Discussion

4.1.2.7.1. *Question: (Dirnagl)* You find that there is a short spreading hypoperfusion before hyperperfusion sets in after K^+ microinjection into the cortex. As the name implies, cortical spreading depression is characterized by a suppression of neuronal activity. May it be that the hypoperfusion is simply caused by the coupling of metabolism and blood flow in the brain: lower neuronal activity leading to lower CBF?

Answer: (Tomita) Yes, I believe so. However, the point was that the spread was preceded by an extremely low flow change, and that the low flow ring belt (less than 100 µm) was far narrower than the diameter of the so-called "microcirculatory unit." This strongly suggested that the capillary flow was directly and time-to-time regulated by the pertinent neurons.

4.1.2.7.2. *Question: (Dreier)* We have reported that cortical spreading depression induces a sharp and short initial hypoperfusion when K^+ is elevated in the subarachnoid space (see Fig. 8 of our article: J. Neurosurg., 93(2000) 658). This might be related to the small ring of hypoperfusion which you found after the application of K^+, using your imaging tool. A similar sharp and short initial hypoperfusion can also be found when K^+ is physiological but NOS is inhibited (Duckrow, Brain Res., 618 (1993) 190). Indeed, such a response was also found in a patient after head trauma (Mayevsky, Brain Res., 740 (1996) 268). If elevated K^+ is combined with an NO-lowering agent such as hemoglobin or nitro-L-arginine, the spreading depression can even induce a long lasting ischemic response in the rat brain (up to 90 min!), the so-called "cortical spreading ischemia" (Dreier, J. Cereb. Blood Flow Metab., 18 (1998) 978; Dreier. J. Neurosurg., 93 (2000) 658; Dreier, J. Physiol., 531 (2001) 515).

Answer: (Tomita) Thank you for your helpful comment. I am sure that you are observing an identical phenomenon to that reported here.

Acknowledgements

This study was supported by a research grant from the New Energy and Industrial Technology Development Organization.

References

[1] I. Schiszler, M. Tomita, Y. Fukuuchi, N. Tanahashi, K. Inoue, New optical method for analyzing cortical blood flow heterogeneity in small animals—validation of the method, Am. J. Physiol. 279 (2000) H1291– H1298.

[2] M. Tomita, F. Gotoh, T. Sato, T. Amano, N. Tanahashi, K. Tanaka, M. Yamamoto, Photoelectric method for estimating hemodynamic changes in regional cerebral tissue, Am. J. Physiol. 235 (1978) H56–H63.

[3] M. Tomita, Y. Fukuuchi, N. Tanahashi, M. Kobari, Y. Tomita, M. Ohtomo, Heterogeneity of microflow changes within a cortical area as small as an LDF probe (abstr), J. Cereb. Blood Flow Metab. 21 (Suppl. 1) (2001) S228.

[4] A. Van Harreveld, Visual concomitants of retinal spreading depression, An. Acad. Bras. Cienc. 56 (4) (1984) 519–523.

[5] R.W. Snow, C.P. Taylor, F.E. Dudek, Electrophysiological and optical changes in slices of rat hippocampus during spreading depression, J. Neurophysiol. 50 (3) (1983) 561–572.

[6] M. Muller, G.G. Somjen, Intrinsic optical signals in rat hippocampal slices during hypoxia-induced spreading depression-like depolarization, J. Neurophysiol. 82 (4) (1999) 1818–1831.

[7] A.S. Obeidat, C.R. Jarvis, R.D. Andrew, Glutamate does not mediate acute neuronal damage after spreading depression induced by O_2/glucose deprivation in the hippocampal slice, J. Cereb. Blood Flow Metab. 20 (2) (2000) 412–422.

[8] C.R. Jarvis, T.R. Anderson, R.D. Andrew, Anoxic depolarization mediates acute damage independent of glutamate in neocortical brain slices, Cereb. Cortex 11 (3) (2001) 249–259.

[9] R.D. Andrew, Imaging and preventing spreading depression independent of cerebral blood flow. In this proceedings.

[10] A.J. Hansen, M. Lauritzen, The role of spreading depression in acute brain disorders, An. Acad. Bras. Cienc. 56 (4) (1984) 457–479.

[11] M. Tomita, F. Gotoh, Cascade of cell swelling (cytotoxic edema): thermodynamic potential discharge of brain cells following membrane injury, Am. J. Physiol. 262 (1992) H603–H610.

[12] I. Schiszler, M. Tomita, K. Inoue, N. Tanahashi, Y. Fukuuchi, Sustained microvascular flow response to functional activation in rat cerebral cortex. In this proceedings.

International Congress Series 1235 (2002) 449–456

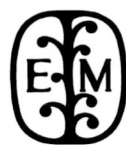

Real-time microcirculatory changes due to spreading depression under focal ischemia

Elisabeth Pinard [a,*], Hélène Nallet [b], Simon Roussel [b],
Eric MacKenzie [b], Jacques Seylaz [a]

[a]*Laboratoire de Recherches Cérébrovasculaires, CNRS UPR 646, 10 Avenue de Verdun, 75010 Paris, France*
[b]*CNRS UMR 6551, Boulevard Henri Becquerel, 14074 Caen, France*

Abstract

Laser-scanning confocal fluorescence microscopy was used to investigate microcirculatory influences of spreading depression (SD)-like depolarizations elicited by occlusion of the rat middle cerebral artery (MCA). Six rats underwent halothane anesthesia and mechanical ventilation. A closed cranial window was implanted over their frontoparietal cortex. They were placed under a Biorad Viewscan confocal microscope and intravenously given fluorescein isothiocyanate (FITC)-Dextran and FITC-labeled erythrocytes. The capillaries were visualized down to 200 μm below the brain surface and the images were video recorded (50/s). The MCA was occluded under the microscope using an intraluminal remotely controlled method and the reperfusion was induced 2 h later. Furthermore, the brains were histologically examined 24 h later. Under ischemia, the erythrocyte velocity through the capillaries was depressed by 35% and venous blood became highly sluggish. The arteriole diameter did not change significantly, however, the direction of arteriolar blood flow was episodically and transiently reversed. During spontaneous SD-like depolarization, the arteriole diameter significantly increased (+19% vs. MCAO) while capillary erythrocyte velocity was further depressed by 15%. This decrease in velocity was more pronounced (25%) when depolarization were associated with transient reversal of arteriolar flow. Following reperfusion, microcirculatory variables rapidly returned to the baseline. All rats exhibited infarcts 24 h after the occlusion. These results indicate that SD-like depolarizations have an adverse influence on penumbral micro-circulation, i.e., a reduction in capillary perfusion by erythrocytes, despite arteriolar dilatation. © 2002 Elsevier Science B.V. All rights reserved.

Keywords: Microcirculation; Focal ischemia; Spreading depression; Confocal microscopy

* Corresponding author. Tel.: +33-1-44-89-77-37; fax: +33-1-44-89-78-25.
E-mail address: pinard@ext.jussieu.fr (E. Pinard).

0531-5131/02 © 2002 Elsevier Science B.V. All rights reserved.
PII: S 0 5 3 1 - 5 1 3 1 (0 2) 0 0 2 1 2 - 1

1. Introduction

Under focal ischemia, spontaneous transient depolarizations occur irregularly in the ischemic border zones. They are very similar to cortical spreading depressions (SD) and are probably due to the spread of increased extracellular K^+ and glutamate from the core of the lesion (for review, see Refs. [1,2]). The duration of these SD-like periinfarct depolarizations is determined by the level of residual blood flow in the periphery of the focal ischemia, since the recovery phase is critically dependent on an increased blood supply to normalize the ionic gradients [3].

Hemodynamic data, all obtained by laser Doppler flowmetry (LDF), suggest that the flow response to these depolarizations in the ischemic penumbra is limited by the hemodynamic capacity of the collateral system [4–6]. Recently, LDF data from Nallet et al. [7] showed that the amplitude of the increase in blood supply is proportional to the residual blood flow. However, regional tissue perfusion reflected by LDF may be dissociated from cerebral capillary perfusion [8]. Since ischemia-induced depolarizations are presumably important factors in the development of cerebral ischemic damage and since their hemodynamic correlates are of crucial importance in the fate of the penumbra, the aim of the present study was to characterize the penumbral microcirculatory changes, in terms of capillary perfusion, associated with these electrophysiological phenomena. To that end, microcirculation was visualized in real-time by laser scanning confocal fluorescence microscopy [9] and DC-potential shifts were measured during 2-h middle cerebral artery occlusion, and 1-h reperfusion in a cortical penumbral area.

2. Materials and methods

2.1. Confocal microscopy

A detailed description of the method has been published [9]. In brief, the rat cortical microcirculation was explored through a closed cranial window, using a BioRad View-scan confocal laser scanning unit attached to a Nikon Optiphot-2 microscope. The light source was an argon–krypton laser. Fluorescein-isothiocyanate (FITC)-Dextran was injected into the blood circulation to visualize the microvessels and delineate their lumen. FITC-labeled erythrocytes were injected via the same route at a tracer dose (<2%) to study capillary perfusion. The images were recorded at video speed (50/s) with a SIT camera and a PAL-VHS video recorder. The images were analyzed off-line to determine the vessel diameter and the velocity and flux of the fluorescent labeled erythrocytes through the capillaries.

2.2. Surgery

The experiments were performed on six male Sprague–Dawley rats (270–300 g) under halothane anesthesia. The rats were intubated and artificially ventilated. The femoral artery and vein were cannulated for blood pressure, blood gas, pH and hematocrit analysis, and for administration of the fluorescent tracers, respectively. Rectal temperature was kept close to 37.5 °C throughout the experiment. A closed cranial window was performed over the right frontoparietal cortex, as previously described [9]. In addition, electrodes were placed to record the DC potential and electrocorticogram (ECoG). Finally, in order to induce reversible focal cerebral ischemia under the confocal microscope, a remotely controlled intraluminal middle cerebral artery (MCA) occlusion [10] was prepared. An enlarged nylon suture was advanced from the external carotid artery (ECA) into the internal carotid artery 5 mm after the external skull base. The portion of the thread remaining outside the ECA stump was inserted into a catheter and secured.

2.3. Experimental protocol

The rat was placed under the confocal microscope and its head was immobilized with a device closely fitting the confocal microscope stage. FITC-Dextran (molecular weight=70,000) diluted in 0.9% NaCl (2.5 mg/ml) was injected intravenously (0.5 ml), followed by FITC-labeled erythrocytes. The whole cranial window was systematically explored with a 10× objective. The most appropriate area of investigation (presence of at least one pial arteriole and a dense capillary network) was then chosen with a 20× objective lens. The intraparenchymal capillaries were visualized by changing the focus from the pial arterioles down to a depth of 200 μm beneath the surface of the brain. Recording sequences were performed during a control period, at the MCA occlusion, for the following 2 h, and when the thread was removed. Additional video recording was performed at the start of each neuronal depolarization seen on the DC potential. At the end of the experiment, all scars were carefully wound; the rat was extubated and returned to its cage. Twenty-four hours later, the brain was removed in order to perform classical histology for quantitative infarct volume measurement corrected for edema.

2.4. Statistical analysis

Statistical analyses were performed by ANOVA using Statview software (Abacus Concepts, USA), followed, when appropriate, by Fisher PLSD post hoc tests. Values are given as means ±S.D. and $p < 0.05$ was accepted as significant.

3. Results

3.1. Histopathology

Four rats had a cortical and subcortical infarct whose volume was $127.0 \pm 14.3 \text{ mm}^3$ (cortex $107.5 \pm 11.3 \text{ mm}^3$, subcortex $19.5 \pm 7.7 \text{ mm}^3$). Two rats exhibited a subcortical infarct only ($18.9 \pm 1.3 \text{ mm}^3$).

3.2. Physiological parameters

Physiological variables were kept within the normal range throughout the experiment. The hematocrit was not significantly modified by the tracer injection.

3.3. MCA occlusion

The advancement of the thread up to the MCA branching induced a reduction of ECoG amplitude, a visible reduction of the flow speed through the microvessels, and frequent changes in the arteriole diameters. The mean diameter of arterioles under investigation was 33 ± 12 μm and it was nonsignificantly increased under ischemia by $107\pm18\%$ (Fig. 1), while the erythrocyte velocity through the capillaries was significantly reduced from 0.51 ± 0.19 to 0.33 ± 0.14 mm/s. In addition, the blood flow was sluggish in the venules. Transient stops in arteriole blood flow or reversals of the flow direction occurred frequently in five ischemic rats. Erythrocyte circulation through the capillaries remained irregular and depressed, but was never completely stopped. Irreversible stops of plasma or erythrocyte flow through capillaries were never observed. A shift of the capillary bed with respect to the surface microvessels was observed as soon as 30 min after the occlusion in four rats, indicating the occurrence of brain edema.

3.4. SD-like depolarization

Spontaneous transient negative DC shifts were recorded in MCA-occluded rats (3–8/rat) over the 2 h of ischemia, with a mean duration of 2.0 ± 1.0 min. These DC shifts were accompanied by a significant transient increase in arteriole diameter by $119\pm23\%$ of the baseline (Fig. 1), and by a further decrease in the velocity of erythrocytes through the

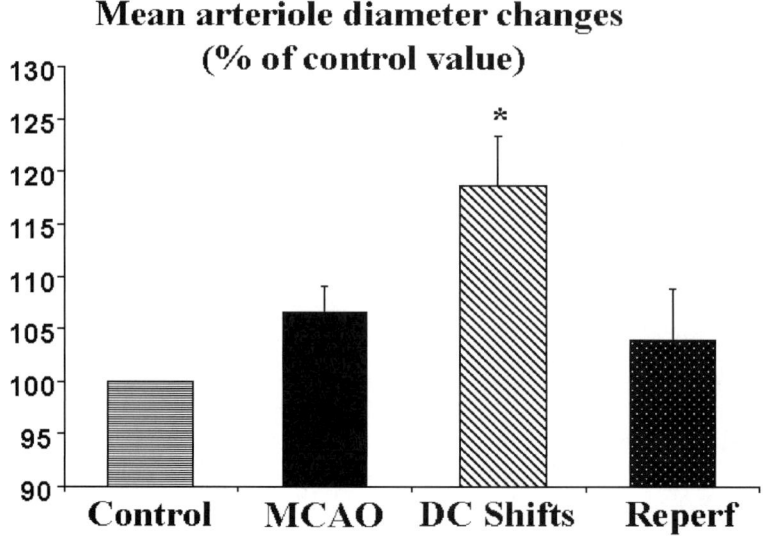

Fig. 1. Mean changes in arteriole diameter under MCA occlusion (MCAO) in the absence of negative DC shifts, during DC shifts (or SD-like depolarizations) spontaneously occurring in ischemic conditions and under reperfusion (Reperf). Values are expressed in percent of the control value (Control), i.e., before the MCA occlusion. *Significantly different from all other values (ANOVA: $p<0.029$; Fisher PLSD: $p<0.047$).

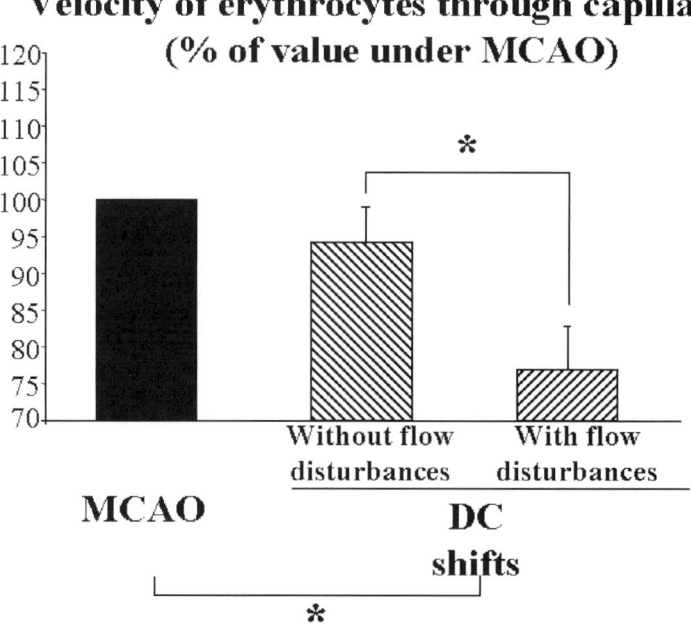

Fig. 2. Mean changes in velocity of fluorescent erythrocytes through capillaries under MCA occlusion (MCAO) and negative DC shifts, depending on the occurrence of transient disturbances in blood flow through the arterioles (arrest or reversal). *Fisher PLSD following a significant ANOVA ($p < 0.021$). In the comparison between with and without flow disturbances indicates a statistical difference at $p < 0.046$. In the comparison between MCAO and DC shifts: $p < 0.031$.

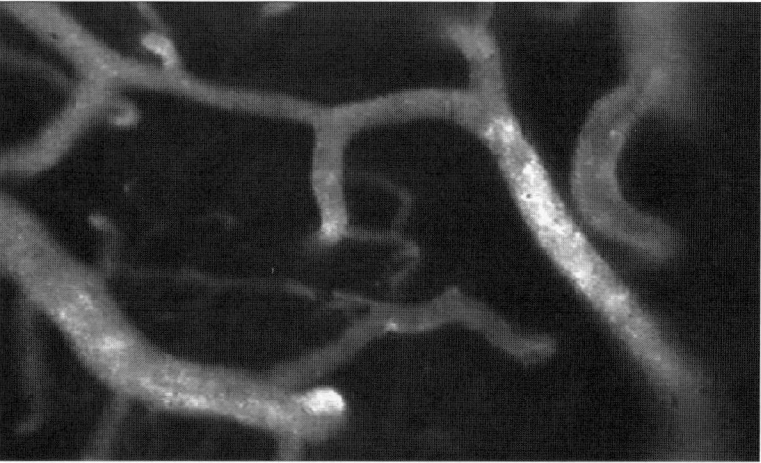

Fig. 3. A typical example of reversal of blood flow direction through an arteriole during a SD-like depolarization under MCA occlusion.

capillaries (Fig. 2). Brief stops or reversals of blood flow in the arterioles were frequent (41%) during SD-like depolarizations (Fig. 3). The comparison of erythrocyte velocity during DC shifts with versus without these hemodynamic disturbances indicated a significant difference between the two groups, with a further reduction ($\sim 20\%$) of the velocity of the erythrocytes through the capillaries when the flow disturbances occurred (Fig. 2).

3.5. Reperfusion

When the thread was removed, blood perfusion through all microcirculatory beds was instantaneously accelerated, without significant changes in arteriole and venule diameters. The velocity of fluorescent erythrocytes through the capillaries returned to its baseline value attaining 0.50 ± 0.24 mm/s. No capillary recruitment (i.e., newly perfused capillaries) was observed. No further DC shifts were recorded and ECoG recovered rapidly, although disturbances reappeared episodically.

4. Discussion

To better discuss the present data, it should be stressed that our exploration of microcirculation was done on very small caliber vessels at the pial level and at the very beginning of the penetrating level, as well as on intraparenchymal capillaries in the upper layers of the cortex by changing the focus of the confocal microscope.

The surrounding penumbra of evolving brain infarcts is known to have a highly dynamic structure. Our video recordings support such a dynamic aspect in terms of tissue perfusion and directly show that the penumbral microcirculatory events are extremely variable and heterogeneous from rat to rat, and also within the same rat. As shown by the histological analysis, the location of the penumbra was not reproducible, i.e., the ischemic lesion did not integrate the cortical penumbra in all rats. This means that our investigation was not devoted to similar parts of the penumbra. In case of striatal infarcts, we were exploring the external zone of the penumbra that will not be part of the infarct, whereas in the case of the cortico-striatal infarcts, we were exploring an inner zone of the penumbra. In the first case, a few SD-like depolarizations occurred, whereas in the second case, a large number of these depolarizations were recorded. Interestingly enough, despite the electrophysiological differences, no clear distinction could be made between these two cases on a microcirculatory point of view. This means that the microcirculatory changes that we have measured are not dependent on the localization of the measurement with respect to the final infarct location.

Transient or prolonged changes in arteriolar blood flow direction support a major role of the changes in perfusion pressure gradients in the regulation of penumbral blood flow. Redistribution of the blood flow seems to be due to mechanical factors such as a decrease in myogenic tone and a decrease in shear stress (shown to induce constrictions in pial arteries) [11] in anastomotic pathways, since both arteriole diameter and capillary erythrocyte velocity came back to their preocclusion level as soon as the thread was withdrawn. At that time, neuronal and glial events were involved in an irreversible process leading to tissue lesion in most rats, thus, suggesting that neither their metabolites nor the neurotransmitters could be the main actors in the regulatory mechanisms. Conversely, vasomotor mechanisms in endothelial and smooth muscle cells were still efficient since all of the arterioles reacted to the return of blood flow. As regards the hypothesized obstacles of capillary perfusion, the variable trajectory and the irregular time-course (with many interruptions) of the erythrocytes through the whole capillary network are not in favor of irreversible obstructions by leukocytes or compression by astrocytic endfeet [12]. Again, our data support a major role of perfusion pressure. Another reason to exclude the swelling of astrocytic endfeet as a cause of troubled capillary perfusion is the persistence of edema after MCA occlusion, while capillary perfusion regained its normal value.

During SD-like depolarizations, when no transient reversal of blood flow direction occurred, an increase in arteriole diameter and a decrease in erythrocyte velocity through the capillaries were measured. However, in case of arrest or reversal of arteriolar blood flow at the same time as the negative DC shift propagated, a further decrease in erythrocyte velocity was measured. This indicates that SD-like depolarizations are deleterious for the tissue, even in the external zone of the penumbra. A possible explanation of this paradoxical microcirculatory event is a "steal phenomenon". As already suggested, K^+ and various metabolites could be involved in arteriole dilatation at the pial level, but without affecting tissue capillary perfusion due to the low level of perfusion pressure and to the changes in pressure gradients.

4.1.3.6. On-Site Discussion

4.1.3.6.1. *Question: (Hotta)* Have you compared changes recorded by LDF metry with your microscopical observation?

Answer: (Pinard) Yes, but not in the same rats. In a recently published paper, Nallet et al. [Brain Res. 879 (2000) 122] reported that blood flow measured by LDF in similar experimental conditions either transiently and moderately increased or did not change during periinfarct depolarizations. This suggests that LDF does not reflect actual tissue blood flow changes under low flow conditions, as already shown by Hudetz et al. [Am. J. Physiol. 274 (1998) H982].

4.1.3.6.2. *Comment: (Strong)* In support of your second hypothesis (steal), we reported in a paper [J. Cereb. Blood Flow Metab. 3 (1983) 86], the observation that hydrogen clearance rate in the cat MCA occlusion penumbra (marginal gyrus, close to the anterior cerebral input) decreases transiently on the middle cerebral side of the interface, and simultaneously increases rearer the anterior cerebral side.

4.1.3.6.3. *Question: (Andrew)* Regarding the vascular effects that you observe in the penumbral region, can you comment on whether these effects are strictly a result of each SD-Iike events, or if these events may also promote continued SD events and ischemic changes?

Answer: (Pinard) It is clear that each transient negative shift in DC current was associated with the microvascular changes I have just described. So, I would say that they are a result of each SD-Iike event. However, it is not because two events occur concomitantly that they are causally related. Definitely, these events never promoted continued neuronal depolarizations in the area under investigation or induced repetitive SD events but, taking into account other data in the literature, we speculate that they contribute to ischemic changes, namely infarct core expansion.

References

[1] K.A. Hossmann, Periinfarct depolarizations, Cereb. Brain Metab. Rev. 8 (1996) 195–208.

[2] T.P. Obrenovitch, The ischaemic prenumbra: twenty years on, Cereb. Brain Metab. Rev. 7 (1995) 297–323.

[3] G. Mies, Blood flow dependent duration of cortical depolarizations in the periphery of focal ischemia of rat brain, Neurosci. Lett. 221 (1997) 165–168.

[4] T. Iijima, G. Mies, K.A. Hossmann, Repeated negative DC deflections in rat cortex following middle cerebral artery occlusion are abolished by MK-801: effect on volume of ischemic injury, J. Cereb. Blood Flow Metab. 12 (1992) 727–733.

[5] T. Back, K.A. Hossman, Cortical negative DC deflections following middle cerebral artery occlusion and KCl-induced spreading depression: effect on blood flow, tissue oxygenation, and electroencephalogram, J. Cereb. Blood Flow Metab. 14 (1994) 12–19.

[6] G. Mies, K. Kohno, K.A. Hossmann, Prevention of periinfarct direct current shifts with glutamate antagonist NBQX following occlusion of the middle cerebral artery in the rat, J. Cereb. Blood Flow Metab. 14 (1994) 802–807.

[7] H. Nallet, E.T. MacKenzie, S. Roussel, Haemodynamic correlates of penumbral depolarization following focal cerebral ischaemia, Brain Res. 879 (2000) 122–129.

[8] A.G. Hudetz, H. Shen, J.P. Kampine, Nitric oxide from neuronal NOS plays critical role in cerebral capillary flow response to hypoxia, Am. J. Physiol. 43 (1998) H982–H989.

[9] J. Seylaz, R. Charbonne, K. Nanri, D. Von Euw, J. Borredon, K. Kacem, P. Meric, E. Pinard, Dynamic in vivo measurement of erythrocyte velocity and flow in capillaries and of microvessel diameter in the rat brain by confocal laser microscopy, J. Cereb. Blood Flow Metab. 19 (1999) 863–870.

[10] S.A. Roussel, N. Van Bruggen, M.D. King, J. Houseman, S.R. Williams, D.G. Gadian, Monitoring the initial expansion of focal ischaemia changes by diffusion-weighted MRI using a remote controlled method of occlusion, NMR Biomed. 7 (1994) 21–28.

[11] R.M. Bryan, M.S. Steenberg, L.A. Schildmeyer, S.P. Marrelli, T.D. Johnson, Integrins mediate shear stress-induced constrictions in rat middle cerebral arteries, Soc. Neurosci. Abstr. 26 (2) (2000) 646.10.

[12] G.J. Del Zoppo, Microvascular changes during cerebral ischemia and reperfusion, Cereb. Brain Metab. Rev. 6 (1994) 47–96.

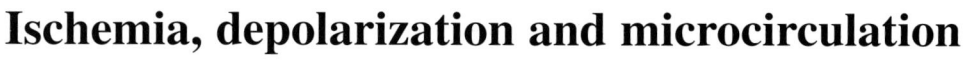

Ischemia, depolarization and microcirculation

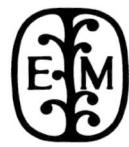

International Congress Series 1235 (2002) 457–464

Functional activation of peri-infarct tissue for prediction of recovery after focal ischemia

W.-D. Heiss*

Max-Planck-Institut für Neurologische Forschung, Gleueler Str. 50, 50931 Cologne, Germany

Abstract

In models of focal cerebral ischemia and in patients with ischemic stroke, functional disturbance and unresponsiveness to activation by specific tasks can be caused by irreversible morphologic destruction of the tissue by functional impairment in the penumbra, or by disconnection from the network by subcortical lesions. These three compartments can be distinguished by electro-physiological measures in the experimental models and by functional neuroimaging modalities in patients after having a stroke. The ability to (re)activate and (re)integrate important portions of a functional network can be tested by activation studies and has an impact on prognosis. Only if centers with a high hierarchy can be involved in a special task recovery will be satisfactory. The predominant activation of the secondary regions, which are usually not involved in task performance, permits only partial improvement, and the outcome is at a lower level. For the involvement of regions close to the damaged primary centers, neuronal plasticity may be responsible, and remote intrahemispheric activation and an interhemispheric shift of the activity to the contralateral network, might be due to the deficiency of collateral and transcallosal inhibition. The reviewed results prove that electrophysiological and neuroimaging studies can be used to assess the functional state of tissue after ischemia and may be of value for prediction of outcome in stroke patients. © 2002 Elsevier Science B.V. All rights reserved.

Keywords: Functional neuroimaging; Estimation of prognosis; Tissue viability; Evoked potentials; Reserve capacity; Functional activation

Recovery of disturbed neurologic function after an ischemic stroke is frequently seen. However, the mechanisms involved are ill defined and may be different in the various stages after the attack. Recovery of function early after the stroke is related to the volume of penumbra tissue that escapes infarction, and the resolution of edema may play a role in

* Tel.: +49-221-4726-220; fax: +49-221-4726-349.
E-mail address: wdh@pet.mpin-koeln.mpg.de (W.-D. Heiss).

this early stage. Later on, recruitment of additional neurons in the vicinity of a lesion and rearrangement of large-scale neural networks involving ipsilateral or even contralateral cortical areas, contribute to long-term improvements of disturbed neurologic function. Furthermore, appropriate training and targeted rehabilitation measures can support these mechanisms. For early prediction of the probability of functional recovery, the distinction between irreversibly damaged and functionally impaired but morphologically preserved tissue is necessary.

1. Experimental ischemia

The function of cortical tissue in ischemia can be disturbed by various pathophysiologic conditions: morphological damage, functional impairment, or disconnection, and deafferentation by subcortical lesions. The cortical function is impaired if the local blood flow decreases below the threshold for maintaining regular neuronal activity, morphologic damage develops if insufficient perfusion persists for a period of time, the duration of which is dependent on the extent of residual blood flow. Tissue perfused between these two limits is coined penumbra, which has the capacity to recover if perfusion is improved within the time window before irreversible damage occurs. Whereas the conditions leading to irreversible damage characterizing functional impairment of morphologically intact tissue (i.e., penumbra) have been studied extensively in animal models and in stroke patients [1–5], the third cause of disturbed cortical function, the disconnection or deafferentation by subcortical lesions, was less investigated and often escapes direct observation. These tissue compartments often exhibit decreased flow and metabolism due to a decreased functional state, which is caused by a lack of excitatory input (functional and metabolic deactivation, often referred to as diaschisis [6]).

Middle cerebral artery occlusion (MCAO) in the cat can be used as a model of ischemia, which clearly exhibits the various mechanisms of disturbed function. Simultaneous measurements of the regional blood flow, and determinations of cortical function by recording of spontaneous neuronal activity and evoked responses, permit the correlation of function to locally or remotely disturbed blood flow and to define thresholds for the maintenance of function. In addition, the transient ischemia model with reperfusion after defined occlusion times, can be used to determine the duration of a tolerable ischemic episode at a certain level of residual perfusion, and to define the time-dependent threshold for morphological integrity. This model was used to determine the effect of residual flow and length of ischemia on the viability of cortical neurons yielding the well-accepted curve, defining the survival threshold for neuronal tissue [7] (modified by Powers [8]) and separating reversible and irreversible ischemic damage.

Within the territory of the MCA, the various tissue compartments affected by the different pathophysiologic mechanisms can be distinguished [9]. In the core of the MCA territory, the ischemia is most severe; this area involves the ectosylvian cortex, and therefore, auditory evoked responses are affected and usually abolished, especially as a consequence of severe blood flow reduction. In this ischemic core, morphologic damage develops after a rather short period, and EP is irreversibly abolished after an occlusion period of 1 h, if residual flow is close to zero during the ischemic period. In areas surrounding the core of ischemia, the local blood flow is less affected during MCAO and is usually maintained at a level of 30–50% of control. In these areas, the pertinent evoked responses—somatosensory from front limb stimulation and visual EPs in posterior regions—disappear with some delay, indicating the progressive functional disturbance of the cortex. This progressive impairment and selective vulnerability of cortical function is also seen in a typical order of EP changes: postsynaptic—neuronal—components of EPs are lost at higher flow levels, whereas afferent—axonal—components are still recorded at lower residual flow [10]. These areas represent the penumbra and reperfusion after 1 h of MCAO, which usually leads to a complete recovery of the EPs, whereas recovery was incomplete after 2 h MCAO. In the area receiving the projections from the hind limb (posterior sigmoid gyrus), flow was not markedly affected by MCAO. However, the EPs disappeared with some delay, indicating ischemic impairment of afferent fiber tracts; in this area the EPs recovered completely after 1 h and to a high extent after 2 h of MCAO. The EPs to all multimodality stimulations persisted in the thalamic relay nuclei, where flow was not affected by MCAO.

Recording the activity of single cortical neurons can further elucidate the functional state of the tissue. In the area with severe ischemia (auditory area), evoked activity ceased within the first 2 min of MCAO, whereas in areas with mild ischemia (visual area, front limb representation) or intact perfusion (hind limb representation), evoked neuronal activity was abolished with a delay of 5–20 min. In contrast, spontaneous neuronal activity ceased only in the ischemic core, but was less affected in the mild ischemia area and unchanged in the non-ischemic region. As proof of selective afferent dysfunction, transcallosaly elicited responses could be recorded [11]. These results clearly demonstrate the different mechanisms-local damage, regionally impaired function, and deafferentation—leading to cortical and neurologic deficit.

2. Ischemic stroke

In patients with ischemic stroke, various tissue compartments can be distinguished early after the attack by functional neuroimaging modalities. In particular, positron emission tomography was instrumental in describing the various patterns and quantifying flow and metabolic changes characterizing irreversibly damaged tissue, functionally impaired but morphologically preserved cortex or intact but deafferented cortex. Usually, multitracer application and arterial blood sampling are necessary for these determinations, limiting their application in clinical routine or when potentially harmful therapeutic strategies, e.g., thrombolysis, are planned. As surrogate markers for tissue damage or penumbra in early stroke MRI procedures, Xe-CT and SPECT can be used (review in Ref. [5]). In the first hours after an ischemic stroke, irreversible morphological damage is indicated by a severe decrease of flow (5–12 ml/100 g/min) and/or of $CMRO_2$ (below 60 µmol/100 g/min), whereas in penumbra tissue, energy metabolism is preserved at a value above the threshold. A marker of neuronal integrity, the benzodiazepine receptor ligand flumazenil, predicts irreversible cortical damage if binding is decreased below 3.4 times the mean of white matter, and this result can be obtained non-invasively [12]. In the vicinity of developing or permanent infarcts, decreased glucose metabolism indicates a functionally deactivated cortex, which is usually preserved at follow-up, however, it may still correlate to neurologic deficits since this region is not integrated into the functional network.

Spontaneous neurologic recovery after a stroke is significantly related to the volume of penumbra tissue that escapes infarction [13,14]. As a consequence of the restoration of this penumbra tissue, functional activation may return in the immediate vicinity of a cortical infarct as observed with fMRI and finger tapping of the recovering hand [15]. However, left motor and sensory areas can also be activated by imagination of movement of the paretic hand, in patients with severe paresis of the right arm after a left striato–capsular lesion, indicating the disconnection of the functional cortex by subcortical damage. In addition to the location and the extent of the ischemic damage, the state of non-infarcted tissue in the hemisphere ipsilateral to the lesion is important for substantial recovery: diffuse damage to the tissue might have occurred previous to or concurrent with the stroke. The resulting neuronal loss, which decreases the reserve capacity of the tissue to cope with the defect, is reflected in a decreased metabolic rate at rest and a reduced response to functional activation [16].

The capacity for functional activation and reintegration into the network is of great importance for recovery of the neurologic deficits. Functional neuroimaging studies have given new insights into the changes of activation patterns, which accompany disturbed function and are responsible and reflect functional improvement [17]. Activation studies during performance or intention to perform impaired functions show the complex alternative routes within the functional network. However, the lack of clear relationships between effective performance and extent of activation of the compensatory routes may point to a hierarchy of the various structures in a network for efficient recovery.

Recruitment of the surviving neurons within the primary cortical area and of additional neurons in the direct vicinity, seems to be the most efficient method for regaining function. This mechanism is evident from electrophysiological studies in experimental models [18], but could also be deducted from investigations of stroke patients with transcranial magnetic stimulation: enlargement and displacement of the motor hand area on the affected hemisphere were seen with improvement of arm paresis after intensive rehabilitation therapy [19,20]. Reintegration of functionally impaired temporal areas was also demonstrated in patients who recovered substantially from post-stroke aphasia [21].

Activation of remote or even contralateral parts of the functional network is less efficient for recovery of the neurologic deficits. Results from activation studies during or after (partial) recovery of the motor function is controversial and still do not reveal a clear pattern. Patients with subcortical infarcts during intended movement, usually show activation of the sensorimotor and premotor cortex to the same extent as the normal [22–24], similar to the one observed when such movements are imagined indicating activation of the disconnected cortex. Bilateral activations of the premotor cortex and the supplementary motor areas were especially marked with recovery of hand function after acute severe hemiparesis [25], and activation was shifted posteriorly and enlarged with a lesion in the left fronto–parieto–temporal cortex [26]. It was interesting to note that activation in the sensorimotor cortex and in the parietal lobes with passive arm movements was significantly increased in patients that had not recovered [24]. Increased activity in the intact motor cortex, ipsilateral to the paretic side with movement of the paretic fingers, was regularly observed after recovery from a stroke [27]. However, the extent of the ipsilateral activation was not related to the functional recovery [28], and was even stronger in non-recovered hemiplegic patients [24].

In recovery from post-stroke aphasia, the involvement of the complex network and the hierarchy of different parts for achieving a satisfactory outcome, were studied in more detail in a group of 23 patients [21]. In the post-acute state with severe language disturbance, the activation during word repetition is shifted to regions of the right hemisphere (temporal and opercular regions) and in patients with temporal lesions also to the left Broca area. The outcome with satisfactory speech performance can only be reached if this shift of activation is reversed, and especially if left temporal areas are reintegrated into the functional network. Persisting activation in areas not involved in this task in normal humans—e.g., the left opercular region and the supplementary motor area—was found in patients achieving the lowest grade of improvement. There was also a difference in patients in whom the infarct was in the frontal or subcortical areas: only those reached a high level of language performance, who reactivated the left temporal areas. If this could not be achieved due to functional disconnection of the morphologically intact temporal gyrus, the outcome was less favorable and severe language dysfunction persisted. These results were confirmed in studies using fMRI to visualize speech-induced activation [29].

Shifts of eloquent regions observed with chronic lesions, e.g., brain tumors, may help to interpret the mechanisms involved in these compensatory processes [30]. With slowly progressing lesions within the left hemisphere, the specific areas activated during language tasks (verb generation) are dislocated, and regions usually not involved in healthy controls are activated in the ipsilateral hemisphere. Additionally, areas homotopic to the frontal and temporal language centers in the contralateral hemisphere can be activated and this interhemispheric shift can be reversed with improvement of language function after surgical removal of the tumor. This means that two different mechanisms are involved: an intrahemispheric and an interhemispheric transfer of activation. The intrahemispheric shift might be due to neuronal plasticity, involving undamaged neurons in the vicinity of the lesion in the performance of a task for which these neurons are usually not necessary (widening of primary areas, as shown in experimental models by Nudo et al. [18]). For the interhemispheric shift of activation, a more complex mechanism might be responsible: for the lateralization of specialized functions—e.g., language—transcallosal inhibition of the corresponding centers in the subdominant hemisphere seems to be necessary, and transcallosal inhibition of cortical areas was described during motor tasks [31] and language performance [32]. If the transcallosal projections are damaged, transcallosal inhibition is impaired [33], and contralateral homotopic areas are activated during language tasks [30,34]. A failure of collateral inhibition can also be responsible for the (re)activation of ipsilateral, more remote, and usually silent portions of a functional network. Both these disinhibition phenomena can be studied by functional neuroimaging in neurologic patients and followed also during rehabilitation by evaluating various therapeutic strategies.

4.2.2.5. On-Site Discussion

4.2.1.5.1. *Question: (Strong)* Are there any data on the influence of different rehabilitation strategies on functional recovery as measured by imaging?

Answer: (Heiss) Data on the effect of different rehabilitation procedures are still scarce. We have done a double-blind controlled study on the effect of adjuvant drug therapy for recovery of posts stroke aphasia. With the drug (Piracetam, 2×2.4 g/day) the extent of activation in the left temporal language areas was significantly higher than in the placebo group—and the drug group also reached higher scores of language performance (Kessler et al., Stroke 2000; 31: 2112).

4.2.1.5.2. *Question: (Ances)* Have you looked at any recovery paradigms that could lead to an increase in activation in the peri-infarct area?

Answer: (Heiss) In addition to the data mentioned in my previous answer (4.2.1.5.1.), we did not test the effect of different rehabilitation procedures on activation patterns, but this would certainly be interesting for testing the effect of "force-induced" motor rehabilitation.

4.2.1.5.3. *Question: (Nemoto)* I noted that in one of your CBF maps by PET, you have indicated at $12-25$ ml/100 g/min range. Is the 12 ml/100 g/min your cut-off or lower limit for the CBF image?

Answer: (Heiss) For the definition of cortical ischemia, we have used two different limits. The lower one—at 12 ml/100 g/min, as the cortical level for ischemic change—but with the clear definition of irreversible change with Flumazenil, this threshold could be set to a lower value. The upper one, the upper limit of penumbra, was set originally to $18-22$ ml/ 100 g/min, but recently could be more clearly defined by a statistical approach (95% probability of survival) to be at 14.1 ml/100 min.

4.2.1.5.4. *Question: (Naritomi)* In the acute phase of stroke, cerebral blood flow and metabolism are completely depressed in the contralateral cerebellar hemisphere or cerebral hemisphere due to diaschisis. In the later phase, these remote areas show high flow or metabolism when the primary ischemic area tries to be activated. The presence or absence of remote area metabolic depression may be related with the extents of functional recovery. How do you think about the relationship between the diaschisis and the functional recovery?

Answer: (Heiss) If an activation is observed during task performance (speaking) in the ipsilateral hemisphere outside the infarct, there is also an activation within the contralateral cerebellum, which was affected by diaschisis. That means, that diaschisis could be reversed with activation—and the activation pattern including the effect on the cerebellum was related to improved recovery.

References

[1] J. Astrup, B.K. Siesjö, L. Symon, Thresholds in cerebral ischemia—the ischemic penumbra, Stroke 12 (6) (1981) 723–725.
[2] W.-D. Heiss, R. Graf, The ischemic penumbra, Curr. Opin. Neurol. 7 (1) (1994) 11–19.
[3] K.-A. Hossmann, Viability thresholds and the penumbra of focal ischemia, Ann. Neurol. 36 (4) (1994) 557–565.
[4] J.-C. Baron, Mapping the ischaemic penumbra with PET: implications for acute stroke treatment, Cerebrovasc. Dis. 9 (1999) 193–201.

[5] W.-D. Heiss, Ischemic penumbra: evidence from functional imaging in man, J. Cereb. Blood Flow Metab. 20 (9) (2000) 1276–1293.

[6] D.M. Feeney, J.C. Baron, Diaschisis, Stroke 17 (1986) 817–830.

[7] W.-D. Heiss, G. Rosner, Functional recovery of cortical neurons as related to degree and duration of ischemia, Ann. Neurol. 14 (3) (1983) 294–301.

[8] W.J. Powers, Hemodynamics and metabolism in ischemic cerebrovascular disease, Neurol. Clin. 10 (1992) 31–48.

[9] K. Kataoka, R. Graf, G. Rosner, W.-D. Heiss, Experimental focal ischemia in cats: changes in multimodality evoked potentials as related to local cerebral blood flow and ischemic brain edema, Stroke 18 (1) (1987) 188–194.

[10] C. Umbach, W.-D. Heiss, H. Traupe, Effect of graded ischemia on functional coupling and components of somatosensory evoked potentials, J. Cereb. Blood Flow Metab. 1 (Suppl. 1) (1981) 198–199.

[11] R. Graf, K. Kataoka, G. Rosner, W.-D. Heiss, Cortical deafferentation in cat focal ischemia: disturbance and recovery of sensory functions in cortical areas with different degrees of cerebral blood flow reduction, J. Cereb. Blood Flow Metab. 6 (5) (1986) 566–573.

[12] W.-D. Heiss, L.W. Kracht, A. Thiel, M. Grond, G. Pawlik, Penumbral probability thresholds of cortical flumazenil binding and blood flow predicting tissue outcome in patients with cerebral ischaemia, Brain 124 (2001) 20–29.

[13] M. Furlan, G. Marchal, F. Viader, J.M. Derlon, J.-C. Baron, Spontaneous neurological recovery after stroke and the fate of the ischemic penumbra, Ann. Neurol. 40 (2) (1996) 216–226.

[14] W.-D. Heiss, L. Kracht, M. Grond, J. Rudolf, B. Bauer, K. Wienhard, G. Pawlik, Early [^{11}C]Flumazenil/H$_2$O positron emission tomography predicts irreversible ischemic cortical damage in stroke patients receiving acute thrombolytic therapy, Stroke 31 (2) (2000) 366–369.

[15] S.C. Cramer, G. Nelles, R.R. Benson, J.D. Kaplan, R.A. Parker, K.K. Kwong, D.N. Kennedy, S.P. Finklestein, B.R. Rosen, A functional MRI study of subjects recovered from hemiparetic stroke, Stroke 28 (12) (1997) 2518–2527.

[16] W.-D. Heiss, J. Kessler, H. Karbe, G.R. Fink, G. Pawlik, Cerebral glucose metabolism as a predictor of recovery from aphasia in ischemic stroke, Arch. Neurol. 50 (9) (1993) 958–964.

[17] K. Herholz, W.-D. Heiss, Functional imaging correlates of recovery after stroke in humans, J. Cereb. Blood Flow Metab. 20 (2000) 1619–1631.

[18] R.J. Nudo, B.M. Wise, F. SiFuentes, G.W. Milliken, Neural substrates for the effects of rehabilitative training on motor recovery after ischemic infarct, Science 272 (5269) (1996) 1791–1794.

[19] P. Cicinelli, R. Traversa, P.M. Rossini, Post-stroke reorganization of brain motor output to the hand: a 2–4 month follow-up with focal magnetic transcranial stimulation, Electroencephalogr. Clin. Neurophysiol. 105 (6) (1997) 438–450.

[20] J. Liepert, W.H. Miltner, H. Bauder, M. Sommer, C. Dettmers, E. Taub, C. Weiller, Motor cortex plasticity during constraint-induced movement therapy in stroke patients, Neurosci. Lett. 250 (1) (1998) 5–8.

[21] W.-D. Heiss, J. Kessler, A. Thiel, M. Ghaemi, H. Karbe, Differential capacity of left and right hemispheric areas for compensation of poststroke aphasia, Ann. Neurol. 45 (4) (1999) 430–438.

[22] C. Weiller, F. Chollet, K.J. Friston, R.J.S. Wise, R.S.J. Frackowiak, Functional reorganization of the brain in recovery from striatocapsular infarction in man, Ann. Neurol. 31 (5) (1992) 463–472.

[23] B. Weder, U. Knorr, H. Herzog, B. Nebeling, A. Kleinschmidt, Y. Huang, H. Steinmetz, H.J. Freund, R.J. Seitz, Tactile exploration of shape after subcortical ischemic infarction studied with PET, Brain 117 (1994) 593–605.

[24] G. Nelles, G. Spiekermann, M. Jueptner, G. Leonhardt, S. Müller, H. Gerhard, H.C. Diener, Reorganization of sensory and motor systems in hemiplegic stroke patients. A positron emission tomography study, Stroke 30 (8) (1999) 1510–1516.

[25] R.J. Seitz, P. Hoflich, F. Binkofski, L. Tellmann, H. Herzog, H.J. Freund, Role of the premotor cortex in recovery from middle cerebral artery infarction, Arch. Neurol. 55 (8) (1998) 1081–1088.

[26] P.M. Rossini, C. Caltagirone, A. Castriota-Scanderbeg, P. Cicinelli, C. Delgratta, M. Demartin, V. Pizzella, R. Traversa, G.L. Romani, Hand motor cortical area reorganization in stroke: a study with fMRI, MEG and TCS maps, NeuroReport 9 (9) (1998) 2141–2146.

[27] F. Chollet, V. Di Piero, R.J.S. Wise, D.J. Brooks, R.J. Dolan, R.S.J. Frackowiak, The functional anatomy of

motor recovery after stroke in humans: a study with positron emission tomography, Ann. Neurol. 29 (1) (1991) 63–71.

[28] Y. Cao, L. D'Olhaberriague, E.M. Vikingstad, S.R. Levine, K.M.A. Welch, Pilot study of functional MRI to assess cerebral activation of motor function after poststroke hemiparesis, Stroke 29 (1) (1998) 112–122.

[29] Y. Cao, E.M. Vikingstad, K.P. George, A.F. Johnson, K.M.A. Welch, Cortical language activation in stroke patients recovering from aphasia with functional MRI, Stroke 30 (11) (1999) 2331–2340.

[30] A. Thiel, Plasticity of language networks in patients with brain tumors, A PET activation study, Ann. Neurol. 50 (2001) 620–629.

[31] T. Kujirai, M.D. Caramia, J.C. Rothwell, B.L. Day, P.D. Thompson, A. Ferbert, S. Wroe, P. Asselman, C.D. Marsden, Corticocortical inhibition in human motor cortex, J. Physiol. 471 (1993) 501–519.

[32] H. Karbe, K. Herholz, M. Halber, W.-D. Heiss, Collateral inhibition of transcallosal activity facilitates functional brain asymmetry, J. Cereb. Blood Flow Metab. 18 (10) (1998) 1157–1161.

[33] B. Boroojerdi, K. Diefenbach, A. Ferbert, Transcallosal inhibition in cortical and subcortical cerebral vascular lesions, J. Neurol. Sci. 144 (1–2) (1996) 160–170.

[34] O.A. Selnes, The ontogeny of cerebral language dominance, Brain Lang. 71 (1) (2000) 217–220.

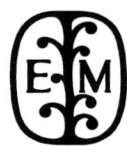

International Congress Series 1235 (2002) 465–474

Ischemic depression of neuronal activity: real time comparison between DC potential changes and alterations of ion and transmitter homeostasis

Rudolf Graf*, Hiroyuki Nozaki, Shingo Toyota, Kouichi Ohta, Mario Valentino, Eiji Kumura, Christian Dohmen, Takayuki Sakaki, Gerhard Rosner, Wolf-Dieter Heiss

Max-Planck-Institut für neurologische Forschung, Gleueler Str. 50, 50931 Cologne, Germany

Abstract

The initial phase of brain ischemia sets the scene for final functional disturbance and tissue damage. Important contributors in the course of early events are tissue depolarization and breakdown of ion and of transmitter homeostasis including transmitter-gated ion channel opening. To relate these events to the severity of cerebral blood flow (CBF) reduction, we used two ischemia models in cats: a global model produced complete ischemia and a focal model produced gradual reductions in the CBF. We employed ion-selective microelectrodes in combination with microdialysis/HPLC to detect direct current (DC) potential and extracellular calcium as well as amino acids and purine catabolites. Additionally, we used amperometric glutamate electrodes for rapid detection of glutamate. Most regions exhibited tissue depolarization and were, therefore, denominated as severely ischemic. An extracellular decrease in calcium and an increase in glutamate were associated with depolarization. The temporal pattern of changes differed among models and regions: the initial phase took less than 10 min in global but up to 30 min in focal ischemia. Since extracellular adenosine as a marker of ATP depletion exhibited similar temporal variability in the various regions, we suggest that minor, not easily detectable, perfusional and metabolic differences are responsible for major differences in the pathophysiology of the initial phase of brain ischemia. © 2002 Elsevier Science B.V. All rights reserved.

Keywords: Cerebral ischemia; Cerebral blood flow; Cortical direct current potential; Calcium ion; Glutamate

* Corresponding author. Fax: +49-221-4726-298.
  E-mail address: rudolf.graf@pet.mpin-koeln.mpg.de (R. Graf).

0531-5131/02 © 2002 Elsevier Science B.V. All rights reserved.
PII: S 0 5 3 1 - 5 1 3 1 (0 2) 0 0 2 1 4 - 5

1. Introduction

After induction of global brain ischemia, as for example, associated with cardiac arrest, higher functions such as consciousness or spontaneous electrical activity are lost within seconds. Soon thereafter, within minutes, metabolism ceases. Ion homeostasis at cellular membranes breaks down and ions distribute more or less according to their electrochemical gradients. Very early in this sequence of events, a negative shift of the cortical direct current (DC) potential is observed, typically referred to as "anoxic depolarization" [1–3]. The DC potential reflects changes in the membrane potentials of the neurons and glial cells surrounding an extracellular electrode [1,4]. As transmitter release and re-uptake are closely coupled to depolarization and transmembrane ion gradients, homeostasis of various neuroactive substances such as glutamate or GABA seems to be disturbed as well, already in the initial phase of ischemia. Studies on the rapid changes of glutamate, however, are rare [5,6], and simultaneous measurements of ion concentrations, e.g., of calcium, are lacking.

Focal ischemia differs from global ischemia in two major aspects [7]. First, cerebral blood flow (CBF) reduction is, in general, less severe than in global ischemia, and the rate of energy depletion may, therefore, differ between the two types of ischemia. Second, it produces spatial gradients of CBF reduction. Ischemia is severe in core regions, moderate in regions adjacent to the core, typically referred to as the ischemic penumbra [8], and mild in more peripheral regions. Penumbral tissue is still viable when reperfused but metabolically compromised, and it may spread out with time to neighboring regions leaving fatal tissue behind [9,10]. As regards gradual reductions of CBF and metabolism, changes of the DC potential and ion gradients have been shown to differ in focal ischemia compared to those in global ischemia [11]. In particular, the course of ischemic shifts and the DC potential of the ions are slowed down.

In the studies reported here, we aimed to determine disturbances of ion and transmitter homeostasis in relation to different degrees of CBF reduction, metabolic derangement, and tissue depolarization. For that purpose, we applied both a global and a focal model of brain ischemia in cats and several techniques were used to simultaneously measure the CBF, DC potential, extracellular calcium ($[Ca^{2+}]_o$), and glutamate in various brain regions.

2. Materials and methods

The studies reported here were approved by the local Animal Care Committee and the Regierungsprasident of Cologne and are in compliance with the German Laws for Animal Protection. The cats were artificially ventilated with a 70%/30% NO_2/O_2 gas mixture. In the global ischemia experiments, they were anesthetized with α-chloralose. Measurements were performed in cortical gray matter (GM) and subcortical white matter (WM). The regional cerebral blood flow (CBF) was measured either by laser Doppler probes (Moor Instruments, UK) placed on the cortical surface or by platinum electrodes that measured hydrogen clearance. Self-manufactured double-barreled ion-selective microelectrodes measured $[Ca^{2+}]_o$ and on the reference channel cortical DC potential. Microdialysis (membranes: 0.4 μm in diameter) in combination with HPLC measured extracellular amino acids and purine catabolites. In additional experiments, a dialysis electrode (Sycopel

International, UK) perfused with artificial cerebrospinal fluid containing glutamate oxidase at a constant flow measured the extracellular glutamate concentration amperometrically [6]. Either a 10-min transient or 1-h permanent global ischemia was induced by bilateral temporary occlusion of the subclavian and common carotid arteries.

In the focal ischemia experiments, the cats were also artificially ventilated; however, this time they were anesthetized with 0.8–1.5% halothane. Measurements were performed similar to those described for global ischemia. The recording sites were different: parallel measurements were regularly obtained from ectosylvian, suprasylvian, or marginal gyri representing regions with a gradual CBF alteration in the ischemic focus. The proximal left middle cerebral artery (MCA) was prepared transorbitally, and a device for remote occlusion was implanted [12]. In the experiments reported here, either permanent or 60-min transient MCA occlusion was applied.

3. Results

We will first describe alterations of the various parameters observed in the initial phase after induction of global ischemia. This model was characterized by an almost complete reduction of CBF. For comparison regarding different rates of metabolic derangement, we

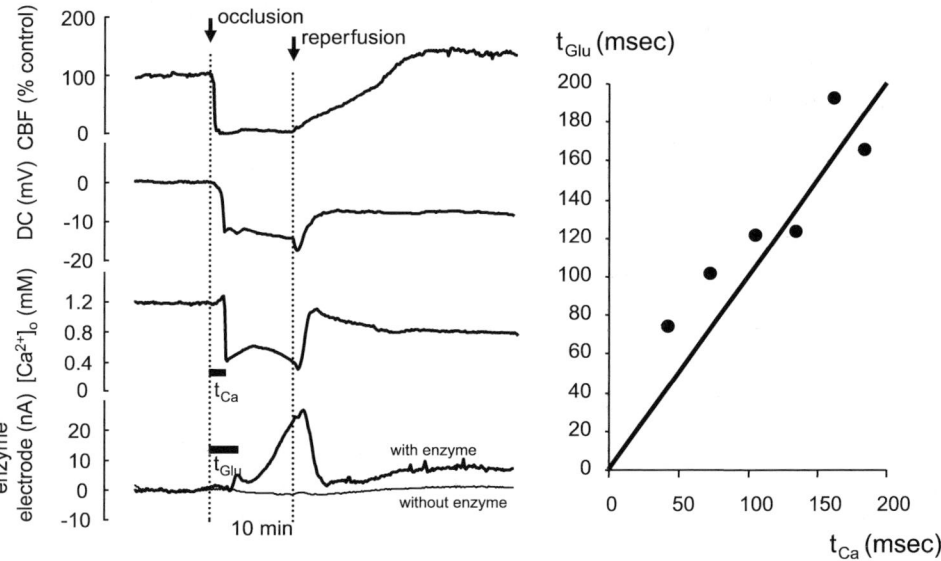

Fig. 1. Left: Actual recordings of CBF, DC potential, $[Ca^{2+}]_o$, and amperogram of glutamate electrodes during 10 min of global ischemia and reperfusion. Glutamate electrode calibration showed good linear correlation between the glutamate concentration and oxidation current (nA) produced by glutamate oxidation. Since the glutamate electrode measures directly in the tissue, time course recordings are without relevant delay compared with recordings of other variables. t_{Ca} and t_{Glu}: time points of early $[Ca^{2+}]_o$ minima and glutamate maxima. Right: Comparison of the exact time points of t_{Ca} and t_{Glu} for single experiments. The time points correlated significantly ($p < 0.05$, Spearman's correlation coefficient).

evaluated in this model both the cortical gray and subcortical white matter compartments. Second, we will describe the results derived from measurements in different regions of focal ischemia.

Just after the induction of transient 10-min global ischemia (Fig. 1, left side), the cortical CBF decreased steeply and the electrocorticogram (not shown) became flat. The DC potential dropped by about 15 mV, and its steep decline was finished about 2 min after occlusion. $[Ca^{2+}]_o$ and glutamate showed biphasic alterations with the first steep decline of $[Ca^{2+}]_o$ preceding the first rise of glutamate and the first minimum of $[Ca^{2+}]_o$ preceding the first little maximum of glutamate by some seconds. A second rise of glutamate starting at about 5 min after occlusion was only paralleled by a small secondary drop of $[Ca^{2+}]_o$. After recirculation, the various parameters were recovered with different time courses. $[Ca^{2+}]_o$, and glutamate recovered first, reaching control levels within about 5 min. CBF recovery was relatively slow in this particular case, and hypoperfusion was seen for about 10–15 min after arterial reopening. Later on, CBF turned into hyperperfusion. Electrocorticogram recovery was also slow and not yet completed at the end of the observation period.

In Fig. 2, the course of the DC potential, $[Ca^{2+}]_o$, and of extracellular glutamate is shown during 120 min of global ischemia in relation to the changes of adenosine, an intermediate

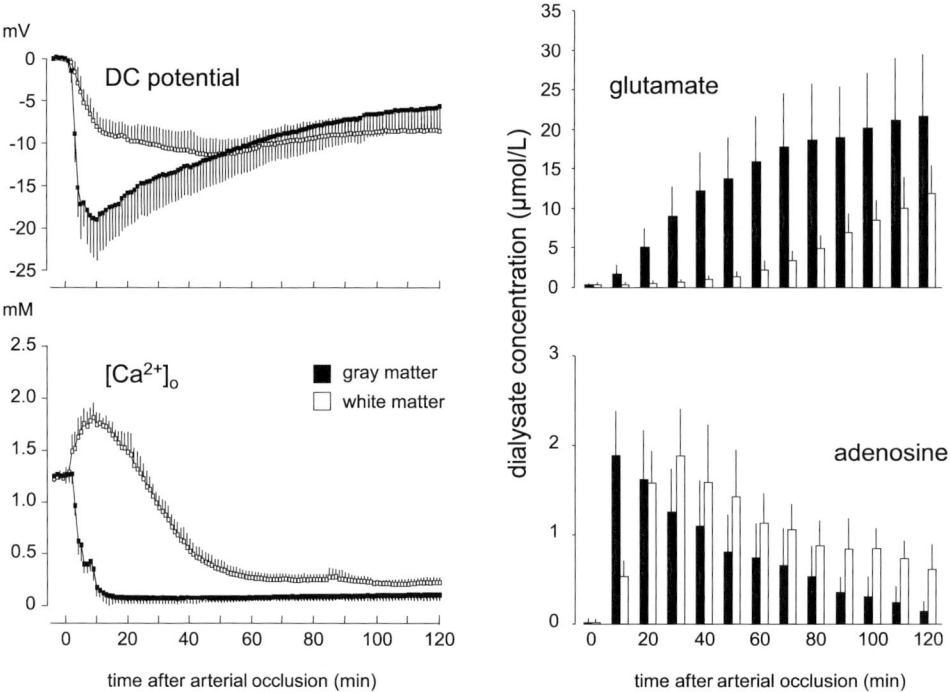

Fig. 2. Changes in the DC potential, $[Ca^{2+}]_o$, extracellular glutamate, and adenosine measured in the cortical gray matter (GM) and subcortical white matter (WM) during 120 min of global ischemia. Data (means±S.D.) were sampled every minute for the DC potential and $[Ca^{2+}]_o$, and every 10 min for glutamate and adenosine. Note the slower course of alteration of all variables after induction of ischemia in the WM compartment and, in particular, the delayed response of $[Ca^{2+}]_o$.

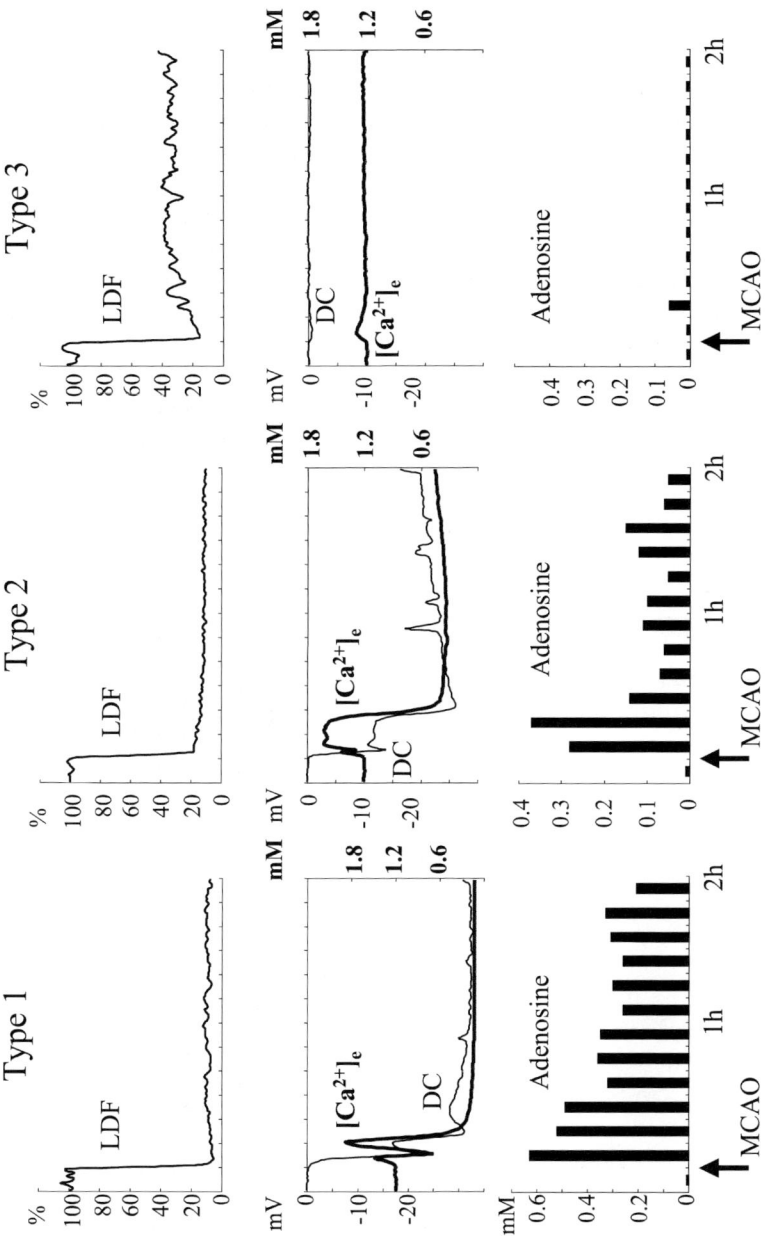

Fig. 3. Three types of initial changes in CBF measured by laser Doppler flowmetry (LDF), direct current (DC) potential, $[Ca^{2+}]_o$ and extracellular adenosine in different regions of an ischemic focus. Actual recordings of type 1 resemble fast responses seen in global ischemia, with adenosine peaking in the first dialysate sample taken after arterial occlusion. In comparison, recordings of type 2 show delayed responses in the DC potential and $[Ca^{2+}]_o$. Adenosine peaks only in the second sample suggesting a slower depletion of ATP, even though LDF does not provide major differences. Even in recordings of type 3, pronounced changes of LDF were obtained, whereas the other variables remained almost unchanged.

product of purine catabolism that served as a rather fast metabolic marker [13]. Comparative measurements in GM and WM revealed the importance of the rate of metabolic decay. After the onset of ischemia, the DC potential rapidly decreased in GM. Thereafter, it tended to shift back to higher values. In WM, the negative shift of the DC potential was slower and smaller. Interestingly, a remarkable change in the rate of depolarization from fast to slow was observed in WM 10 min after the onset of ischemia. After reaching the minimum, the DC potential in WM tended to shift back, too; however, the values remained lower than in GM. $[Ca^{2+}]_o$ steeply declined in GM during the first minutes of ischemia, reaching minimal levels already 15 min after occlusion. In contrast, $[Ca^{2+}]_o$ in WM increased during the early period of ischemia, reaching a maximum 10 min after occlusion. It decreased slowly thereafter and fell below the control values only 30 min after the occlusion and reached its final level after about 60 min. Ischemic extracellular accumulation of glutamate was immediate in GM and delayed by almost 1 h in WM. The slope of the glutamate increase was steeper in the early phase of ischemia and reached a plateau almost 1 h after the induction of ischemia, whereas the accumulation rate of glutamate in WM was continuous until the end of the observation period. Adenosine reached a maximum in GM after 10 min of ischemia and returned roughly to the control levels over the following 2 h of ischemia. In WM, adenosine started to increase promptly after the onset of ischemia, too; however, the slope of this increase was not as steep.

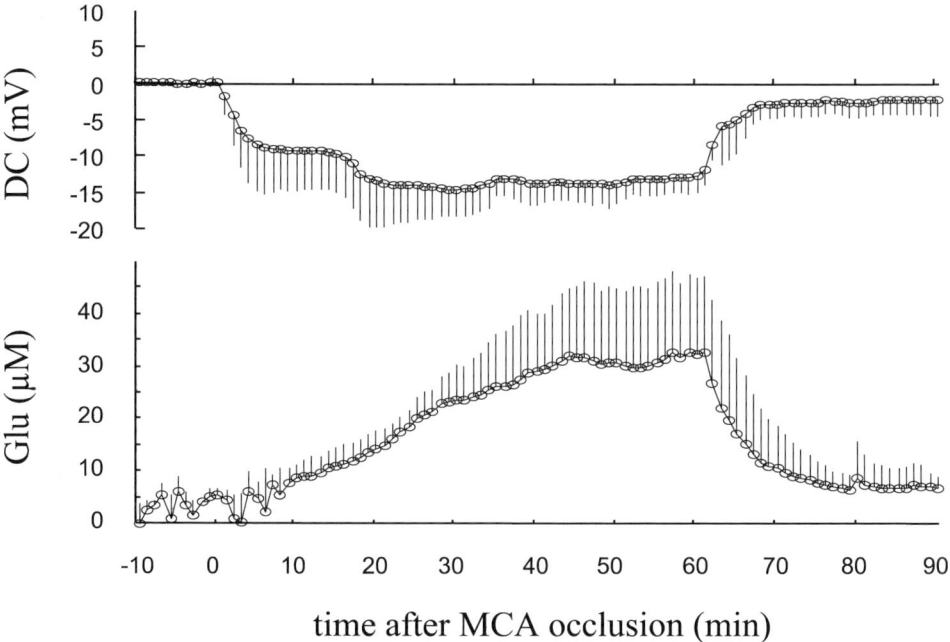

Fig. 4. Changes in the direct current (DC) potential and extracellular glutamate measured in the cortex (ectosylvian gyrus) during 60 min of focal ischemia and reperfusion. Data (means±S.D.) were sampled every minute. Extracellular concentrations of glutamate have been recalculated according to in vitro calibration of amperographic recordings with the glutamate electrode. Note the biphasic course of the negative shift of the DC potential and the somewhat delayed increase of glutamate.

A maximum concentration was only reached in the 30-min sample. Following this peak, the concentration slowly declined, staying well above GM values until the end of the observation period.

In comparison with global ischemia, ischemic alterations of the various parameters varied in focal ischemia depending on the recording site and on the severity of CBF reduction. In Fig. 3, this variability is documented by showing three representative sets of recordings. In type 1, immediate responses after the onset of ischemia are fast, resembling the responses described for global ischemia. The biphasic decay of the DC potential and of $[Ca^{2+}]_o$, however, is more pronounced. Adenosine peaks in the dialysate sample were taken in the first 10 min after arterial occlusion. In comparison, recordings of type 2 show delayed responses in DC potential and $[Ca^{2+}]_o$. The delayed $[Ca^{2+}]_o$ response is of particular interest since it resembles the delayed response seen in global, complete ischemia in the WM compartment (see Fig. 2). Obviously, tissue under conditions of type 2 is less compromised than that of type 1. This is underlined by measurements of adenosine, which peaks only in the second 10-min sample suggesting a slower depletion of ATP, even though alterations of laser Doppler flowmetry (LDF) seem to be very similar in the two presented examples. Even in recordings of type 3, pronounced changes of LDF were obtained. However, in this example, the other variables showed only minor changes documenting a subcritical stage of energy depletion that did not result in an immediate loss of ion homeostasis.

In Fig. 4, biphasic DC potential changes of type 2 during 60-min MCA occlusion and subsequent reperfusion were summarized and compared with extracellular glutamate changes obtained with glutamate electrodes. A biphasic response of glutamate was not as obvious as in the global ischemia experiments. Particularly, the first glutamate peak was not regularly seen. This may derive from the larger heterogeneity among regions in an ischemic focus. Even the small distances between insertion sites of ion-selective and glutamate electrodes may have added to higher variability. A pronounced steady rise of glutamate started only around 10 min after occlusion and continued thereafter throughout the ischemic episode. Upon reperfusion, both $[Ca^{2+}]_o$ and glutamate concentrations recovered almost to baseline levels.

4. Discussion

The early phase of brain ischemia may initiate later loss of function and damage of tissue. According to studies in global ischemia and anoxia, it is known that the early or initial phase takes only several minutes. Changes in the cortical DC potential have been described to develop in three phases [14]. In the first phase, the DC potential may show either a hyper- or hypopolarizations [14–19]. Second, a dramatic phase of steep negative deflection follows, which is usually denominated as anoxic depolarization [14]. It is followed by a third phase, which is characterized by a slower decrease in the DC potential before a final state of depolarization is reached. It has been revealed by ion-selective microelectrode recordings that these three phases of DC potential changes are accompanied by three phases of changes in $[K^+]_o$ and $[Ca^{2+}]_o$: in the first phase, $[K^+]_o$ and $[Ca^{2+}]_o$ show slow and small increases; in the second phase, $[K^+]_o$ manifests a rapid and large increase and $[Ca^{2+}]_o$ shows an abrupt drop; and finally, $[K^+]_o$ gradually increases and $[Ca^{2+}]_o$ gradually decreases in the third phase.

Our findings in global ischemia indicate that in the early sequence of events, glutamate follows a biphasic course as has been shown before [6,20]. This biphasic change is thought to reflect synaptic release followed by the reversal of glutamate re-uptake [6]. Evidence for the synaptic release is presented by our findings of a very close relationship between early extracellular decline in $[Ca^{2+}]_o$ and a rise in glutamate because $[Ca^{2+}]_o$ influx is thought to induce synaptic vesicular release of glutamate. Since the second large rise in glutamate is not correlated with any further $[Ca^{2+}]_o$ decrease, we speculate that this is mainly caused by nonsynaptic mechanisms including reversal of glutamate uptake. Evidence for this speculation could be provided, e.g., by measurement of other ion activities since glutamate uptake is coupled to transmembrane ion gradients, in particular, that of Na^+ and K^+. Negative DC potential shifts measured in the study are highly indicative of such ion gradient changes. The secondary rise of $[Ca^{2+}]_o$ and glutamate may be additionally explained by other factors, e.g., shrinkage of extracellular space, which has been demonstrated to play a role in early ischemia [21]. The results obtained in cerebral WM during global ischemia document that differences in the rate of metabolic decay may be the main causes for the differences in the course of events, i.e., the faster ATP depletion in areas in which metabolic markers such as adenosine appear faster in the extracellular space.

Our findings in focal ischemia indicate that the time course of changes in the initial phase is more variable than those in global ischemia. They also confirm the notion that differences in the rate of ATP depletion as deducible from extracellular changes of adenosine (or other purine catabolites not shown here) are relevant for the various courses. Three types of DC potential alteration and concomitant changes of $[Ca^{2+}]_o$ have been defined [11]. Type 3 was found in the cortex if the CBF reduction stayed above the upper CBF threshold of the ischemic penumbra [8,22]. Absence of ion-homeostasis disturbances is verified by stable DC potential and $[Ca^{2+}]_o$. Types 1 and 2 are observed in the core of focal ischemia with residual CBF below 20% of the control, documenting that even in the core of focal ischemia, considerable variations exist with regard to the progression of ion-homeostasis disturbances.

The second phase of type 1 DC potential change is quite similar to that described for anoxic depolarization in anoxia and global ischemia. The latency from the onset of ischemia to this phase and the final extent of negative deflection are similar to those reported for anoxic depolarization in the rat and cat brain [17–19,23]. A concurrent rapid decrease in $[Ca^{2+}]_o$ as shown in type 1 is also a typical finding in anoxic depolarization [14,16,18]. In type 2, a more modest or delayed decline of the DC potential and also of $[Ca^{2+}]_o$ was typical, paralleled by a later peak of extracellular adenosine. It is, however, important to note that the course of these responses is quite variable, presumably reflecting minor differences in residual perfusion and metabolism.

Tissue depolarization is a multicellular expression of microscopic cellular alterations in the tissue [24]. It may be determined as a function of the number of depolarized cells as well as the membrane potential of each cell. Therefore, a sudden negative shift of the DC potential in the second phase of type 1 indicates that most of the cells in the region have started to depolarize at this time point. This abrupt change seems to distinguish type 1 from type 2. In type 2, the number of depolarized neurons and/or glia seems to increase more gradually and more slowly than that in type 1. In conclusion, the results of our studies show that the initial phase of brain ischemia is more variable than one would think from studies of anoxia or global ischemia alone. The variations in the course of tissue depolarization and of ion or transmitter homeostasis breakdown seem to depend mainly on minimal differences in the disturbance of tissue perfusion and tissue metabolism.

4.2.2.7. On-Site Discussion

4.2.2.7.1. *Question: (Kempski)* What do you exactly mean by 'terminal depolarization'? Is it spontaneously reversible?

Answer: (Graf) Terminal (delayed) depolarization was observed in experiments with permanent MCA occlusion. The earliest time point of this type of depolarization was about 6 h after onset of ischemia. We never reperfused in such cases.

4.2.2.7.2. *Question: (Strong)* (1) Can delay in the microdialysis system account for the delay you describe between electrophysiological depolarization and glutamate release of 30–40 ms? (2) Could change in plasma glucose account for variation in the rate of decline in EEG recovery from PIDs?

Answer: (Graf) (1) The glutamate electrode system does not really have much of a time delay since the electrode is in the tissue. Diffusion into the microdialysis system, however, may account for some delay. So, the glutamate may be somewhat earlier but most probably not before the first steep decrease in extracellular Ca^{2+}. (2) We have not measured plasma glucose.

4.2.2.7.3. *Question: (Greenberg)* How were the animals divided into type I, type II, and type III? Was there a threshold of flow that led to change in ion flux, such as calcium?

Answer: (Graf) Animals were divided by the DC potential response. Type I showed an immediate negative DC potential response. Type II a delayed shift, and type II showed either no shift or transient (periinfarct) depolarizations.

Acknowledgements

The glutamate oxidase was donated by Dr. Hitoshi Kusakabe (Yamasa, Japan). The authors would like to thank Dipl. Ing. B. Radermacher and Mrs. Paula Gabel for their excellent technical assistance.

References

[1] A.J. Hansen, Effect of anoxia on ion distribution in the brain, Physiol. Rev. 65 (1985) 101–148.
[2] R.L. Martin, H.G.E. Lloyd, A.I. Cowan, The early events of oxygen and glucose deprivation. Setting the scene for neuronal death? Trends Neurosci. 17 (1994) 251–257.
[3] M. Erecinska, I.A. Silver, Ions and energy in mammalian brain, Prog. Neurobiol. 43 (1) (1994) 37–71.

[4] J. O'Leary, S. Goldring, D-C potentials of the brain, Physiol. Rev. 44 (1964) 91–125.

[5] T.P. Obrenovitch, J. Urenjak, D.A. Richards, Y. Ueda, G. Curzon, L. Symon, Extracellular neuroactive amino acids in the rat striatum during ischaemia. Comparison between penumbral conditions and ischaemia with sustained anoxic depolarisation, J. Neurochem. 61 (1993) 178–186.

[6] S. Asai, Y. Iribe, T. Kohno, et al., Real time monitoring of biphasic glutamate release using dialysis electrode in rat acute brain ischemia, NeuroReport 7 (1996) 1092–1096.

[7] B.K. Siesjö, Pathophysiology and treatment of focal cerebral ischemia: Part I. Pathophysiology, J. Neurosurg. 77 (1992) 169–184.

[8] J. Astrup, L. Symon, N.M. Branston, N.A. Lassen, Cortical evoked potential and extracellular K^+ and H^+ at critical levels of brain ischemia, Stroke 8 (1977) 51–57.

[9] W.-D. Heiss, R. Graf, The ischemic penumbra, Curr. Opin. Neurol. 7 (1994) 11–19.

[10] W.-D. Heiss, R. Graf, K. Wienhard, J. Löttgen, R. Saito, T. Fujita, G. Rosner, R. Wagner, Dynamic penumbra demonstrated by sequential multitracer PET after middle cerebral artery occlusion in cats, J. Cereb. Blood Flow Metab. 14 (1994) 892–902.

[11] K. Ohta, R. Graf, G. Rosner, W.-D. Heiss, Profiles of cortical tissue depolarization in cat focal cerebral ischemia in relation to calcium ion homeostasis and nitric oxide production, J. Cereb. Blood Flow Metab. 17 (1997) 1170–1181.

[12] R. Graf, K. Kataoka, G. Rosner, W.-D. Heiss, Cortical deafferentation in cat focal ischemia: disturbance and recovery of sensory functions in cortical areas with different degrees of CBF reduction, J. Cereb. Blood Flow Metab. 6 (1986) 566–573.

[13] C. Dohmen, E. Kumura, G. Rosner, W.-D. Heiss, R. Graf, Adenosine in relation to calcium homeostasis: comparison between gray and white matter ischemia, J. Cereb. Blood Flow Metab. 21 (2001) 503–510.

[14] A.J. Hansen, T. Zeuthen, Extracellular ion concentrations during spreading depression and ischemia in the rat brain cortex, Acta Physiol. Scand. 113 (1981) 437–445.

[15] F. Vyskocil, N. Kríz, J. Bures, Potassium-selective microelectrodes used for measuring the extracellular brain potassium during spreading depression and anoxic depolarization in rats, Brain Res. 39 (1972) 255–259.

[16] C. Nicholson, G. ten Bruggencate, R. Steinberg, H. Stöckle, Calcium modulation in brain extracellular microenvironment demonstrated with ion-selective micropipette, Proc. Natl. Acad. Sci. U. S. A. 74 (1977) 1287–1290.

[17] W.F. Blank Jr., H.S. Kirshner, The kinetics of extracellular potassium changes during hypoxia and anoxia in the cat cerebral cortex, Brain Res. 123 (1977) 113–124.

[18] R.J. Harris, L. Symon, Extracellular pH, potassium, and calcium activities in progressive ischaemia of rat cortex, J. Cereb. Blood Flow Metab. 4 (1984) 178–186.

[19] Y. Xie, E. Zacharias, P. Hoff, F. Tegtmeier, Ion channel involvement in anoxic depolarization induced by cardiac arrest in rat brain, J. Cereb. Blood Flow Metab. 15 (1995) 587–594.

[20] E. Zilkha, T.P. Obrenovitch, A. Koshy, et al., Extracellular glutamate: on-line monitoring using micro-dialysis coupled to enzyme-amperometric analysis, J. Neurosci. Methods 60 (1995) 1–9.

[21] I. Vorísek, E. Syková, Ischemia-induced changes in the extracellular space diffusion parameters, K^+, and pH in the developing rat cortex and corpus callosum, J. Cereb. Blood Flow Metab. 17 (1997) 191–203.

[22] W.-D. Heiss, T. Hayakawa, A.G. Waltz, Cortical neuronal function during ischemia. Effects of occlusion of one middle cerebral artery on single-unit activity in cats, Arch. Neurol. 33 (1976) 813–820.

[23] A.J. Hansen, The extracellular potassium concentration in brain cortex following ischemia in hypo- and hyperglycemic rats, Acta Physiol. Scand. 102 (1978) 324–329.

[24] Q. Chen, M. Chopp, G. Bodzin, H. Chen, Temperature modulation of cerebral depolarization during focal cerebral ischemia in rats. Correlation with ischemic injury, J. Cereb. Blood Flow Metab. 13 (1993) 389–394.

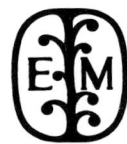

International Congress Series 1235 (2002) 475–479

Ischemic energy failure and ions shifts are smaller and slower in white matter than in gray matter

Eiji Kumura [a,b,*], Christian Dohmen [b], Rudolf Graf [b],
Toshiki Yoshimine [c], Wolf-Dieter Heiss [b]

[a]*Nakakawachi Medical Center of Acute Medicine, Osaka, Japan*
[b]*Max-Planck-Institut für neurologische Forschung, Köln, Germany*
[c]*Department of Neurosurgery, Osaka University Graduate School of Medicine, Japan*

Abstract

Brain ischemia causes rapid energy depletion resulting prominent ion shifts which are responsible for tissue damage. In the present study, we measured extracellular concentrations of ions and adenosine, a determinant of ATP degradation, in gray and white matter during global ischemia. In eight cats, global ischemia was induced by extracranial arteries occlusion. Extracellular levels of Na^+, K^+, Ca^{2+} and pH were measured with microelectrodes, and levels of adenosine were determined by microdialysis-HPLC in gray and white matter. After the arterial occlusion, extracellular K^+ concentration ($[K^+]o$) increased, $[Na^+]o$ and pH decreased. Except for $[Ca^{2+}]o$, changes of ion concentrations in white matter were comparable to those in gray matter, although the speed and the magnitude of change were much slower and smaller. In gray matter, $[Ca^{2+}]o$ started to decrease at 1 min after and reaching minimum at 15 min. $[Ca^{2+}]o$ in white matter was increased during initial 30 min, and reached minimum at 120 min. In both regions, extracellular adenosine levels increased significantly, however, the peak in white matter was delayed by 20 min compared to that in gray matter. The present study demonstrated slower and smaller ion shifts and ATP breakdown in white matter ischemia than those in gray matter ischemia. © 2002 Elsevier Science B.V. All rights reserved.

Keywords: Cerebral ischemia; Calcium; White matter; Adenosine; Extracellular ions

1. Introduction

Brain ischemia causes rapid energy depletion resulting prominent ion shifts, which are responsible for tissue damage. The ionic movements across neuronal membranes are

* Corresponding author. Nakakawachi Medical Center of Acute Medicine, 3-4-13, Nishi-Iwata, Higashio-saka, Osaka 578-0947, Japan. Tel.: +81-6-6785-6166; fax: +81-6-6785-6165.
E-mail address: ekumura@nyc.odn.ne.jp (E. Kumura).

0531-5131/02 © 2002 Elsevier Science B.V. All rights reserved.
PII: S 0 5 3 1 - 5 1 3 1 (0 2) 0 0 2 1 5 - 7

substantial for the understanding of anoxic or ischemic injury [1]. In gray matter, the ion shifts largely depend on transmitter-gated ion channel opening. While white matter consists of axons and glia but not synapses, ischemic ion shifts are likely to be mediated by non-synaptic mechanisms. In the present study, we simultaneously measured extracellular concentrations of ions and adenosine, a determinant of ATP degradation [2], during global cerebral ischemia in gray and white matter regions of the cat brain.

2. Materials and methods

Eight adult cats were anesthetized with α-chloralose under artificial ventilation of 70% N_2O and 30% O_2. Both common carotid arteries and both proximal subclavian arteries were exposed. To form snare ligatures, nylon sutures were placed around each exposed artery [3]. For extracellular measurements of sodium, potassium, calcium and pH (hydrogen ion) concentrations ($[Na^+]o$, $[K^+]o$, $[Ca^{2+}]o$, pH, respectively), double-barreled ion-selective microelectrodes were used. Platinum iridium electrodes were used to measure cerebral blood flow by hydrogen clearance method. Two burr holes were made above the temporal auditory cortex and above the frontal cortex. Assemblies of multiple microelectrodes, a microdialysis probe and a platinum electrode were inserted at the middle ectosylvian gyrus site 1 mm deep into cortex (gray matter), and at the marginal gyrus site, 9 mm deep into the corona radiata (white matter). Thermocouples were inserted adjacent to the assemblies. Body and brain temperatures were controlled separately at 37.0 °C. Microdialysis probes (CMA/12, Carnegie Medicin, Sweden) were perfused continuously with artificial CSF at a flow rate of 2 μl/min. Ten-minute samples of dialysate were used for HPLC measurements. Determination of adenosine concentrations was described previously [4]. Global cerebral ischemia was initiated and kept for 2 h by occluding the four extracranial arteries.

3. Results

Immediately after the induction of ischemia, all cats showed flat electrocorticogram and significant blood flow reduction (<3 ml/ 100 g/minute) in both gray and white matter. Fig. 1A summarizes ion changes during arterial occlusion. Except for Ca^{2+}, changes of ion concentrations in white matter were comparable to those in gray matter, although the speed and magnitude of change were much slower and smaller. In gray matter, $[Ca^{2+}]o$ (preischemic control 1.3±0.1 mM) started to decrease 1 min after the occlusion, and reached 0.1±0.1 mM at 30 min after occlusion. In contrast, $[Ca^{2+}]o$ in white matter (preischemic control: 1.2±0.1 mM) was initially increased reaching 1.7±0.1 mM at 15 min after occlusion. The levels, thereafter, decreased gradually and slowly reaching 0.3±0.1 mM at 60 min after occlusion.

Extracellular adenosine levels determined by microdialysis revealed early, but significant elevations in both gray and white matter (Fig. 1B). Basal levels of adenosine did not differ significantly between gray and white matter. In gray matter, adenosine rose immediately after the induction of ischemia and reached a maximum concentration already after 10 min of ischemia. After this transient increase, adenosine gradually decreased following 2 h of

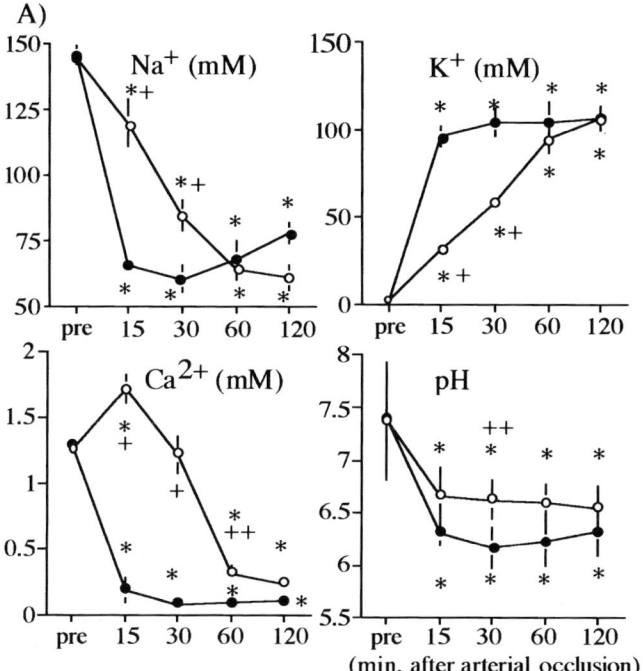

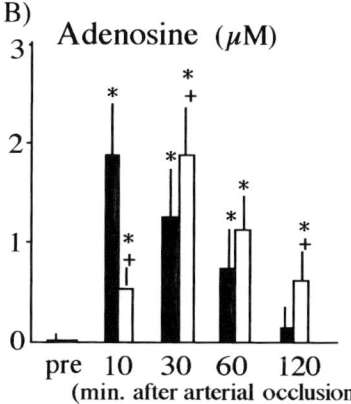

Fig. 1. (A) Changes in extracellular ions concentrations measured in gray and white matter before and during global cerebral ischemia. Open circles indicate ion concentrations in white matter, and close circles indicate in gray matter. Data are mean±SD (pre, preischemic control; *, $p < 0.01$: significantly different from preischemic control; +, $p < 0.01$, ++, $p < 0.05$: significantly different from gray matter). (B) Changes in extracellular adenosine concentrations measured in gray and white matter before and during global cerebral ischemia. Open bars indicate adenosine concentrations in white matter, and close bars in gray matter. Dialysate was sampled for 10 min preceding the times indicated. Data are mean±SD (pre, preischemic control; *, $p < 0.05$: significantly different from preischemic control; +, $p < 0.05$: significantly different from gray matter).

ischemia. In white matter, adenosine started to increase promptly after the induction of ischemia, however, the peak of adenosine was delayed by 20 min compared to that in gray matter (Fig. 1B). Following this peak, the concentration slowly declined staying well above that of gray matter throughout the experiment period.

4. Discussion

The present study firstly demonstrated ischemic change in extracellular Na^+, K^+, Ca^{2+}, and pH in white matter. Except for Ca^{2+}, ionic shifts across the cell membrane during cerebral ischemia are considerably smaller than in gray matter, when blood flow is equally reduced in both regions. Among ion fluxes during early course of ischemia, changes in $[Ca^{2+}]o$ clearly differed between gray and white matter. During the initial 30 min after the induction of ischemia, $[Ca^{2+}]o$ in white matter showed transient increase, whereas $[Ca^{2+}]o$ in gray matter showed a steep decrease. In gray matter, this steep decrease was attributable to the opening of voltage-gated and N-methyl-D-aspartate receptor-mediated Ca^{2+} channels [5]. Ca^{2+} influx via these Ca^{2+} channels is hardly expected in white matter, because white matter lacks synapses. Therefore, early rise in $[Ca^{2+}]o$ in white matter may have to be explained by two pathophysiological processes that occurred simultaneously. First, ischemic shrinkage of the extracellular space should elevate $[Ca^{2+}]o$ without affecting net content of calcium ion. The shrinkage affected both gray and white matter, and the degree of ischemic shrinkage was similar in gray and white matter [6]. Second, little or no change of transmembrane Ca^{2+} conductance occurred during early course of white matter ischemia. A biphasic axonal $[Ca^{2+}]$ rise was reported in in vitro anoxic axon [7]. A first increase immediately after the anoxia was ascribed to Ca^{2+} release from internal store, and a second steep increase began about 40 min later due to a reverse operation of Na^+–Ca^{2+} exchanger. The second process required membrane depolarization and increased Na^+ level in axon [7]. Taken these evidences as a basis, transmembrane Ca^{2+} conductance may not be changed during early course of white matter ischemia.

At 30 min after the induction of ischemia, $[Ca^{2+}]o$ in white matter started to decrease steeply (Fig. 1A). Decrease in $[Na^+]o$ in white matter also became prominent after 30 min of ischemia. After this phase, when axoplasm Na^+ already increases through its nodal channel may result Ca^{2+} influx by reverse action of Na^+–Ca^{2+} exchanger in ischemic axon. Glia also has Na^+–Ca^{2+} exchanger, so that delayed decrease in $[Ca^{2+}]o$ in white matter may ,namely, be ascribed to the reverse action of this exchanger.

In response to energy depletion induced by hypoxia or ischemia, extracellular adenosine is dramatically elevated [8]. Adenosine is mainly formed intracellularly due to massive and rapid ATP catabolism and transported out of the cell via a nucleoside transporter. In the present study, extracellular levels of adenosine in gray matter already peaked at 10 min after ischemia induction (Fig. 1B). The peak in white matter was delayed for 20 min compared to that in gray matter, although the peak value was almost the same between two regions. The slow rise in adenosine levels in white matter can be explained by slower breakdown of ATP in this region than that in gray matter, which clearly related to small and slow alterations of transmembrane ion shifts. In addition, spreading depression usually seen in ischemic gray matter can increase energy consumption, which may further promote ATP degradation in gray matter. Not only as a degraded ATP by-product, but also as a neuroprotective substance, adenosine has been studied extensively [2,8]. Adenosine blocks presynaptic Ca^{2+} influx and hyperpolarizes postsynaptic membrane by increasing K^+ and Cl^- conductance [2]. In white matter, adenosine confers partial protection against ischemia by PKC dependent down-regulation of Na^+ channels and Na^+–Ca^{2+} exchanger [9]. Slower decline of extracellular adenosine levels in white matter (Fig. 1B) after 30 min of ischemia, therefore, might act as reducing Ca^{2+} influx in white matter.

The present study demonstrated slower and smaller extracellular ions shift and ATP breakdown in white matter ischemia than that in gray matter ischemia. Since white matter is involved more than 80% of strokes, further studies are necessary to clarify specific pathophysiology and insight into the effective treatments of white matter ischemia.

References

[1] A.J. Hansen, Effect of anoxia on ion distribution in the brain, Physiol. Rev. 65 (1985) 101–148.

[2] K.A. Rudolphi, P. Schubert, F.E. Parkinson, B.B. Fredholm, Adenosine and brain ischemia, Cerebrovasc. Brain Metab. Rev. 4 (1992) 346–369.

[3] E. Kumura, R. Graf, C. Dohmen, G. Rosner, W.D. Heiss, Breakdown of calcium homeostasis in relation to tissue depolarization: comparison between gray and white matter ischemia, J. Cereb. Blood Flow Metab. 19 (1999) 788–793.

[4] K. Matsumoto, R. Graf, G. Rosner, N. Shimada, W.D. Heiss, Flow thresholds for extracellular purine catabolite elevation in cat focal ischemia, Brain Res. 579 (1992) 309–314.

[5] B.K. Siesjö, Pathophysiology and treatment of focal cerebral ischemia: Part 1. Pathophysiology, J. Neurosurg. 77 (1992) 169–184.

[6] I. Vorísek, E. Syková, Ischemia-induced changes in the extracellular space diffusion parameters, K^+, and pH in the developing rat cortex and corpus callosum, J. Cereb. Blood Flow Metab. 17 (1997) 191–203.

[7] P.K. Stys, Anoxic and ischemic injury of myelinated axons in CNS white matter: from mechanistic concepts to therapeutics, J. Cereb. Blood Flow 18 (1998) 2–25.

[8] H. Hagberg, P. Andersson, J. Lacarewicz, I. Jacobson, S. Butcher, M. Sandberg, Extracellular adenosine, inosine, hypoxanthine, and xanthine in relation to tissue nucleotides and purines in rat striatum during transient ischemia, J. Neurochem. 49 (1987) 227–231.

[9] R. Fern, S.G. Waxman, B.R. Ransom, Modulation of anoxic injury in CNS white matter by adenosine and interaction between adenosine and GABA, J. Neurophysiol. 72 (1994) 2609–2615.

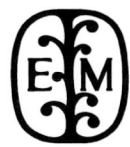

International Congress Series 1235 (2002) 481–486

Temporal profile of gene induction after venous ischemia accompanied by spreading depression as compared to spreading depression alone

Takanobu Kaido [a], Cara Heers [b], Daniela Bartsch [b], Axel Heimann [a], Oliver Kempski [a,*]

[a]Institute for Neurosurgical Pathophysiology, Johannes Gutenberg-University Mainz, Langenbeckstr 1, 55101, Mainz, Germany
[b]Jansen Research Foundation, Neuss, Germany

Abstract

The occlusion of two adjacent cortical veins is followed by a widespread reduction of rCBF and the occurrence of small infarcts, which become larger if spreading depression (SD) occurs. The model appears to be useful for studying penumbra pathophysiology. Here, the time course of gene expression in the penumbra was compared to those induced by the SD alone. In an experiment involving rats, an occlusion of two cortical veins was induced by i.v. rose bengal and fiberoptic illumination. Ten SDs were induced at 7-min intervals. Changes of the gene expression after 2, 8, 24 and 72 h were analysed for 13 genes by RT-PCR. The housekeeping gene glyceraldehyde-3-phosphate dehydrogenase (GAPDH) was used for normalization, and expression patterns were studied by cluster analysis. c-*fos*, cox-2 and bcl-2 responded early (2 h) and far more after the two-vein occlusion with plus SD than after the experiment with SD alone. Secondly, HO-1 and c-*myc* were increased 24 h after SD was carried out in animals without ischemia. These increases were specific for SD. bcl-xL, bad and bax had minor and late increases. Cyclin D1 showed a moderately increased expression 72 h after ischemia. A cluster analysis confirmed the related expression patterns of (a) HO-1 and c-*myc* 24 h after SD, and (b) c-*fos* and cox-2 early after two-vein occlusion was carried out. © 2002 Elsevier Science B.V. All rights reserved.

Keywords: Heme oxygenase-1; Cyclooxygenase-2; Penumbra; Gene expression; Spreading depression

---

* Corresponding author. Tel.: +49-6131-173636; fax: +49-6131-176640.
E-mail address: kempski@nc-patho.klinik.uni-mainz.de (O. Kempski).

0531-5131/02 © 2002 Elsevier Science B.V. All rights reserved.
PII: S0531-5131(02)00234-0

1. Introduction

Treatment of a stroke is to a large part an attempt to save the ischemic penumbra [1], which when left untreated, will sooner or later die. In the rat MCA-occlusion model, most of the penumbra turned into infarct within 6 h [2]. A possible reason for this secondary decay is an increase in the metabolic needs of the tissue as a consequence of metabolic activation by periinfarct depolarizations, spreading depression (SD) which go along with a complete breakdown of the ion gradients and, hence, increased metabolic demands for ion pumping and propagate tissue decay [3,4]. Another cause might be the persisting low flow conditions in the penumbra which are tolerated for several hours; however, it might then be insufficient to further support tissue survival. The individual significance of both mechanisms, persisting low flow and metabolic activation, remains to be determined.

The occlusion of two adjacent cortical veins is followed by a more widespread reduction of the regional CBF than after MCA occlusion and the occurrence of comparatively small infarcts, which also become larger if SD occurs spontaneously or is induced [5]. Therefore, the model appears useful for studying the processes which occur in the penumbra zones, and mechanisms of secondary tissue damage in the penumbra, in particular. One way to detect such mechanisms is to study changes in the expression of potentially harmful or protective genes. The aim of the current study, therefore, was to determine the time course of gene expression changes in the ischemic/periischemic low blood flow zone, as compared to respective changes induced by spreading depression alone.

2. Materials and methods

Male Wistar rats were anesthetized with chloral hydrate. The rectal temperature was kept close to 37.0 °C throughout the experiment by a feedbackcontrolled heating pad. Poly-ethylene catheters were inserted into the right femoral artery and vein for continuous registration of the mean arterial pressure, for arterial blood gas sampling and for administration of fluid and drugs. Also, the rats were mounted in a stereotaxic frame. After a 2.0-cm midline skin incision, a right frontoparietal cranial window was made for access to the brain surface. An occlusion of two adjacent cortical veins was induced by i.v. rose bengal and fiberoptic illumination for 10 min [5–8]. The diameter of the occluded veins was approximately 100 mm. Rose bengal (50 mg/kg body wt.) was injected slowly without effect on the systemic arterial pressure, and care was taken to avoid illumination of the tissue and other vessels near the target vein. The vein was illuminated for 10 min via the micromanipulator-assisted light guide. To occlude the second selected vein, half of the initial rose bengal dose was injected intravenously before the illumination was repeated with the new target. After the two-vein occlusion, ten SDs were induced with cortical microinjections of KCl (150 mM) at 7-min intervals. The spreading depressions were monitored by cortical impedance measurements using a precision LCR monitor (4282A; Hewlett-Packard, USA). After 2, 8, 24 or 72 h, the cortical tissue was dissected immediately (ipsi- vs. contralateral tissue between the two occluded veins, i.e., in the territory with low rCBF) and frozen in liquid nitrogen. Three to five animals were investigated for each condition. The mRNA levels were determined by semiquantitative RT-PCR for the following genes: heme oxygenase-1 (HO-1), the immediate early genes c-*fos*, c-*jun* and c-*myc*, the bcl-2 family members bcl-2, bcl-xL, bax and bad, superoxide dismutases 1 and 2, and the cell cycle related gene cyclin D1. The housekeeping gene glyceraldehyde-3-phosphate dehydrogenase (GAPDH) was used for normalization. The ratio of the relative amounts of mRNA (normalized to GAPDH) from the operated to the contralateral side was calculated. The related expression patterns were evaluated by cluster analysis [9].

3. Results

There were no statistical differences in the physiological data, which were all within the normal range. Venous occlusion evolved with the well-described typical time course [6–8]. We were able to relate selected genes to four major groups because of their different expression patterns in the tissue. First, we found a group of genes, which responded early (2 h) and strongly, but far more were found after two-vein occlusion plus SD than after SD alone (c-*fos* and cox-2). Cox-2 was stimulated 13.6-fold by vein occlusion plus SD; however, only 1.55-fold by SD alone. The mean stimulation of the c-*fos* expression was 69.4-fold, whereas with SD alone, the stimulation was more moderate (10.8-fold); furthermore, these effects were transient. After 24 h, there was a strong decrease in the mRNA level, which was significantly lower than in SD animals. Similarly, not very strong changes were observed in the bcl-2 expression, which was also elevated (2.7-fold) 2 h after the two-vein occlusion and then normalized again. Secondly, we could detect changes in gene expression 24 h after the induction of SD in animals without vein occlusion (HO-1, c-*myc*). These increases (19.0-fold and 5.4-fold, respectively) were specific for SD, whereas a combination of the two-vein occlusion plus SD after an initial moderate stimulation led to a suppression at that time point. Later on, i.e., 72 h after vein occlusion, these genes again developed moderately increased expression patterns. The third group comprises of the remaining tested members of the bcl-2 family (bcl-xL, bad and bax). In general, these expression changes were small: bax, bad and bcl-xL increased late, 72 h after two-vein occlusion. Finally, cyclin D1 showed a moderately (5.6-fold) increased expression late (72 h) after ischemia.

In addition, cluster analysis revealed related expression patterns of (a) HO-1 and c-*myc* 24 h after SD, and (b) c-*fos* and cox-2, and also bcl-2 early after two-vein occlusion in combination with SD.

4. Discussion

We present here a model, which permits to discriminate changes in gene expression in the vicinity of focal ischemia from those elicited by spreading depression, which is known to occur spontaneously in the ischemic penumbra, and tends to worsen the metabolic situation as well as the outcome [3,4]. On the other hand, SD is known to precondition the brain, i.e., to induce tolerance for a subsequent episode of ischemia [10]. Therefore, the current study and others to follow can help to discriminate tolerance inducing from damaging alterations. Among the changes observed, many have been described before in other models (e.g., immediate early gene induction after ischemia). It was also known that SD and also hypoxia (which can also induce tolerance) induce HO-1 [11,12]. Other authors have described an increase of the HO-1 protein by focal and global ischemia [13,14]. However, a direct comparison between focal ischemia and SD so far has not been made. Our data clearly indicate that only SD, but not ischemia (here even in combination with SD), caused an enhanced expression of HO-1. Moreover, HO-1 is interesting as a potentially beneficial gene/protein since animals over expressing the protein have a better outcome from focal ischemia [15], and the neurons from those animals resist oxidative stress mediated from cell death [16]. HO-1 inhibits inflammatory reactions (selecting expression [17]) and catalyzes the formation of the vasodilator CO and, thereby, also suppresses the hypoxic induction of the gene encoding plasminogen activator inhibitor-1 (PAI-1) [18]. Further research is necessary in order to evaluate the role of HO-1 in tolerance induction. The lack of HO-1 upregulation in subacute stages of the penumbra may contribute to its decay.

Another significant result of this study was the early and more than moderate increase of the COX-2 expression after venous ischemia but not after SD. COX-2 not only catalyzes the production of vasoactive prostaglandins from arachidonic acid, but also the formation of free radicals during that process. COX-2 is also blamed for a potentiation of excitotoxicity [19]. Hence, in the increased expression of COX-2, mRNA may reflect an attempt of the penumbra tissue to improve collateral perfusion by vasodilation, e.g., by prostacyclin formation [20], which may be accompanied by the cited deleterious side effects of an increased production of reactive oxygen species and aggravation of excitotoxicity via COX-2 in the penumbra.

In conclusion, we have presented evidence that mechanisms initiated by brain activation by SD, as well as the loss of CBF control in the penumbra, can be adequately studied by assessing gene expression changes in the two-vein occlusion model. The potentially protective nature of HO-1 as well as the postulated unfavorable role of COX-2 are supported by our data.

4.24.6. On-Site Discussion

4.2.4.6.1. **Question: (Seylaz)** (1) I have a question about your model of ischemia based on venous occlusion. Can you comment of the pressure induced in capillaries and in the occluded veins? Does the maneuver induce an increase of cerebral blood volume? (2) The early expression of c-*fos* you showed 2 h after ischemia is very interesting. Is there any data for an earlier expression of c-*fos* following ischemia?

Answer: (Kempski) (1) Model is described in our article (Otsuka et al. Exp. Neurol. 2000; 162:201). We did not measure intravenous pressure, but I expect it to be increased compared to normal. (2) Early c-*fos* has been described before. However, Sharp et al. (Cereb. Blood Flow Metab. 2000; 20(7):1011) have postulated c-*fos* to increase due to spreading depression. We can now show that the increase from ischemia is far larger than that by SD alone.

4.2.4.6.2. **Question: (Tamura)** What is the physiological significance for such large amount of gene induction?

Answer: (Kempski) We try to find typical patterns of gene expression for ischemia as compared to SD alone at different time parity in order to find that significance.

4.2.4.6.3. *Question: (Strong)* Which of the genes you described might initiate the inflammatory cascade after ischemia?

Answer: (Kempski) Many of the immediate early genes might be involved. However, more studies are needed to further elucidate that question.

References

[1] J. Astrup, B.K. Siesjö, L. Symon, Thresholds in cerebral ischemia—the ischemic penumbra, Stroke 12 (1981) 723–725.

[2] M.D. Ginsberg, Injury mechanisms in the ischemic penumbra—approaches to neuroprotection in acute ischemic stroke, Cerebrovasc. Dis. 7 (Suppl. 2) (1997) 7–12.

[3] T. Back, M. Ginsberg, W.D. Dietrich, B.D. Watson, Induction of spreading depression in the ischemic hemisphere following experimental middle cerebral artery occlusion: effect on infarct morphology, J. Cereb. Blood Flow Metab. 16 (1996) 202–213.

[4] G. Mies, T. Iijima, K.-A. Hossmann, Correlation between periinfarct DC shifts and ischemic neuronal damage in rat, NeuroReport 4 (1993) 709–711.

[5] H. Otsuka, K. Ueda, A. Heimann, O. Kempski, Effects of cortical spreading depression on cortical blood flow, impedance, DC-potential, and infarct size in a rat venous infarct model, Exp. Neurol. 162 (2000) 201–214.

[6] H. Nakase, A. Heimann, O. Kempski, Local cerebral blood flow in a rat cortical occlusion model, J. Cereb. Blood Flow Metabol. 6 (1996) 720–728.

[7] H. Nakase, O. Kempski, A. Heimann, T. Takeshima, J. Tintera, Microcirculation following cerebral venous occlusions assessed by laser Doppler scanning, J. Neurosurg. 87 (1997) 307–314.

[8] H. Nakase, K. Nagata, H. Otsuka, T. Sakaki, O. Kempski, Local cerebral blood flow autoregulation following asymptomatic cerebral venous occlusion in the rat, J. Neurosurg. 89 (1998) 118–124.

[9] M.B. Eisen, P.T. Spellman, P.O. Brown, D. Botstein, Cluster analysis of genome-wide expression patterns, PNAS 95 (1998) 14863–14868.

[10] S. Kobajashi, V.A. Harris, F.A. Welsh, Spreading depression induces tolerance of cortical neurons to ischemia in rat brain, J. Cereb. Blood Flow Metab. 15 (1995) 721–727.

[11] P. Garnier, C. Demougeot, N. Bertrand, A. Prigent-Tessier, C. Marie, A. Beley, Stress response to hypoxia in gerbil brain: HO-1 and Mn SOD expression and glial activation, Brain Res. 893 (2001) 301–309.

[12] J. Koistinaho, S. Pasonen, J. Yrjänheikki, P.H. Chan, Spreading depression-induced gene expression is regulated by plasma glucose, Stroke 30 (1999) 114–119.

[13] J.W. Geddes, L.C. Pettigrew, M.L. Holtz, S.D. Craddock, M.D. Maines, Permanent focal and transient global cerebral ischemia increase glial and neuronal expression of heme oxygenase-1, but not heme oxygenase-2, protein in rat brain, Neurosci. Lett. 210 (1996) 205–208.

[14] T. Nimura, P.R. Weinstein, S.M. Massa, S. Panter, F.R. Sharp, Heme oxygenase-1 (HO-1) protein induction in rat brain following focal ischemia, Mol. Brain Res. 37 (1996) 201–208.

[15] N. Panahian, M. Yoshiura, M.D. Maines, Overexpression of heme oxygenase-1 is neuroprotective in a model of permanent middle cerebral artery occlusion in transgenic mice, J. Neurochem. 72 (3) (1999) 1187–1203.

[16] K. Chen, K. Gunter, M.D. Maines, Neurons overexpressing heme oxygenase-1 resist oxidative stress-mediated cell death, J. Neurochem. 75 (1) (2000) 304–313.

[17] T.J. Vachharajani, J. Work, A.C. Issekutz, D.N. Granger, Heme oxygenase modulates selectin expression in different regional vascular beds, Am. J. Physiol.: Heart Circ. Physiol. 278 (2000) H1613–H1617.

[18] T. Fujita, K. Toda, A. Karimova, S.F. Yan, Y. Naka, S.F. Yet, D.J. Pinsky, Paradoxical rescue from ischemic lung injury by inhaled carbon monoxide driven by derepression of fibrinolysis, Nat. Med. 7 (5) (2001) 598–604.

[19] K.A. Kelley, L. Ho, D. Winger, J. Freire-Moar, C.B. Borelli, P.S. Aisen, G.M. Pasinetti, Potentiation of excitotoxicity in transgenic mice overexpressing neuronal cyclooxygenase-2, Am. J. Pathol. 155 (3) (1999) 995–1004.
[20] O. Kempski, E. Shohami, D. von Lubitz, J.M. Hallenbeck, G. Feuerstein, Postischemic production of eicosanoids in gerbil brain, Stroke 18 (1987) 111–119.

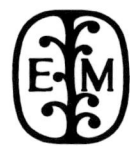

International Congress Series 1235 (2002) 487–492

Ischemia caused by inverse coupling between neuronal activation and cerebral blood flow in rats

Jens P. Dreier*, Olaf Windmüller, Gabor Petzold, Ute Lindauer,
Karl M. Einhäupl, Ulrich Dirnagl

Department of Neurology, Charité Hospital, Humboldt University, 10098 Berlin, Germany

Abstract

Cortical spreading depression (CSD) typically leads to cortical spreading hyperemia followed by cortical spreading oligemia in rats. This physiological response can be experimentally inverted so that the neuronal activation leads to ischemia [cortical spreading ischemia (CSI)]. It has been proposed that CSI may be related to clinical conditions such as migraine-induced stroke and delayed ischemic neurological deficits after subarachnoid hemorrhage. The underlying change of the vascular reactivity to CSD is achieved by superfusion of artificial cerebrospinal fluid (ACSF) containing an elevated K^+ concentration together with an NO-lowering agent. The NO-lowering agent may either be an NO-scavenger such as oxyhemoglobin (oxy-Hb) or an NO synthase (NOS)-inhibitor such as N-nitro-L-arginine (L-NNA). In the present study, we compared the potency of oxy-Hb and L-NNA to induce CSI. CSI was significantly longer in the presence of oxy-Hb. This may either be due to scavenging of blood-derived NO by oxy-Hb or NO-independent vasoconstrictive properties of oxy-Hb. © 2002 Elsevier Science B.V. All rights reserved.

Keywords: Spreading depression; Vasospasm; Subarachnoid hemorrhage; Migraine; Hemoglobin

1. Introduction

Supply with energy substrates is a necessary presupposition for neuronal functioning. As an example, if brain slices become hypoxic, at first, neurons hyperpolarize and astrocytes depolarize [1]. The next electrophysiological event in the ischemic/hypoxic cascade occurs only one or a few minutes later, when a steep neuronal and astroglial

---

* Corresponding author. Fax: +49-30-450-560932.
E-mail address: jens.dreier@charite.de (J.P. Dreier).
URL: http://www.charite.de/ch/neuro/.

0531-5131/02 © 2002 Elsevier Science B.V. All rights reserved.
PII: S 0 5 3 1 - 5 1 3 1 (0 2) 0 0 2 3 5 - 2

depolarization starts at a spot in the tissue. This depolarization propagates as a wave in the gray matter both in vivo [2] and in vitro [3].

A similar but transient depolarization wave can also be induced at a physiological cerebral blood flow (CBF) and tissue oxygen level by local stimuli such as K^+ [= cortical spreading depression (CSD)]. CSDs represent a special type of neuronal activation. Hence, CSDs are coupled to a rise in CBF under physiological conditions [= cortical spreading hyperemia (CSH)] [4].

To any rule, there are exceptions. We have discovered a K^+-induced CSD-like depolarization, which triggered ischemia due to inverse coupling between neuronal activation and CBF in rats [5]. Thus, the abovementioned fundamental processes appeared to be turned upside down: Firstly, neuronal activation did not induce vasodilatation but vasoconstriction under this special condition. Secondly, a neuronal depolarization wave was not triggered by ischemia but ischemia was triggered by a neuronal depolarization wave. As a result, the ischemia propagated in the cerebral cortex together with the depolarization wave [= cortical spreading ischemia (CSI)].

Cortical spreading ischemia (CSI) occurs when a CSD-like depolarization travels through a cortical area exposed to an NO-lowering agent and elevated K^+. In the present study, we compared the efficacy of the NO synthase (NOS)-inhibitor N-nitro-L-arginine (L-NNA) and the NO-scavenger oxy-hemoglobin (oxy-Hb) to induce CSI.

2. Materials and methods

2.1. Surgery

The experiments were approved by the Landesamt für Arbeitsschutz, Gesundheits-schutz und technische Sicherheit Berlin (G 0346/98). Male Wistar rats ($n = 69$; 250–380 g) were anesthetized with thiopental sodium intraperitoneally, tracheotomized and artificially ventilated. The mean arterial pO_2 (PaO$_2$), PaCO$_2$ and pH were monitored. A closed cranial window was implanted as previously described (Fig. 1A) [5]. The cortical surface at the window was continuously superfused with artificial cerebrospinal fluid (ACSF). The composition of the ACSF in millimolar was: Ca^{2+} 1.5; Mg^{2+} 1.2; HCO_3^- 24.5; Cl^- 135; glucose 3.7; urea 6.7. The K^+ concentrations in the ACSF ([K^+]$_{ACSF}$) (3, 20 mM) determined the Na^+ concentrations (152, 135 mM). The ACSF was equilibrated with a gas mixture comprising 6.6% O_2, 5.9% CO_2, and 87.5% N_2. Hemoglobin (Hb) was freshly prepared from citrate blood of Wistar rats and transferred to the ACSF by gel chromatography as previously reported [5]. Ninety percent of the total Hb was oxy-Hb in this preparation as measured by a radiometer (ABL system 625, radiometer, Copenhagen, Denmark).

2.2. Experimental setup

In addition to the closed window, a second open cranial window was laterally implanted to elicit CSD by a droplet of KCl (Fig. 1A). The neuronal/astroglial depolarization wave spread from the open to the closed window where the CBF was measured by

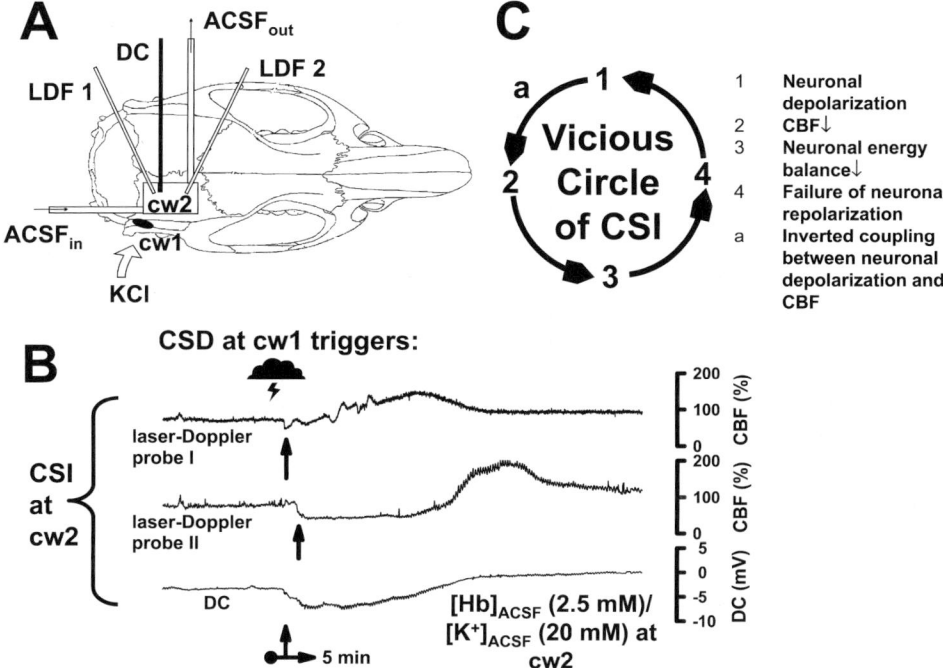

Fig. 1. (A) Experimental setup. cw1 = open cranial window; cw2 = closed window. KCl elicited CSD at cw1. From cw1, the spreading neuronal activation propagated to cw2 at which the CBF response was inverted. $ACSF_{in}$ = inflow; $ACSF_{out}$ = outflow tube; LDF1/2 = laser Doppler flow probes; DC = Ag–AgCl electrode. (B) Original recording of a cortical spreading ischemia (CSI) at cw2 which was triggered in the presence of ACSF containing hemoglobin ($[Hb]_{ACSF}$) at 2.5 mM and K^+ ($[K^+]_{ACSF}$) at 20 mM, when a spreading neuronal activation arrived from cw1. Note the propagation of CSI from laser Doppler probes I–II. (C) Vicious circle underlying CSI. The spreading neuronal activation induces vasoconstriction (inverted coupling between neuronal metabolism and CBF). Thereby, the neuronal supply with energy substrates is reduced leading to a failure of neuronal repolarization so that the vasoconstriction persists.

laser Doppler flow probes (Perimed, Järfälla, Sweden), and the DC potential by an Ag–AgCl electrode. At the closed window, the CBF response to the spreading neuronal activation was locally inverted due to an NO-lowering agent [either L-NNA (1 mM, Sigma, Deisenhofen, Germany), $n = 54$ or Hb (2.5 mM), $n = 15$] combined with an elevated K^+ concentration (20 mM) in the ACSF so that CSI instead of CSH occurred (Fig. 1B).

2.3. Data analysis

Data were analyzed by comparing the relative changes in CBF and the absolute changes of the DC potential. The CBF changes were calculated in relation to the baseline at the onset of the experiment (100%). Mean value comparisons were made by the Mann–Whitney U-test. All data in text, tables and figures are given as mean values ± S.D.

3. Results

The systemic variables remained within physiological limits during the experiments. Topical superfusion of the NO-lowering agents and elevated $[K^+]_{ACSF}$ decreased the resting CBF to $85 \pm 20\%$ (L-NNA) and $74 \pm 34\%$ (Hb), respectively. During the first CSI, the CBF fell to $35 \pm 18\%$ (L-NNA) and $35 \pm 25\%$ (Hb). The hypoperfusion lasted for 7.6 ± 12.9 min (L-NNA) and 31.3 ± 36.0 min (Hb) ($p < 0.01$). It was followed by a hyperperfusion ($183 \pm 73\%$ [L-NNA] vs. $129 \pm 63\%$ [oxy-Hb], $p < 0.05$). The negative DC shift was -6.9 ± 2.7 mV and -7.5 ± 2.6 mV, respectively. It lasted for 11.6 ± 13.7 min (L-NNA) vs. 35.2 ± 33.7 min (Hb) ($p < 0.001$). The duration of the negative DC shift and hypoperfusion were positively correlated ($r = 0.98$, $p < 0.01$), while the duration of the hypoperfusion and the level of the hyperperfusion were negatively correlated ($r = -0.50$, $p < 0.01$) ($n = 69$). No significant difference was detected between the first and second CSI.

4. Discussion

4.1. CSI in the presence of topical oxy-Hb was longer than in the presence of topical NOS inhibition

This effect was possibly related to scavenging of blood-derived NO [6] by the subarachnoid oxy-Hb, while this source of NO was not reduced by brain topical NOS inhibition leading to a shorter ischemic response under L-NNA.

An alternative explanation is related to NO-independent vasoconstrictive properties of oxy-Hb e.g. mediated by the induction of oxygen radical species: In the CSI, the CBF response to CSD is inverted so that local vasoconstriction is induced instead of vaso-dilatation. The vasoconstriction reduces the neuronal supply with energy substrates, thereby, preventing the neuronal repolarization. Since the neuronal depolarization produces the vasoconstriction, a vicious circle results leading to prolonged ischemia (Fig. 1C) [7]. However, if the resting CBF is increased by either NO-dependent or NO-independent vasodilators, the hypoperfusion starts from a higher CBF level. Thus, the CBF level during the hypoperfusion is higher in the presence of the vasodilator than in its absence. Hence, more energy is provided for the neuronal repolarization process during the hypoperfusion phase, thereby breaking the vicious circle [7]. This unspecific influence of vascular tone on the expression of CSI is likely to work in both directions. As an example, if the NO-lowering agent possesses additional NO-independent vasoconstrictive properties such as oxy-Hb, the CSI would be more pronounced.

4.2. Clinical implication

Oxyhemoglobin is the protein (~ 20 mM) and K^+ the ion (~ 100 mM) with the highest concentration in red blood cells. These factors accumulate in the subarachnoid clot in temporal correlation with hemolysis after subarachnoid hemorrhage (SAH) [8,9]. Therefore, we proposed a possible link between CSI and the delayed ischemic neuro-logical deficits (DINDs) after SAH [5]. This link was supported by the pathoanatomy of the ischemic lesions after CSI corresponding with the characteristic pattern of bell-shaped and band-like cortical infarcts associated with DINDs in man [9]. Cortical spreading ischemia was originally described being induced by NOS inhibition and elevated $[K^+]_{ACSF}$ [10]. The present study indicates that oxy-Hb more potently induces CSI than NOS inhibition.

4.2.5.7. On-Site Discussion

4.2.5.7.1. *Question: (ladecola)* What is the evidence that propagation of the spreading depression waves between the two windows was not due to diffusion of KCL rather than propagation of the spreading depression wave?

Answer: (Dreier) Spreading depression is elicited by a drop of KCL at a small window several millimeters distant from a closed cranial window. Passive diffusion of K^+ is limited to a large degree by glial buffering so that the depolarization wave arriving at the closed window can not be related to passive diffusion of K^+ but to the cascade of events related to spreading depression. We have also direct evidence that a simple passive diffusion of K^+ is not responsible since we measured K^+ in the tissue at the second window using a K^+-sensitive microelectrode. The characteristics K^+ signal is a steep rise to approximately 60 mM, which is not preceded by a slow K^+ increase. This is typical of spreading depression but not passive diffusion of K^+. The ischemic CBF response occurs either simultaneously with or with a short delay after the arrival of the spreading neuronal activation at the closed cranial window. Thus, it appears that the spreading neuronal activation induces the ischemic CBF response.

4.2.5.7.2. *Queston: (Jones)* I am concerned about the effect of NOS inhibition with superfused LNNA, as some effects of NOS inhibition need very long periods of super-fusion to become evident. If NOS inhibition was not effective, locally produced NO could still be present in the brain, and your conclusion that blood delivered NO is the only contributing factor to the length of ischemia could be incorrect. Even 91% inhibition, as assessed from your in vitro assay, and 90 min of LNNA superfusion might leave enough uninhibited NOS in the correct anatomical location to provide a shortened duration of ischemia from locally produced NO. To protect your final conclusion that nonlocal NO is responsible, a functional assay of NOS inhibition using both endothelial independent agents such as superfused acetylcholine or inhaled CO_2, would be useful.

Answer: (Dreier) In principle, both LNNA and hemoglobin effectively induce cortical spreading ischemia in combination with elevated K^+. That L-NNA similar to hemoglobin induces cortical spreading ischemia indicates that NO-lowering is the predominant function by which hemoglobin produces cortical spreading ischemia since L-NNA and hemoglobin are otherwise factors of a completely different nature. However, the duration of the ischemic CBF response is longer when hemoglobin is used. This is of pathophysiological interest because extracellular hemoglobin being a natural NO-lowering agent is the relevant factor in the pathogenesis of delayed ischemic neurological deficits (DINDs) after subarachnoid hemorrhage (SAH). The potent effect of hemoglobin supports the link between animal model and clinical syndrome. We offered two possible explanations for the stronger effect of hemoglobin compared with L-NNA: (1) Scavenging of blood derived

NO or (2) NO-independent vasoconstrictive effects of hemoglobin e.g. mediated by generation of oxygen radical species. However, incomplete suppression of local endothelially or neuronally derived NO by L-NNA may still contribute to the smaller effect of LNNA in comparison with that of hemoglobin.

Acknowledgements

The DFG-SFB 507 A1, and the Hermann and Lilly Schilling foundation supported this study.

References

[1] M. Müller, G.G. Somjen, Na^+ and K^+ concentrations, extra- and intracellular voltages, and the effect of TTX in hypoxic rat hippocampal slices, J. Neurophysiol. 83 (2000) 735–745.

[2] A.A.P. Leão, Further observations on the spreading depression of activity in the cerebral cortex, J. Neurophysiol. 10 (1947) 409–414.

[3] P.G. Aitken, G.C. Tombaugh, D.A. Turner, G.G. Somjen, Similar propagation of SD and hypoxic SD-like depolarization in rat hippocampus recorded optically and electrically, J. Neurophysiol. 80 (1998) 1514–1521.

[4] M. Lauritzen, Pathophysiology of the migraine aura, the spreading depression theory [Review], Brain 117 (1994) 199–210.

[5] J.P. Dreier, K. Körner, N. Ebert, A. Görner, I. Rubin, T. Back, U. Lindauer, T. Wolf, A. Villringer, K.M. Einhäupl, M. Lauritzen, U. Dirnagl, Nitric oxide scavenging by haemoglobin or nitric oxide synthase inhibition by N-nitro-L-arginine induce cortical spreading ischaemia when K^+ is increased in the subarachnoid space, J. Cereb. Blood Flow Metab. 18 (1998) 978–990.

[6] L. Jia, C. Bonaventura, J. Bonaventura, J.S. Stamler, S-nitrosohaemoglobin: a dynamic activity of blood involved in vascular control, Nature 380 (1996) 221–226.

[7] J.P. Dreier, G. Petzold, K. Tille, U. Lindauer, G. Arnold, U. Heinemann, K.M. Einhäupl, U. Dirnagl, Ischaemia triggered by spreading neuronal activation is inhibited by vasodilators in rats, J. Physiol. 531 (2001) 515–526.

[8] R.M. Pluta, J.K. Afshar, R.J. Boock, E.H. Oldfield, Temporal changes in perivascular concentrations of oxyhemoglobin, deoxyhemoglobin, and methemoglobin after subarachnoid hemorrhage, J. Neurosurg. 88 (1998) 557–561.

[9] J.P. Dreier, N. Ebert, J. Priller, D. Megow, U. Lindauer, R. Klee, U. Reuter, Y. Imai, K.M. Einhäupl, I. Victorov, U. Dirnagl, Products of hemolysis in the subarachnoid space inducing spreading ischemia in the cortex and focal necrosis in rats: a model for delayed ischemic neurological deficits after subarachnoid hemorrhage? J. Neurosurg. 93 (2000) 658–666.

[10] J. Dreier, K. Körner, T. Back, T. Wolf, A. Görner, U. Lindauer, A. Villringer, U. Dirnagl, Cortical spreading ischemia (CSI): a novel phenomenon induced by cortical spreading depression (CSD), NOS inhibition and elevated extracellular potassium, Soc. Neurosci. Abstr. 21 (1995) 225.

Regulatory factors and microcirculation

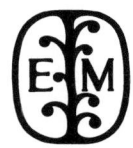

International Congress Series 1235 (2002) 493–500

Tumor necrosis factor-α, heme oxygenase-1 and manganese superoxide dismutase immunostaining of vessels and perivascular brain cells provides evidence for cyclic activation and inactivation of brain vessel segments

Christl A. Ruetzler, Kazuhide Furuya, Hidetaka Takeda, John M. Hallenbeck*

Stroke Branch, National Institute of Neurological Disorders and Stroke, National Institutes of Health, 36 Convent Drive MSC 4128, Building 36/Room 4A03, Bethesda, MD 20892-4128, USA

Abstract

The present work explores the possibility that several mediators of local hemostasis, inflammation and reactivity in blood vessels contribute to cyclic activation and inactivation of individual segments of the brain microvascular tree. Immunohistochemistry was performed with anti-manganese superoxide dismutase (MnSOD), anti-heme oxygenase-1 (HO-1), and antitumor necrosis factor-α (TNF-α) in five different strains of rats and in rats that received lipopolysaccharide to activate their vessels. In both normal and activated brain vessels, immunoreactivity was present as concentric perivascular rings involving vessel wall and surrounding parenchyma that appeared to coincide with one another in serial sections. The ring patterns suggested radial expansion from the vessel lumen into the surrounding parenchyma in cyclic waves. The average number of vessels per high power field (HPF) (mean ± SD) with perivascular cuffs of immunoreactive MnSOD increased from 51 ± 28 in Wistar, 72 ± 46 in Wistar-Kyoto, and 84 ± 30 in Sprague–Dawley rats (no spontaneous strokes) to 184 ± 72 in spontaneously hypertensive stroke-prone rats (SHR-SP) (spontaneous strokes). Perivascular immunoreactive cuffs are also increased in spontaneously hypertensive rats (SHR) by the induction of cytokine expression by lipopolysaccharide (64 ± 15 vs. 131 ± 32/HPF). The findings are interpreted to indicate that focal hemostatic balance normally fluctuates in brain vessels and influences surrounding parenchymal cells. Perivascular immunor-

---

* Corresponding author. Fax: +1-301-402-2769.
E-mail address: Hallenbj@ninds.nih.gov (J.M. Hallenbeck).

0531-5131/02 © 2002 Elsevier Science B.V. All rights reserved.
PII: S 0 5 3 1 - 5 1 3 1 (0 2) 0 0 2 3 7 - 6

eactive cuffs representing this process are more frequent in animals with LPS-induced endothelial activation or genetic stroke-proneness. © 2002 Elsevier Science B.V. All rights reserved.

Keywords: Microvessels; MnSOD; Heme oxygenase; TNF-α; Activation

---

1. Introduction

A number of powerful enzyme and cell signaling systems operate at the blood-endo-thelial interface and can influence the initiation and course of brain ischemia [1]. These systems are usually subject to rigorous control. With respect to hemostasis, potent anti-thrombotic factors that are induced in endothelial cells concurrently with the activation of prothrombotic factors provide the mutual regulation necessary to maintain fluid blood within the circulation [2]. An overall effect of this form of feedback control is systemic fluctuations in thrombogenic potential. Examples include early morning hours reduced capacity for fibrinolysis [3], increased platelet aggregability [4] and a corresponding tendency for strokes to occur preferentially at this time [5].

The concept that hemostatic balance can also fluctuate focally within vessel beds is a relatively recent postulate that owes its origins to dramatic increases in understanding of endothelial cell biology in the last 20 years [6]. According to this model, various ex-tracellular signals and cellular responses in different regions of the vascular tree are integrated by local endothelium. These diverse environmental cues would include cyto-kines, chemokines, nitric oxide, endothelin, growth factors, hemodynamic forces, cell-to-cell signaling, and signaling associated with integrins and other adhesion molecules. Transduction of these signals by endothelium is regulated in space and time. The net effect of these variables is to cause differential expression of endothelial cell-derived procoagu-lant and anticoagulant activities focally throughout the vascular tree.

The distribution patterns of immunoreactivity of several indicators of inflammatory and oxidative stress as well as that of a key antioxidant enzyme have been studied in brain sections. The aim of the current work was to characterize the perivascular expression of the proinflammatory marker tumor necrosis factor-α (TNF-α), the oxidative stress marker heme oxygenase-1 (HO-1), and the antioxidant manganese superoxide dismutase (MnSOD) in brain vessels of several rat strains and to evaluate the role of endothelial activation by LPS in the modulation of the expression of these proteins.

2. Materials and methods

2.1. Animals

Male (12–14 week) spontaneously hypertensive rats (SHR) (Taconic Farms, German-town, NY, USA) and Wistar rats (Charles River Labs, Wilmington, MA, USA) were studied as were male and female (18 week) spontaneously hypertensive stroke-prone rats (SHR-SP) (Kyoto University, Japan). The NIH Animal Care and Use Committee approved all procedures in animals.

2.2. Histology

The following untreated rats were used in the histologic study: SHR ($n=4$), Wistar ($n=3$), and SHR-SP ($n=4$). Additional SHRs received LPS ($n=10$) or saline ($n=5$) intravenously (i.v.). The animals were anesthetized with 0.8% halothane in 30% oxygen and 70% nitrous oxide. Bacterial LPS (*Escherichia coli* 0111: B4 phenol extract; Sigma, St Louis, MO, USA) was suspended in 0.5 ml of sterile 0.9% saline and 0.9 mg/kg was administered intravenously (i.v.). Control animals received saline i.v. After transcardial perfusion with 4% buffered paraformaldehyde (pH 7.43) under deep pentobarbital anesthesia (65 mg/kg intraperitoneal (IP) injection), brains were postfixed for 4 h in 4% paraformaldehyde and paraffin embedded. Sections (7 μm) were cut on a rotary micro-tome, mounted on Probe On Plus Microscope Slides (Fisher Scientific, Pittsburgh, PA, USA), and stained with hematoxylin and eosin for morphologic evaluation. Adjacent sections were used for immunohistochemistry.

2.3. Immunohistochemistry

Briefly, sections were deparaffinized, rehydrated, and permeabilized with 0.3% Triton in phosphate-buffered saline (PBS) for 1 h and rinsed. The slides were immersed in a solution of 3% hydrogen peroxide in 10% methanol/PBS. Slides were washed in PBS 4×5 min and incubated for 2 h in 5% normal goat or 5% normal donkey serum in PBS. Sections were incubated with one of the following primary antibodies diluted in 2% goat serum/PBS overnight at 4 °C: rabbit anti-MnSOD in a concentration of 1:200 (a gift from Dr. Kato, Department of Biochemistry, Institute for Developmental Research, Aichi, Prefectual Colony, Kamiya, Kaugai, Aichi 480-03, Japan), rabbit anti-HO-1, 1:100 (StressGen, Victoria, Canada), and goat anti-TNF-α diluted 1:40 in 2% rat serum/PBS (R&D Systems, Minneapolis, MN, USA). After washing in PBS 4×10 min, sections were incubated with the appropriate biotinylated secondary antibody, goat anti-rabbit or donkey anti-goat (Jackson Immuno Research Labs, West Grove, PA, USA) in a concentration of 1:1000 for 1 h at room temper-ature. Slides were washed as before and incubated for 1 h in an avidin–biotin–peroxidase complex (ABC-Elite Kit, Vector Laboratories, Burlingham, CA, USA) at room temperature. Antigen antibody binding was visualized with diaminobenzidine (DAB Kit, Sigma). For the assessment of nonspecific staining, primary antibodies were omitted or replaced by normal rabbit or goat immunoglobulin G (IgG). TNF-α staining was abolished by the absorption of antibody with a 50-fold excess of recombinant rat TNF-α.

2.4. Quantification of perivascular manganese superoxide dismutase expression

Brain sections were analyzed with a Zeiss Axioplan microscope (Carl Zeiss, Jena, Germany). Images of four different regions (left and right hippocampus, left and right thalamus) were acquired at $50 \times$ magnification with the Metamorph Image Processing System (Universal Imaging, West Chester, PA, USA) and the number of vessels expressing immunoreactive MnSOD cuffs was counted per field of view (393,216 μm^2).

3. Results

3.1. Manganese superoxide dismutase immunohistochemistry

Expression of manganese superoxide dismutase was found in the brains of all animals in a pattern of clearly defined cuffs and rings around blood vessels of all sizes. The number of vessels per high power field (HPF) with MnSOD perivascular cuff expression was variable among untreated rats of different strains. Wistar rats showed the lowest levels of perivascular MnSOD immunoreactivity/HPF (51 ± 28, mean $\pm$ SD) and SHR-SP showed the highest levels (184 ± 72). Untreated SHR had 64 ± 15 vessels/HPF with perivascular immunoreactivity and these levels increased to 131 ± 32 after LPS stimulation in these animals. The difference between perivascular immunoreactivity in Wistar and SHR-SP was significant at $P < 0.001$ and the difference between naïve SHR and LPS-stimulated SHR was significant at $P < 0.02$.

MnSOD expression was most prominent around vessels of the hippocampus, striatum, and thalamus, but could be found throughout the brain. Consistent with the mitochondrial location of MnSOD, the staining was granular. It followed several different staining patterns (Fig. 1). Some vessels were surrounded by tightly packed, intensely staining cuffs that did not extend far beyond the vessel wall. Other vessels were surrounded by thick cuffs of large diameter relative to the central vessel. The staining intensity of these latter cuffs varied from dense to faint. In other vessels, the inner area of the cuff was completely

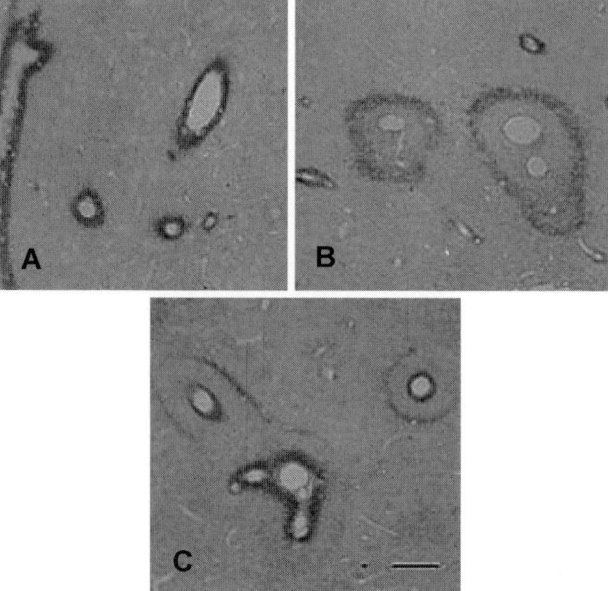

Fig. 1. Immunostaining for MnSOD around thalamic brain vessels of SHR-SP. (A) Perivascular cuff tightly adjacent to lumen. (B) Ring some distance away from lumen with clearing around vessel. (C) Second ring appearing close to lumen within the expanded first ring. Scale bar = 100 μm.

unstained adjacent to the vessel wall with only an outer ring staining for MnSOD. These larger cuffs, which appear to have expanded radially from the central vessel, could extend to an outer diameter of about 50 µm and within some of these expanded cuffs, a nascent ring within a ring could be observed. In this pattern, the smaller inner ring hugged the vessel wall and stained intensely for MnSOD whereas the larger outer ring stained weakly and surrounded tissue in which the MnSOD immunoreactivity was faint or absent. When the MnSOD primary antibody was omitted, the perivascular cuff staining was eliminated. These patterns were inferred to indicate that MnSOD is induced in wave upon wave originating at the vessel wall and spreading radially from there into the surrounding parenchymal tissue. Cells with the morphology of endothelium, pericytes and astrocytes were positive for MnSOD and the staining for MnSOD was most prominent in neurons.

3.2. HO-1 immunohistochemistry

The HO-1 immunoreactivity pattern in the brains of all experimental animals corresponded to the perivascular MnSOD pattern. The staining was robust and coincident with that of MnSOD, but was not as strong. Brains of untreated SHR-SP showed pronounced cuffing as did SHR that received intravenous injections of LPS. Wistar rats showed occasional lightly stained cuffing. The enzyme was expressed in cells with the morphology of endothelium, microglia and astrocytes, and perivascular macrophages.

3.3. Tumor necrosis factor-α immunohistochemistry

The cuffing pattern around vessels of all sizes for tumor necrosis factor-α was the same as that described previously for MnSOD and HO-1, but the staining was weaker. Where it was expressed, its distribution coincided closely with the spatial distribution of HO-1 and MnSOD. However, its distribution was less extensive and its intensity was lower. Tumor necrosis factor-α was expressed in cells with the morphology of endothelium, pericytes, astrocytes and some neurons.

3.4. Hematoxylin and eosin staining

No pathologic changes or abnormalities were noted in this series. Even the brains and blood vessels of animals that showed strong staining for MnSOD such as SHR-SP and LPS-stimulated SHR showed no obvious pathology.

4. Discussion

The current study shows that immunoreactive MnSOD surrounds scattered intraparenchymal brain vessels in normal rats from several different strains. The distribution patterns of the immunoreactivity suggest that within scattered microvessel segments, an endogenous stimulus for up-regulation of MnSOD repeatedly develops. These stimuli then expand centrifugally in cyclic waves. Immunoreactivity patterns for HO-1 and TNF-α suggest that they are part of the same process (Fig. 2).

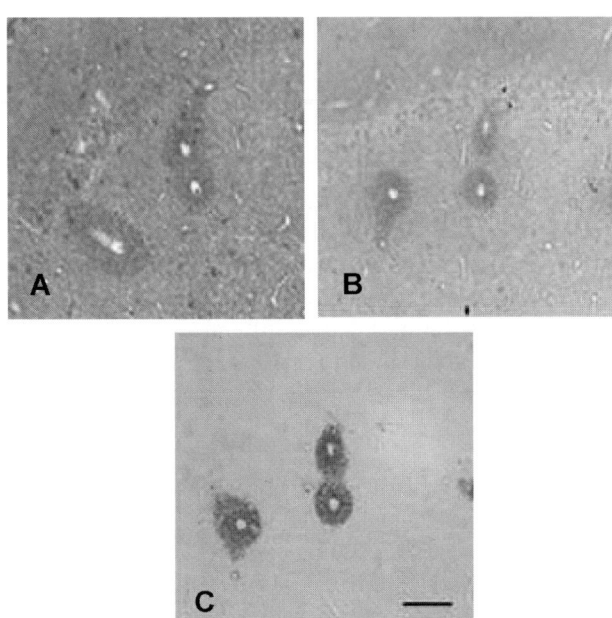

Fig. 2. Immunostaining around blood vessels in adjacent hippocampal sections of naïve SHR-SP. Cuffs around vessels staining positive for (A) TNF-α, (B) HO-1 and (C) MnSOD. Scale bar = 50 μm.

TNF-α expression has been detected in a number of different cell types in the brain under various experimental conditions. This cytokine has a number of proinflammatory and procoagulant effects on endothelium [1,6]. TNF-α can also directly stimulate production of HO-1 and MnSOD [7]. There are three known isoforms of heme oxygenase. HO-1 is inducible, HO-2 is constitutive and there is also a recently identified isoform, HO-3 [8]. In response to stressful stimuli particularly reactive oxygen species (ROS), endothelium [9], astrocytes, and neurons [10] produce HO-1. In addition to providing a signal that indicates preceding cellular stress [11], HO-1 also serves as an antioxidant. MnSOD is a mitochondrial antioxidant enzyme that can be induced by cytokines such as TNF-α or by ROS [12].

A glimpse of the dynamism involved in focal hemostatic balance in the brain is provided by the current findings. Based on the observations herein, the authors propose that under normal conditions, scattered intraparenchymal brain vessels randomly undergo cyclic fluctuation in proinflammatory and prothrombotic potential alternating with anti-inflammatory and antithrombotic potential. These cyclic fluctuations originate within the vessels and spread radially outward to involve parenchymal cells and their processes within a perivascular circumference of approximately 50 μm. The hemostatic balance of vessel segments tilts in a proinflammatory and prothrombotic direction with the local release of TNF-α and generation of ROS. In response, vascular and perivascular cells exposed to these stimuli synthesize HO-1 and MnSOD to help restore hemostatic balance. These cyclic fluctuations occur under normal circumstances within a homestatic range and local circulatory disturbances and tissue damage do not occur. If the fluctuations become larger and exceed some threshold, however, they could predispose local segments to thrombosis or hemorrhage.

4.3.1.6. On-Site Discussion

4.3.1.6.1. *Question: (Kuschinsky)* Is this an on–off phenomenon? It looks like starting and stopping rather suddenly. Did you find a time course?

Answer: (Hallenbeck) We really cannot be precise about the kinetics with this static approach. Once expressed, the biologic half-lives of these proteins are measured in hours.

4.3.1.6.2. *Question: (Kent)* (1) You never saw any local neutrophil/macrophage reaction—how do you explain this? (2) The regulation of a MnSOD is well known at a transcriptional level—have you investigated whether these are mediating your findings?

Answer: (Hallenbeck) (1) We did not stain for it and in these sections, it is easy to miss adherent cells. Also, this seems to occur in a "homeostatic range" and firm adhesion may not occur. (2) We have not investigated this but it is a good idea.

4.3.1.6.3. *Question: (Dirnagl)* What is the evidence that you are looking at a truly oscillatory phenomenon, and what might be the length of one cycle?

Answer: (Hallenbeck) The interesting exercise would be to try to come up with an alternative explanation for the patterns I have just described. Proof of oscillation would, of course, require a different experimental approach. Based on the biologic half-lives of the proteins involved, I would suggest that the duration of a cycle would be measured in hours.

4.3.1.6.4. *Question: (Kempski)* Do the "cuffs" show a variation during the clay, i.e., if animals are killed at different times of the day, is the picture different?

Answer: (Hallenbeck) Because of known diurnal variation, this is very interesting question. Unfortunately, we do not have the data to answer it.

4.3.1.6.5. *Question: (Gaehtgens)* Do you think that what you describe as the balance between pro- and anti-thrombotic properties can be considered as a true homeostatic phenomenon in the sense that it would have a set point, an error signal and a mechanism to return the system to the set point once it has been moved "out of balance"? Are there any ideas what the error signal could be and how it could be deleted?

Answer: (Hallenbeck) It is apparent that we should not describe this as homeostatic balance defined by these rigorous criteria since we do not know the data to satisfy the definition. What we show is an interplay between agonists and antagonists that does not become deviation amplifying and lead to thrombosis.

4.3.1.6.6. *Question: (Hamel)* How did you inject LPS?

Answer: (Hallenbeck) It was injected intravenously.

4.3.1.6.7. *Comment: (Hamel)* There is similarity with reaction/activation of brain capillary endothelial cells following systemic/local injection of LPS in the rat forelimb by S. Rivest and colleagues. They have similarly found that they may be particularly reactive to inflammation, even a reaction initiated locally in the periphery.

References

[1] J.M. Hallenbeck, Inflammatory reactions at the blood endothelial interface in acute stroke, in: B.K. Siesjo, T. Wieloch (Eds.), Advances in Neurology, Cellular and Molecular Mechanisms of Ischemic Brain Damage, vol. 71, Lippincott-Raven, Philadelphia, 1996, pp. 281–300.

[2] D.R. Rosenberg, W.C. Aird, Vascular-bed-specific hemostatic and hypercoagulable states, N. Engl. J. Med. 340 (1999) 1555–1564.

[3] P. Angleton, W.L. Chandler, G. Schmer, Diurnal variation of tissue-type plasminogen activator and its rapid inhibitor (PAI-1), Circulation 79 (1989) 101–116.

[4] A. Jovicic, V. Ivanisevic, R. Nicolajevic, Circadian variations of platelet aggregability and fibrinolytic activity in patients with ischemic stroke, Thromb. Res. 64 (1991) 487–491.

[5] J.R. Marler, T.R. Price, G.L. Clark, J.E. Muller, T. Robertson, J.P. Mohr, D.B. Hier, P.A. Wolf, L.R. Caplan, M.A. Foulkes, Morning increase in onset of ischemic stroke, Stroke 20 (1989) 473–476.

[6] J.S. Pober, R.S. Cotran, Cytokines and endothelial cell biology, Physiol. Rev. 70 (1990) 427–451.

[7] C.M. Terry, J.A. Clikeman, J.R. Hoidal, K.S. Callahan, TNF-α and Il-1α induce heme oxygenase-1 via protein kinase C, Ca^{2+}, and phospholipase A2 in endothelial cells, Am. J. Physiol. 276 (1999) H1493–H1501.

[8] W.K. McCoubrey Jr., T.J. Huang, M.D. Maines, Isolation and characterization of a cDNA from the rat brain that encodes hemoprotein heme oxygenase-3, Eur. J. Biochem. 247 (1997) 725–732.

[9] C.M. Terry, J.A. Clikeman, J.R. Hoidal, K.S. Callahan, Effect of tumor necrosis factor-α and interleukin-1α on heme oxygenase-1 expression in human endothelial cells, Am. J. Physiol. 274 (1998) H883–H891.

[10] B.E. Dwyer, R.N. Nishimura, S.-Y. Lu, Differential expression of heme oxygenase-1 in cultured cortical neurons and astrocytes determined by the aid of a new heme oxygenase antibody. Response to oxidative stress, Mol. Brain Res. 30 (1995) 37–47.

[11] D.K. Poss, S. Tonegawa, Reduced stress defense in heme oxygenase 1-deficient cells, Proc. Natl. Acad. Sci. U. S. A. 94 (1997) 10925–10930.

[12] G.H.W. Wong, D.V. Goeddel, Induction of manganese superoxide dismutase by tumor necrosis factor: possible protective mechanism, Science 242 (1988) 941–944.

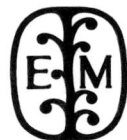

International Congress Series 1235 (2002) 501–507

Control of flow on the microvascular level

Wolfgang Kuschinsky*, Johannes Vogel

*Department of Physiology and Pathophysiology, University of Heidelberg,
Im Neuenheimer Feld 326, D-69120 Heidelberg, Germany*

Abstract

The finding of a permanent perfusion of all brain capillaries under normal conditions raises the question of "How is cerebral blood flow distributed to the different capillaries?" Experiments, in which an intravascular dye was injected and its distribution to the brain capillaries was measured, have shown a heterogeneous capillary perfusion under normal conditions and a more homogeneous capillary perfusion during conditions of increased cerebral blood flow such as hypercapnia and whisker barrel stimulation. With such a mechanism, it is possible that, an enhanced exchange of blood gases and metabolic fuels and waste products is obtained, without the need of recruitment of previously non-perfused capillaries. © 2002 Elsevier Science B.V. All rights reserved.

Keywords: Capillary perfusion; Flow heterogeneity; Capillary recruitment; Non-perfused capillaries; Cerebral blood flow

1. Do non-perfused capillaries exist in the brain?

It is now generally accepted that, under physiological conditions, all capillaries are perfused in the brain. This conclusion is based on the following findings: when an intravascular marker, such as Evans blue, is injected i.v., it can be detected a few seconds later in all brain capillaries [1]. This indicates a complete and instantaneous filling of all brain capillaries after injection of an intravascular marker. The complete filling of all brain capillaries is verified by a double staining of the capillary vessel wall, in addition to the detection of the intravascular marker (Fig. 1). The principle of a complete perfusion of all the capillaries in the brain is only disturbed during extreme pathophysiology. During brain ischemia after occlusion of the middle cerebral artery, areas of slow capillary perfusion

---

* Corresponding author. Tel.: +49-6221-544033; fax: +49-6221-544561.
E-mail address: wolfgang.kuschinsky@pio1.uni-heidelberg.de (W. Kuschinsky).

0531-5131/02 © 2002 Elsevier Science B.V. All rights reserved.
PII: S 0 5 3 1 - 5 1 3 1 (0 2) 0 0 2 3 9 - X

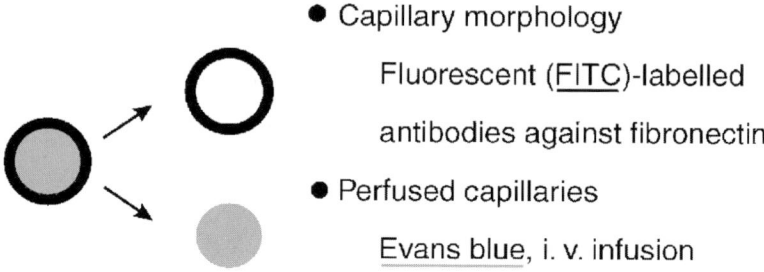

Fig. 1. Flourescent double stain.

evolve. Within hours and days, parts of the slowly perfused areas are converted to non-perfused areas [2]. Such non-perfused areas show an extremely low blood flow, indicating the existence of nonviable tissue when capillary perfusion is stopped. These data show that capillary perfusion is maintained even at low blood flow in the brain, and non-perfused capillaries only arise during ischemia.

2. How is the blood flow distributed to the different capillaries?

If a continuous perfusion of all the capillaries exists, how is the blood flow distributed to the different capillaries? In principle, there are two possibilities: the blood flow can be either evenly or unevenly distributed to the capillaries. In other words, the velocity of flow could be either identical or different in the various capillaries. Taking into account the variations in length of the capillaries in any given network, it appears reasonable to expect a heterogeneous perfusion velocity in the capillary networks of the brain. We have addressed this question in the following way [3]: a bolus of Evans blue is injected i.v. in either conscious or anesthetized rats. Within 3–4 s, the bolus has filled all of the brain capillaries. At this moment, the animal is decapitated. In cryosections of the brain, the intensity of the fluorescence in a capillary is an indicator of the velocity of flow in this capillary since the bolus filled, at this point, more intensely the rapidly perfused than the slowly perfused capillaries. These experiments have shown an extreme heterogeneity of fluorescent intensity under normal physiological conditions in conscious and anesthetized rats. This indicates an extreme heterogeneity of the perfusion velocity in different capillaries of the brain. Fig. 2 shows the results of such measurements. The degree of heterogeneity is given for four brain structures as a coefficient of variation (S.D./mean·100). It is evident that the heterogeneity of the microflow is about the same in the different brain structures although blood flow varies by a factor of about five. The explanation is based upon the fact that capillary density is also different between the brain structures by a factor of about five. Therefore, the amount of blood flow per capillary is identical for each capillary, irrespective of the brain structure investigated as indicated in Fig. 2. These results indicate identical perfusion patterns in the different parts of the brain. Furthermore, these patterns are not influenced by the basal flow in this brain structure.

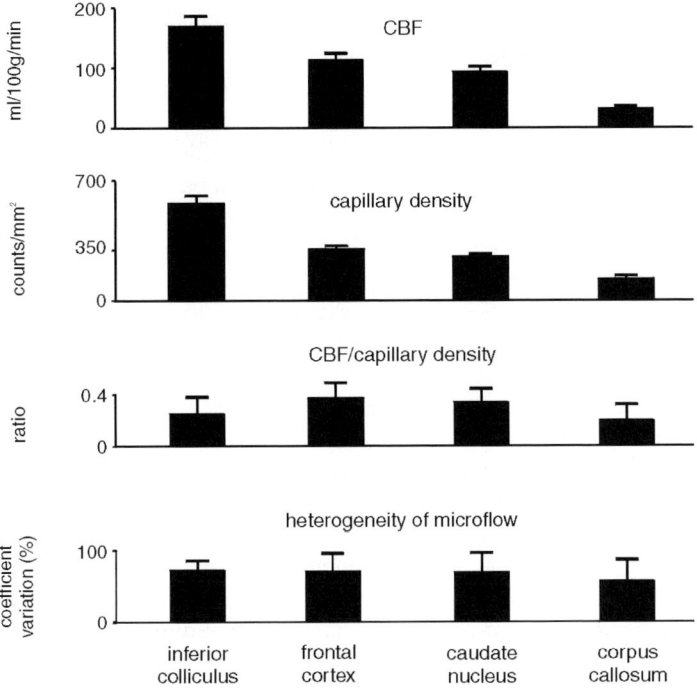

Fig. 2. Relationship between cerebral blood flow, capillary density and flow heterogeneity.

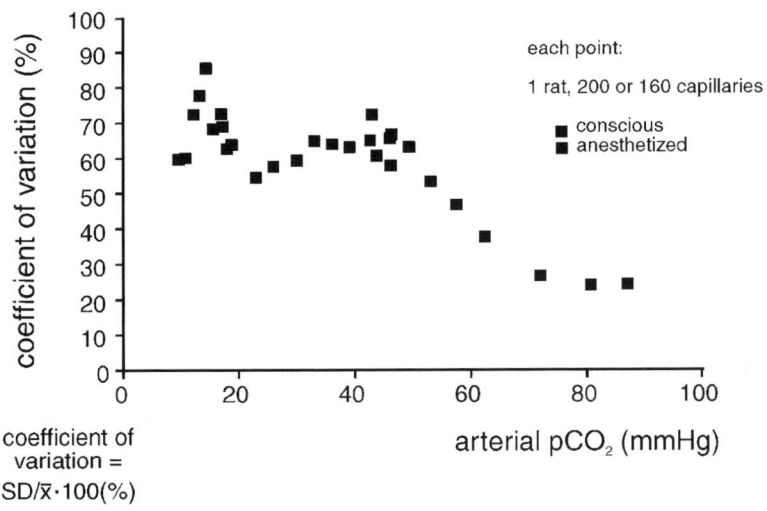

coefficient of
variation =
SD/x̄·100(%)

Fig. 3. Variations of intercapillary Evans blue concentration.

After resting conditions, a heterogeneous capillary perfusion is shown, and the question arises how the pattern of microvascular perfusion is influenced during an increased cerebral blood flow. In principle, the heterogeneity could either be maintained due to an increased velocity in all capillaries, or the hereogeneity could be decreased by an enhanced flow preferentially in the slowly perfused capillaries. In order to investigate this question, two types of experiments were performed: the cerebral blood flow was increased either by inhalation of CO_2 or by stimulation of the rats' whiskers. The results of the variations in pCO_2 are shown in Fig. 3. The main finding in these experiments is the decrease in heterogeneity of the microvascular blood flow during increases in arterial pCO_2, which are known (and have also been verified in these experiments) to increase cerebral blood flow. The conclusion drawn from these experiments is that an increased blood flow results in a more homogeneous microvascular flow pattern, which is based on an increased velocity of perfusion, preferentially in the slowly perfused capillaries.

The second approach to increase cerebral blood flow was to stimulate the whiskers of the rats for an induction of functional hyperemia. The heterogeneity of capillary flow was determined in the corresponding brain cortex [4].

The results are shown in Fig. 4. The reciprocal relationship between blood flow and flow hetereogeneity shows that the heterogeneity of microflow is decreased during functional hyperemia. Apparently, it is not important whether the cerebral blood

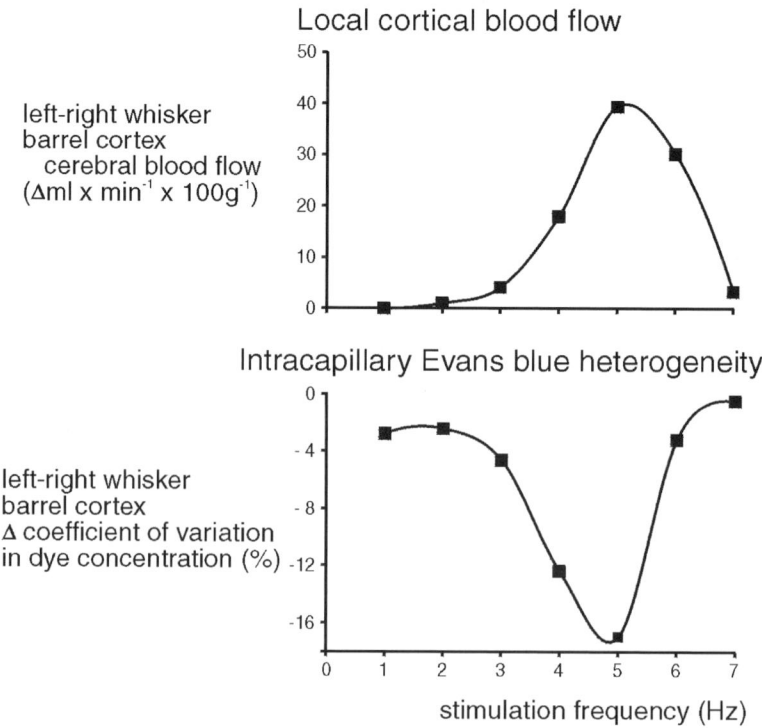

Fig. 4. Whisker stimulation.

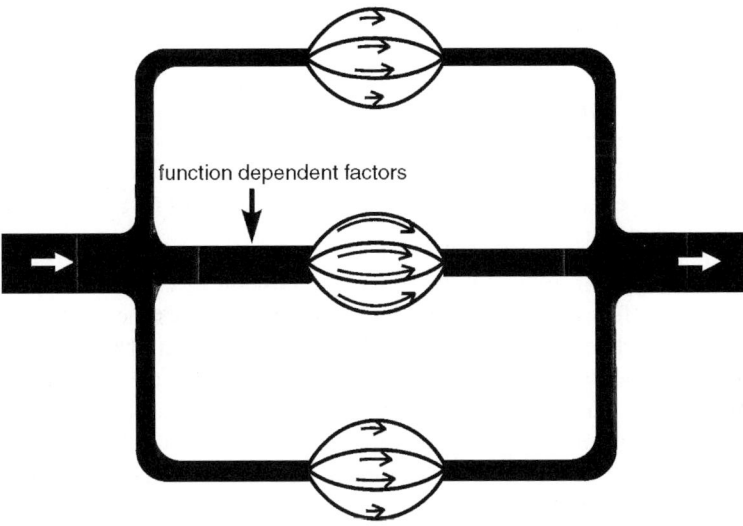

Fig. 5. Brain capillary networks during local functional activation—hypothesis.

flow is increased by functional activation or by CO_2: the result is a decrease in perfusion hetereogeneity.

3. Can these findings lead to a unifying concept of microvascular regulation during brain activation?

From these findings, the following concept of vascular and microvascular regulation during brain activation can be derived. Brain activation induces, by unknown and known (K^+, H^+, adenosine, NO) mechanisms, a dilation of the arterioles which supply one or several capillary units. Three such units are shown schematically in Fig. 5. The vasodilation results in an increased perfusion of the capillary units. As outlined, the increased perfusion induces a more homogeneous perfusion of the capillary units, and as a result of this change in the perfusion pattern, an enhanced exchange of blood gases, metabolic fuels and waste products can take place.

4.3.2.5. On-Site Discussion

4.3.2.5.1. *Question: (Gaehtgens)* This is a very interesting study and very convincing data. However, there is one observation which needs additional explanation: why is the heterogeneity in the absence of red cells at high PCO_2 greater than in the presence of red cells?

Answer: (Kuschinsky) This is indeed a puzzling finding. Certainly, there is a basic heterogeneity due to the fact that the different capillaries in the networks have a different length resulting in different resistances within the network. The flow heterogeneity found after blood exchange should reflect this structural heterogeneity which is not influenced by flow changes.

4.3.2.5.2. *Question: (Paulson)* I am pleased to see heterogeneity of capillary perfusion confirmed. But I have still a critical question. With increased flow, the linear flow rate in larger as well as smaller vessels increases. Therefore, the time 4 s from dye injection to decapitate during hypercapnia might correspond to an interval of 6–8 s during rest. Should this influence your results?

Answer: (Kuschinsky) In principle, this might be possible if cardiac output is doubled. However, such an effect is prevented by the design of the experiments. By a continuous measurement of blood conductance during and after the injection of Evans blue, we know the arterial concentration changes at any moment. Decapitation always is performed during the ascending part of the concentration (i.e. conductance) curve. In addition, we observe also a decrease in heterogeneity of microflow in the whisker barrel cortex during whisker stimulation. In this case, the changes in flow are local and there is certainly no change in the flow rate in the larger feeding vessels.

4.3.2.5.3. *Comment: (Paulson)* According to your theory, the decreased heterogeneity during high flow situations is due to a more equal and homogeneous red cell compared to plasma flow. This implies that the tissue hematocrit should increase and be closer to the systemic hematocrit. Also, the transit time through the cerebrovascular bed of erythrocytes should be closer to that of plasma.

Response to comment (Kuschinsky) Yes, I agree.

4.3.2.5.4. *Question: (Tanifuji)* Hiro Fukuda and Seong-Gi Kim suggested that changes in CBF or CBV have 100-μm level precision. If there is no active mechanism of capillary control, then how can we explain this high precision of changes in CBF and CBV during neuronal activation?

Answer: (Kuschinsky) In my opinion, passive mechanisms are sufficient to explain the results of a decreased heterogeneity during increases in flow, but this doesn't exclude the possibility that an active mechanism on the single capillary level may exist. If such a mechanism has been convincingly demonstrated, it could add to the mechanism postulated here. Anyway, a precision of about 100 μm as you mentioned could be completely congruent with the proposed mechanism. According to this mechanism, one capillary unit consisting of a small number of capillaries (e.g. 10) is supplied by one precapillary arteriole. Any change in the resistance of this arteriole will affect the perfusion of all capillaries in this unit. Right now, we do not know the size of such a unit, but it could have the size of 100 μm.

4.3.2.5.5. *Question: (Watanabe)* During induced hyperemia, we observed much more capillaries compared to the normal state. Can this be called the recruitment of capillaries? (Compared to the normal state, we observe much more capillaries during induced hyperemia. That means that, in the control state, there are many capillaries containing no red blood cells, only plasma. How does this apply to your model?)

Answer: (Kuschinsky) What you observed is exactly what one would expect from our model. In a nonactivated brain area, you will see rather few erythrocytes in the microcirculation. With increasing blood flow, the number of visible erythrocytes should increase. This increased number of erythrocytes is the consequence of a more homogeneous perfusion of the capillary bed.

4.3.2.5.6. *Question: (Busch)* Until recently, stroke was treated by lowering the hematocrit. Do you think we should increase it now?

Answer: (Kuschinsky) The question as to what is the "optimal" hematocrit has never convincingly been answered. The reason is that we cannot exactly define the perfusion conditions in the microcirculation: the blood viscosity is not known locally because the shear stress to which the erythrocytes are locally exposed is not known. But we do know that an increased hematocrit results in an increased viscosity of the blood. That such an increased hematocrit can be detrimental in the clinical situation is demonstrated by the disease polycythemia, in which patients, due to their high hematocrit, have an increased risk to suffer from ischemic diseases. So there is no reason to increase the hematocrit above normal values in patients suffering from ischemic diseases.

References

[1] U. Göbel, H. Theilen, W. Kuschinsky, Congruence of total and perfused capillary network in rat brains, Circ. Res. 66 (1990) 271–281.
[2] J. Vogel, A. Hermes, W. Kuschinsky, Evolution of microcirculatory disturbances after permanent middle cerebral artery occlusion in rats, J. Cereb. Blood Flow Metab. 19 (1999) 1322–1328.
[3] R. Abounader, J. Vogel, W. Kuschinsky, Patterns of capillary plasma perfusion in brains of conscious rats during normo- and hypercapnia, Circ. Res. 76 (1995) 120–126.
[4] J. Vogel, W. Kuschinsky, Decreased heterogeneity of capillary plasma flow in the rat whisker barrel cortex during functional hyperemia, J. Cereb. Blood Flow Metab. 16 (1996) 1300–1306.

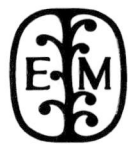

International Congress Series 1235 (2002) 509–514

Response of cerebral neocapillaries to acetylcholine: an intravital microscopic observation

Kolammal Nageswari, Takashi Yamakawa, Hideyuki Niimi *

Department of Vascular Physiology, National Cardiovascular Center Research Institute, Osaka 565 8565, Japan

Abstract

The purpose of this study was to examine the response of cerebral neocapillaries to acetylcholine (ACh) in mice. Wild type male mice were used. After anesthesia, a small area of the bone over the parietal cortex was removed to expose the cerebral cortex. The gel–nylon mesh sandwich system was placed over the exposed area. The growth factors bFGF and PDGF were used at a concentration of 6 ng/ml. After the surgical area was covered with a polyurethane biomembrane, the skin was closed with sutures. After 28 days of incubation, the neocapillaries were topically suffused with ACh and the responses of the vascular diameter and red blood cell (RBC) velocity were evaluated using intravital video microscopy. A control group was included to examine the responses of the pial vessels to ACh. A significant increase in vascular diameter and RBC velocity was observed in the control group, while the neocapillaries failed to show anything significant in the bFGF group. However, a significant increase in RBC velocity from the baseline value was observed in the PDGF group. It is suggested that the neocapillaries might have matured in the PDGF group with the formation of pericytes/smooth muscle cell function (SMC), leading to relaxation via the cGMP pathway. © 2002 Elsevier Science B.V. All rights reserved.

Keywords: Cerebral neocapillary; Acetylcholine; Intravital microscopy

1. Introduction

The blood supply to cerebral tissue is continuously regulated to meet the varying demands of the tissue [1]. Up to now, there has been no report available on vasomotor responses of the cerebral neocapillaries, though vasomotor responses of newly developed

* Corresponding author. Tel.: +81-6-6833-5012; fax: +81-6-6872-7485.
E-mail addresses: nages@jsc.ncvc.go.jp (K. Nageswari), niimi@ncvc.go.jp (H. Niimi).

coronary collateral vessels and endothelial function in well-developed canine coronary collateral vessels have been reported [2–4].

Quite recently, we have developed a model to study cerebral angiogenesis [5]. The cerebral angiogenesis was induced by growth factors bFGF and PDGF at various concentrations in mice. We observed the cerebral neocapillary development and its remodeling on different days after incubation, from 1 week to 1 month. In this paper, using our mice model, a pilot study is carried out to examine the response of the cerebral neocapillaries to acetylcholine (ACh), which is an important regulator of cerebral blood flow (CBF) [6,7]. We evaluated the changes in red blood cell (RBC) velocity and diameter after the topical application of ACh, based on the observed images using intravital video microscopy.

2. Materials and methods

2.1. Preparation of nylon mesh, biomembrane system

This system was used to stimulate the cerebral angiogenesis. A ready-made kit of collagen for tissue culture (Cellmatrix, Nitta Gelatin, Japan) was used to prepare the gel for incorporating the growth factors bFGF and PDGF-BB, which were obtained from Sigma, USA. The growth factors in bovine serum albumin (BSA, Sigma) were used at the concentration of 6 ng/ml. The collagen with growth factor was placed on a square piece of nylon mesh (5×5-mm width; Nylon Mesh Screen No. 230, Japan). The nylon mesh is 50 μm in thickness and 60×60 μm in mesh size. Another square piece of nylon mesh was placed over the gel mixture and completed the nylon mesh sandwich system. The thickness between the two meshes is approximately 20 μm. A small piece of nylon mesh sandwich sheet was used to place the exposed area of the cerebral cortex.

2.2. Implantation of the nylon mesh sandwich system

Animal experiments were conducted in conformity with the "Guiding Principles in the Care and Use of Animals". Wild type male mice (CB57/6J, 8–10 weeks old) were used for this study. A mouse was anesthetized with pentobarbital sodium (50 mg/kg body weight). A small area over the parietal cortex was removed using a drill to expose the cerebral cortex. The dura was separated and the gel–nylon mesh sandwich system was placed over the exposed cortex. The surgical area was covered with a polyurethane biomembrane and the skin was closed with silk thread (4–0). The animal was allowed to recover in the cage with the usual supply of food and water.

2.3. Animal preparation

After incubation for 28 days, the animal was anesthetized with pentobarbital sodium (50 mg/kg body weight, i.p.) and mechanically ventilated. A polyethylene cannula was inserted into the right common carotid artery to inject the FITC labeled RBCs [8], and the animal head was fixed in a surgical head holder. Furthermore, the skin above the cerebral cortex was incised and the biomembrane was separated.

2.4. In vivo observation

The neocapillaries on the upper surface of the nylon mesh were observed under the fluorescence video microscope (Nikon CFI 60, Japan). The images were recorded on a video tape recorder, which was running at 30 frames per second. Based on the video images, the RBC velocity (dual window method) and diameter were calculated [8]. The neocapillary with the diameter 11 to 16 µm ($n=6$ in each group) was chosen for the observation of the vasodilatory changes after suffusion with ACh. After the initial recordings for 15 to 30 min, the neocapillaries were topically suffused with ACh (acetylcholine chloride 5×10^{-3} M) for 60 s. The changes in RBC velocity and diameter were recorded. A control group was included in this study to monitor the responses of the pial microvessels to ACh.

3. Results

Figs. 1 and 2 show the response of RBC velocity and diameter to Ach, respectively. An increase in RBC velocity from the basal value was significant for the control group (pial vessels) and PDGF group (neocapillaries). However, the bFGF group did not show any significant increase in RBC velocity after the topical application of ACh. The percentage of increase in the RBC velocity of PDGF was significant as compared to bFGF. On the other hand, the diameter changes were significant for the control group.

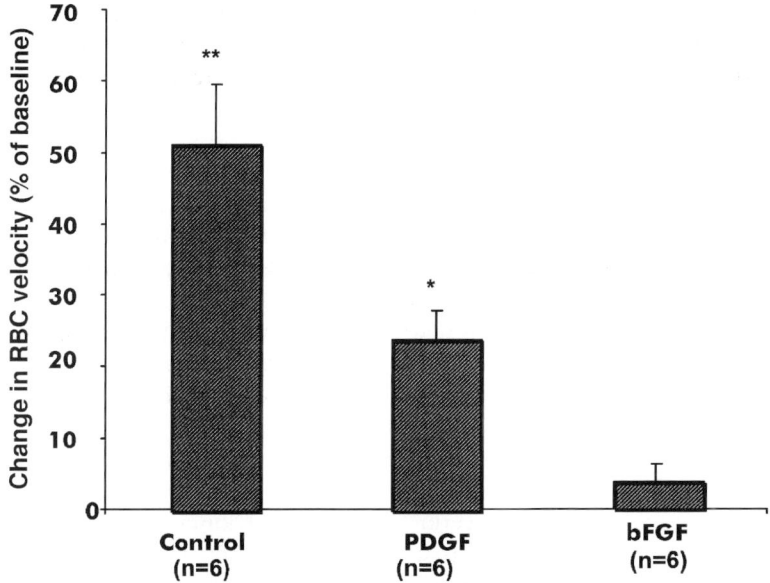

Fig. 1. Response of RBC velocity to ACh. The vessels with a diameter 11 to 16 µm were chosen for this study. Number of vessels studied is given in parentheses. Data are means±SE from each group. Statistical analysis was done using Student's *t*-test. **$P<0.001$ as compared to PDGF and bFGF. *$p<0.001$ as compared to bFGF.

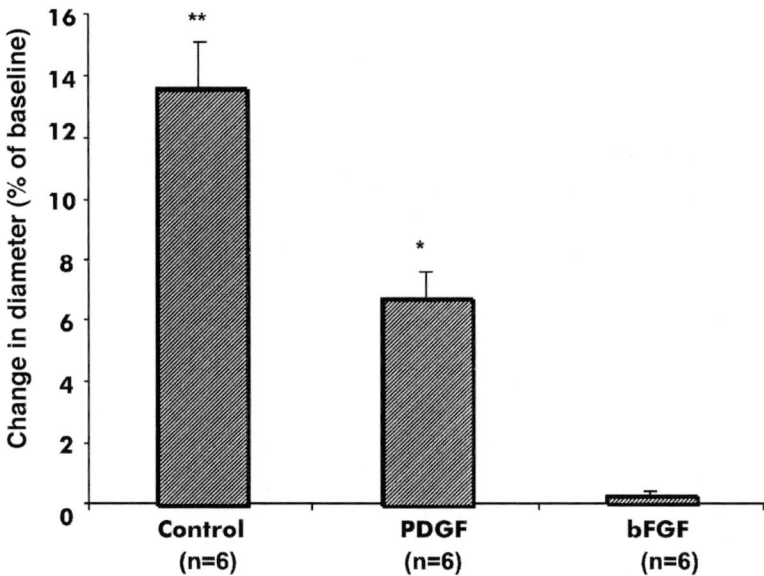

Fig. 2. Response of diameter to ACh. The vessels with a diameter 11 to 16 μm were chosen for this study. Number of vessels studied is given in parentheses. Data are means±SE from each group. Statistical analysis was done using Student's *t*-test. **P<0.001 as compared to PDGF and bFGF. *p<0.001 as compared to bFGF.

There was no alteration in diameter in the bFGF group after the topical application of ACh. However, the PDGF group showed about a 7% increase in the diameter from its baseline value.

4. Discussion

Cholinergic mechanisms have been implicated in the control of the cerebral arterial system and microvasculature [9,10]. Cholinergic-mediated increases in the local CBF have been observed in the frontal and parietal subdivisions of the cerebral cortex on stimulation of basal forebrain cholinergic neurons and muscarinic ACh receptors (mAChR), some of which are presumably associated with the local microcirculation, and have been implicated in this response [7]. The present study showed an increase in RBC velocity as well as in the diameter, after applying ACh topically on mouse cerebral vessels, which support the previous findings. Altman et al. [3] and Flynn et al. [11] reported that well-developed canine collateral vessels studied 6–12 months after coronary occlusion, underwent vasodilation in response to nitroglycerin, Ach and bradykinin. Vasoconstriction of the collateral vessels in response to angiotensin II, serotinin, or the thromboxane A2 analogue U-46619 was reported by Wright et al. [12]. Kinn et al. [2] have reported that as early as 2 weeks after coronary artery occlusion, the developing collateral vessels are capable of substantial vasomotor activity. However, in the present study a significant increase was observed in the RBC velocity in the cerebral neocapillaries from the base line value in the

PDGF group, while the bFGF group failed to show any change. The intracerebral cholinergic mechanisms, which participate in the regulation of local or global blood flow, also involve muscarinic cholinergic receptors [13]. It has been reported by an in vitro study that pericytes have muscarinic binding sites that might respond to ACh [14]. This supports our findings that the RBC velocity and diameter increased after the application of ACh in the PDGF group. Pericytes have been attributed a variety of roles including regulation of permeability, mediation of contractility, maintenance of integrity, and smooth muscle cell function (SMC) [15]. In addition, pericytes are reported to regulate the migration and proliferation of endothelial cells during angiogenesis [15]. The localization in pericytes of cGMP-dependent protein kinase [16] and contractile elements including actin [17] and myosin [18] supports their proposed involvement in microvascular contractility. Pericytes express PDGF receptors and respond to PDGF in vitro [19].

Although bFGF have also been reported as a candidate for involvement in SMC/pericyte-precursor recruitment, and also enhances endothelium-dependent relaxation of the collateral-perfused coronary microcirculation, the present results did not show any change in RBC velocity/diameter after the application of ACh. Our study showed that immuno-histochemical staining by alpha-SMA was stronger in PDGF rather than bFGF (data not shown). It is conjectured that the failure of increase in RBC velocity/diameter in the bFGF group may be due to the immature/absence of SMC/pericytes in the newly developed vessels or due to the tortuous nature of neocapillaries developed in the bFGF group.

4.3.3.6. On-Site Discussion

4.3.3.6.1. *Question: (Tomita)* How do you think that the velocity of RBC is regulated in the newly generated capillaries without supporting parenchymal cells?

Answer: (Nageswari) We believe that pericytes control flow.

4.3.3.6.2. *Question: (Hamel)* Do you believe that the immature pericytes will respond to other vasoactive substances, like vasoconstrictors such as serotonin?

Answer: (Nageswari) In the present study, we observed the RBC velocity and diameter respond to acetylcholine in PDGF group while bFGF group failed to show any change. But it is not sure that pericytes/smooth muscle cells are matured or immatured in PDGF group. But it showed a positive staining for immunohistochemical staining with L-SMA. As I said earlier, the failure of increase in RBC velocity/diameter in bFGF group may be due to its tortuous nature of neocapillaries or may be absence/immature nature of pericytes. We will be carrying out more studies with different vasoactive agents to test the response of cerebral neocapillaries to vasoactive substances.

4.3.3.6.3. *Question: (Maiese)* With your application of bFGF or PDGF to stimulate neocapillary growth, did you observe any anatomical or functional differences between capillaries treated with bFGF or PDGF since these trophic factors employ some independent cellular mechanisms which can promote vascular growth?

Answer: (Nageswari) Yes, the neocapillary density that we observed for bFGF group was very tortuous compared to PDGF group. On the other hand, hemodynamic characteristics did not show significant difference.

References

[1] H. Niimi, Microcirculatory control in the brain tissue, in: T. Kamada, T. Shiga, R.S. MaCuskey (Eds.), Tissue Perfusion and Organ Function. Ischemia/Reperfusion Injury, Elsevier, Amsterdam, 1996, pp. 49–59.

[2] J.W. Kinn, J.D. Altman, M.W. Chang, R.J. Bache, Vasomotor responses of newly developed coronary collateral vessels, Am. J. Physiol. 271 (2) (1996) H490–H497.

[3] J. Altman, D. Dulas, T. Pavek, D.D. Laxson, D.C. Homans, R.J. Bache, Endothelial function in well-developed canine coronary collateral vessels, Am. J. Physiol. 264 (2) (1993) H567–H572.

[4] P.V. Hautamaa, X.Z. Dai, D.C. Homans, R.J. Bache, Vasomotor activity of moderately well-developed canine coronary collateral circulation, Am. J. Physiol. 240 (1981) H890–H897.

[5] H. Niimi, K. Nageswari, G. Ranade, S. Yamaguchi, T. Yamakawa, Microcirculatory characterization of cerebral angiogenesis in mice using intravital videomicroscopy, Clin. Hemorheol. Microcirc. 23 (2–4) (2000) 293–301.

[6] F. Dauphin, E.T. MacKenzie, Cholinergic and vasoactive intestinal polypeptide innervation of the cerebral arteries, Pharmacol. Ther. 67 (1995) 385–417.

[7] A. Sato, Y. Sato, Cholinergic neural regulation of regional cerebral blood flow, Alzheimer Dis. Assoc. Disord. 9 (1995) 28–38.

[8] S. Yamaguchi, T. Yamakawa, H. Niimi, Red cell velocity and microvessel diameter measurement by a two fluorescent tracer method under epifluorescence microscopy: application to cerebral microvessels of cats, Int. J. Microcirc. 11 (1992) 403–416.

[9] S.P. Arneric, M.A. Honig, T.A. Milner, S. Greco, C. Iadecola, D.J. Reis, Neuronal and endothelial site of acetylcholine synthesis and release associated with microvessels in rat cerebral cortex: ultrastructural and neurochemical studies, Brain Res. 454 (1988) 11–30.

[10] S.P. Duckles, Cholinergic innervation of cerebral arteries, in: C. Owman, J.E. Hardebo (Eds.), Neuronal Regulation of Brain Circulation, Elsevier, Amsterdam, 1986, pp. 235–243.

[11] N.M. Flynn, D. Kenny, R. Pelc, D.C. Warltier, Z.J. Bosnjak, J.P. Kampine, Endothelium-dependent vaso-dilation of canine coronary collateral vessels, Am. J. Physiol. 261 (1991) H797–H801.

[12] L. Wright, D.C. Homans, D.D. Laxson, X.Z. Dai, R.J. Bache, Effect of serotinin and thromboxane A2 on blood flow through moderately well developed coronary collateral vessels, J. Am. Coll. Cardiol. 19 (1992) 687–693.

[13] C. Iadecola, M.D. Underwood, D.J. Reis, Muscarinic cholinergic receptors mediate the cerebrovascular elicited by stimulation of the cerebellar fastigial nucleus in rat, Brain Res. 368 (1986) 375–379.

[14] G. Ferrari-Dileo, E.B. Davis, D.R. Anderson, Cholinergic binding sites in pericytes isolated from retinal capillaries, Blood Vessels 28 (1991) 542–546.

[15] R.F. Nicosia, S. Villaschi, Rat aortic smooth muscle cells become pericytes during angiogenesis in vitro, Lab. Invest. 73 (5) (1995) 658–666.

[16] N.C. Joyce, P. DeCamilli, J. Boyles, Pericytes, like smooth muscle cells, are immunocytochemically positive for cyclic GMP-dependent protein kinase, Microvasc. Res. 26 (1984) 5013–5017.

[17] N.C. Joyce, M.F. Haire, G.E. Palade, Contractile proteins in pericytes: I. Immunoperoxidase localization of tropomyosin, J. Cell Biol. 100 (1985) 1379–1386.

[18] N.C. Joyce, M.F. Haire, G.E. Palade, Contractile proteins in pericytes: I. Immunocytochemical evidence for the presence of two isomyosins in graded concentrations, J. Cell Biol. 100 (1985) 1387–1395.

[19] L.R. Bernstein, H. Antoniades, B.R. Zetter, Migration of cultured vascular cells in response to plasma and platelet-derived factors, J. Cell Sci. 56 (1982) 71–82.

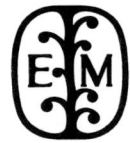

International Congress Series 1235 (2002) 515–524

Imaging synchronization and propagation of intracellular calcium oscillation during non-synaptic seizure-like neuronal activity in rat

Yoko Takiyama [a,*], Kunio Kato [b,1], Takafumi Inoue [c],
Fumihiko Sakai [a], Katsuhiko Mikoshiba [b,c,d]

[a]Department of Internal Medicine, Kitasato University School of Medicine,
1-15-1 Kitasato, Sagamihara, Kanagawa 2288555, Japan
[b]Mikoshiba Calciosignal Net Project, Exploratory Research for Advanced Technology (ERATO),
Japan Science and Technology Corporation (JST), Bunkyo, Tokyo 1130021, Japan
[c]Department of Molecular Neurobiology, The Institute of Medical Science,
The University of Tokyo, Minato, Tokyo 1080071, Japan
[d]Developmental Neurobiology Laboratory, Brain Science Institute,
The Institute of Physical and Chemical Research (RIKEN), Wako, Saitama 3510198, Japan

Abstract

Electrophysiological studies have shown that decreases in extracellular Ca^{2+} concentration and increases in extracellular K^+ concentration cause non-synaptic seizure-like neuronal activity in the hippocampus. Using the calcium imaging technique, we investigated the role of intracellular Ca^{2+} concentration in the cause of non-synaptic seizure-like neuronal activity. Rat hippocampal slice culture was loaded with calcium indicator dye. Non-synaptic seizure-like neuronal activity was induced by low Ca^{2+}/high K^+ solution. The calcium imaging, with a confocal laser scanning microscope and extracellular field recording were made simultaneously. Pharmacological inhibitors were used to examine the mechanism of the intracellular Ca^{2+} changes. As a result, intracellular Ca^{2+} oscillation occurred in neurons in a nonuniform fashion after replacing the solution, and then, gradual massive synchronization occurred in the large population. This massive synchronized Ca^{2+} oscillation propagated transversely through the CA1 area at a velocity of 4.2–6.8 mm/min. A negative shift, which reflects seizure-like neuronal activity, was observed in extracellular field recording, corresponding to the synchronized intracellular Ca^{2+} oscillation. Voltage-dependent calcium channel blocker and gap junction blocker inhibited this synchronization and the propagation.

---

* Corresponding author. Tel.: +81-42-778-8136; fax: +81-42-778-6400.
E-mail address: yokotaki@kitasato-u.ac.jp (Y. Takiyama).
[1] Present address: Department of Neuropsychiatry, Kochi Medical School, Kohasu, Oko-cho, Nankoku 783-8505, Japan.

0531-5131/02 © 2002 Elsevier Science B.V. All rights reserved.
PII: S 0 5 3 1 - 5 1 3 1 (0 2) 0 0 2 4 1 - 8

In conclusion, using the calcium-imaging technique, we demonstrated dynamic changes in synchronization and propagation of intracellular Ca^{2+} oscillation, which corresponded to non-synaptic epileptiform activity. The role of gap junction as a contributing mechanism was speculated. © 2002 Elsevier Science B.V. All rights reserved.

Keywords: Calcium imaging; Intracellular Ca^{2+} oscillation; Non-synaptic seizure-like neuronal activity; Gap junction; Glia

1. Introduction

As a main hypothesis of epilepsy, the abnormality of balance between excitatory and inhibitory neurotransmission has been revealed. On the other hand, an extracellular ion-dependent mechanism without synaptic transmission has been known for epilepsy. Ionic changes in the extracellular space, such as decreases in extracellular Ca^{2+} concentration ($[Ca^{2+}]_o$) and increases in extracellular K^+ concentration ($[K^+]_o$), cause non-synaptic epileptogenesis (seizure-like neuronal activity) in the hippocampus [1–3]. A negative shift, which reflects ionic changes induced by synchronized excitability of neurons, was observed using extracellular field recording in electrophysiological studies, and this method is also used as the epileptic model in vitro [2,3]. However, intracellular calcium changes during this seizure-like neuronal activity have not been well investigated. The purpose of this study was to use the calcium imaging technique to investigate the changes of intracellular Ca^{2+} concentration and the relation with non-synaptic seizure-like neuronal activity in the pyramidal neurons.

2. Materials and methods

2.1. Organotypic slice cultures

The slice cultures were prepared using the interface method as described previously [4] with some modification. Briefly, the hippocampi were removed from 13- to 16-day-old Sprague–Dawley rats under anesthesia and cut into 300-μm horizontal sections. The slices were transferred onto membrane inserts in culture plates. The culture medium consisted of 50% Eagle's minimum essential medium (MEM), 25% heat-inactivated horse serum, 25% Hank's balanced salt solution (HBSS), supplemented with glucose (6.5 g/l), penicillin (50 U/ml), streptomycin (100 μg/ml), and Ara-C (5×10^{-6} M). The slice cultures were maintained more than 7 days in a 5% CO_2 gas mixture incubator at 35 °C. Slices corresponding to P21-33 were used for the experiment.

2.2. Calcium imaging

Slice cultures were treated at 20–21 °C with 10 μM Calcium Green-1 acetoxymethyl-ester form (Calcium Green-1/AM). One slice was transferred to an 800-μl recording chamber and superfused continuously with artificial cerebrospinal fluid (ACSF), which was composed of (in mM): NaCl, 124; $CaCl_2$, 2.0; KCl, 3.0; $MgSO_4$, 2.0; D-glucose, 10; NaH_2PO_4, 1.25; $NaHCO_3$, 22; pH 7.4, and then it was bubbled with a mixture of 95% O_2 and 5% CO_2, kept at 31 ± 1.5 °C, at a flow rate of 1.2 ml/min. Calcium images under the standard solution (ACSF) and low Ca^{2+}/high K^+ solution were recorded and compared. The low Ca^{2+}/high K^+ solutions were composed of: NaCl, 124; $CaCl_2$, 0.2; KCl, 6.0; $MgSO_4$, 4.0; D-glucose, 10; NaH_2PO_4, 1.25; $NaHCO_3$, 22; pH 7.4. The Ca^{2+} free /high K^+ solutions were also used in some cases. Pharmacological agents were added to this superfusing solution.

Fluorescence images (excitation at 488 nm; emission at 510–700 nm) in the CA1 area were obtained using a confocal laser microscope system, through a $5 \times$ objective lens (NA 0.10) and a $40 \times$ water-immersion objective lens (NA 0.80). Ca^{2+} transients were recorded by 512×512 pixel images at the interval of 700 ms.

When the electrophysiological recordings were performed simultaneously, calcium images (excitation at 488 nm; emission at 516–700 nm) in the CA1 area were recorded using a cooled-CCD camera, adapted to an upright microscope through a $40 \times$ water-immersion objective lens (NA 0.80), with a confocal laser scanning unit. Ca^{2+} transients were recorded by binned-pixel images (binning 3×3) at the interval of 700 ms.

The whole slice fluorescence images (excitation at 470–490 nm, emission at 515–550 nm) were obtained using a cooled-CCD camera, adapted to an inverted microscope through a $4 \times$ objective lens (NA 0.16). The Ca^{2+} transients were recorded by binned-pixel images (binning 3×3) at the interval of 700 ms.

In addition, the homemade software produced by Takafumi Inoue, running on a computer, controlled all the electrophysiological apparatus, the laser source, the camera, and data recording.

2.3. Electrophysiological recording

Extracellular field recordings were performed with calcium imaging in the CA1 area. The 3 M NaCl-filled glass microelectrode (10–15-$M\Omega$ resistance) was placed on the pyramidal cell layer. Electrophysiological data were recorded through an amplifier in the current-clamp mode, and filtered at 1 kHz with homemade software at the interval of 100 ms.

2.4. Materials

Some pharmacological agents were used to examine the mechanism of the changes in intracellular Ca^{2+} concentration as follows: NMDA (N-methyl-D-aspartate) type ionotropic glutamate receptor antagonist: D (−)-2-amino-5-phosphonopentanoic acid (D-AP5); AMPA (α-amino-3-hydroxy-5-methyl-4-isoxazolepropionic acid) type ionotropic glutamate receptor antagonist: 6-cyano-7-nitroquinoxaline-2,3-dione (CNQX); metabotropic glutamate receptor antagonist: (RS)-α-methyl-4-carboxyphenylglycine (MCPG); voltage-dependent calcium channel blocker: $NiSO_4$; and gap junction blocker: 1-Octanol.

3. Results

3.1. Development of synchronized intracellular Ca^{2+} oscillation and propagation under perfusing low Ca^{2+}/high K^{+} solution

Under perfusing low Ca^{2+}/high K^{+} solution, synchronization and propagation of intracellular Ca^{2+} oscillation in the neurons was observed. Initially, intracellular Ca^{2+} transients from the neurons occurred in a nonuniform fashion after replacing the solution (Fig. 1, 0–400 s). They gradually changed to rhythmical and regular transients, which were called Ca^{2+} oscillation. Finally, the Ca^{2+} oscillation became synchronized in a population of neurons (Fig. 1, 400–900 s). Under perfusion with Ca^{2+} free/high K^{+} solution, the synchronized Ca^{2+} oscillation was repeated regularly for a certain period and then damped gradually in time ($n = 12$). Under perfusion with low Ca^{2+}/high K^{+} solution, the synchronized Ca^{2+} oscillation continued to be repeated. The initial interval of the oscillation was 16.1 ± 1.20 s (mean $\pm$ S.D., $n = 10$), a half width of the calcium transient was 4.8 ± 0.32 s (mean $\pm$ S.D., $n = 10$). Afterwards, those intervals and half widths tended to increase with time (Fig. 1, 900–1400 s).

In observation of the wide visual field, a massive synchronized intracellular Ca^{2+} transient, in the large population of the neurons, propagated transversely through the CA1 area as shown in Fig. 2. The directions of propagation were toward CA2 and/or subiculum. They were observed continuously with regular intervals (Fig. 2C, 0–14.0 and 15.4–22.4 s).

3.2. Relation of intracellular Ca^{2+} oscillation and seizure-like neuronal activity

By simultaneous recording of calcium imaging and the extracellular field potential, we investigated the relationship between the intracellular Ca^{2+} oscillation and seizure-like neuronal activity. As shown in Fig. 3A and B, initially, the Ca^{2+} transient randomly

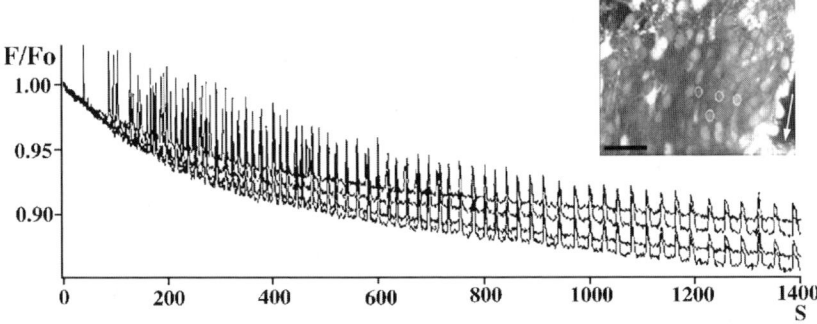

Fig. 1. Development of synchronized intracellular Ca^{2+} oscillation under perfusing low Ca^{2+}/high K^{+} solution. The panel shows fluorescence image of the CA1 area staining with 10 μM Calcium Green-1/AM. White ellipses indicate regions where time courses of fluorescence intensities were plotted below. Arrow shows an insert point of the extracellular field-recording pipette. Time courses of fluorescence intensities are plotted after normalized by the first frame values (Fo). Scale bar = 50 μm.

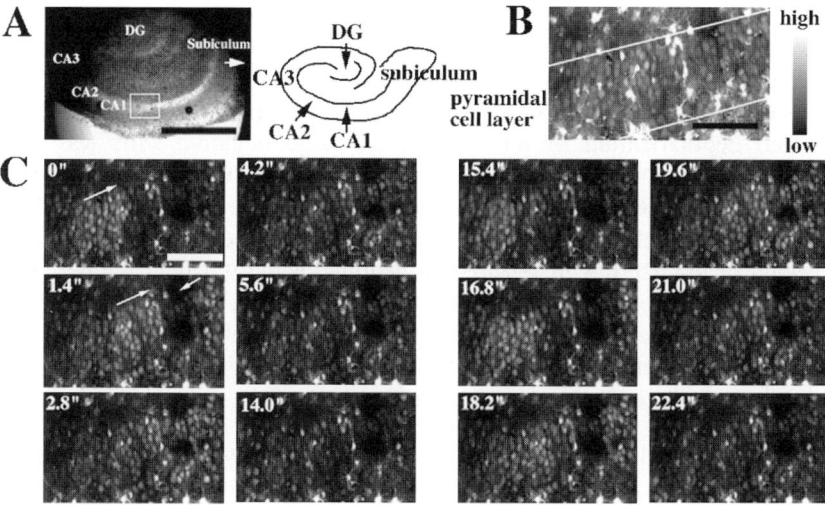

Fig. 2. Massive synchronized intracellular Ca^{2+} transient propagated through the CA1 area under perfusing low Ca^{2+}/high K^+ solution. (A) Low power image of organotypic hippocampal slice culture. Schema is depicted beside. Box indicates observed CA1 area. Scale bar = 1 mm. (B) High power fluorescence image by calcium indicator dye, showing stacked neurons in the area corresponding to the box in (A). Scale bar = 100 μm. (C) The elapsed times from the first panel are indicated. Arrows show the directions of propagation. Scale bar = 100 μm.

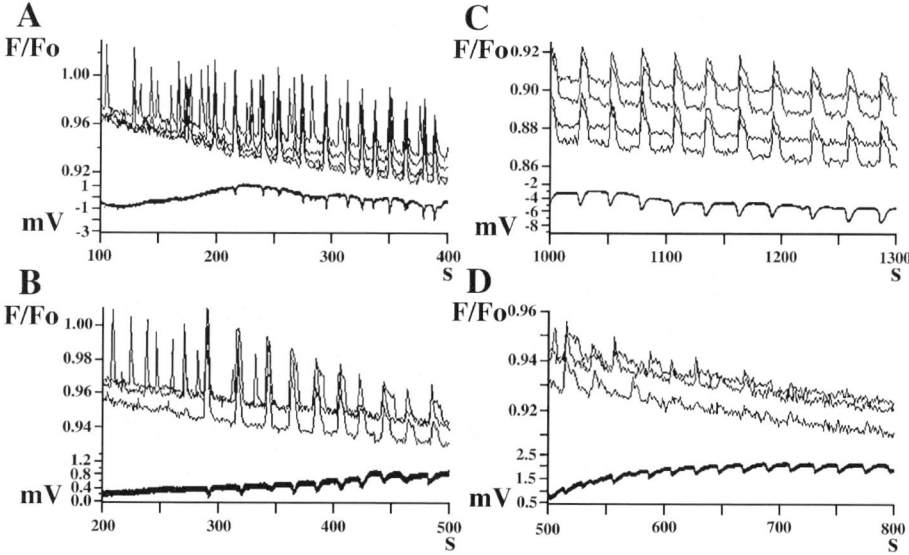

Fig. 3. Relation of intracellular Ca^{2+} oscillation and seizure-like neuronal activity. (A and C) Under perfusing low Ca^{2+}/high K^+ solution. (B and D) Under perfusing Ca^{2+} free /high K^+ solution. Upper traces show fluorescence intensities indicated as F/Fo. Lower traces show field potential.

occurred because each neuron might have a different threshold for excitability and preceded a small irregular negative shift, which reflected depolarization in some of the neurons. When the Ca^{2+} oscillation gradually developed to synchronize, a small irregular negative shift changed to a regular large negative shift, which reflected massive synchronized depolarization of the neurons. A large negative shift was observed, corresponding to the synchronized intracellular Ca^{2+} oscillation (shown in Fig. 3B and C, $n = 10$). In other words, a process of development in the synchronized intracellular Ca^{2+} oscillation was well consistent with the formation of a negative shift, which reflects depolarization of the neurons in seizure-like neuronal activity. Under the perfusion with Ca^{2+} free/high K^+ solution, synchronized intracellular Ca^{2+} oscillation gradually decreased and disappeared. However, the negative shift continued to be repeated at regular intervals (shown in Fig. 3D, $n = 3$). A persistency of the negative shift was not dependent on the intracellular Ca^{2+} concentration.

3.3. Ca^{2+} changes in a whole slice under perfusing low Ca^{2+}/high K^+ solution

During observation of a whole slice (shown in Fig. 4), a massive Ca^{2+} transient, which indicated the synchronized intracellular Ca^{2+} transient in the large population of cells, propagated transversely through the whole CA1 area at an approximate velocity of 4.2– 6.8 mm/min ($n = 7$), not observed in CA3 and the dentate gyrus.

Starting points of the propagation (trigger) existed in particular subareas in CA1, which were near the subiculum and/or adjacent to CA2. Representative directions of propagation were from the CA1-near subiculum toward the subiculum, from the CA1-near subiculum toward CA2, and from CA2 toward the subiculum.

As shown in Fig. 5, the massive synchronized Ca^{2+} oscillation started in the subarea in CA1, which was adjacent to CA2 (region 1), then propagated through regions 2 and 3 along the CA1 pyramidal cell layer. Propagation continued to repeat with regular intervals.

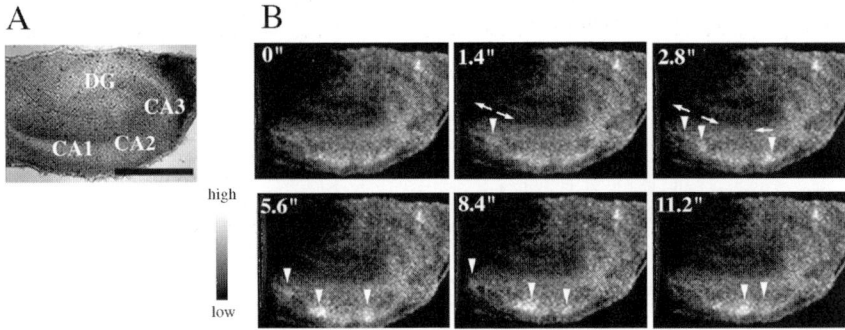

Fig. 4. Ca^{2+} Changes in a whole slice under perfusing low Ca^{2+}/high K^+ solution. (A) A whole slice image by transmitted light. (B) Fluorescence images of a whole slice. The elapsed times from the first panel are indicated. Arrowheads indicate the region of massive synchronized Ca^{2+} oscillation. Arrows indicate the direction of propagation. Scale bar = 1 mm.

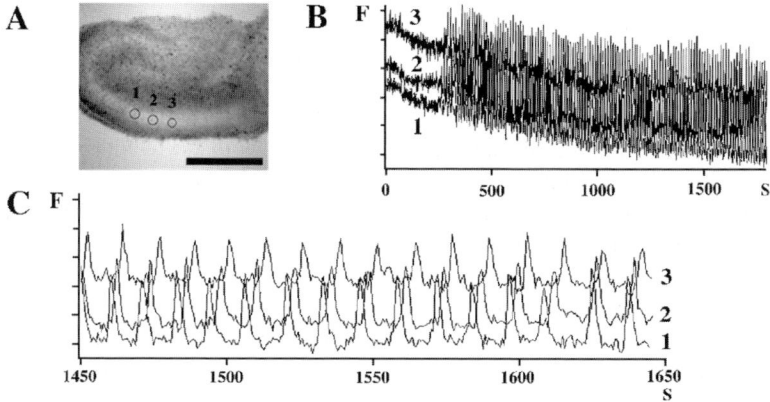

Fig. 5. Massive synchronized Ca^{2+} oscillation started at the particular subareas in the CA1 area. (A) A whole slice image by transmitted light. The circles with numerals indicate regions where the time courses of fluorescence intensities were obtained. Scale bar = 1 mm. Region 1: starting point of the propagation in CA1. Regions 2 and 3: passing points in CA1. (B) Time courses of fluorescence intensities in three regions. (C) Expanded time courses of fluorescence intensities in (B).

3.4. Effects of pharmacological agents to massive synchronized Ca^{2+} oscillation

Some pharmacological inhibitors, which blocked Ca^{2+} influx into cells, were used to examine a mechanism of the changes in intracellular Ca^{2+} concentration. As shown in Fig. 6, the synchronization (regions 1 and 2) and propagation (region 3) in a population of neurons did not change by NMDA and AMPA type ionotropic glutamate receptor

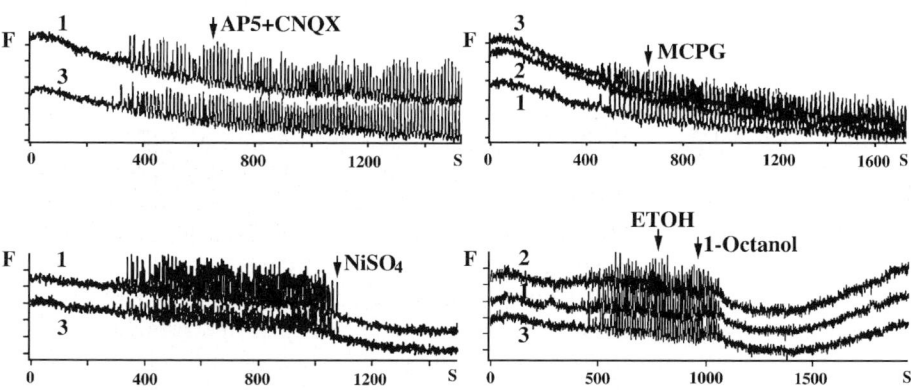

Fig. 6. Effects of pharmacological inhibitors on massive synchronized Ca^{2+} oscillation. Regions 1 and 2: subareas near the subiculum and/or adjacent to CA2 where massive synchronized Ca^{2+} oscillation started in the CA1. Region 3: another subarea in the CA1 (passing region). Pharmacological agents were administrated at the time shown by the arrows.

antagonist (50 μM D-AP5 and 20 μM CNQX, $n = 5$), and metabotropic glutamate receptor antagonist (500 μM/1 mM MCPG, $n = 7$). These findings suggested that those synchronizations and propagations occurred without chemical synaptic transmission, because the glutamates were the main neurotransmitters in excitatory synaptic transmission in the hippocampus. On the other hand, voltage-dependent calcium channel blocker (1 mM $NiSO_4$, $n = 3$) and gap junction blocker (2 mM 1-Octanol, $n = 3$) completely inhibited the synchronization and subsequent propagation.

4. Discussion and conclusion

Under perfusing low Ca^{2+}/high K^+ solution, the synchronization of the intracellular Ca^{2+} oscillation in the large population of neurons reflected seizure-like neuronal activity, which occurred not through synaptic transmission, but through the voltage-dependent calcium channel. We could directly visualize a process of synchronization of the changes in $[Ca^{2+}]_i$ with a negative shift in the extracellular field potential. The fact that persistency of a negative shift was not dependent on changes in $[Ca^{2+}]_i$ in this study demonstrated that dynamic changes in $[Ca^{2+}]_i$ were not integral for non-synaptic seizure-like neuronal activity. Indeed, it has been revealed that a greater rise in $[K^+]_o$ accompanied by the occurrence of a negative shift [1–3] is suggesting the uptake of K^+ into the glial cells, causing a negative shift during seizure-like neuronal activity [1]. Our results were in accordance with those facts in previous studies.

The gap junction blocker completely inhibited synchronization of intracellular Ca^{2+} oscillation and subsequent propagation, suggesting not only the changes in $[Ca^{2+}]_o$ and $[K^+]_o$ but also gap junction played a role in synchronization of intracellular Ca^{2+} oscillation. Interactions through gap junctions between neuron and glial cell, among neurons or glial cells is speculated under non-synaptic seizure-like neuronal activity. It was already revealed that neuronal coupling was increased 2.3 times by gap junction in hippocampal CA1 neurons under the low $[Ca^{2+}]_o$ model [5].

Recently, many intercellular Ca^{2+} waves being observed in glial cells [6] and neurons [7] under various stimuli were discussed with the possible association with spreading depression (SD) [8]. SD is classically characterized as a slowly propagating wave (1–6 mm/min or 20–80 μm/s) of evoked or spontaneous silence in neuronal fast electrical activity, which is associated with a large negative DC potential [8,9], a redistribution of ions, shrinkage of the extracellular space, and an increase in energy metabolism [10]. Intercellular glial Ca^{2+} waves have characteristics similar to SD. For example, intercellular glial Ca^{2+} waves propagate at approximately the same velocity with SD [6], accompanied with gap junctional communication [11]. Intercellular neuronal Ca^{2+} waves (> 100 μm/s) propagating faster than the propagation velocity of SD [7] have not fulfilled the electrophysiological criteria of SD. Meanwhile, gap junctions between neurons [12,13] and glial cells[11] may play important roles in SD. In our study, the characteristics of intercellular neuronal Ca^{2+} waves were similar to SD regarding propagation velocity, consisting of a negative shift, and blocking of synaptic transmission and involvement of gap junction. Further investigation needs to be carried out regarding the SD-like neuronal Ca^{2+} waves.

4.3.4.6. On-Site Discussion

4.3.4.6.1. **Question: (Lauritzen)** Did you observe communication in terms of Ca^{2+} signaling between neurons and glial cells, or was the signal transduction only from glial to glial cells and neuron to neurons?

Answer: (Takiyama) We did not observe directly the communication between neurons and glial cells, neurons and neurons, glial cells and glial cells, but, using a certain inhibitor of glial function, neuronal synchronization and propagation were blocked completely. Therefore, I think communication between neurons and glial cells was existing at least. Glial cells are necessary to synchronize the population of neurons in this study. As preliminary and in complete data, injecting of Lucifer-yellow into neurons under perfusing low Ca^{2+}/high K^+ solution, I observed neuronal coupling was increased in fluorescence image (maybe through gap junction), but experiment was incomplete. I cannot give you a definite answer.

4.3.4.6.2. **Question: (Andrew)** The putative uncoupler octanol might cause damage to the organotypic slice. Did the synchronizing effect of low Ca^{2+} return after octanol was washed off? If not, there are more selective and less noxious gap junction blockers that can be obtained and tested. These are noted in recent papers by C. Naus and co-workers.

Answer: (Takiyama) We probably checked synchronization returned after octanol was washed out. And using a certain inhibitor of glial function, neuronal synchronization and propagation were blocked completely. Therefore, I think communication between neurons and glial cells were existing at least. Glial cells are necessary to synchronize the population of neurons in this study.

References

[1] U. Heinemann, E. Claudia, L. Antje, Epilepsy, in: H. Kettenmann, B.R. Ransom (Eds.), Neuroglia, Oxford Univ. Press, New York, 1995, pp. 936–949.

[2] A. Konnerth, U. Heinemann, Y. Yaari, Nonsynaptic epileptogenesis in the mammalian hippocampus in vitro: I. Development of seizurelike activity in low extracellular calcium, J. Neurophysiol. 56 (1986) 409–423.

[3] A. Leschinger, J. Stabel, P. Igelmund, U. Heinemann, Pharmacological and electrographic properties of epileptiform activity induced by elevated K^+ and lowered Ca^{2+} and Mg^{2+} concentration in rat hippocampal slices, Exp. Brain Res. 96 (1993) 230–240.

[4] L. Stoppini, P.A. Buchs, D. Muller, A simple method for organotypic cultures of nervous tissue, J. Neurosci. Methods 37 (1991) 173–182.

[5] J.L. Perez-Velazquez, T.A. Valiante, P.L. Carlen, Modulation of gap junctional mechanisms during calcium-free induced field burst activity. A possible role for electrotonic coupling in epileptogenesis, J. Neurosci. 14 (1994) 4308–4317.

[6] A.C. Charles, Intercellular calcium waves in glia, GLIA 24 (1998) 39–49.

[7] A.C. Charles, S.K. Kodali, R.F. Tyndale, Intercellular calcium waves in neurons, Mol. Cell. Neurosci. 7 (1996) 337–353.

[8] A.A.P. Leao, Spreading depression of activity in the cerebral cortex, J. Neurophysiol. 7 (1944) 359–390.

[9] P.E. Kunkler, R.P. Kraig, Calcium waves precede electrophysiological changes of spreading depression in hippocampal organ cultures, J. Neurosci. 18 (1998) 3416–3425.

[10] C. Nicholson, R.P. Kraig, The behavior of extracellular ions during spreading depression, in: T. Zeuthen (Ed.), The Application of Ion-Selective Microelectrodes, Elsevier, Amsterdam, 1981, pp. 217–238.

Y. Takiyama et al. / International Congress Series 1235 (2002) 515–524

[11] M. Nedergaard, A.J. Cooper, S.A. Goldman, Gap junctions are required for the propagation of spreading depression, J. Neurobiol. 28 (1995) 433–444.

[12] G.G. Somjen, P.G. Aitken, G.L. Czeh, O. Herreras, J. Jing, J.N. Young, Mechanism of spreading depression: a review of recent findings and a hypothesis, Can. J. Physiol. Pharmacol. 70 (1992) S248–S254.

[13] C. Largo, G.C. Tombaugh, P.G. Aitken, O. Herreras, G.G. Somjen, Heptanol but not fluoroacetate prevents the propagation of spreading depression in rat hippocampal slices, J. Neurophysiol. 77 (1997) 9–16.

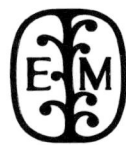

International Congress Series 1235 (2002) 525–532

Therapeutic efficacy of transcranial magnetic stimulation for amyotrophic lateral sclerosis and spinocerebellar degeneration

Masahiro Horiuchi [a,*], Futaba Maki [a], Toshiyuki Yanagisawa [a], Hiroshi Sugihara [a], Yoichi Takahashi [a], Kenjiro Ohashi [b], Kaoru Sasaka [b], Yasuo Nakajima [b]

[a]*Division of Neurology, Department of Internal Medicine, St. Marianna University School of Medicine, 2-16-1 Sugao, Miyamae-ku, Kawasaki 216-8511, Japan*
[b]*Department of Radiology, St. Marianna University School of Medicine, 2-16-1 Sugao, Miyamae-ku, Kawasaki 216-8511, Japan*

Abstract

We treated four patients with amyotrophic lateral sclerosis (ALS) and nine patients with spinocerebellar degeneration (SCD) using transcranial magnetic stimulation (TMS) with an SMN-1200 transcranial magnetic stimulator. The stimulus strength was below 1.5 T and the interpulse interval was greater than 5 s. The stimulus coil was placed on P3, P4 and the bilateral cervical and lumbar root in the ALS patients, and tangentially over Iz, 4 cm lateral to the right from Iz and 4 cm lateral to the left from Iz in the SCD patients. Ten consecutive pulses were delivered to each region in the ALS patients and 15 in the SCD patients. Transcranial magnetic stimulation (TMS) was applied for a total of 20 days for in-patients and once or twice a week as ongoing therapy for outpatients. Patients with ALS were assessed according to the Barthel index, and a respiratory function test was performed before and after TMS. Patients with SCD were neurologically assessed according to the International Cooperative Ataxia Rating Scale (ICARS). In addition, the patients were evaluated for regional cerebral blood flow (rCBF) by $^{99\,m}$Tc-ECD SPECT using a modified Patlak-plot method before and after the TMS trial. No change in the Barthel index or rCBF was observed in patients with ALS. The respiratory function test results improved in one patient in the ALS group. The ICARS rating of seven

* Corresponding author. Tel.: +81-44-977-8111; fax: +81-44-976-8516.
E-mail address: horiuchi@mrg.biglobe.ne.jp (M. Horiuchi).

patients with SCD improved after TMS. The rCBF of patients with SCD in the bilateral cerebellar hemispheres was significantly faster compared to their flow rate before TMS. These data suggest the potential usefulness of TMS as a therapeutic tool for ALS and SCD. © 2002 Elsevier Science B.V. All rights reserved.

Keywords: Transcranial magnetic stimulation; Amyotrophic lateral sclerosis; Spinocerebellar degeneration; Regional cerebral blood flow

1. Background

Transcranial magnetic stimulation (TMS) has been shown to have clear clinical benefits for depression, Parkinson's disease [1] and SCD [2]. We performed TMS therapy for patients with amyotrophic lateral sclerosis (ALS) and spinocerebellar degeneration (SCD).

2. Methods

Four patients (60.8±3.7 years old) (Table 1) with ALS and nine patients with SCD (55.8±11.3 years old) (Table 2) were enrolled in this study. The transcranial magnetic stimulator was an SMN-1200 (Nihon-koden, Tokyo) model with a 14.1-cm circular coil. The stimulus strength was below 1.5 T and the interpulse interval greater than 5 s. The stimulus coil was placed on P3, P4 (international 10–20 system) and the bilateral cervical and lumbar root in the ALS patients and tangentially over Iz, 4 cm lateral to the right from Iz and 4 cm lateral to the left from Iz in the SCD patients. Ten consecutive pulses were delivered to each region in the ALS patients and 15 to the SCD patients.

Transcranial magnetic stimulation (TMS) was performed for a total of 20 days for the in-patients and as ongoing therapy at once or twice a week for the outpatients. Patients with ALS were assessed according to the Barthel index [3] and a respiratory function test was performed before and after TMS. Patients with SCD were neurologically assessed according to the International Cooperative Ataxia Rating Scale (ICARS) [4]. The regional cerebral blood flow (rCBF) was evaluated in patients with ALS in the bilateral frontal lobes, and in patients with SCD in the bilateral cerebellar hemispheres, and pontine base by 99 m Tc-ECD SPECT using a modified Patlak-plot method both before and after the TMS trial.

3. Results

No change in the Barthel index or rCBF was observed in the ALS patients. The respiratory function test results of patient 4 in the ALS group improved after TMS (Fig. 1).

Table 1

No.	Age	Sex	Diagnosis	Onset	Group	Start of TMS	Barthel index (points)		rCBF (before)	Right frontal lobe (ml/100 g/min)	Left frontal lobe (ml/100 g/min)	rCBF (after)	Right frontal lobe (ml/100 g/min)	Left frontal lobe (ml/100 g/min)	Medicine
							Before	After							
1	58	F	ALS (bulbar)	August 1999	Out to In to Out	September 2000	80	80	5 October 2000	49.75	45.15	16 November 2000	50.19	40.55	
2	58	F	ALS	February 2000	Out-patient	November 2000	45	45	9 November 2000	59.82	56.3	25 January 2001	57.78	52.97	Riruzole
3	60	F	ALS	July 1999	Out-patient	October 2000	30	30	5 October 2000	48.62	54.36	7 December 2000	53.73	57.54	Riruzole
4	67	F	ALS	July 2000	In to Out to In	December 2000	85	70	22 November 2000	57.33	60.66	14 December 2000	60.62	61.59	Riruzole

Table 2

No.	Age	Sex	Diagnosis	Onset	Group	Start of TMS	Improvement of ICARS	Before (points)	After
1	53	F	OPCA	1998	In-patient	September 2000	Dysarthria	67	65
2	67	F	OPCA	1995	Outpatient	November 2000		65	65
3	65	M	OPCA	1998	In-patient	October 2000	Truncal ataxia	53	52
4	61	F	OPCA	1998	In to Out	December 2000	Dysarthria	40	38
5	36	M	MJD	1986	In to Out	October 2000	Gait disturbance, nystagmus	34	29
6	54	F	SCA6	1984	Outpatient	December 2000		40	40
7	37	M	MJD	1986	In-patient	February 2001	Gait disturbance, dysarthria	28	20
8	65	M	OPCA	1998	In-patient	February 2001	Gait disturbance, ataxia	40	37
9	64	F	SCA6	1992	In-patient	February 2001	Gait disturbance, ataxia, dysarthria, nystagmus	49	40

The ICARS rating of seven patients with SCD improved after TMS (Fig. 2). The rCBF of patients with SCD in the bilateral cerebellar hemispheres was higher than before TMS (Fig. 3).

4. Discussion

In Parkinson's disease patients, Davis et al. [5] assessed the changes in rCBF and Parkinsonian symptoms during disruption of globus pallidus (GPi) activity with high frequency stimulation delivered through implanted brain electrodes. Positron emission tomography (PET) revealed an increase in rCBF in ipsilateral premotor cortical areas, which improved rigidity and bradykinesia. These results suggest that disrupting excessive inhibitory input of the basal ganglia reverses Parkinsonism, via a thalamic relay, by activation of brain areas involved in the initiation of movement.

In the present study, the respiratory function test result of patient 4 in the ALS group improved after TMS, suggesting that TMS may be an effective therapy for patients with ALS. The underlying mechanism responsible for this improvement remains to be determined.

rCBF (before)	Right cerebellum (ml/100 g/min)	Left cerebellum (ml/100 g/min)	Pontine base	rCBF (after)	Right cerebellum (ml/100 g/min)	Left cerebellum (ml/100 g/min)	Pontine base	Medicine
7 September 2000	40.62	43.6		21 March 2001	37.51	41.28		Ceredist
9 November 2000	47.16	42.28		25 January 2001	47.25	47.79		Ceredist
19 October 20000	39.83	39.77		7 February 2001	45.14	43.89		Ceredist
30 November 2000	49.45	47.05		20 December 2000	50.88	51.77		Ceredist
20 December 2000	63.24	60.08	39.27	22 February 2001	68.46	72.95	54.25	Ceredist
14 December 2000	60.19	59.34		22 February 2001	63.51	67.13		Ceredist
31 January 2001	52.64	53.8		21 March 2001	59.24	63.91		Ceredist
15 February 2001	47.45	46.34	40.54	14 March 2001	45.6	41.26	27.78	Ceredist
21 February 2001	56.69	62.77		15 March 2001	66.97	63.77		Hirtonin

The rCBF of the cerebellar hemisphere of patients with SCD significantly increased during the TMS trial. Transcranial magnetic stimulation (TMS) improved the micro-circulation of the brain with accompanying clinical improvements. Although the exact mechanism by which TMS improved ataxia remains unknown, we speculate that increased blood flow in the cerebellum played a role in this improvement.

5. Conclusions

These findings indicate the potential usefulness of TMS as a therapeutic tool for ALS and SCD.

References

[1] H. Shimamoto, M. Shigemori, Therapeutic effect of repetitive transcranial magnetic stimulation on Parkinson disease, Neurol. Med. 51 (1999) 419–425.

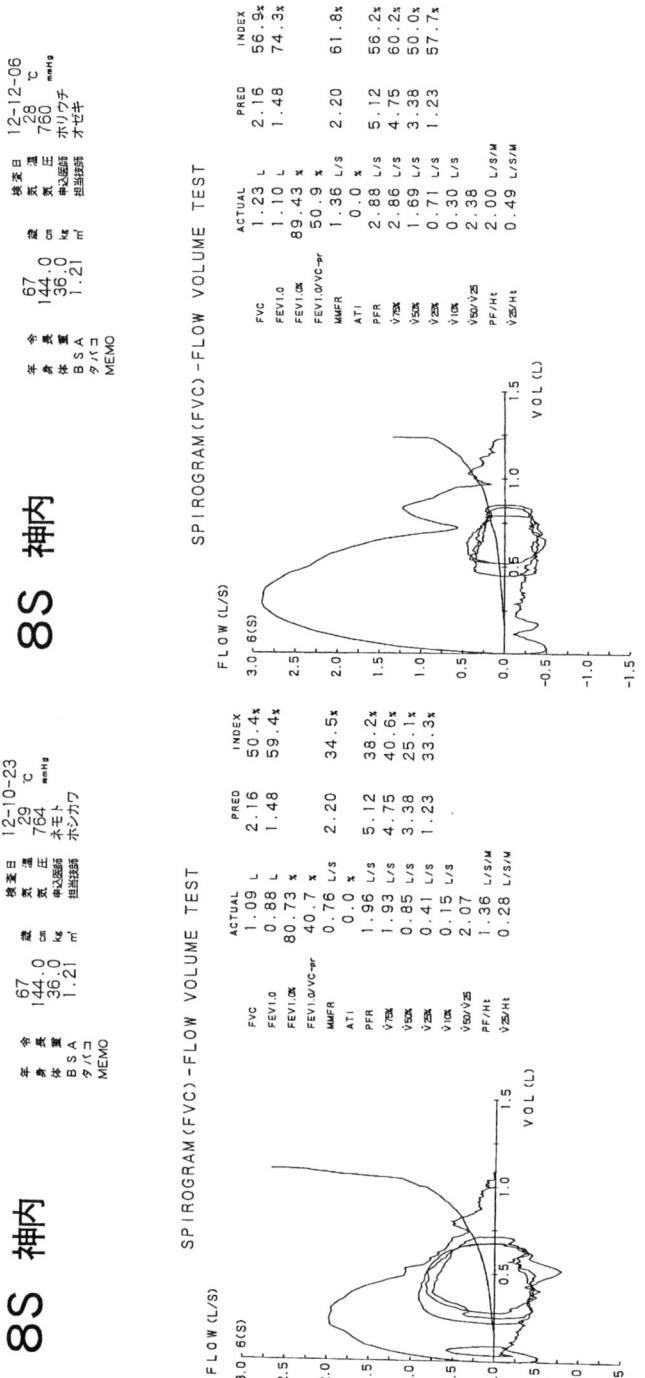

Fig. 1. The respiratory function test results of Patient 4 in the ALS group improved following TMS therapy.

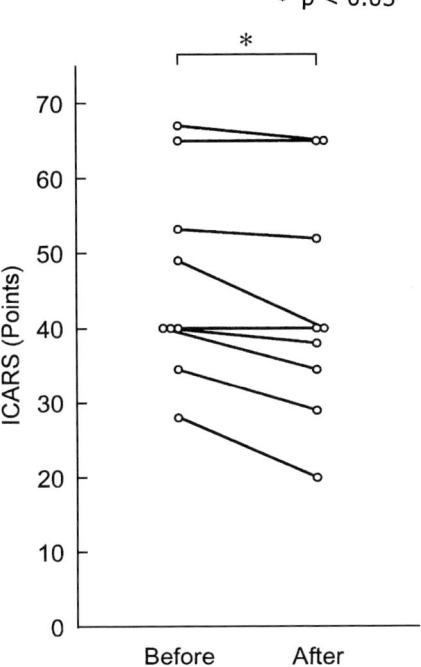

Fig. 2. The ICARS rating of seven patients with SCD improved after TMS.

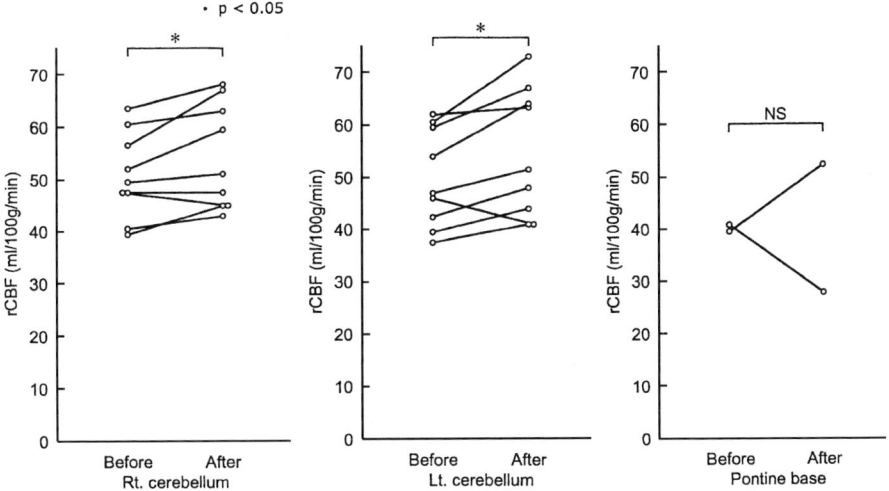

Fig. 3. The rCBF of patients with SCD in the bilateral cerebellar hemispheres was higher compared to before TMS.

[2] H. Shimizu, T. Tsuda, Y. Shiga, K. Miyazawa, Y. Onodera, M. Matsuzaki, M. Nakashima, K. Furukawa, M. Aoki, H. Kato, T. Yamazaki, Y. Itoyama, Therapeutic efficacy of transcranial magnetic stimulation for hereditary spinocerebellar degeneration, Tohoku J. Exp. Med. 189 (1999) 203–211.

[3] F.I. Mahoney, D.W. Barthel, Functional evaluation: the Barthel index, Maryland St. Med. J. 14 (1965) 61–65.

[4] P. Trouillas, T. Takayanagi, M. Hallet, R.D. Currier, S.H. Subramony, K. Wessel, A. Bryer, H.C. Diener, S. Massaquoi, C.M. Gomez, P. Coutinho, M.B. Hamida, G. Campanella, A. Filla, L. Schut, D. Tiemann, J. Honnorat, N. Nighoghossian, B. Manyam, International cooperative ataxia rating scale for pharmacological assessment of cerebellar syndrome, J. Neurol. Sci. 145 (1997) 205–211.

[5] K.D. Davis, E. Taub, S. Houle, A.E. Lang, J.O. Dostrovsky, R.R. Tasker, A.M. Lozano, Globus pallidus stimulation activities the cortical motor system during alleviation of Parkinsonian symptoms, Nat. Med. 3 (1997) 671–674.

Author index

Keyword index